W9-ABH-608

SALEM HEALTH

INFECTIOUS DISEASES & CONDITIONS

SALEM HEALTH

INFECTIOUS DISEASES & CONDITIONS

Volume 2

Editor
H. Bradford Hawley
Wright State University

SALEM PRESS, INC.
Ipswich, Massachusetts   Hackensack, New Jersey

Note to Readers

The material presented in *Salem Health: Infectious Diseases and Conditions* is intended for broad informational and educational purposes. Readers who suspect that they or someone they know has any disorder, disease, or condition described in this set should contact a physician without delay. This set should not be used as a substitute for professional medical diagnosis. Readers who are undergoing or about to undergo any treatment or procedure described in this set should refer to their physicians and other health care providers for guidance concerning preparation and possible effects. This set is not to be considered definitive on the covered topics, and readers should remember that the field of health care is characterized by a diversity of medical opinions and constant expansion in knowledge and understanding.

Library of Congress Cataloging-in-Publication Data

Infectious diseases and conditions / editor, H. Bradford Hawley.
    p. ; cm. – (Salem health)
  Includes bibliographical references and indexes.
  ISBN 978-1-58765-776-4 (set : alk. paper) — ISBN 978-1-58765-777-1 (v. 1 : alk. paper) —
ISBN 978-1-58765-778-8 (v. 2 : alk. paper) — ISBN 978-1-58765-779-5 (v. 3 : alk. paper)
  1. Communicable diseases–Encyclopedias. I. Hawley, H. Bradford. II. Series: Salem health (Ipswich, Mass.)
  [DNLM: 1. Communicable Diseases–Encyclopedias–English. WC 13]
  RC112.I4577 2012
  616.003–dc23

2011020526

Contents

Contents

Complete List of Contents

Volume 1

Volume 2

Volume 3

SALEM HEALTH

INFECTIOUS DISEASES
& CONDITIONS

F

Facial palsy. *See* Bell's palsy.

Fasciitis

CATEGORY: Diseases and conditions
ANATOMY OR SYSTEM AFFECTED: Skin,tissue
ALSO KNOWN AS: Uncomplicated or non-necrotizing infective fasciitis

DEFINITION

Fasciitis is the inflammation of fibrous connective tissues of the body (fascia) associated with bacterial infection.

CAUSES

Skin and soft tissue infections (SSTIs), including fasciitis, can potentially develop from any damage to the skin that allows bacterial entry. Such damage includes cuts (accidental and surgical), scratches, bites, penetration of the skin by objects (such as needles), wounds (such as ulcers or chickenpox sores), and burns. Fasciitis develops when an infection, such as cellulitis, reaches deep enough in the tissue layers under the skin to spread along the underlying fascia.

RISK FACTORS

Persons with diabetes mellitus, liver or kidney disease, or vascular problems, or who are critically ill, of advanced age, or have reduced immune function, are at an increased risk for developing SSTIs. Exposure to organisms through contact with water or animals or as the result of bite wounds or injectable-drug abuse can also increase the risk for SSTI development.

SYMPTOMS

SSTI symptoms include damage associated with the route by which the infecting organisms entered the skin and the inflammation caused by the body's response to the presence of the organisms and toxins they may release. Local symptoms include warmth, redness, swelling, tenderness and pain, and possibly dysfunction of the affected tissues. Persons may also present with general symptoms of infection, including fever, low blood pressure, and a rapid heart rate. In severe cases, persons may exhibit altered mental status.

SCREENING AND DIAGNOSIS

The symptoms and the appearance of the affected tissues are the primary basis for diagnosis. Further assessment may include culturing samples collected through tissue swab, needle aspiration, or blood samples. High white-blood-cell counts and low serum sodium concentrations are more commonly associated with necrotizing forms of fasciitis. X ray, ultrasound, computed tomography (CT), or magnetic resonance imaging (MRI) may be used to asses the depth and extent of the infection.

For the evaluation of fasciitis, differentiation of uncomplicated from necrotizing forms is essential to determine how aggressively to treat the infection. Ultrasound is useful for detecting the degree of fascia involvement, and a CT and an MRI may be used to detect signs of necrosis in the deep tissues.

TREATMENT AND THERAPY

Once it has been determined that a case of fasciitis is uncomplicated and non-necrotizing, doctors will order antibiotic therapy (usually intravenous) as the primary course of treatment. Empiric treatment should be directed against staphylococcal and streptococcal species, with coverage against additional organisms, and follow treatment algorithms based on the location of infection and route of organism entry.

PREVENTION AND OUTCOMES

To prevent the development of fasciitis, one should avoid damage to skin and should treat minor SSTIs to prevent the progression of disease to involvement of the fascia.

Rebecca Stadolnik

FURTHER READING

May, A. K. "Skin and Soft Tissue Infections." *Surgical Clinics of North America* 89 (2009): 403.

Vincent, Ki, and Coleman Rotstein. "Bacterial Skin and Soft Tissue Infections in Adults: A Review of Their Epidemiology, Pathogenesis, Diagnosis, Treatment, and Site of Care." *Canadian Journal of Infectious Diseases and Medical Microbiology* 19 (2008): 173-184.

Wall, Derek, et al. "A Simple Model to Help Distinguish Necrotizing Fasciitis from Nonnecrotizing Soft Tissue Infection." *Journal of the American College of Surgeons* 191 (2000): 227-231.

WEB SITES OF INTEREST

American Academy of Dermatology
http://www.aad.org

Todar's Online Textbook of Bacteriology
http://www.textbookofbacteriology.net

See also: Bacterial infections; Cellulitis; *Enterobacter*; Gangrene; Group A streptococcal infection; *Mycobacterium*; Necrotizing fasciitis; Osteomyelitis; Skin infections; Streptococcal infections; Wound infections.

Fatal familial insomnia

CATEGORY: Diseases and conditions
ANATOMY OR SYSTEM AFFECTED: Brain, central nervous system, muscles, musculoskeletal system

DEFINITION

Fatal familial insomnia (FFI) is a rare, genetic prion disease transmitted as an autosomal dominant trait. The responsible mutation causes prions (proteins found extensively in the body) to assume abnormal shapes and thereby become pathogenic. A nongenetic form of the disease, sporadic fatal insomnia, also exists.

CAUSES

The cause of FFI has been identified as a mutation at codon 178 of the prion-protein gene (PRNP) on chromosome 20. Disease characteristics, such as duration, are determined by a polymorphism at codon 129 of the PRNP gene.

RISK FACTORS

Each offspring of an affected parent has a 50 percent risk of inheriting the mutant gene, which is highly penetrant; as far as is known, those persons who inherit the gene will express the disease. Sporadic cases have no known risk factors.

SYMPTOMS

Insomnia is the hallmark of this disease, although it is not invariably present in the earliest stages. Symptoms are best understood in the context of the histopathology of FFI, primarily involving degeneration and loss of neurons in the thalamus. The thalamus has a crucial integrative function in the brain, relaying all manner of sensory information to the cerebral cortex. A role for the thalamus in regulating autonomic functions and key circadian rhythms is consistent with prominent FFI symptoms. Twenty-four-hour circadian patterns comprise not only the sleep-wake cycle but also the normal ebb and flow of hormone secretions.

Other symptoms include severely impaired motor functions, uncoordinated and jerky muscle movements, and difficulty in speaking and swallowing. The autonomic dysregulation also manifests as fever and sweating. Affected persons are often described as inattentive, restless, and unable to concentrate. Cognition may also be affected.

Secretion of adrenocortical hormones is increased. These hormones are involved in the body's stress reaction, and those affected experience chronic stress. The insomnia that characterizes this disease is progressive and untreatable, leading to the ultimate absence of any sleep patterns or responses.

The first reported case, in 1986, was that of a fifty-three-year-old man. The onset of FFI is most often in middle to late adulthood, although it has been reported in some patients in their early twenties. The duration of the disease, from less than one year to several years, largely depends on genetic factors.

SCREENING AND DIAGNOSIS

Neither careful clinical examination nor standard tests of sleep responses can identify carriers of the FFI mutation before symptoms become apparent. Findings of routine laboratory tests are generally normal. Positron emission tomography, however, which can measure the brain's consumption of glucose, has shown thalamic changes in an asymptomatic gene carrier. Postmortem examination confirms the diagnosis.

TREATMENT AND THERAPY

Palliative treatment has been the only reported treatment. Attempts to alter the disease course with medications have been unsuccessful. Fatal familial insomnia is considered untreatable.

PREVENTION AND OUTCOMES

There is no known way to prevent the disease in a carrier. Prenatal diagnosis is theoretically possible.

Judith Weinblatt, M.S., M.A.

FURTHER READING

Bosque, Patrick J., and Kenneth L. Tyler. "Prions and Prion Diseases of the Central Nervous System (Transmissible Neurodegenerative Diseases)." In *Mandell, Douglas, and Bennett's Principles and Practice of Infectious Diseases,* edited by Gerald L. Mandell, John F. Bennett, and Raphael Dolin. 7th ed. New York: Churchill Livingstone/Elsevier, 2010.

Brown, David R., ed. *Neurodegeneration and Prion Disease.* New York: Springer, 2005.

Max, Daniel T. *The Family That Couldn't Sleep: A Medical Mystery.* New York: Random House, 2007.

_____. "The Secrets of Sleep." *National Geographic,* May, 2010, pp. 74-93.

Prusiner, Stanley B. "The Prion Diseases." *Scientific American* 272, no. 1 (January, 1995): 48-57.

_____, ed. *Prion Biology and Diseases.* 2d ed. Cold Spring Harbor, N.Y.: Cold Spring Harbor Laboratory Press, 2004.

Rowland, Lewis P., and Timothy A. Pedley, eds. *Merritt's Textbook of Neurology.* 12th ed. Philadelphia: Lippincott Williams & Wilkins, 2010.

WEB SITES OF INTEREST

Centers for Disease Control and Prevention
http://www.cdc.gov/ncidod/dvrd/prions

FFI Families Association
http://www.afiff.org

Genetic and Rare Diseases Information Center
http://rarediseases.info.nih.gov/gard

National Institute of Neurological Disorders and Stroke
http://www.ninds.nih.gov

National Organization for Rare Disorders
http://www.rarediseases.org

See also: Creutzfeldt-Jakob disease; Gerstmann-Sträussler-Scheinker syndrome; Guillain-Barré syndrome; Kuru; Prion diseases; Prions; Variant Creutzfeldt-Jakob disease.

Fatigue. *See* Chronic fatigue syndrome.

Fecal-oral route of transmission

CATEGORY: Transmission

DEFINITION

Fecal-oral transmission involves the acquisition of bacteria, viruses, fungi, and parasites from feces through the mouth, either by ingestion or absorption through the oral mucosa.

INTRODUCTION

In fecal-oral transmission, *Escherichia coli* and other enteric bacteria, viruses, and parasites are transmitted when the feces of a person or animal are inadvertently swallowed. This may occur when hands are not washed after using a toilet, after changing a diaper, after working in dirt or soil, after petting animals, and after cleaning up animal waste. Surfaces in day-care centers and public restrooms may be invisibly covered with such microbes.

Fecal-oral transmission also may occur through eating unwashed or improperly washed raw fruits and vegetables that have been grown in (or have been otherwise in contact with) manure-fertilized soil. For example, one enteric disease outbreak was caused by ingesting unpasteurized cider made from unwashed apples that had fallen to the ground. One study has shown that organic lettuce has one of the highest rates of fecal contamination, more than 22 percent. Fecally contaminated irrigation water is another source of pathogens on raw foods.

Such foods may also become contaminated when harvesters or food preparers handle them with unwashed, stool-contaminated hands. Raw, unpasteurized milk may contain fecal contaminants introduced in the milking process. Food handlers should keep their hands washed with antibacterial soap and should use disposable gloves appropriately. Cutting boards must also be kept disinfected. Cooking food at a high temperature for a sufficient length of time kills these bacteria and parasites.

Fecal-oral transmission may also result from swallowing swimming pool water that has not been sufficiently chlorinated. Similarly, lake or river water may be contaminated with animal feces and should not be consumed. To ensure safe drinking water when camping, water may be boiled, filtered, or chemically treated.

AGENTS OF FECAL-ORAL DISEASE

E. coli contamination in the drinking water of developing countries is the underlying cause of travelers' diarrhea. *Shigella* and *Yersinia* bacteria are also frequently found in contaminated water samples. Norovirus and rotavirus are commonly spread following the changing of diapers, including those of adults. *Giardia* cysts and *Cryptosporidium* oocytes in contaminated river water are parasites of fecal-oral transmission.

Gastroenteritis caused by fecal-oral transmission occurs most commonly in the summer. This may be related to increased activities of gardening and farming, animal handling, and recreation in lakes, rivers, and swimming pools. Underlying bacterial causes are most prevalent in the summer, while viral causes are most prevalent in the spring. Underlying bacterial causes are most prevalent in homes and restaurants, while viral causes are most prevalent in housing for the elderly and in hospitals.

IMPACT

Children and the elderly are most likely to experience severe disease and serious complications as a result of enteric infections because of their fragile nutritional and immune states. Additionally, the rate of fecal-oral transmission is two to four times higher among children in day care compared with preschool-age children raised at home. However, the increased use of alcohol-containing hand sanitizers and sanitary wipes is gradually compensating for infrequent or inadequate handwashing.

The U.S. Food and Drug Administration and the U.S. Department of Agriculture are concerned with identifying fecal contamination of foods. Hyperspectral fluorescence imaging systems are emerging to scan crops such as strawberries and cantaloupes and poultry carcasses for fecal contamination.

To minimize fecal-oral transmission, one should wash hands thoroughly with an antibacterial soap, not only when hands are visibly soiled but also, and especially, before eating and preparing food. Disposable gloves should be worn by commercial food handlers when preparing uncooked foods such as salads and sandwiches. Gloves should be changed immediately after handling raw meats. Gloves should be discarded upon leaving the workstation, when contaminated by sneezing or coughing, when stained or torn, and after being worn continuously for four hours.

For body fluid contamination of recreational water venues, calculation tables are available to check the concentration of chlorine and the disinfection time necessary to kill *Giardia* from solid stools and *Cryptosporidium* from liquid stools (diarrhea) at a pH (acid level) of 7.5 and a temperature of 77° Fahrenheit. Public water parks and pools will soon be able to test for human fecal contamination that is not readily apparent with a commercial kit that uses human secretory immunoglobulin A as an indicator. This form of testing is rapid, specific, and cost-effective.

Bethany Thivierge, M.P.H.

FURTHER READING

Centers for Disease Control and Prevention. *Morbidity and Mortality Weekly Report*: "Communitywide Cryptosporidiosis Outbreak—Utah, 2007." *Journal of the American Medical Association* 300 (2008): 1754-1756. This is a case study of an outbreak of chlorine-resistant *Cryptosporidium* in treated recreational water venues causing gastrointestinal distress.

_____. "Cryptosporidiosis Outbreaks Associated with Recreational Water Use—Five States, 2006." *Journal of the American Medical Association* 298 (2007): 1507-1509. This study reports factors for reducing the fecal-oral transmission of *Cryptosporidium* in public recreational water venues.

_____. "Foodborne Transmission of Hepatitis A—Massachusetts, 2001." *Journal of the American Medical Association* 290 (2003): 186-188. This is a case study of a food handler who spread the hepatitis A virus through fecal-oral transmission.

Pajan-Lehpaner, Gordana, and Olivera Petrak. "A One-Year Retrospective Study of Gastroenteritis Outbreaks in Croatia: Incidences and Etiology." *Collegium Antropologicum* 33 (2009): 1139-1144. This study determined differences between bacterial and viral causes of gastroenteritis through fecal-oral transmission.

Van, Rory, et al. "The Effect of Diaper Type and Overclothing on Fecal Contamination in Day-Care Centers." *Journal of the American Medical Association* 265 (1991): 1840-1844. This study determined the differences between plastic diapers and cloth diapers with plastic "overpants" on fecal contamination of toys and commonly handled items.

WEB SITES OF INTEREST

Center for Science in the Public Interest
http://cspinet.org/foodsafety

Centers for Disease Control and Prevention: Foodborne Diseases Active Surveillance Network
http://www.cdc.gov/foodnet

Clean Hands Coalition
http://www.cleanhandscoalition.org

EcoliHub
http://ecolihub.org

See also: Bacteria: Classification and types; Bacterial infections; Developing countries and infectious disease; *Escherichia coli* infection; Food-borne illness and disease; Hygiene; Intestinal and stomach infections; Norovirus infection; Oral transmission; Rotavirus infection; Soilborne illness and disease; Transmission routes; Travelers' diarrhea; Waterborne illness and disease.

Fever

CATEGORY: Diseases and conditions
ANATOMY OR SYSTEM AFFECTED: All
ALSO KNOWN AS: Pyrexia

DEFINITION

A fever is a sustained elevated body temperature. The average normal body temperature in humans is 98.6° Fahrenheit (37° Celsius). A person is considered febrile (to have a fever or to be feverish) when his or her body temperature reaches beyond the upper limits of a normal range, usually 100° F (37.8° C).

Key Terms: Fever

- *Antipyretic drugs.* Fever-reducing drugs, such as sodium salicylate, indomethacin, and acetaminophen

- *Ectotherms.* Organisms that rely on external temperature conditions to maintain their internal temperature

- *Endotherms.* Organisms that control the internal temperature of their bodies by the conversion of calories to heat

- *Febrile.* To have a fever or to be feverish

- *Febrile response.* An upward adjustment of the thermoregulatory set point

- *Metabolic rate.* A measurement of the calories (kilocalories) that are converted into heat energy to maintain body temperature or for physical exertion, or both

- *Pyrogens.* Protein substances that appear at the outset of the process that leads to a fever reaction

- *Thermoregulatory set point.* The ultimate neural control that maintains the normal human internal body temperature at 98.6° Fahrenheit (37° Celsius) and can either raise or lower it

---

CAUSES

A fever is a common symptom of many diseases. It is the body's immune-system reaction to an imbalance or unbalance in the system. Usually this unbalance is caused by the invasion of bacteria, viruses, or other pathogens (disease-causing organisms). The immune system responds to the invasion by increasing metabolism (body processes) to promote healing and by increasing the production of white blood cells to destroy invading pathogens; this, in turn, raises body temperature.

Other internal factors, including cancers such as leukemia, can cause fever because of increased numbers of white blood cells that disrupt the normal temperature balance. Sun and heat overexposure and drugs or drug withdrawal can also cause a fever.

RISK FACTORS

Because fever is such a common response to disease, all persons experience a fever at one time or another. The largest risk factor for fever is exposure to pathogens, especially bacteria and viruses. People who have had cancer and people with chronic illnesses such as human immunodeficiency virus (HIV) infection should monitor for fever, especially fevers that do not resolve with treatment; this can be a sign that disease is progressing. Sun exposure and dehydration (lack of adequate fluids in the body) are also risk factors for fever. Young children and older adults have more difficulty with regulating body temperature and often experience more fevers than do other age groups.

SYMPTOMS

In addition to having a temperature higher than 100° F, people who have a fever often have a general feeling of malaise (aches, weakness, irritability) and headache, shivering, sweating, appetite loss, increased thirst, and dehydration. Very high fevers (103° F, or 39.4° C, and higher) can cause confusion, hallucinations, seizures, and convulsions.

SCREENING AND DIAGNOSIS

Different types of thermometers can be used to determine if a person has an abnormally high body temperature. Thermometers are designed to obtain an accurate temperature from a particular area of the body, such as the mouth, rectum, axilla (armpit), or forehead. These tools range in complexity from a simple plastic strip that changes colors to indicate fever when placed on the forehead to electronic digital devices that are used either in the ear or in the mouth. Basic clinical thermometers are slender glass tubes filled with colored alcohol or mercury that reacts to heat.

TREATMENT AND THERAPY

Usually, treatment of fever involves treating the underlying cause. Rest and light blankets will help to keep the feverish person comfortable until the fever passes. Increasing the intake of cool liquids, such as water and juice, will help the person to avoid dehydration. Aspirin, acetaminophen (such as Tylenol), and ibuprofen (such as Advil) are nonprescription drugs that reduce fever and aches.

PREVENTION AND OUTCOMES

Because fever is a natural immune process, it is impossible to prevent. However, persons with a fever, especially the very young and the old, should be closely monitored because very high fevers can cause tissue damage, organ failure, and death.

Laura J. Pinchot, B.A.

FURTHER READING

Cohen, Barbara J. *Memmler's The Human Body in Health and Disease.* 10th ed. Philadelphia: Lippincott Williams & Wilkins, 2005.

El-Radhi, Sahib, James Caroll, and Nigel Klein, eds. *Clinical Manual of Fever in Children.* New York: Springer, 2009.

Mackowiak, Philip A., ed. *Fever: Basic Mechanisms and Management.* 2d ed. Philadelphia: Lippincott-Raven, 1997.

Parkham, Peter. *The Immune System.* 2d ed. New York: Garland Science, 2005.

WEB SITES OF INTEREST

See also: Bacterial infections; Fever of unknown origin; Hospitals and infectious disease; Iatrogenic infections; Immune response to bacterial infections; Immune response to fungal infections; Immune response to viral infections; Infection; Viral infections.

Fever of unknown origin

CATEGORY: Diseases and conditions
ANATOMY OR SYSTEM AFFECTED: All
ALSO KNOWN AS: Pyrexia of unknown origin

DEFINITION

A high body temperature without a clear cause is a fever of unknown origin, or FUO. An FUO is an intermittent temperature of a minimum 101° Fahrenheit (38-39° Celsius) and more than three weeks in duration. The FUO also is marked as such if a minimum of one week has passed in attempting to find its cause.

CAUSES

There are many rare causes of a high temperature. The following list includes a few of the uncommon causes: unusual infections, extrapulmonary tuberculosis, atypical tuberculosis, tropical diseases in temperate climates/latitudes (malaria, dengue fever, yellow fever), rare organisms (fungi, viruses, uncommon bacteria), obscure infections, prostatitis, sinusitis, hidden abscesses, collagen vascular (connective tissue, autoimmune) diseases, rheumatoid arthritis, systemic lupus erythematosus, inflammatory diseases, sarcoidosis, Crohn's disease (regional ileitis), cancer, lymphoma (Hodgkin's and non-Hodgkin's), leukemia, kidney cancer, liver cancer, drug reactions, antibiotics, epilepsy medications, immunoglobulin, antipsychotic drugs (Thorazine, Haldol), antihistamines, hereditary metabolic diseases, hormone disturbances, hyperthyroidism, brain disorders that affect temperature regulation, tumors, and strokes.

RISK FACTORS

The factors that increase the chance of developing an FUO include foreign travel, especially to developing and tropical countries; current medications (both prescription and over-the-counter); cancer or brain tumor; collagen vascular disease (an autoimmune disorder of connective tissue); human immunodeficiency virus (HIV) infection; acquired immunodeficiency syndrome (AIDS); current or recent hospitalization; and similar problems in the patient's family.

SYMPTOMS

One should not assume these symptoms are caused by an FUO. A fever is a common indication of many problems. These problems can be both serious and trivial. One should consult a doctor if experiencing any of the following symptoms: elevated temperature by thermometer reading, sweats, chills, and widespread body aches.

SCREENING AND DIAGNOSIS

A doctor will ask about symptoms and medical history and will perform a physical exam. The patient can help the doctor by taking his or her own temperature several times a day. The doctor may refer the patient to a specialist.

The first efforts after the usual evaluation will be to narrow the possibilities. This is done by examining the circumstances under which the fever began. The doctor will ask questions about traveling abroad, hospitalization, any damage to the immune system (for example, by AIDS), and current medications.

Many different tests may be indicated at some point. These tests include exhaustive studies of blood, urine, and all other bodily products; exhaustive imaging studies, such as X rays, computed tomography (CT)

and magnetic resonance imaging (MRI) scans, and ultrasound examinations; nuclear medicine studies; endoscopies (lungs, stomach and intestines, sinuses); and biopsies (samples taken by knife or needle) of suspect tissues.

TREATMENT AND THERAPY

There is no treatment for an FUO until the underlying disease is identified. When the fever's cause is discovered, treatment will follow.

PREVENTION AND OUTCOMES

There are many causes for an FUO. Prevention includes everything one does to stay healthy. One should take all preventive measures recommended by public health departments when traveling to developing countries or countries in tropical regions.

Ricker Polsdorfer, M.D.; reviewed by Rosalyn Carson-DeWitt, M.D.

FURTHER READING

Amin, K., and C. A. Kauffman. "Problem Infections in Primary Care: Fever of Unknown Origin—A Strategic Approach to this Diagnostic Dilemma." *Postgraduate Medicine* 114, no. 3 (September, 2003).

Beers, M. H., and R. Berkow. "Biology of Infectious Disease." In *The Merck Manual Home Health Handbook*, edited by Robert S. Porter et al. 3d ed. Whitehouse Station, N.J.: Merck Research Laboratories, 2009.

Gelfand, J. A., and M. V. Callahan. "Fever of Unknown Origin." In *Harrison's Principles of Internal Medicine*, edited by Anthony Fauci et al. 17th ed. New York: McGraw-Hill, 2008.

Roth, A. R., and G. M. Basello. "Approach to the Adult Patient with Fever of Unknown Origin." *American Family Physician* 68 (2003): 2223-2229. Available at http://www.aafp.org/afp/20031201/2223.html.

Torpy, J. "Fever in Infants." *Journal of the American Medical Association* 291 (2004): 1284.

WEB SITES OF INTEREST

American Academy of Pediatrics
http://www.healthychildren.org

Centers for Disease Control and Prevention
http://www.cdc.gov

Public Health Agency of Canada
http://www.phac-aspc.gc.ca

See also: Bacterial infections; Developing countries and infectious disease; Diagnosis of fungal infections; Fever; Fungal infections; Hospitals and infectious disease; Iatrogenic infections; Infection; Tropical medicine; Viral infections.

Fifth disease. *See* Erythema infectiosum.

Filariasis

CATEGORY: Diseases and conditions
ANATOMY OR SYSTEM AFFECTED: Lymphatic system, tissue
ALSO KNOWN AS: Lymphatic filariasis

DEFINITION

Filariasis is an infection with microscopic, threadlike worms transmitted from person to person by repeated mosquito bites. The adult worm lives and reproduces in the lymph system and produces microscopic worms known as microfilariae. These microfilariae circulate throughout the blood vessels of the body. When a mosquito bites an infected person and moves on to the next person, the microfilariae are deposited into the skin and move to the lymphatic system. The disease is often referred to as lymphatic filariasis, especially when symptoms occur.

CAUSES

The mosquito is the vector or disease-carrying insect that transmits filariasis from person to person. In Africa, the *Anopheles* mosquito is the most common vector. The *Culex quinquefasciatus* mosquito in the Americas and the *Mansonia* mosquito in Asia and the Pacific Rim transmit the infection.

Three species of worms cause lymphatic filariasis. Most infections are caused by *Wuchereria bancrofti*, but in Asia the infection filariasis is also caused by *Brugia malayi* and *B. timori*. The adult worms live up to seven years. Multiple mosquito bites over time are needed before symptoms of the disease occur.

RISK FACTORS

Living in a subtropical or tropical area where the infection is common is the greatest risk factor. Exposure to repeated mosquito bites increases the risk.

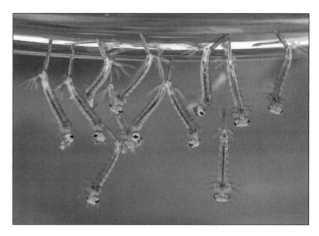

Larvae of the disease-causing Culex mosquito. (CDC)

Persons with occasional, short visits to tropical or subtropical countries with a history of the disease are at very low risk. There have been no reported cases originating in the United States in recent years.

SYMPTOMS

The worm that causes filariasis damages the lymph system. Persons who are infected may have no symptoms or may never develop clinical symptoms. Lymphedema, or lymph fluid collection in the tissues, is the primary symptom. Lymphedema is swelling that may be seen in the legs, arms, breasts, and genitalia. Swelling of the scrotum in men may occur due to infection with one of the causative worms. There is a decreased function of the lymph system, making it difficult for the body to fight infection. Hardening of the skin from bacterial infection may also be a symptom. In Asia, pulmonary filarial infection may cause a cough, wheezing, and difficulty breathing.

SCREENING AND DIAGNOSIS

There is no screening test for filariasis. The diagnosis is made with a blood smear that is stained and viewed under a microscope. The microfilariae circulate in the blood at night, so blood collection is more accurate when done at night. A serology test for immunoglobulin G4 may show elevated levels. Because lymphedema symptoms may occur many years after infection, laboratory tests may be negative.

TREATMENT AND THERAPY

Certain drugs may be used to kill the microfilariae and the adult worms. However, if clinical symptoms such as lymphedema are present, drugs are not used because an active infection is rarely present. A lymphedema therapist will provide help with skin care, exercise, and treatments to manage symptoms. Surgery may be indicated for infection of the scrotum.

PREVENTION AND OUTCOMES

To prevent infection, one should avoid mosquito bites in tropical and subtropical areas of the world by sleeping in an air-conditioned room or under a mosquito (sleeping) net, wearing long sleeves and pants, and using mosquito repellent, especially between dusk and dawn.

Patricia Stanfill Edens, R.N., Ph.D., FACHE

FURTHER READING

Jong, Elaine C., and Russell McMullen, eds. *Travel and Tropical Medicine Manual*. 4th ed. Philadelphia: Saunders/Elsevier, 2008. A useful reference manual with advice on preventing, evaluating, and managing diseases that can be acquired in tropical environments and countries outside the United States.

Lu, S., et al. "Localized Lymphedema (Elephantiasis): A Case Series and Review of the Literature." *Journal of Cutaneous Pathology* 36 (2009): 1-20.

McDowell, Julie, and Michael Windelsprecht. *The Lymphatic System*. Santa Barbara, Calif.: Greenwood Press, 2004.

Marquardt, William C., ed. *Biology of Disease Vectors*. 2d ed. New York: Academic Press/Elsevier, 2005. This textbook is geared to graduate students and researchers, but most of the information is accessible to general readers.

Muller, Ralph. *Worms and Human Disease*. 2d ed. New York: CABI, 2002. An advanced-student textbook that covers all human worm infections with emphasis on diagnosis, treatment, clinical manifestations, pathogenesis (disease development), epidemiology, and control.

WEB SITES OF INTEREST

Centers for Disease Control and Prevention
http://www.cdc.gov/parasites

Microbiology and Immunology On-line: Parasitology
http://pathmicro.med.sc.edu/book/parasit-sta.htm

Neglected Tropical Diseases Coalition
http://www.neglectedtropicaldiseases.org

Partners for Parasite Control
http://www.who.int/wormcontrol

See also: Arthropod-borne illness and disease; Bubonic plague; Developing countries and infectious disease; Disease eradication campaigns; Elephantiasis; Hookworms; Insect-borne illness and disease; Lymphadenitis; Mosquitoes and infectious disease; Onchocerciasis; Parasites: Classification and types; Parasitic diseases; Pathogens; Plague; Skin infections; Tropical medicine; Vectors and vector control; Worm infections.

Filoviridae

CATEGORY: Pathogen
TRANSMISSION ROUTE: Direct contact

DEFINITION

The Filoviridae is a family of nonsegmented, negative-sense, ribonucleic acid (RNA) viruses, distinguished from other members of the order Mononegavirales by having filamentous virus particles. The two known genera, Ebola virus and Marburg virus, cause virulent hemorrhagic fevers in humans and other primates.

Taxonomic Classification for Filoviridae

Kingdom: Unassigned
Phylum: Vira
Subphylum: Ribovira
Class: Ribohelica
Order: Mononegavirales
Family: Filoviridae
Genera:
Ebolavirus
Marburgvirus

NATURAL HABITAT AND FEATURES

The natural habitat of the Ebola virus and the Marburg virus, whose existence was unknown before 1967, has been a subject of much speculation and intense investigation. The first human cases of Marburg infection occurred in Germany but resulted from exposure to primates imported from central Africa, where sporadic direct transmission to humans also occurs. Loci of Ebola are found in Zaire, the southern Sudan, and the Ivory Coast in West Africa. Another species of Ebola, not pathogenic to humans, causes outbreaks in monkeys in the Philippines.

Extensive serological testing of likely reservoir species in affected areas has pinpointed a common fruit bat, *Rousettus aegyptiacus*, as a carrier for Marburg. Fruit bats are strongly suspected in Ebola. They have been confirmed as carriers of two other emergent lethal viral illnesses in the Mononegavirales order: nipah virus infection (Southeast Asia) and hendra virus infection (Australia). In fruit bats these viruses are either asymptomatic or cause mild illnesses.

Negative-strand RNA viruses, having penetrated a cell, serve as templates for positive strands of RNA that co-opt the cellular machinery of the cell to synthesize viral proteins. Transcription begins at a promoter site and may stop at boundaries between genes, producing positive strands coding only for certain proteins. As infection proceeds, the transcription process ignores gene boundaries and produces complete positive copies, which in turn serve as templates for the entire virus genome. Genome and proteins self-assemble into virions that bud off from the host cell membrane. Viruses of this type have high mutation rates because of an absence of proofreading ability in the enzyme that governs viral synthesis.

PATHOGENICITY AND CLINICAL SIGNIFICANCE

Members of the Filoviridae cause some of the most virulent viral illnesses known, with mortality rates of up to 90 percent, even in modern hospital settings. This virulence, coupled with moderate infectivity and the potential for human-to-human transmission, make Ebola and Marburg viruses matters of utmost concern for epidemiologists. These viruses are considered class-four hot pathogens. Their equally devastating effect on nonhuman primates constitutes a grave threat to rare species in central Africa. An ongoing epidemic among lowland gorillas may lead these magnificent animals to extinction.

Aside from Marburg virus in fruit bats, no active zoonosis attributed to Filoviridae in mammals other than primates has been identified, despite extensive searching. However, paleoviruses representing infections with genetically similar viruses occur in rodents and insectivores, and in bats, in central Africa. A paleovirus is a genetic marker, either a portion of the virus, incorporated into host deoxyribonucleic acid (DNA), or genes encoding for specific resistance, which has been passed through geologic time and can be used to trace the infection history of entire lineages of animals.

The extreme pathogenicity of Ebola and Marburg viruses dictate stringent quarantine measures and extreme care in the protection of researchers and medical and veterinary personnel to prevent their coming in contact with the pathogen. Since the time of the outbreaks in Marburg and in a primate facility in Reston, Virginia, screening and quarantine procedures for the legal movement of primates used for research have become much more rigorous, but illegal trade in monkeys from the Eastern Hemisphere remains a concern. No endemic infections attributable to Filoviridae are known from the Western Hemisphere or from outside the tropics.

Identification of an active case of either disease warrants immediate isolation of the infected person in a hospital setting. In this setting, intensive care can be provided with minimal contact with health care providers, recent contacts can be traced and isolated for observation, and the source of the infection can possibly be identified. Although the prospects for finding an effective therapeutic agent or developing a vaccine do not appear promising, identifying the animal reservoir opens an avenue for modifying human behavior to minimize exposure.

DRUG SUSCEPTIBILITY

No drugs have been identified that show promise in treating either Marburg or Ebola virus infections. One study showed some inhibition by S-adenosylhomocysteine hydrolase inhibitors in vitro and in a lethal mouse model. Any antiviral agent would need to be specific to the genomes and replication strategies of negative-sense single-strand RNA viruses. No common antiviral drug is effective against any member of the Mononegavirales.

Martha A. Sherwood, Ph.D.

FURTHER READING

Dimmock, N. J., A. J. Easton, and K. N. Leppard. *Introduction to Modern Virology.* 6th ed. Hoboken, N.J.: Wiley-Blackwell, 2007. A textbook for medical students and graduate students in biology, with a detailed section on the structure and replication of negative-sense single-strand RNA viruses.

Huffman, Michael, and Colin Chapman, eds. *Primate Parasite Ecology: The Dynamics and Study of Host-Parasite Relationships*. New York: Cambridge University Press, 2009. Contains an account of Ebola epidemics among gorillas and chimpanzees and speculations on how the disease shapes social structure.

Kahn, Alan J., ed. *RNA Viruses: A Practical Approach*. New York: Oxford University Press, 2000. A technical multiauthored book aimed primarily at research virologists, emphasizing genetics and molecular biology.

Mahanty, Siddhartha, and Mike Bray. "Pathogenesis of Filoviral Haemorrhagic Fevers." *The Lancet: Infectious Diseases* 4 (2004): 487-498.

Norkin, Leonard. *Virology: Molecular Biology and Pathogenesis*. Washington, D.C.: ASM Press, 2010. Using the framework of the Baltimore classification scheme, the author provides a detailed account of virus structure and replication and of the basis for disease pathology.

Preston, Richard M. *The Hot Zone*. New York: Random House, 1994. The best-selling journalistic account of outbreaks of Ebola, Ebola-Reston, and Marburg viruses, with much information on pathogenesis, symptoms, and quarantine measures.

WEB SITES OF INTEREST

Centers for Disease Control and Prevention
http://www.cdc.gov

International Committee for Taxonomy of Viruses
http://www.ictvdb.org

Virus Pathogen Database and Analysis Resource
http://www.viprbrc.org/brc

World Health Organization
http://www.who.int/csr/disease/ebola

See also: Arenaviridae; Ebola hemorrhagic fever; Hemorrhagic fever viral infections; Lassa fever; Marburg hemorrhagic fever; Primates and infectious disease; Viral infections; Viruses: Structure and life cycle; Viruses: Types.

Fleas and infectious disease

CATEGORY: Transmission

DEFINITION

Fleas are insects belonging to the order Siphonoptera, which includes 2,380 described species with 15 families and 238 genera. All are obligatory, hematophagous (blood-eating) parasites of warm-blooded mammals and birds. Fleas are wingless and are laterally compressed in shape; they have helmet-shaped heads and simple eyes. They range from light yellow to jet black and from 1 to 5 millimeters. Fleas are remarkably mobile; some can jump as far as 32 centimeters (as much as two hundred times their body length).

Flea species are found on all continents and have adapted to regions as diverse as equatorial deserts and Arctic tundra. The highest diversity of flea species is found in the subtropical to temperate regions of Eurasia. Flea lifestyles are diverse too; fleas can live as nest parasites, waiting to take a meal until the host returns for a rest. Some species, cat fleas (*Ctenocephalides felis*), for example, live most of their time on the host. In one genus of fleas, the *Tungidae*, the females become endoparasites by burrowing into human skin of the feet to feed. Although they tend to prefer one or a few host species, most fleas are opportunistic and will feed on what is available.

Fleas are reproductively prolific: *C. felis* can lay twenty to fifty eggs per day. The wormlike, free-living larvae hatch within two to five days. The larvae feed on adult feces, consisting of partly digested blood. Flea larvae develop into adults by passing through a cocoon-like pupae phase. Development occurs faster in environments with a humidity level of about 75 percent and in places with warm temperatures, optimally between 70° and 90° Fahrenheit. Conversely, eggs and larvae can remain viable at cooler temperatures for as long as twelve months.

NATURAL HISTORY AND RISK FACTORS

As blood feeders, fleas are efficient vectors for disease because they inject and ingest pathogens directly into and from new hosts. Their mobility means they have a large range, which provides for widespread transmission. Also, as opportunistic feeders, they can spread disease among different host species too. Fleas transmit pathogens to their progeny transovarially; that is, female fleas pass pathogens directly into their

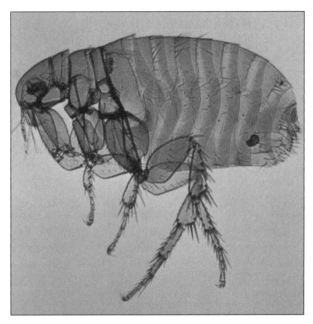

Microscopic image of Xenopsylla cheopis, the oriental rat flea. (CDC)

eggs. Because fleas can persist for long periods in environments that are not ideal, the pathogens they carry are likely to find new, susceptible hosts to infect. The result can be waves of recurring epidemics and epizootics.

As parasites, fleas are resilient and persistent, and they have developed resistance to insecticides. Those species that live in the environment can avoid insecticides on the host; those that live on the host avoid insecticides in the environment. As human parasites they are annoying, at minimum, and can cause skin infection and allergies. Some domestic animals can become overwhelmingly infested and suffer anemia that can be fatal.

FLEAS AS VECTORS

Fleas are vectors for the most devastating human disease in history, plague. Fleas also transmit murine typhus and can infect children with tapeworms of the family Diphylidium; fleas also might be reservoirs for cat scratch fever.

Plague. The oriental rat flea, *Xenopsylla cheopis*, is the principle vector for *Yersinia pestis*, the bacterial pathogen that causes plague. The disease takes three forms: bubonic, septicemic, and pneumonic. Bubonic plague is so called because lymph nodes swell and

blacken and become buboes. The fatality rate for untreated bubonic plague is as high as 75 percent. Septicemic and pneumonic forms are even more likely to be fatal, especially if antibiotic therapy is not started promptly.

Historically, plague caused three major pandemics: the Justinian plague in the sixth century, which spread around the Mediterranean region; the Black Death that started in Europe in the fourteenth century and continued intermittently for three hundred years; and a more recent pandemic that started in China in the mid-nineteenth century. The most notorious pandemic, the Black Death, is estimated to have killed 40 to 60 percent of Europe's population. The disease is also blamed for igniting the persecution of whole groups and populations, such as foreigners and Jews. The injustice of the disease also led the general population to doubt the authority of the Roman Catholic faith and of established authority, such as the land-owning nobility.

The Black Death was spread when rats were transported by ship and over land on trade routes. The rats died of the disease and the fleas left the rats to find new hosts, often humans, and transmitted *Y. pestis.* Once established in a host, *Y. pestis* can also be spread between humans either directly through respiratory droplets or through flea bites.

The disease reservoir for plague is in wild rodents, such as ground squirrels and prairie dogs. Rats and domestic animals can carry infected fleas to humans, and humans can be exposed directly from proximity to wild animals.

Murine typhus. Fleaborne, or murine, typhus is caused by rickettsial pathogens. *Rickettsia* are microorganisms between virus and bacteria in size and lifestyle; they are small and can survive only as intracellular parasites. Murine typhus causes flulike symptoms, such as headache, muscle aches, and fever, but symptoms can include a rash similar to that of measles. Although it is rarely (less than 2 percent) fatal, murine typhus can cause severe disease in the elderly and in immunocompromised persons.

Internationally, murine typhus is associated with indoor rats and *X. cheopis.* In the United States, the pathogen is more likely to be found in *C. felis.* Investigations of recent outbreaks in the Los Angeles region and in southern Texas revealed that the pathogen is more likely to be found associated with opossums and cats than with rodents.

Cat scratch fever. Cat scratch fever is caused by the bacterium *Bartonella henselae* and is transmitted to people who have been scratched by infected cats. Symptoms include fever and swollen lymph nodes. Although fleas do not appear to transmit the disease to people directly, they do appear to transmit it between cats; fleas also act as a reservoir for the organism.

Diplydium tapeworms. Fleas harbor tapeworm eggs in their gut and transmit the parasite to domestic animals when the domestic animals ingest the fleas as they groom. Children who ingest fleas also can be infected. The parasite is easily treated and does not cause serious disease.

PREVENTION AND CONTROL

Fighting flea infestations requires using insecticides on hosts and in the environment; intensive, adequate sanitation also is necessary. As common and annoying parasites of domestic animals, fleas have inspired considerable research into new insecticides that are less toxic and more effective. Modern innovations use arthropod hormones that interfere with larval development.

IMPACT

The World Health Organization estimates that thousands of people die every year from plague, mostly contracted from exposure to wildlife fleas. Similarly, murine typhus affects thousands of people worldwide.

Cynthia L. Mills, D.V.M.

FURTHER READING

Atkinson, P. W., ed. *Vector Biology, Ecology, and Control.* New York: Springer Science, 2010. This book is a good source for the reader who needs a detailed study of vectors and latest methods for effective vector control.

Azad, Abdu F., et al. "Flea-Borne Rickettsioses: Ecological Considerations." *Emerging Infectious Diseases* 3 (1997): 319-327. Review updating fleaborne murine typhus and environmental risk factors around the world.

_____. "Rickettsial Pathogens and Their Arthropod Vectors." *Emerging Infectious Diseases* 4 (1998): 179-186. Review of rickettsial diseases.

Marquardt, William C., ed. *Biology of Disease Vectors.* 2d ed. New York: Academic Press/Elsevier, 2005. Textbook on the biology of the vectors, including fleas, of disease in humans.

Stenseth, Nils, et al. "Plague: Past, Present, and Future." *PLoS Medicine* 5 (2008): 9-13. History and latest status of plague, describing its world distribution.

WEB SITES OF INTEREST

Fleas of the World
http://fleasoftheworld.byu.edu

Tree of Life Web Project
http://tolweb.org

See also: Arthropod-borne illness and disease; Cats and infectious disease; Dogs and infectious disease; Flies and infectious disease; Insect-borne illness and disease; Insecticides and topical repellants; Mites and chiggers and infectious disease; Mosquitoes and infectious disease; Parasitic diseases; Pathogens; Rat-bite fever; Rodents and infectious disease; Ticks and infectious disease; Transmission routes; Vectors and vector control; Viral infections.

Flesh-eating bacteria. *See* Necrotizing fasciitis.

Flies and infectious disease

CATEGORY: Transmission

DEFINITION

Flies can transmit more than sixty-five infectious diseases to humans and can carry more than one hundred species of pathogens. They spread disease either by biting directly into the skin (biological transmission) or by carrying disease-causing agents (pathogens) on their feet, mouths, or bodies and depositing them on humans; this process is called mechanical transmission.

Flies have been implicated in contaminating food with food-borne pathogens, such as *Escherichia coli*, which can be found on the mouths or in the feces of common houseflies. Flies can also leave disease-causing agents such as bacteria on or near areas such as wounds or mucous membranes, areas that allow the bacteria to enter the body and flourish. Most of the infectious diseases occurring from fly transmission in the Northern Hemisphere appear as relatively

Fly Facts

TAXONOMIC CLASSIFICATION

Kingdom: Animalia
Subkingdom: Bilateria
Phylum: Arthopoda
Subphylum: Uniramia
Class: Insecta
Order: Diptera
Suborder: Brachycera, thirty-five families

Geographical location: Every continent
Habitat: Grasslands, forests, and areas near rivers and lakes
Gestational period: Eggs hatch in two to seven days; adulthood occurs in one to six weeks
Life span: One to six months
Special anatomy: Six legs; compound eyes; one pair of wings, antennae, proboscises; and pulvilli

mild stomach upset; these diseases often go undiagnosed and rarely require medical intervention. For this reason, the causes of many flyborne illnesses are difficult to verify or identify.

Specific types of flies have been shown to transmit certain diseases in particular geographic areas and in particular developing populations. Female sandflies are associated with the transmission of leishmaniasis, a parasitic infection, and black flies are responsible for the spread of worm larvae, which causes onchocerciasis (also known as river blindness).

TRANSMISSION

Many types of flies feed off the blood of humans and animals. The flies are able to sense the potential availability of their next meal by the movement, warmth, moisture, and carbon dioxide emission of a nearby body. In warmer climates, humans tend to expose most of their skin, thereby increasing the potential for fly bites. Flies pierce the skin with their mouths and inject a small amount of saliva. This saliva contains an anticoagulant that prevents blood from clotting, allowing a fly to consume the blood. Any bacteria or parasites, such as worm larvae, contained in the saliva of the fly are injected into the bitten body, beginning the infection process.

Other diseases, such as trachoma or strep infection,

do not require an actual bite from a fly to be transmitted. A single fly can carry more than 33 million bacteria in its mouth or on its body, including its feet. The fly acts as a vector, carrying bacteria from a pathogen source or from one infected person to another. For example, after landing on the nasal or ocular discharge of a trachoma-infected child, a fly, now carrying the infectious agent, can directly deposit that agent into the eyes of other children. Young children and infants are often not able to brush flies away, which is why infection rates are so high for this age group.

PREVENTION AND OUTCOMES

Research has shown that fly control programs have significantly reduced the transmission and infection rates of some diseases. Insecticide treatment of an area or community can decrease the number of flies, but environmental and hygiene improvements are also implemented to limit fly contact.

Changes to the methods a community uses to manage waste and keep livestock can reduce fly populations near living spaces. The World Health Organization has been active in the development and support of insecticide spraying programs to reduce the breeding of flies and in education programs to teach people how to reduce fly populations.

IMPACT

The transmission of disease by flies is most common in tropical regions and in developing areas, where there are limited resources to control fly populations or to treat disease. Also, areas that are minimally affected by fly-transmitted diseases may find that risks increase during environmental disasters, such as flooding or tsunamis. Water increases the chance for flies to reproduce; clean water sources, following a disaster, often become contaminated with pollutants. This combination of water availability (for reproducing) and water pollution drastically increases the risk of infection in humans.

Fly population changes are strongly influenced by climate and weather patterns too. Predictive models suggest that fly populations are expected to increase because of climate change. Further studies will forecast fly population levels and ensure the effective implementation of control measures to manage future public health risks and disease.

April Ingram, B.S.

FURTHER READING

Fernando, Ranjan, et al. *Tropical Infectious Diseases: Epidemiology, Investigation, Diagnosis, and Management.* London: Greenwich Medical Media, 2001. Provides detailed information and pictures describing the treatment and management of tropical diseases, including those carried or transmitted by flies and in which regions around the world they are commonly found.

Graczyk, Thaddeus, et al. "The Role of Non-biting Flies in the Epidemiology of Human Infectious Diseases." *Microbes and Infection* 3 (2001): 231-235. A thorough review article that describes the spread of disease by flies in developing countries and discusses the transmission of infection in the home and in hospital environments.

Marquardt, William, ed. *Biology of Disease Vectors.* 2d ed. Burlington, Mass.: Academic Press/Elsevier, 2005. An excellent reference for understanding the roles of flies and other insects in the transmission of infectious disease. Discusses prevention and control strategies and future implications.

Shaffer, Julie, et al. "Filthy Flies? Experiments To Test Flies as Vectors of Bacterial Disease." *American Biology Teacher* 69 (2007): e28-e31. Provides background information on and a step-by-step outline for an experiment that demonstrates the behavior and disease vectoring ability of flies.

WEB SITES OF INTEREST

Centers for Disease Control and Prevention
http://www.cdc.gov/parasites

World Health Organization
http://www.who.int

See also: Arthropod-borne illness and disease; Blood-borne illness and disease; Developing countries and infectious disease; Fleas and infectious disease; Insect-borne illness and disease; Insecticides and topical repellants; Mites and chiggers and infectious disease; Mosquitoes and infectious disease; Parasitic diseases; Pathogens; Saliva and infectious disease; Ticks and infectious disease; Transmission routes; Tropical medicine; Vectors and vector control.

Flu. *See* Influenza.

Flukes

CATEGORY: Pathogen
TRANSMISSION ROUTE: Ingestion

DEFINITION

Flukes are leaf-shaped parasitic flatworms (trematodes) that adhere with their suckers to the internal organs of a host. More than six thousand species of flukes are found worldwide; they have a life cycle that is dependent on at least two or more hosts. Flukes are classified by the organ location they infest (such as blood, liver, lung, and intestines). Flukes in the families of Schistosmatidae, Echinostomatidae, Fasciolidae, Opisthorchioidea, Heterophyidae, and Paragonimidae are known to infect humans.

Taxonomic Classification for Flukes

Kingdom: Animalia
Subclass: Digenea
Phylum: Platyhelminthes
Class: Trematoda
Order: Strigeatida, Echinostomida, Opisthorchiida, Plagiorchiida
Family: Schistosmatidae, Echinostomatidae, Fasciolidae, Opisthorchioidea, Heterophyidae, Paragonimidae
Genera: *Schistosoma, Echinostoma, Fasciolopsis, Opisthorchis, Heterophyes, Paragonimus*
Species:
S. haematobium
S. intercalatum
S. japonicum
S. mansoni
S. mekongi
E. trivolvis
F. hepatica
F. buski
O. felineus
O. viverrini
H. heterophyes
P. westermani

NATURAL HABITAT AND FEATURES

Flukes are obligate parasites because they are dependent on their hosts for nourishment. They are also considered endoparasites because their life cycle

Flatworm (Fluke) Facts

Geographical location: Worldwide

Habitat: The larvae of Monogenea (ectoparasitic flukes) and Trematoda (endoparasitic flukes) may be found in streams, but adults live within the body of a host

Gestational period: Varies among flatworm species, but most species lay eggs within a few days after fertilization; eggs usually hatch within a few days to a few weeks after being deposited

Life span: Varies among species, but can be up to thirty years in some flukes

Special anatomy: Elongated, bilateral invertebrates without appendages, have neither a true body cavity nor a circulatory system; parasitic species have specially adapted mouth parts for attaching to the tissues of the host

is dependent on the internal environment of a minimum of two different hosts. The host animal of adult flukes tends to be a predatory vertebrate. Flukes that infect humans are found in all countries, but their geographic distribution is dependent on the availability of needed intermediate hosts, such as mollusks found in fresh-water environments. Their natural habitat is therefore dependent on the various stages of their complex life cycle and on the environment of the required host.

Flukes range in size from microscopic to large, depending on the species. Liver, lung, and intestinal flukes may enter the final host through ingestion, and blood flukes enter the host through penetration of skin. Flukes in human hosts will reside in various internal organs and will feed off those organs. Eggs of the various species are produced by adult worms and passed through feces or sometimes through sputum. Feces-containing eggs that end up in fresh-water supplies, and the presence of the necessary intermediate host, will restart the life cycle. Once in fresh water, the eggs hatch into a larval state (miracidum) and seek the necessary intermediate host, typically a snail. Once inside the intermediate host, the fluke morphs into a second larval state known as cercariae. The cercariae exit the intermediate host to find secondary hosts, such as aquatic plants, crustaceans, or fish, where they will form a cyst (mesocercaria) until ingested by the final host; here they can mature to adults in the de-

sired internal organ. Blood flukes will enter a human host through skin penetration as cercariae in fresh water. Once the adult stage is reached, production of eggs begins. Many species of flukes have the ability to reproduce both sexually and asexually.

PATHOGENICITY AND CLINICAL SIGNIFICANCE

Flukes are responsible for two neglected tropical diseases (NDT): food-borne trematodiases (FBT), from eating certain types of raw or undercooked food (aquatic vegetation, crustaceans, and fish), and schistosomiasis. Liver flukes, lung flukes, and intestinal flukes are linked to FBT, whereas blood flukes cause schistosomiasis. Schistosomiasis ranks second to malaria as one of the most prevalent parasitic infections in the world.

Symptoms of fluke infestation include allergic responses, rash (swimmer's itch), fever, weakness, inflammation, abdominal pain, nausea, and diarrhea. Movement of flukes and their eggs through internal organs results in blockage, swelling, and lasting organ damage that may lead to additional immune responses, inflammation, cirrhosis, anemia, hepatomegaly, or cancer. Fluke infections are often misdiagnosed, resulting in irreparable internal organ damage. Diagnosis is confirmed by examination of eggs in a stool sample or from a tissue sample through biopsy. Prevention of fluke parasitism is possible through improved water sanitation and avoidance of eating raw or undercooked foods.

DRUG SUSCEPTIBILITY

Drug therapy for most flukes includes praziquantel, triclabendazole, oxamniquine, and bithionol. Drug resistance is an increasing concern, and scientists have made progress on vaccines against flukes.

Susan E. Thomas, M.L.S.

FURTHER READING

"Blood Trematodes: Schistosomes." In *Diagnostic Medical Parasitology*, edited by Lynne Shore Garcia. 5th ed. Washington, D.C.: ASM Press, 2007.

Davis, Andrew. "Schistosomiasis." In *Manson's Tropical Diseases*, edited by Gordon C. Cook and Alimuddin I. Zumla. 22d ed. Philadelphia: Saunders/Elsevier, 2009.

Despommier, Dickson D., et al. *Parasitic Diseases.* 5th ed. New York: Apple Tree, 2006.

Fried, Bernard, and Amy Abruzzi. "Food-Borne Trematode Infections of Humans in the United States of America." *Parasitology Research* 106 (2010): 1263-1280.

"Intestinal Trematodes" In *Diagnostic Medical Parasitology*, edited by Lynne Shore Garcia. 5th ed. Washington, D.C.: ASM Press, 2007.

"Liver and Lung Trematodes." In *Diagnostic Medical Parasitology*, edited by Lynne Shore Garcia. 5th ed. Washington, D.C.: ASM Press, 2007.

Sithithaworn, Paiboon, et al. "Food-Borne Trematodes." In *Manson's Tropical Diseases*, edited by Gordon C. Cook and Alimuddin I. Zumla. 22d ed. Philadelphia: Saunders/Elsevier, 2009.

WEB SITES OF INTEREST

Animal Diversity Web, University of Michigan Museum of Zoology
http://animaldiversity.ummz.umich.edu

Centers for Disease Control and Prevention
http://www.cdc.gov/parasites

Microbiology and Immunology On-line: Parasitology
http://pathmicro.med.sc.edu/book/parasit-sta.htm

See also: Ascariasis; Cholera; Clonorchiasis; Developing countries and infectious disease; Dracunculiasis; Food-borne illness and disease; Giardiasis; Hookworms; Intestinal and stomach infections; Malaria; Parasitic diseases; Pinworms; Roundworms; Schistosomiasis; Tapeworms; Trichinosis; Tropical medicine; Waterborne illness and disease; Whipworm infection; Worm infections.

Food-borne illness and disease

CATEGORY: Transmission
ALSO KNOWN AS: Enteric diseases, food poisoning

DEFINITION

Food-borne illnesses and diseases, or enteric diseases, are transmitted to humans from infectious organisms in food and water, generally resulting in gastrointestinal symptoms that vary in severity and duration. Enteric diseases may be caused by viruses, bacteria, or parasites. Technically, the phrase "food poisoning" refers to ingestion of food-borne toxins rather than infectious agents such as bacteria and viruses.

Enteric diseases are thought to cause about 70 percent of cases of diarrhea. Often, what is referred to as a stomach bug or a twenty-four-hour flu is actually the result of a food-borne illness. It is usually difficult to pinpoint the cause of stomach upset because of the long incubation periods for most infectious agents and because exposure occurs several times each day. As a result, epidemiologists believe that for every known case of food-borne illness, dozens more go unreported.

To be confirmed as a case of enteric disease, the illness must lead a person to seek medical care. A stool specimen must be collected and sent to a laboratory, which tests the sample for multiple organisms. If the lab confirms a specific pathogen, it must report the case to the local health department or to the Centers for Disease Control and Prevention (CDC), or both. An outbreak is said to occur when two or more cases can be traced to the same source, as when multiple people become ill after eating the same food at a picnic.

CHARACTERISTICS

Symptoms associated with enteric diseases vary according to the pathogen responsible, but often include diarrhea, nausea, abdominal pain, vomiting, and fever. Generally, food-borne illness results in a temporary, uncomfortable period of stomach upset. A health care provider should be consulted, however, if the patient has trouble keeping liquids down or has diarrhea that persists for more than three days and is accompanied by a fever of more than 101.5° Fahrenheit, is bloody, and leads to dehydration. In addition, an estimated 15 percent of people who experience acute gastroenteritis develop reactive arthritis within four weeks of infection with *Campylobacter, Salmonella, Shigella, Yersinia*, or, occasionally, *Escherichia coli* O157:H7. Symptoms of this type of arthritis include lower extremity stiffness and pain.

The most common cause of food-borne illness in the United States is the family of noroviruses (Norwalk virus being the best known). The incubation period is twelve to forty-eight hours and the illness lasts for twelve to sixty hours. Symptoms include nausea, vomiting, abdominal cramping, diarrhea, fever, muscle pain, and headache. Common sources

Top Ten Pathogens Causing Foodborne Illnesses in the United States (2009)

Pathogen	Estimated Cases	Hospitalizations	Deaths
Noroviruses	21 million	20,000	124
Campylobacter species	1.9 million	10,539	99
Salmonella species	1.3 million	16,102	536
Clostridium perfringens	248,520	41	7
Giardia intestinalis (also known as *G. lamblia*)	200,000	500	1
Staphylococcus	185,060	1,753	2
Escherichia coli (all forms)	173,107	2,785	78
Toxoplasma gondii	112,500	2,500	375
Shigella species	89,648	1,246	14
Yersinia enterocolitica	86,731	1,105	2

include shellfish and other foods (such as those in salad bars) contaminated by infected persons.

Campylobacter infections result in the onset of symptoms two to five days after the consumption of contaminated raw or undercooked poultry, unpasteurized milk, or contaminated water. Symptoms, including diarrhea (sometimes bloody), cramps, fever, and vomiting, last two to ten days.

Salmonella spp. are commonly found in eggs, poultry, unpasteurized milk and juice, cheese, raw fruits and vegetables (such as sprouts and melons), and streetvended foods. Most strains of *Salmonella* cause symptoms that include diarrhea, fever, cramps, and vomiting. Certain strains result in typhoid fever, with fever, headache, constipation, malaise, chills, and myalgia. Symptoms appear after an incubation period of one to three days and typically last four to seven days.

Clostridium perfringens infections have an incubation period of eight to sixteen hours after ingestion of a contaminated food, such as meat, poultry, or gravy; and after ingestion of dried or precooked foods or foods left out of a refrigerator or freezer (at room temperature or higher) for too long. Symptoms include watery diarrhea, nausea, and cramping, which last twenty-four to forty-eight hours.

Giardia is a parasite that causes symptoms one to two weeks after consumption of contaminated water, uncooked food, or food handled by an ill person after cooking. Diarrhea, stomach cramps, and gas can last days or weeks.

Staphylococcus aureus infections commonly result in the sudden onset of severe nausea and vomiting and cramps (and sometimes diarrhea and fever), one to six hours after eating contaminated foods, such as unrefrigerated or improperly stored meats, mayonnaisebased salads, pastries containing cream or cheese, and other prepared foods. Symptoms last twenty-four to forty-eight hours.

E. coli has several forms, most of which are harmless and all of which are common in the digestive tracts of warm-blooded animals (including humans). Enterotoxigenic *E. coli* (ETEC) is a common cause of travelers' diarrhea (also known colloquially as Montezuma's revenge, Delhi belly, and yalla yalla). ETEC infection typically has a one-to-three-day incubation period, after which the infected person experiences watery diarrhea, cramps, and vomiting for three days to one week or more. ETEC is associated with fecalcontaminated water or food.

Less common, but more serious, forms of *E. coli* are known as enterohemorrhagic *E. coli* (EHEC), which include *E. coli* O157:H7 and other Shiga toxin-producing *E. coli* (STEC). These forms of *E. coli* result in severe and often bloody diarrhea, abdominal pain, and vomiting and are more common in children under age four years. Illness manifests one to eight days after con-

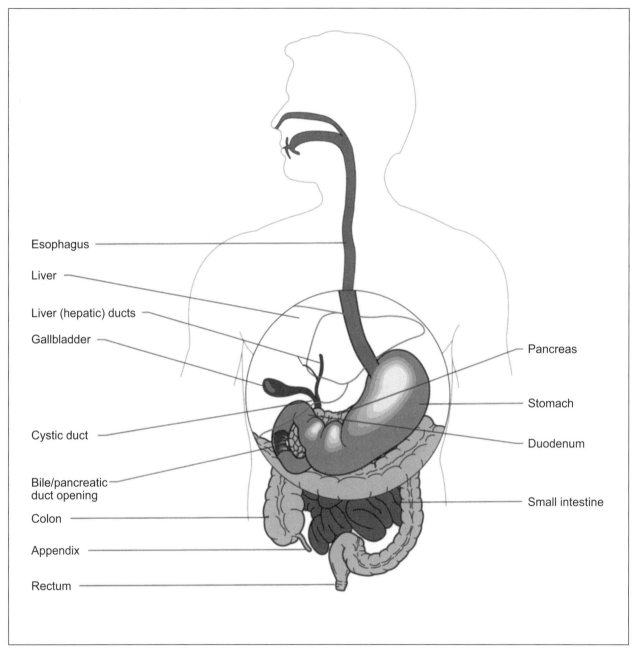

Esophagus

Liver

Liver (hepatic) ducts

Gallbladder

Cystic duct

Bile/pancreatic duct opening

Colon

Appendix

Rectum

Pancreas

Stomach

Duodenum

Small intestine

Food-borne illness and disease involve a variety of body organs and systems, from the mouth to the rectum.

sumption of undercooked beef, especially hamburger, unpasteurized milk and juice, raw fruits and vegetables, and contaminated water. EHEC-associated symptoms generally last five to ten days. About 2 to 7 percent of persons infected with *E. coli* O157:H7 (mostly children and the elderly) develop hemolytic-uremic syndrome, and of those, about one-third develop chronic kidney disease and 3 to 5 percent die. *E. coli* transmitted from infected poultry and pork products is thought to be a significant cause of the six to eight million urinary tract infections (UTIs) that occur each year in the United States.

Toxoplasma gondii is a parasite that infects humans through the ingestion of unwashed fruits and vegetables contaminated by animal feces or the ingestion of raw and partially cooked meat (especially pork, lamb, and venison). The incubation period is five to twenty-three days and symptoms, which are present only in about 20 percent of infected persons, include flulike illness or swollen lymph nodes (or both), which can last months.

Shigella infections result in symptoms of abdominal cramps, fever, and diarrhea about twenty-four to forty-eight hours after contact with contaminated food and last four to seven days. *Shigella* is associated with fecal-oral transmission, often spread from an infected food worker to ready-to-eat foods such as raw vegetables, salads, and sandwiches.

Yersinia infections cause symptoms including diarrhea, vomiting, fever, abdominal pain, and, sometimes, a red rash. *Yersinia* is associated with undercooked pork, unpasteurized milk, tofu (soy), and contaminated water. Symptoms appear twenty-four to forty-eight hours after infection and last one to three weeks. Rarely, *Yersinia* can result in a bloodstream infection.

In addition to the foregoing common causes of food-borne illnesses, certain others are tracked by the CDC, often because they can be deadly. *Listeria* is one such pathogen. Although only three persons in every one million persons get the disease, it is fatal in 25 percent of those infected and is especially harmful to fetuses. *Listeria* can survive refrigeration for weeks, but cooking kills the bacteria. Raw milk, undercooked or raw foods such as smoked salmon, and soft cheeses are the most common food sources. *Listeria* is responsible for an estimated 2,300 hospitalizations and 500 deaths each year.

TREATMENT

Initial treatment for persons with food-borne illnesses generally focuses on rehydration, because both vomiting and diarrhea tend to lead to potentially dangerous dehydration. Antibiotic therapy is necessary only in cases of invasive bacterial infections, such as *Shigella*. In persons with mild to moderate *Salmonella* infection, antibiotic therapy may not be helpful and may actually be harmful; it can lead to the person being a long-term asymptomatic carrier who can easily spread the bacteria to others. Antibiotics should never be used for persons with suspected STEC infec-tion because of the increased risk for development of hemolytic-uremic syndrome, which is fatal 5 to 10 percent of the time and leads to chronic kidney disease in another 10 percent. Similarly, antibiotic therapy in persons with *C. difficile* infection increases the risk of developing toxic megacolon, with a 20 percent mortality rate. Antibiotic treatment is ineffective in cases caused by viruses.

RISK FACTORS

The risk factors associated with food-borne illnesses range from those at the kitchen level to those in the food system as a whole. Raw and undercooked foods, inadequate home canning, cross-contamination (in which bacteria is transmitted by, for example, the use of unwashed cutting boards), insufficient hygiene by food service workers, and foods kept at the wrong temperatures are all examples of risk factors at the consumer level.

At the producer level, food system issues include widespread consolidation, industrialization, and globalization, all risk factors for the spread of food-borne illnesses because they can lead to a lack of oversight and inspection and to problems with tracing foods that are produced on an industrial scale. For example, one infected cow can contaminate large amounts of ground beef because meat from many animals is often mixed during the processing of the ground beef.

Labor and economic development issues also can play a role in the spread of food-borne diseases. For example, a large percentage of fresh fruits and vegetables comes from countries without chlorinated water supplies. Contaminated water that is used to irrigate fields or wash produce after harvest can lead to *Salmonella* and *E. coli* infections inside the tissue of the produce itself, where it cannot be washed off. Farm workers, food service workers, and meat workers without appropriate access to toilets or facilities for handwashing can contaminate food too.

Industrial-scale, concentrated or confined animal-feeding operations (CAFOs) are sources of nearly all the meat, poultry, and eggs in the United States. CAFOs generate enormous amounts of animal waste, which is often disposed of by being spread (as raw manure) on agricultural fields. Runoff from these fields can contaminate drinking water. CAFOs are also blamed for increasing the development of antibiotic-resistant bacteria by the routine use of low doses of antibiotics in herds, which cause the animals to grow faster. The close contact of thousands of confined animals also facilitates the spread of pathogens among those animals.

PREVENTION AND OUTCOMES

In home kitchens, consumers can reduce their risk of food-borne illnesses by practicing four principles of safe food handling: clean, separate, cook, and chill. "Clean" means washing hands and food-preparation surfaces thoroughly and often. "Separate" means keeping items that are used for animal products separate from items used for other foods, and keeping animal products separate from other items in one's grocery cart, grocery bags, and refrigerator. "Cook" refers to cooking foods to a high enough internal temperature to kill pathogens and staying away from raw or partially cooked foods, such as rare steaks or sauces containing raw eggs. "Chill" refers to refrigerating leftover food promptly in a refrigerator kept at 40° Fahrenheit or lower. Consumers should also practice the so-called 2-2-4 rule for safe handling of leftovers: no more than two hours should pass between cooking the food and refrigerating leftovers; store food in shallow containers (no more than two inches deep) so it cools quickly once refrigerated; and use or freeze the food within four days.

Consumers also can reduce their food-borne disease risk through their food choices. Avoiding or minimizing consumption of animal products is one way to minimize risk, as meat, poultry, seafood, eggs, and dairy are the primary sources of food-borne diseases in the United States. Free-range eggs are less likely to carry *Salmonella* than are eggs from hens kept in battery cages, and organic eggs are even safer than free-range eggs. Meat and poultry from animals raised on smaller farms, on pasture, and (for cattle) on eating grass rather than corn is less likely than factory-farmed meat and poultry to carry *E. coli* and other pathogens.

Only one-quarter of food-borne illnesses originate from improper home food-handling, with the remainder caused by problems at the source or somewhere along the chain before food reaches the eater. Regulatory oversight of food in the United States is fragmented among multiple departments and agencies. The U.S. Department of Agriculture (USDA) inspects meat, poultry, and pasteurized and processed eggs, whereas the U.S. Food and Drug Administration (FDA) regulates all other foods. Regulatory fragmentation and resource and budget constraints on inspec-

tion processes may be further systemic causes of the ongoing problems related to food safety in the United States.

IMPACT

The CDC estimates that food-borne illnesses are responsible for at least 76 million illnesses, 325,000 hospitalizations, and 5,000 deaths in the United States each year. About 5 percent of the population may be affected at any one time, of whom about 20 percent will seek medical care.

Food-borne illnesses cost the U.S. economy billions of dollars each year. Costs are incurred by patients and the health care system for treatment. Patients may lose wages, and their illnesses are a drain on productivity. One estimate of the costs associated with just six bacterial pathogens and one parasite was $6.5 billion to $34.9 billion annually.

Outbreaks also lead to food recalls and associated costs. For example, in 2008, Westland/Hallmark recalled more than 143 million pounds of beef after the USDA deemed the beef unfit for human consumption. In 2009, the Peanut Corporation of America recalled more than 3,900 different bulk peanut-butter products from roughly 360 different companies because of suspected *Salmonella* contamination. The USDA reported fifty-two recalls of meat contaminated with *E. coli* O157:H7 between 2007 and 2009. In addition, food-borne illnesses also lead to an intangible cost: the loss of trust in the food system. In a 2009 survey, less than 20 percent of respondents said they trusted food companies to develop and sell safe foods.

Lisa M. Lines, M.P.H.

FURTHER READING

American Medical Association. "Diagnosis and Management of Foodborne Illnesses: A Primer for Physicians and Other Health Care Professionals." Available at http://www.cdc.gov/mmwr/preview/mmwrhtml/rr5304a1.htm. A comprehensive guide to diagnosis and treatment of common food-borne diseases, with patient scenarios.

Flint, James A., et al. "Estimating the Burden of Acute Gastroenteritis, Foodborne Disease, and Pathogens Commonly Transmitted by Food: An International Review." *Clinical Infectious Diseases* 41 (2005): 698-704. An international review of the wide-ranging burden (incidence, hospitalizations, and mortality) associated with food-borne illnesses.

Gaman, P. M., and K. B. Sherrington. *The Science of Food: An Introduction to Food Science, Nutrition, and Microbiology.* 4th ed. Boston: Butterworth-Heinemann/Elsevier, 2008. Examines food composition and microbiology. Includes good bibliographical references and an index.

Hickmann, Meredith A. ed. *The Food and Drug Administration (FDA).* Hauppauge, N.Y.: Nova Science, 2003. Explains how the FDA is responsible for ensuring the safety of foods, drugs, medical devices, cosmetics, and other products.

Iwamoto, Martha, et al. "Epidemiology of Seafood-Associated Infections in the United States." *Clinical Microbiology Reviews* 23 (2010): 399-411. An updated review of seafood-related infections and diseases in the United States.

Jay, James M., Martin J. Loessner, and David A. Golden. *Modern Food Microbiology.* 7th ed. New York: Springer, 2005. This excellent textbook summarizes the state of knowledge of the biology and epidemiology of the microorganisms that cause food-borne illness.

Lynch, M. F., et al. "The Growing Burden of Food-borne Outbreaks Due to Contaminated Fresh Produce: Risks and Opportunities." *Epidemiology and Infection* 137 (2009): 307-315. Focuses on food-borne diseases associated with fresh produce. Includes suggestions for preventive approaches.

Mead, Paul S., et al. "Food-Related Illness and Death in the United States." *Emerging Infectious Diseases* 5 (1999): 607-625. The source of frequently cited estimates of the number of cases, hospitalizations, and deaths attributable to food-borne diseases in the United States each year.

Nestle, Marion. *Safe Food: The Politics of Food Safety.* Updated ed. Berkeley: University of California Press, 2010. Examines the policy and politics associated with food safety issues.

Pigott, David C. "Foodborne Illness." *Emergency Medicine Clinics of North America* 26 (2008): 475-497. Provides a review of the epidemiology, etiology, and treatment for infections caused by most of the common pathogens.

WEB SITES OF INTEREST

American College of Gastroenterology
http://www.acg.gi.org

Center for Food Safety and Applied Nutrition
http://www.fda.gov/food

Center for Science in the Public Interest: Food Safety
http://cspinet.org/foodsafety

Centers for Disease Control and Prevention: Foodborne Diseases Active Surveillance Network
http://www.cdc.gov/foodnet

Clean Hands Coalition
http://www.cleanhandscoalition.org

FoodSafety.gov
http://www.foodsafety.gov

National Center for Home Food Preservation
http://www.uga.edu/nchfp

Partnership for Food Safety Education
http://www.fightbac.org

U.S. Department of Agriculture, Food Safety and Inspection Service
http://www.fsis.usda.gov

See also: *Campylobacter*; *Clostridium*; Developing countries and infectious disease; *Escherichia*; Fecal-oral route of transmission; *Giardia*; Intestinal and stomach infections; *Listeria*; Oral transmission; *Salmonella*; *Shigella*; *Staphylococcus*; Transmission routes; Travelers' diarrhea; Tropical medicine; Waterborne illness and disease; *Yersinia*.

Francisella

CATEGORY: Pathogen
TRANSMISSION ROUTE: Blood, direct contact, inhalation

DEFINITION

Francisella are small, nonmotile, gram-negative coccobacilli that are found in water, soil, plants, and mammals. The bacteria may be vectored by ticks, flies, or mosquitoes. The clinical manifestations of infection vary greatly depending upon the portal of entry, virulence of the strain, and host immunity.

Taxonomic Classification for *Francisella*

Kingdom: Bacteria
Phylum: Proteobacteria
Class: Gammaproteobacteria
Order: Thiotricales
Family: Francisellaceae
Genus: *Francisella*
Species:
F. tularensis
F. philomiragia

NATURAL HABITAT AND FEATURES

The bacteria of the *Francisella* genus are found in the natural environment. They have been isolated from soil, water, and plants. Mammalian natural reservoirs include rodents (muskrats, voles, and lemmings), lagomorphs (rabbits and hares), and insectimorphs (shrews, moles, and hedgehogs). Humans, wild animals (such as deer and foxes), and domestic animals (such as dogs and cats) also serve as hosts. Blood-feeding arthropods and insects serve as vectors. In the United States, there is a summer peak in cases associated with tick bites and a smaller peak in the winter associated with hunting.

The tiny coccobacilli comprising the *Francisella* genus are only weakly gram-negative, as they take up the safranin counterstain poorly. They are nonmotile, aerobic, non-spore-forming organisms that are weakly catalase positive and that ferment only a few sugars. Each possesses a capsule that is rich in fatty acids and that functions as a major virulence factor.

Francisella bacteria are fastidious, and nearly all strains require supplementation with sulfhydryl compounds, such as cysteine, cystine, or thiosulphate, to grow on artificial media. The organisms grow slowly with a generation time of one hour, and cultures usually take three to five days for colonies to appear when incubated aerobically at 95° to 98.6° Fahrenheit (35° to 37° Celsius). The bacteria are potentially infectious for laboratory workers, either by inoculation through small breaks in the skin or by inhalation. All specimens and cultures must be handled in a biological safety cabinet using gloves. *Francisella* have been isolated from skin ulcers, biopsies of skin and internal organs, lymph node aspirates, sputum, bone marrow, and blood.

There are four subspecies of *F. tularensis* that are identified by biochemical, cultural, and molecular methods. *F. tularensis* sub. *tularensis* is the most common subspecies in North America and is also the most virulent. *F. tularensis* sub. *holarctica* is also found in North America and is the usual species identified in Europe and Asia. The live vaccine strain of *F. tularensis* is derived from subspecies *holarctica*, and there is also a variant, biovar *japonica*, which is found in Japan. The subspecies *novicida* is of lower virulence and is associated with disease in immunocompromised persons and in persons who nearly drowned in fresh-water sources. Subspecies *mediasiatica* is found only in Kazakhstan and Turkmenistan.

F. philomiragia is an uncommon opportunistic pathogen that infects the immunocompromised human host and persons who have survived a drowning in salt-water sources. A closely related bacterium causes granulomatous disease in salt-water fish such as the Atlantic cod.

PATHOGENICITY AND CLINICAL SIGNIFICANCE

F. tularensis is a virulent pathogen that can infect a suitable host with a dose of only ten to fifty bacteria when injected into the skin or inhaled into the lungs. Infection through the gastrointestinal tract from ingestion requires a much larger dose. The most common route of infection is cutaneous inoculation, which allows the organism to multiply at the site and produce a papule that matures into an ulcer in about one week. The organism then spreads to the regional lymph glands.

Further dissemination to multiple organs may occur through the lymphatics and blood vessels. This form of infection is called ulceroglandular tularemia and usually results from contaminated tick or other insect bites and from direct contact with an infected animal or animal product. The host responds with an acute inflammatory reaction to both the organism and the necrotic tissue produced by the infection. Antibody is produced, but is insufficient to resolve the infection. Neutrophils and macrophages are able to ingest, but not kill, this facultative intracellular pathogen. Indeed, *F. tularensis* not only is able to survive macrophage ingestion; the pathogen also proliferates intracellularly, killing the cell and releasing progeny. Development of an adequate cell-mediated immune response is necessary for recovery.

The inhalation of *F. tularensis* as an aerosol or in an aqueous milieu, such as occurs in near-drowning, usually results in pneumonia. The acute inflammatory response is much the same as occurs in cutaneous inoculation, and the neutrophilic response may further damage the lung. Again, the ability of the organism to survive and multiply after ingestion by alveolar macrophages allows for progression of the infection and for systemic spread.

The combination of virulence and a small minimal-infecting dose makes *F. tularensis* an ideal agent for bioterrorism. Additionally, virtually an entire targeted population would be susceptible to infection. While a live vaccine strain was developed in the mid-twentieth century, there have been many problems with vaccine development. No vaccine is available for general use.

Diagnosis of the illnesses caused by *Francisella* still depends largely on clinical suspicion with serology, culture, and the polymerase chain reaction test. Before the existence of antibiotics, tularemia mortality was as high as 60 percent; it is now less than 4 percent. In the United States, tularemia is an uncommon illness; it occurs at a rate of only 0.05 cases per 100,000 persons.

DRUG SUSCEPTIBILITY

Francisella bacteria are susceptible to many classes of antibiotics, including aminoglycosides, tetracyclines, chloramphenicol, fluoroquinolones, macrolides, rifamycins, and some cephalosporins. However, the efficacy of these agents in treating the diseases caused by these organisms has been demonstrated only with a few agents. The aminoglycosides, streptomycin and gentamicin, are bactericidal and provide effective treatment. Bacteriostatic agents, such as doxycycline and chloramphenicol, are less efficacious. Fluoroquinolones have been shown to provide good therapy.

H. Bradford Hawley, M.D.

FURTHER READING

Guillemin, Jeanne. *Biological Weapons.* New York: Columbia University Press, 2005. Covers the history of terrorist- and state-sponsored development of biological weapons.

Hodges, Lisa S., and Robert L. Penn. "*Francisella tularensis* (Tularemia) as an Agent of Bioterrorism." In *Mandell, Douglas, and Bennett's Principles and Practice of Infectious Diseases*, edited by Gerald L. Mandell, John F. Bennett, and Raphael Dolin. 7th ed. New York: Churchill Livingstone/Elsevier, 2010. A discussion of the history and potential use of this organism as an agent of attack.

Penn, Robert L. "*Francisella tularensis* (Tularemia)." In *Mandell, Douglas, and Bennett's Principles and Practice of Infectious Diseases*, edited by Gerald L. Mandell, John F. Bennett, and Raphael Dolin. 7th ed. New York: Churchill Livingstone/Elsevier, 2010. A complete description of tularemia and the causative bacterium.

Staples, J. Erin, et al. "Epidemiologic and Molecular Analysis of Human Tularemia, United States, 1964-2004." *Emerging Infectious Diseases* 12 (2006): 1113-1118. An analysis of organisms from 316 human cases of tularemia from thirty-nine U.S. states.

Wenger, Jay D., et al. "Infection Caused by *Francisella philomiragia* (Formerly *Yersinia philomiragia*): A Newly Recognized Human Pathogen." *Annals of Internal Medicine* 110 (1989): 888-892. A comprehensive review of this unusual organism and infection in fourteen persons.

World Health Organization. *WHO Guidelines on Tularemia.* Geneva: Author, 2007. An extensive monograph on tularemia around the world that includes a discussion of the infectious organism.

WEB SITES OF INTEREST

Todar's Online Textbook of Bacteriology
http://www.textbookofbacteriology.net

U.S. Army Medical Research Institute of Infectious Diseases
http://www.usamriid.army.mil

See also: Anthrax; Arthropod-borne illness and disease; Bacterial infections; Biological weapons; Blood-borne illness and disease; Insect-borne illness and disease; Pathogens; Soilborne illness and disease; Ticks and infectious disease; Tularemia; Vectors and vector control; Waterborne illness and disease.

Fungal infections

CATEGORY: Diseases and conditions
ANATOMY OR SYSTEM AFFECTED: All
ALSO KNOWN AS: Mycoses

DEFINITION

Fungal infections are those infections in which a host is colonized by pathogenic (disease-causing) fungi.

The words "infection" and "disease" are often treated as synonyms, but it is important to clarify the distinction between these two terms. An infection is an invasion of the body by pathogenic microbes, and the term "disease" is used to describe the abnormal state of health caused by the infection (or the pathogen).

CAUSES

Fungal infections are typically caused by the some of the pathogenic members of the simple, heterotrophic, eukaryotic kingdom called Fungi. Fungi lead a saprophytic existence, whereby they obtain nutrition from their substrate (or host) by the process of extracellular digestion. Fungal infections are widely seen in humans, nonhuman animals, and various species of plants. Fungal pathogens such as *Pneumocystis* are included on the World Health Organization's list of emerging eukaryotic pathogens.

RISK FACTORS

Fungi make spores during their reproductive cycles, whether that cycle is sexual or asexual. Because fungal spores are airborne, fungal infections usually start in the lungs or on the skin. Typically, fungal infections are not serious unless they infect a host who has a weakened immune system. Therefore, some risk factors for fungal infections include having acquired immunodeficiency syndrome, extensive burns, lung disorders such as emphysema, and diabetes. Other risk factors include the use of immunosuppressant drugs (such as corticosteroids), cancer chemotherapy, and drugs that block host rejection in organ transplants.

SYMPTOMS

Any type of fungal infection is called mycosis (plural mycoses) and is typically chronic in nature. Five groups of mycoses have been classified on the basis of target tissue and mode of entry of the pathogen.

Systemic mycosis typically affects tissues and organs deep inside the body. These infections, which are caused by fungi that live in soil, include respiratory infections such as histoplasmosis (caused by *Histoplasma capsulatum*). This disease resembles tuberculosis, so clinical symptoms include lung lesions.

Subcutaneous mycosis targets tissue beneath the skin and includes candidiasis (caused by *Candida albicans*). Symptoms of candidiasis include patchy, white oral lesions accompanied with cracking at the ends of the lips and a swollen and painful tongue. Fungal infections of the epidermis are caused by fungi called dermatophytes and are classified as cutaneous mycoses. Examples include ringworm (tinea) infection, commonly known as athlete's foot and typically marked by itchy, scaly patches that may blister in body parts that are warm and moist.

Superficial mycoses affect outermost layers of skin and hair and thus commonly colonize hair shafts and nails, primarily in tropical regions of the world. Opportunistic fungi that are normally harmless can become a serious threat in an immunocompromised host. An example of an opportunistic mycosis is mucormycosis, which is caused by *Rhizopus* and *Mucor*. Symptoms of mucormycosis include pain, fever, eye inflammation, oral blisters, and black patches on the affected area.

SCREENING AND DIAGNOSIS

Once a preliminary diagnosis has been made, the diagnosis for fungal infections is often done using one or more of the following methods, depending on the target organ and the symptoms produced therein. For multisymptom fungal diseases such as histoplasmosis, recommended tests include fungal cultures, fungal stains, and urine and blood tests. These tests often are followed by chest X rays, computed tomography (CT) scans, and bronchoscopy. In a bronchoscopy, a thin, flexible tube is inserted into the airway to study abnormalities of the respiratory system. In suspected fungal infections, bronchoscopy also can be used to obtain a small section of tissue for a lung biopsy. Fungal cultures can take up to four weeks to grow and analyze; a faster alternative is detecting antigens or antibodies in blood and urine samples. A CT scan is especially helpful for diagnosing complications produced by histoplasmosis. To diagnose most other fungal diseases, fungal cultures and fungal stains usually suffice. However, in systemic diseases such as blastomycosis, sputum cultures are helpful too.

TREATMENT AND THERAPY

Because fungal growth is extremely slow, months and years often pass before a person seeks medical treatment. A number of antifungal drugs are available for those persons who do seek treatment.

Antifungal drugs typically act in one of the following ways: targeting the fungal membrane (by destroying the sterols therein), blocking cell-wall or nucleic-acid synthesis, or inhibiting mitotic microtubules. Antifungals that attack fungal sterols include oral drugs such as amphotericin B and ketoconazole (used to treat systemic infections) and topical ointments such as clotrimazole (for cutaneous infections such as athlete's foot). Tolnaftate is a drug used to treat athlete's foot and griseofulvin is an antifungal used to treat cutaneous mycoses (fungal skin infections).

PREVENTION AND OUTCOMES

Fungi and fungal spores are everywhere in the environment, making avoidance of fungal infections difficult. However, it can help to maintain good hygiene. For example, to help prevent athlete's foot, one should ensure that feet are dry and well aerated.

Studies indicate that since the beginning of the twenty-first century, an increase in numbers of fungal infections has been seen worldwide, and most of these infections are occurring either as nosocomial (hospital acquired) infections or as opportunistic infections in persons with compromised immune systems. Under these circumstances, a first step in preventing the spread of fungal diseases is awareness of these types of infections.

Sibani Sengupta, Ph.D.

FURTHER READING

Harrison, S., and W. F. Bergfeld. "Diseases of the Hair and Nails." *Medical Clinics of North America* 93 (2009): 1195-1209. A detailed article that summarizes some of the most commonly seen fungal infections.

Jacobs, P., and L. Nall. *Fungal Disease: Biology, Immunology, and Diagnosis.* New York: Marcel Dekker, 1997. A great resource for readers new to the study of fungal diseases.

Tortora, Gerard J., Berdell R. Funke, and Christine L. Case. *Microbiology: An Introduction.* 10th ed. San Francisco: Benjamin Cummings, 2010. A good reference on the pathogenicity and usefulness of microorganisms.

Webster, John, and Roland Weber. *Introduction to Fungi.* New York: Cambridge University Press, 2007. An introductory textbook for biology majors, in which fungi types are clearly presented and illustrated.

WEB SITES OF INTEREST

Centers for Disease Control and Prevention, Division of Foodborne, Bacterial, and Mycotic Diseases
http://www.cdc.gov/nczved/divisions/dfbmd

Microbiology and Immunology On-line: Mycology
http://pathmicro.med.sc.edu/book/mycol-sta.htm

Systematic Mycology and Microbiology Laboratory
http://www.ars.usda.gov

See also: Antifungal drugs: Mechanisms of action; Antifungal drugs: Types; Aspergillosis; Athlete's foot; Blastomycosis; Candidiasis; Chromoblastomycosis; Coccidiosis; Diagnosis of fungal infections; Fungi: Classification and types; Fungi: Structure and growth; Histoplasmosis; Immune response to fungal infections; Infection; Jock itch; Melioidosis; Mold infections; Mucormycosis; Mycetoma; Mycoses; Opportunistic infections; Prevention of fungal infections; Treatment of fungal infections.

Fungi: Classification and types

CATEGORY: Pathogen
ALSO KNOWN AS: Fungal systematics

DEFINITION

The term "fungi" refers to eukaryotic, heterotrophic organisms that digest organic matter by secreting enzymes into the extracellular environment, assimilating nutrients, including fixed carbon, by osmosis.

GENERAL CHARACTERISTICS

Except in unicellular forms, the basic growth pattern of fungi consists of filamentous hyphae (slender tubes that are the basic building blocks of fungi), with little cellular differentiation in vegetative tissues. Reproduction, both sexual and asexual, is by means of spores, usually microscopic.

Biologists formerly included fungus as the phylum Mycota within the plant kingdom, but beginning in the 1960's they adopted a five kingdom classification; one of the kingdoms was reserved for fungi. With increasing knowledge of ultrastructure and physiological processes at the molecular level, it became evident that the fungi were not monophyletic. Sequencing of ribosomal deoxyribonucleic acid (DNA) confirmed this. It also helped clarify the probable taxonomic position of fungal species (including some important human pathogens) without diagnostic morphological features. Sequencing also aided taxonomists in constructing a more natural system reflecting phylogeny and actual biological affinity. From a practical point of view, the better a taxonomic system, the more useful it is for making identifications critical to diagnosis and for predicting what therapies are most promising.

Ribonucleic acid (RNA) sequencing and a form of mathematical analysis known as cladistics have identified dozens of distinct evolutionary lines among the eukaryotes, most of them consisting of obscure groups of protozoa. The Myxomycetes (slime molds), included with fungi in older classifications, are now considered to be animals closely related to one group of amoeboid protozoa. An important group of aquatic fungi organisms, the Oomycetes or Oomycota, are now placed in the kingdom Straminipila with several phyla of algae, including kelp and diatoms, that have the same flagellar structure and cell wall chemistry. The remaining fungi fall on that portion of the tree of life that also includes Metazoa (multicellular animals), vascular plants and green algae, and some protozoa.

The clade (group consisting of an organism and all its descendants) including the Zygomycota, Ascomycota, and Basidiomycota, sometimes termed Eumycota, consists of overwhelmingly terrestrial organisms that lack motile spores or any vestige of a flagellar base. Most are haploid except for the zygote, which immediately undergoes meiosis before formation of spores. Several orders formerly included in the Zygomycetes may be distinct enough to warrant recognition at a higher taxonomic level. The Microsporidia, a group of obligate animal parasites formerly regarded as primitive or degenerate protozoa, groups with the Eumycota. The Chytridiomycota encompasses aquatic forms with zoospores equipped with a whiplash 9+2 flagellum, cell walls containing chitin, and, in a number of species, regular alternation between haploid and diploid generations. Many species are parasitic on algae.

OOMYCOTA (KINGDOM STRAMINIPILES)

The diagnostic feature of this small but economically important phylum of organisms is a motile zoospore bearing two flagella, one of the "tinsel" type, with numerous lateral fibrils (mastigonemes). Other ultrastructural and biochemical features distinguishing them from the Eumycota include cellulose rather than chitin as the principal cell wall component, tubular rather than flattened cristae in the mitochondria, and a starchlike cellular storage product, mycolaminarin.

The name "Oomycete" comes from the sexual phase of the life cycle, which involves production of specialized hyphal outgrowths of markedly unequal sizes, the oogonium and antheridium, in which meiosis takes place. These fuse, leading to karyogamy (fusion of nuclei) within the oogonium; one or more diploid resting oospores then develop. Upon germination, a mass of diploid nonseptate hyphae are produced. Most species also produce spores asexually in sporangia.

There are two well-marked classes within the Oomycota, the Peronosporomycetidae and the Saprolegniamycetidae. The first, including the Peronosporales, Rhypdiales, and Lagenidiales, consists mainly of biotrophic parasites of terrestrial plants. There is one oospore per oogonium. In many genera, the sporangia are wind-disseminated as a unit and may germinate on the host without production of zoospores. *Phytophthora infestans*, the cause of potato blight, belongs to the Peronosporales. The Saprolegniamycetidae, including the Saprolegniales and Leptomitales, consists of aquatic fungi with sporangia releasing zoospores directly into the environment. Oogonia produce multiple oospores.

Some Saprolegniales are important pathogens of fish and other aquatic animals. *Pythium insidiosum* attacks domestic animals in tropical regions and has been confirmed as a rare agent of human disease. It may be more common, as the clinical symptoms and morphology of the fungus suggest zygomycosis and a firm diagnosis require DNA sequencing of the pathogen.

EUMYCOTA: PHYLUM CHYTRIDIOMYCOTA

In older classifications, Chytridiomycetes were grouped with the Oomycetes in a general category, Phycomycetes, or algal-like fungi. The diagnostic feature is a zoospore with a single 9+2 flagellum, the same type found in plants and multicellular animals. Sexual reproduction is through fusion of zoospores to form a zygote. Some chytrids form extensive mycelium (mass of hyphae), while in others the vegetative body consists of a single cell anchored to the host by rhizoids that converts to a zoosporangium. Growth and asexual reproduction can take place in both the haploid and diploid phases.

Based on DNA sequencing, there are three distinct phyletic groups of fungi with uniflagellate zoospores: the Chytridiomycota, including the Chytridiales,

Spizellomycetales, and Rhizophydiales; the Blasto-cladiomycota, which are mainly parasites on soil and freshwater invertebrates; and the Neocallimastigomy-cota, a small group of anaerobes inhabiting the stomachs of ruminants. There have been no known reports of human disease caused by Chytridiomycota, but *Batrachochytrium dendrobalis* causes a devastating disease of frogs and other amphibians.

EUMYCOTA: PHYLUM ZYGOMYCOTA

The Zygomycota are characterized by the absence of motile stages in the life cycle and by nonseptate hyphae, cell walls containing chitin, production of non-motile sexual spores in sporangia, and fusion of hyphal outgrowths of equal size to form a diploid zygospore, often thick-walled and ornamented, that serves as a resting spore. About nine hundred species are known, amounting to approximately 1 percent of the total number of described fungi.

Based on DNA sequencing and morphology and host relationships, the Zygomycota have been divided into four classes, the Mucormycotina, Kickxellomycotina, Entomophthoramycotina, and Zoopagomycotina. Additionally, the Glomeromycetes, an ancient group of obligately mycorrhizal fungi symbiotic on the roots of higher plants, and the Microsporidia, specialized animal pathogens formerly classified as protozoa, appear to be more closely related to the Zygomycetes than to other Eumycota.

The Mucormycotina, comprising the Mucorales, Endogonales, and Mortierellales, includes fast-growing saprophytes with abundant asexual reproduction, including the familiar black bread-mold *Rhizopus stolon-ifera*. Species of *Mucor* and several other genera cause rare but extremely dangerous fulminating infections in immunocompromised persons.

Most members of the Kickxellomycotina and Zoopagomycotina are specialized parasites or commensals on invertebrate animals and other fungi. They have not been implicated in human disease. The Entomophthoromycota, which includes a number of insect pathogens used as agents of biological control, is characterized by conidia that are actively discharged. Several species of *Conidiobolus* and *Basidiobolus ranarum* infect humans, usually immunocompromised persons, producing chronic skin ulcers and polyps. The classification of *Basidiobolus* in the Entomophthorales has been questioned; its DNA sequence suggests affinity with the Chytridiomycetes.

Microsporidia, which cause chronic infections in many vertebrate animals, including humans, were originally thought to be protozoa and to be near the base of the eukaryotic family tree based on small cell size, small genomes, and a lack of mitochondria. A unique feature of the cell is a triggered filament that aids in penetration of host cells. DNA analysis suggests the simple structure is not primitive but instead evolved in the parasitic habitat.

EUMYCOTA: SUBKINGDOM DIKARYA

The subkingdom Dikarya is a well-defined clade composed of the Ascomycota and Basidiomycota and includes more than 90 percent of the species described as fungi. These predominantly terrestrial fungi lack motile spores and have chitinous cell walls. An extensive mycelium composed of regularly septate hyphae is usually present. The distinctive feature defining this clade is a life-cycle stage between plasmogamy (fusion of cells) and karyogamy (fusion of nuclei), during which the cells are binucleate, with a complete set of chromosomes from each parent. In Ascomycota, the binucleate stage is confined to the actual sexual fruit body, but in Basidiomycota it constitutes the main vegetative thallus—persisting, in some genera of wood-destroying fungi, for decades or even centuries.

Older classifications sometimes formally recognized a third class, the Deuteromycetes or Fungi Imperfecti, for fungi with septate hyphae and no known sexual cycle. Manuals for identifying these fungi still group them in a form-class for convenience. Some morphologically defined form-genera of asexually reproducing fungi, such as *Penicillium* and *Alternaria*, represent distinct biological entities connecting to genera defined by the sexual stage, while others do not. The trend in recent years has been to use biochemistry of metabolites to classify yeasts, which are very simple morphologically and represent a growth phase of many human pathogens. With the advent of DNA sequencing, it has become possible to correctly classify any organism of interest.

Phylum Ascomycota. These organisms have a vegetative thallus, except in yeasts, that comprises haploid septate hyphae, cells that are generally uninucleate. Asexual reproduction is by means of conidia—unicellular to multicellular spores, typically airborne and often produced abundantly. Sexual reproduction in most families is initiated by fertilization of a specialized enlarged cell, the ascogonium, with small airborne conidia known as spermatia, followed by limited proliferation of binucleate cells. Karyogamy and meiosis take place inside a saclike cell called an ascus, within which ascospores (usually eight) are delimited.

The Ascomycota is the largest and most diverse natural phylum of Eumycota and includes the majority of species of medically important fungi and the majority of plant pathogens. Between one-quarter and one-third of the known species form symbiotic lichen associations with algae and cyanobacteria.

For the most part, the division of the Ascomycota into classes and orders, proposed in the mid-twentieth century and based on the structure and development of ascocarps and asci, agrees with the division based on DNA sequencing. However, the old subclass Hemiascomycetes—defined by the absence of fruit bodies and including the Taphrinales, mainly obligate biotrophic parasites of higher plants, and the Saccharomycetales (ascomycetous yeasts with no or limited mycelial growth)—becomes the subphyla Taphrinomycota and Saccharomycota.

Molecular studies have shown that the important human pathogen *Pneumocystis carinii*, which occurs as undifferentiated yeastlike cells in host tissue and has not been successfully cultured, is a member of the Taphrinomycota. Another important pathogen, *Candida albicans*, is a representative member of the Saccharomycota, which also includes brewer's yeast. The yeast growth form is characterized by single cells that bud off multiple daughter cells from undifferentiated loci on the cell surface. Some yeasts, including *C. albicans*, have a diploid vegetative state.

The old class Euascomycetes, renamed subphylum Pezizomycotina, includes fifty-eight recognized orders of Ascomycetes producing asci in distinct fruiting bodies. They are grouped in seven well-defined classes, plus four orders in classes by themselves. The most important divisions are Pezizomycetes, Eurotiomycetes, Laboulbeniomycetes, Lecanoromycetes, Leotiomycetes, and Sordariomycetes.

Pezizomycetes are fungi with disc-shaped fruit bodies (apothecia) and operculate asci, related hypogeous gastroid forms, the true truffles, Dothideomycetes, fungi with enclosed fruit bodies (perithecia), ascostromatic development, and bitunicate asci. This group includes many plant pathogens. Abundantly sporulating asexual stages are common allergens, and a few species are opportunistic human pathogens.

Eurotiomycetes are fungi with enclosed, aporate, often reduced fruit bodies, and simple thin-walled asci. Asexual stages of Eurotiales include the genera *Penicillium* and *Aspergillus*. This class includes the majority of true human pathogens and agents of food spoilage that produce toxins and carcinogens. The dermatophyte genera *Trichophyton* and *Microsporon* and the serious pathogens *Histoplasma* and *Paracoccidioides* belong to the order Onygenales.

Laboulbeniomycetes are specialized ectoparasites of arthropods, with very reduced thalli. Lecanoromycetes are Lichen mycobionts and saprophytes with apothecia and complex (but not functionally bitunicate) asci. Leotiomycetes are plant parasites that have unitunicate asci, apothecia, and ascohymenial development. Sordariomycetes have a perithecium fruit body, ascohymenial development, and unitunicate asci. This diverse group includes many important plant pathogens. *Fusarium* and *Sporothrix* are conidial stages of Sordariomycetes.

Phylum Basidiomycota. These organisms have a vegetative thallus, except in yeasts, comprised of haploid dikaryotic septate hyphae. Production of asexual spores is infrequent in Hymenomycetes but a regular part of the life cycles of Uredinomycetes (rusts) and Ustilagomycetes (smuts). Sexual reproduction is initiated by fusion of undifferented haploid mycelial cells (Hymenomycetes) or pycniospores functioning as spermatia (Uredinomycetes). Karyogamy and meiosis take place inside a clublike structure called a basidium, Basidiospores, produced externally, are forcibly discharged. Basidiomycetes are most important in nature as decomposers of wood, plant pathogens (rusts and smuts), and mycorrhizal symbionts of forest trees. Subphyla are Puccinomycotina, Ustilagomycotina, and Agaricomycotina.

From a human perspective, the most important groups in the subphylum Puccinomycotina are the Pucciniales (rusts), obligate biotrophic plant parasites with complex life cycles, and the Sporidiobolales, the main group of basidiomycetous yeasts. Of particular interest to medical mycologists is *Cryptococcus (Filobasidiella) neoformans*, in which multiple mitotic divisions follow meiosis in the basidium and basidiospores are budded off in chains.

The subphylum Ustilagomycotina consists of mainly obligate plant parasites with complex life cycles, divided into two classes, the Ustilagomycetes (smuts) and Exobasidiomycetes (leaf curl diseases and some smuts). There is one human parasite, the dermato-phyte yeast *Melasseza.*

As the name implies, the subphylum Agaricomyco-tina includes the familiar edible mushroom *Agaricus campestris.* Also called Hymenomycetes, members of this group have a life cycle including a limited undif-ferentiated mycelial haploid phase followed by hyphal fusion establishing a dikaryon. Dikaryotic hyphae have characteristic clamp connections and complex dolipore septa. Basidia are typically borne in a layer (the hymenium) on complex fruit bodies. Basidia are septate in the Tremellomycetes (jelly fungi) and uni-cellular in the Agaricales (mushrooms), Polyporales (woody pore fungi), and Phallales (stinkhorns). The orders of Agaricomycotina have long been defined by microanatomy and chemistry rather than gross fruit-body form, and present classifications based on DNA analysis closely approximate older treatments. This subphylum contains no important human pathogens.

IMPACT

Having an accurate system of classification for fungi or any other group of organisms that have a signifi-cant impact on humans is critical to identifying spe-cies and devising methods of control that are tailored to the particular organism. In a clinical setting, health care providers need to identify the agent causing the disease to initiate appropriate therapies. In research laboratories, the development of effective therapies depends on understanding the biochemistry and life cycle of the target pathogen, a process greatly aided by being able to classify it with a biologically related species.

Human pathogenic fungi have always presented a challenge to medicine because fungi are more closely related to humans than are bacteria and most pro-tozoa. Drugs that inhibit fungal growth are therefore likely to be toxic to humans. Most common fungal in-fections are superficial or localized and can be treated topically. However, growing populations of immuno-compromised persons, including those with human immunodeficiency virus (HIV) infection, transplant recipients, and persons undergoing chemotherapy, have led to the emergence of a number of systemic, life-threatening mycoses.

DNA sequencing is a great aid in identifying and treating fungal diseases. It has established the taxo-nomic position and, therefore, the most promising avenues for therapy for morphologically ambiguous

pathogens such as Microsporidia and *Pneumocystis.* DNA sequencing is becoming available as a clinical di-agnostic tool for establishing the identity of a pathogen in tested persons.

Martha A. Sherwood, Ph.D.

FURTHER READING

Hibbet, David S., et al. "A Higher-Level Phylogenetic Classification of the Fungi." *Mycological Research* 111 (2007): 509-547. A comprehensive review of mo-lecular taxonomy, with an extensive bibliography.

Larone, Davise H. *Medically Important Fungi: A Guide to Identification.* 4th ed. Washington, D.C.: ASM Press, 2003. Includes an outline classification, descrip-tions and illustrations of human pathogenic spe-cies in tissue samples and culture, and a guide to common cultural contaminants.

Priest, Fergus G., and Michael Goodfellow, eds. *Applied Microbial Systematics.* Boston: Kluwer Academic, 2000. This volume focuses on mycorrhizal fungi and insect pathogens. Includes a good treatment of the molecular systematics of entomopathogenic Zygo-mycota.

Webster, John, and Roland Weber. *Introduction to Fungi.* New York: Cambridge University Press, 2007. A text-book for college biology majors, in which fungi clas-sification is clearly presented and illustrated. Incor-porates updated gene sequencing and cladistics.

WEB SITES OF INTEREST

British Mycological Society
http://fungionline.org.uk

GenBank
http://www.ncbi.nlm.nih.gov/taxonomy

National Fungus Collections
http://www.ars.usda.gov/is/np/systematics/usfungu.htm

Tree of Life
http://tolweb.org/tree

See also: Antifungal drugs: Mechanisms of action; An-tifungal drugs: Types; Diagnosis of fungal infections; Fungal infections; Fungi: Structure and growth; Im-mune response to fungal infections; Mold infections; Mycoses; Prevention of fungal infections; Treatment of fungal infections.

Fungi: Structure and growth

CATEGORY: Pathogen

DEFINITION

Fungi share certain characteristics: eukaryotic cells with membrane-bound nuclei and cellular organelles; a filamentous growth form (unicellular in some species) with limited vegetative differentiation; a protoplast surrounded by a rigid cell wall; characteristic storage products including trehalose, glycogen, sugar alcohols, and lipids; sexual and asexual reproduction by means of microscopic spores; and lack of chlorophyll. All are chemoheterotrophic, using preexisting sources of organic carbon and the energy from chemical reactions for growth and energy. Most are haploid in the vegetative state.

GENERAL CHARACTERISTICS

Fungi organisms belong to two distinct evolutionary lines, the Kingdom Straminopiles, which includes water molds of the phylum Oomycota, and the Eumycota, including most terrestrial fungi. This discussion pertains principally to those Eumycota that lack flagellated zoospores—the Mucormycota or Zygomycetes, Ascomycota, and Basidiomycota. With the exception of a few rare opportunistic infections, this encompasses all medically important fungi.

STRUCTURE: CELLULAR ULTRASTRUCTURE

Fungal cells are eukaryotic, with one or more membrane-bound nuclei containing chromosomes. Instead of centrioles, the cells possess a simpler structure, the spindle pole body, which serves to divide replicated chromosomes during cell division. The nuclear envelope remains intact during mitosis and meiosis. Fungal chromosomes are small and few. The small genome and predominantly haploid life cycle are correlated with the absence of centrioles; Oomycota and Chytridiomycota, which possess them, have diploid vegetative states and genomes comparable in size to eukaryotic algae.

Fungal mitochondria are typically elongate and have distinctive flattened cristae. Other cellular components include endoplasmic reticulum, ribosomes, Golgi bodies, and vacuoles that serve as storage area for cellular byproducts. The cell is bound by a proteinaceous plasma membrane, outside of which is a rigid cell wall. The cell wall itself consists of a network

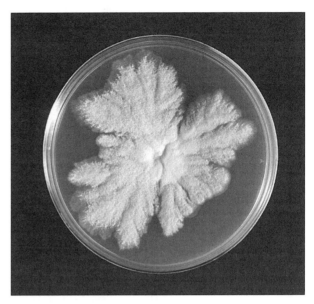

A laboratory culture of growing colonies of a species of the fungus Trichophyton. (CDC)

of fibrils composed of chitin, an insoluble nitrogen-containing polysaccharide, within a matrix of soluble polysaccharides.

STRUCTURE: HYPHAE AND VEGETATIVE STRUCTURES

The basic building block of a fungus is the hypha, a slender tube divided by septa. In aggregate, a mass of hyphae is called a mycelium. In Zygomycota, septa are infrequent except in fruiting structures; the mycelium is coenocytic and cells have numerous nuclei. In Ascomycota and Basidiomycota, septa occur at regular intervals. Ascomycete septa have simple pores large enough for nuclei and other organelles to pass through, allowing for limited internal transport within a thallus. Many Basidiomycetes have a specialized dolipore septum surrounded by parenthosomes (membranous caps). During cell division in the dikaryophase, Basidiomycetes produce a septal structure called a clamp connection that allows the two parent nuclei to divide in tandem. Clamp connections and dolipore septa are evident even in fragmentary material and can be useful in clinical diagnosis or evaluation of microfossils.

Hyphal branching is usually sympodial, initiated at some distance behind the growing tip. The assimilative phase of a fungus consists of undifferentiated branched hyphae growing in a loose network on or within the substrate.

Some fungi, including many human pathogens, have a yeast growth form, with isolated single cells that reproduce by budding. The mechanisms for bud formation mirror those for formation of asexual conidia in filamentous forms. They vary among yeasts, reflecting their diverse taxonomic affiliations. A number of human pathogens are thermally dimorphic, producing true hyphae at lower temperatures and yeast cells at body temperature.

Vegetative structures exhibiting cellular differentiation include rhizomorphs, stromata, and sclerotia. Rhizomorphs, produced by wood-decaying Basidiomycetes, are long bundles of hyphae with an outer cortex of thick-walled, melanized cells. Stromata are cushionlike plates of solid mycelium. Sclerotia are multicellular resting bodies, also with a rind of thick-walled cells. The tissue, in common with sterile portions of many fruit bodies, may be composed of pseudoparenchyma (of tightly packed isodiametric cells). Ontogenetically, fungal pseudoparenchyma originates from closely septate tubular hyphae rather than from a meristematic cell that divides in three planes.

Many biotrophic plant parasites produce specialized appresoria for attaching to plant surfaces and penetrating host cuticle. Among the Ascomycota, two exceptions to the general rule of undifferentiated vegetative structures may be noted. The thalli of lichens, whose form is determined by the mycobiont, are often quite complex, and hyphal types and specialized structures among tropical leaf-inhabiting Loculoascomycetes are very diverse.

Cellular differentiation in fungi is generally reversible, with any viable cell being capable, given the right growing conditions, of reconstituting the entire organism.

STRUCTURE: SPOROCARPS AND SPORES

Most diversity in fungal morphology is associated with the production of spores, both sexual and asexual. Asexual spores, the product of mitotic division of haploid nuclei, may be produced by internal cleavage within a sporangium (sporangiospores, characteristic of Zygomycota, and zoospores, characteristic of Chytridiomycota and Oomycota) or by extrusion from a more or less modified hyphal cell (conidia, characteristic of Ascomycota, and uredospores and teliospores in the Basidiomycota). Sexual spores are the immediate product of either fusion of nuclei called karyogamy (Oomycota, Zygomycota) or karyogamy followed by meiosis (Asomycota, Basidiomycota). In the latter two, sometimes grouped in the Subkingdom Dikarya, they are often produced on highly differentiated sporocarps, of which mushrooms are a conspicuous example.

Among the Zygomycetes, human pathogens are found in the Mucorales and Entomophthorales. Both groups have isolated zygospores, often thick-walled and ornamented. Meiosis occurs upon zygospore germination, and the immediate product is either a germ sporangium or haploid mycelium. Typical Mucorales produce stalked sporangia containing numerous unicellular asexual spores. In the Entomophthorales, spores are solitary and are actively discharged. The Glomales, mycorrizal zygospore-forming fungi whose evolutionary affinities may be closer to the Dikarya, produce zygospores in hypogeous gastroid sporocarps.

The asexual stages of Ascomycota are classified according to means of spore production, type of sporocarp (if any), and morphology of the spores themselves. Spore production may be through hyphal fragmentation at the septa or, more commonly, through extrusion from specialized conidiogenous cells borne on conidiophores. A common type of conidiogenesis, found in *Aspergillus* and *Penicillium*, involves flask-shaped cells called phialides that produce long chains of spores. In *Aspergillus*, the phialides are clustered on a swollen cell at the apex of a long multicellular conidiophore.

In addition to condiophores on undifferentiated mycelium, asexual sporulation may also involve fruit bodies consisting of hyphae aggregated to form a stalk with a spore-bearing head (synnemata), flattened structures with an exposed sporulating surface (sporodochia), and flask-shaped structures with pores (pycnidia). Pycnidia may bear appendages or be embedded in stromatic tissue.

Conidia may be unicellular or multicellular, smooth or ornamented, and pigmented or unpigmented. Aquatic freshwater forms are often branched or coiled to aid flotation.

The diagnostic feature of an Ascomycete is the ascus, a saclike structure in which karyogamy and meiosis take place. Following meiosis, and usually one or more mitotic divisions, membranes delimit ascospores. When fully mature, turgor pressure builds up and ascospores are actively discharged through an apical pore. Some groups have rings or other structures associated with the pore, and one large class, the Loculoascomycetes, has bitunicate asci with an inner separable wall that extrudes during discharge.

The Saccharomycetales (yeasts) and Taphrinales lack fruit bodies. Remaining orders of Ascomycota may have cleistothecia (enclosed bodies with no defined opening), apothecia (cup-shaped structures with an exposed hymenium), or perithecia (flask-shaped bodies with a preformed pore). Perithecia may be imbedded in a stroma. The majority of true human pathogens belong to the cleistothecial orders Eurotiales and Onygenales. Sexual states of these species, if known, are only produced in culture. In contrast, plant-pathogenic species often fruit abundantly on the host. One apothecial group, the Pezizales, has given rise through increasing convolutions of the hymenium to both the morels and to true truffles, in which the hymenium is entirely enclosed and spores are passively dispersed by animals. The human pathogens *Sporothrix* and *Fusarium* are asexual states of perithecial fungi.

Ascospores may be unicellular or septate, hyaline or pigmented, with ornaments, mucilaginous sheaths, and appendages. The diagnostic feature of a Basidiomycete is a basidium, a club-shaped or filamentous structure within which karyogamy and meiosis take place. Basidiospores are produced externally and are actively discharged. The Agaricomycotina, the largest subphylum, have club-shaped basidia bearing basidiospores, usually four, on peglike sterigmata. A tremendous variety or sporocarps are produced, with a common design feature of presenting the largest possible surface area of hymenium to the air while protecting it from the elements. In gill fungi (Agaricales) and pore fungi (Polyporales), the basidia are arranged on the surface of closely packed cavities spaced so that the actively discharged basidiospore just clears the hymenium and falls vertically to the air space below the stalked or laterally attached fruit body. In gastroid forms, the hymenium is permanently enclosed. Sporocarps in some species may weigh several kilograms and produce millions of spores. Some soil-inhabiting and root-parasitic agarics form so-called fairy rings—the visible manifestation, in fruiting season, of an underground mycelium that can extend for hundreds of feet.

The core of the subphylum Pucciniomycotina consists of plant rusts, specialized parasites of higher plants that alternate between hosts, producing different spore types on each. Of more interest to medicine are the Sporidiobolales, the Basidiomycetous yeasts, whose deoxyribonucleic acid (DNA) places them close to Puccinia and other plant rusts. The one important human pathogen, *Cryptococcus (Filobasidiella) neoformans*, produces unique basidia within which multiple mitotic divisions following meiosis support production of chains of basidiospores on the sterigmata.

GROWTH: HYPHAL ELONGATION AND DIFFERENTIATION

Fungal hyphal growth takes place at the apex, with little or no elongation as a result of the addition of wall material to older cells and no secondary thickening as a result of lateral division. When fungal structures expand from the addition of tissue, this expansion comes from the initiation of lateral branches along existing hyphae.

Close to the tip of a growing hypha is a region of dense vesicles containing the precursors for cell wall formation, synthase enzymes to catalyze polymerization, and lytic enzymes to break down existing cell wall to allow for insertion of additional material. The apex of a hypha is in a state of dynamic equilibrium that maintains rigidity and structural integrity while allowing for expansion.

Nutrient depletion and release of inhibitory compounds suppress branching, controlling the density of vegetative mycelium. Hyphal tips may be geotropic, chemotropic, or, rarely, phototropic. Germination and growth of parasitic species may be stimulated by specific compounds produced by the host. Hyphae will grow along a nutrient gradient and also toward mycelia of a compatible mating type.

Growth rates vary widely. Under optimal conditions in the laboratory, *Neurospora crassa* and a few saprophytic Mucorales can increase biomass by 60 percent in an hour. In nature, such species rapidly deplete substrates of nutrients and survive by producing durable resting stages. At the other extreme, some lichenized fungi in harsh environments grow less than a millimeter a year.

Dikaryotic mycelia of Agaricales, apparently originating from a single hyphal fusion, can be impressively large and long-lived. The current record appears to be an individual colony of *Armillaria ostryae*, a wood-destroying mushroom, in Malheur County, Oregon. The colony is 3.5 miles in diameter, at least 2,400 years old, and genetically uniform.

GROWTH: ASSIMILATION AND NUTRITION

Fungi obtain nutrients by secreting enzymes that break down complex organic molecules into simple soluble fragments that are absorbed through the cell wall. Parasitic forms may also excrete compounds that alter host metabolism to produce simpler compounds. Eumycota are among the few eukaryotes that can degrade cellulose. The ability to degrade lignin, the main structural component of woody plants, is restricted to Basidiomycota.

Most fungi are aerobic. A few, including the familiar brewer's yeast, are facultative anaerobes. The facultative anaerobes are most likely to be implicated in life-threatening human infections, because in all of these the fungus invades only dead tissue, which is no longer oxygenated. Most fungi require a moist environment for active growth, but many can persist for long periods under very dry conditions. Some are resistant to high osmotic tension and can live in saline environments.

As a group, fungi have enormous biosynthetic capabilities that are extensively exploited for industrial purposes. Some can synthesize the complete range of essential amino acids from inorganic sources of nitrogen, sulfur, and phosphorus. Fungal protein is better balanced for human nutrition than is protein from green plants, one of the reasons that fermentation of grain for human consumption has been a human practice since the Stone Age.

There is an extensive literature on the specific nutrient requirements of fungal species of interest to humans. In general, obligate parasites, whether of humans or of their crop plants, have very specific requirements, while opportunistic invaders do not.

IMPACT

Probably the greatest impact that fungi have on human infectious diseases is not in their role as agents of mycoses but as allies is the fight against infections caused by other organisms. Since the discovery, in 1928, of the first form of penicillin, a secondary metabolite of *Penicillium notatum* (now called *P. chrysogenum*) and other species, scientists have identified a host of clinically useful antimicrobial compounds produced by fungi in nature, as well as enzymes, vita-

mins, and other organic compounds useful in therapy. With the advent of genetic engineering, it has become possible to insert genes from diverse parts of the plant and animal world into a fungal genome, using the genetically engineered fungus as a factory to manufacture complex biologically active compounds. Fungi are ideal for this purpose because the technology for growing them in bioreactors on an industrial scale is well established.

As laboratory organisms, fungi have contributed a great deal to the basic understanding of eukaryotic biochemistry and genetics. The simplicity, short generation time, and ease of manipulation of fungi make them ideal subjects for basic research. Such research rarely translates directly into clinical practice but is vital to the development of modern highly targeted disease therapies that depend on understanding host-parasite interactions at the molecular level.

Human pathogenic fungi have always presented a challenge to medicine, because fungi are more closely related to humans than are bacteria and most protozoa. Until recently, however, most common fungal infections seen in clinical practice in the developed world were superficial or localized and thus could be treated topically. However, growing populations of immunocompromised persons, including those infected with the human immunodeficiency virus (HIV), transplant patients, and persons undergoing chemotherapy, have led to the emergence of a number of systemic, life-threatening mycoses as growing threats to human health. Responding to this challenge will require understanding fungal growth and metabolism at the molecular level.

Martha A. Sherwood, Ph.D.

FURTHER READING

Alexopoulos, Constantine J., C. W. Mims, and M. Blackwell. *Introductory Mycology*. New York: John Wiley & Sons, 1996. A standard textbook for college biology majors, covering general ultrastructure and metabolism and the morphology of various taxa.

Kendrick, Bryce. *The Fifth Kingdom*. 3d ed. Newburyport, Mass.: Focus, 2000. A strength of this book on fungi are the numerous line drawings illustrating the structure and development of all major fungal groups.

Larone, Davise H. *Medically Important Fungi: A Guide to Identification*. 4th ed. Washington, D.C.: ASM Press,

2003. Includes an outline classification, descriptions and illustrations of human pathogenic species in tissue samples and culture, and a guide to common cultural contaminants.

Webster, John, and Roland Weber. *Introduction to Fungi.* New York: Cambridge University Press, 2007. A textbook for college biology majors that clearly classifies and illustrates fungi. Also incorporates gene sequencing and cladistics.

WEB SITES OF INTEREST

British Mycological Society
http://fungionline.org.uk

National Fungus Collections
http://www.ars.usda.gov/is/np/systematics/usfungu.htm

See also: Antifungal drugs: Mechanisms of action; Antifungal drugs: Types; Diagnosis of fungal infections; Fungal infections; Fungi: Classification and types; Immune response to fungal infections; Mold infections; Mycoses; Prevention of fungal infections; Treatment of fungal infections.

Fusarium

CATEGORY: Pathogen
TRANSMISSION ROUTE: Direct contact, inhalation

DEFINITION

Fusarium are widely distributed plant pathogens that can cause skin, wound, lung, and invasive infections in humans. *Fusarium* also produce many allergens and mycotoxins.

NATURAL HABITAT AND FEATURES

Fusarium are widely distributed fungi (molds) that grow on a variety of substrates, including plants (and their roots), food, soil, and wet, indoor environments. *Fusarium* tend to produce fast-growing, woolly to cottony, flat-spreading cultures and come in many colors, including white, gray, red, cinnamon, pink, yellow, and purple.

Fusarium are present mainly in the anamorphic or asexual phase. Some *Fusarium* species also have a telemorphic phase and produce ascospores. Some of the

---

Taxonomic Classification for *Fusarium*

Kingdom: Fungi
Phylum: Ascomycota
Class: Sordariomycetes
Order: Hypocreales
Family: Nectariaceae
Genus: *Fusarium*
Species:
F. acuminatum
F. avenaceum
F. chlamydosporum
F. culmorum
F. equisti
F. graminearum
F. incarnatum
F. moniliforme
F. oxysporum
F. poae
F. proliferatum
F. sacchari
F. solani
F. subglutinans
F. verticillioides

---

more common *Fusarium* ascospore forms are *Gibberella avenacea, intricans, zea, subglutinans,* and *moniformis;* these are the telomorphic forms of *F. avenaceum, equiseti, graminearum, subglutinans,* and *verticilloides,* respectively. *Haematonectria* spp. are teleomorphic forms of *F. solani.*

Fusarium often produce two types of asexual spores, including macroconidia, borne on long sickle or banana-shaped structures, and microconidia, borne on chains. Many species of *Fusarium* also produce chlamydospores, which are thick-walled resting spores that can survive long periods in unfavorable conditions, such as drought.

Like most fungi, *Fusarium* are usually identified by macroscopic and microscopic features, although molecular methods such as 28S rRNA (ribosomal ribonucleic acid) gene-sequencing may also be used.

PATHOGENICITY AND CLINICAL SIGNIFICANCE

Fusarium exposure can adversely affect human health by three mechanisms: infection (fusariosis), exposure to allergens, and exposure to toxics produced by *Fusarium. Fusarium* frequently invade the skin, especially if the skin is damaged by trauma, burns, or diabetic ulcers. *Fusarium* also can invade the eyes (endophtalmitis), nasal sinuses, and lungs. Localized *Fusarium* infections may disseminate through the bloodstream to become life-threatening infections.

Invasive disseminated *Fusarium* infections commonly occur in immunocompromised persons, such as those with leukemia, lymphoma, or HIV infection; those who are malnourished or neutropenic; persons suffering from burns or other skin trauma; and persons taking immunosuppressive drugs following bone or organ transplantation. Invasive *Fusarium* infections can spread through blood vessels and cause tissue infarction (tissue death).

The rate of *Fusarium* invasive infection is on the rise and now makes up 1 to 3 percent of all invasive fungal infections. Disseminated invasive *Fusarium* infections have high mortality rates that range from about 30 to 90 percent.

F. solani is the most common cause of skin and disseminated invasive *Fusarium* infections (about 50 percent), followed by *oxysporum* (about 20 percent) and *verticillioidis* and *monilforme* (about 10 percent each).

Fusarium also produce a variety of toxins (mycotoxins), including fumonisins, trichothecenes, and zearalenones. Domestic animals and humans have become acutely ill after eating foods contaminated with *Fusarium* mycotoxins.

Fumonisins can increase the risk of some cancers, can damage the immune system, and can cause respiratory problems. Trichothecenes damage the immune and nervous systems, block cell protein synthesis, and cause vomiting. Zearalenones are estrogen-mimicking chemicals that can cause early female puberty, infertility, and spontaneous abortion in humans and other mammals. Human studies have linked consumption of *Fusarium*-contaminated corn (maize) with higher rates of early female puberty. Exposure to airborne *Fusarium* spores can also worsen asthma and sinus problems.

DRUG SUSCEPTIBILITY

Fusarium infections are sometimes difficult to diagnose in their early and less serious stages. Infections can often be diagnosed by culturing *Fusarium* from the blood and from skin lesions. High resolution computed tomography (CT) scans of the chest are often useful in diagnosing fusariosis. Polymerase chain reaction (PCR) blood tests also are used to diagnose *Fusarium* infections.

Localized *Fusarium* skin infections can often be treated with topic antifungal drugs such as natamycin and voriconazole. Disseminated *Fusarium* infections are often difficult to treat because few antifungals are consistently effective against many *Fusarium* species. Amphotericin B is often used as a first-line drug against *Fusarium*; however, roughly 50 percent of *Fusarium* isolates, including many *solani* and *verticilloides*, are resistant to amphotericin B. Some *Fusarium* strains are susceptible to voriconazole and posaconazole, while few *Fusarium* isolates are susceptible to itraconazole. Most *Fusarium* strains are resistant to the new echinocandin drugs (anidulafungin, caspofungin, and micafungin). These chinocandin drugs are generally effective in treating disseminated *Aspergillus* and *Candida* infections.

Other treatments that may be helpful in some cases of fusariosis include surgical debulking of *Fusarium*-infected tissue, removal of contaminated catheters, and using granulocyte-colony-stimulating factors.

The best method for controlling *Fusarium* infections is avoidance of the mold. Medical experts recommended that immunocompromised persons who are hospitalized be placed in rooms with positive air pressure, air filtration, sterile water, and adequately cleaned surfaces, sinks, and showers to reduce the risk of *Fusarium* infection. Any water damage or visible mold growth in hospital rooms should be cleaned immediately. To significantly reduce exposure to *Fusarium* and their mycotoxins in the home, persons should keep dry, clean, and refrigerated all stored food, such as grains, fruits, vegetables, and animal feeds.

Luke Curtis, M.D.

FURTHER READING

Marom, Edith M., et al. "Imaging of Pulmonary Fusariosis in Patients with Hematologic Malignancies." *American Journal of Roentgenology* 190 (2008): 1605-1609.

Nucci, Marcio, and Elias Anaissie. "Fusarium Infections in Immunocompromised Patients." *Clinical Microbiology Reviews* 20 (2007): 695-704.

Patridge-Hinckley, Kimberly, et al. "Infection Control Measures to Prevent Invasive Mould Diseases in Hematopoietic Stem Cell Transplant Recipients." *Mycopathologica* 168 (2009): 329-337.

Samson, Robert, Ellen Hoesktra, and Jens Frisvad. *Introduction to Food and Airborne Fungi.* 7th ed. Utrecht, the Netherlands: Central Bureau for Fungal Cultures, 2004.

Stanzani, Marta, et al. "Update on the Treatment of Disseminated Fusariosis: Focus on Voriconazole." *Therapeutics and Clinical Risk Management* 3 (2007): 1165-1173.

Webster, John, and Weber, Roland. *Introduction to Fungi.* New York: Cambridge University Press, 2007.

Web Sites of Interest

British Mycological Society
http://fungionline.org.uk

Systematic Mycology and Microbiology Laboratory
http://www.ars.usda.gov

See also: Airborne illness and disease; Allergic bronchopulmonary aspergillosis; Antifungal drugs: Types; Aspergillosis; *Aspergillus*; Blastomycosis; Chromoblastomycosis; *Coccidioides*; Coccidiosis; Fungal infections; Fungi: Classification and types; Histoplasmosis; Mucormycosis; Mycetoma; Mycoses; Paracoccidioidomycosis; Pathogens; Respiratory route of transmission; Soilborne illness and disease; Wound infections.

G

Gangrene

CATEGORY: Diseases and conditions
ANATOMY OR SYSTEM AFFECTED: Circulatory system, skin, tissue
ALSO KNOWN AS: Dry gangrene, gas gangrene, organ death, tissue death, wet gangrene

DEFINITION

Gangrene is the death of an organ or of body tissue. When the blood supply is cut off, the tissue does not get enough oxygen and begins to die. If the gangrene is widespread, shock can occur.

There are three main types of gangrene: dry gangrene, in which a lack of blood supply causes the tissue to dry up and slough off; wet gangrene, which usually occurs when the tissue is infected with bacteria and the tissue becomes moist and breaks down; and gas gangrene, in which a particular type of bacteria (*Clostridium*) produces gas bubbles in the tissue.

CAUSES

Causes of gangrene include infection, especially after surgery or injury; diabetes; or any condition that blocks blood flow to the tissues (such as atherosclerosis).

RISK FACTORS

The factors that increase that chance of developing gangrene include smoking; alcohol use; traumatic injury, especially crushing injuries; wound infection after surgery; frostbite; burns; atherosclerosis; diabetes; Raynaud's disease; blood clots; ruptured appendix; hernia; and intravenous (IV) drug use.

SYMPTOMS

Symptoms of gangrene include swelling; pain, followed by numbness when the tissue is dead; sloughing off of skin; color changes, ranging from white, to red, to black; shiny appearance to skin; frothy, clear, watery discharge; fever and chills; and nausea and vomiting.

SCREENING AND DIAGNOSIS

A doctor will ask about symptoms and medical history and will perform a physical exam. Tests for gangrene may include blood tests, tests of the discharge and the tissue; X rays; a magnetic resonance imaging (MRI) scan (a scan that uses radio waves and a powerful magnet to produce detailed computer images); and a computed tomography (CT) scan (a detailed X-ray picture that identifies abnormalities of fine tissue structure).

TREATMENT AND THERAPY

Treatment of gangrene includes antibiotics, given through an IV in a potent form; blood thinners, given to prevent blood clots; debridement, a surgical procedure to cut away dead and dying tissue to keep gangrene from spreading; amputation, or the removal of a severely affected body part; and hyperbaric oxygen therapy, exposure of the affected tissue to oxygen at high pressure.

PREVENTION AND OUTCOMES

If the patient has diabetes, he or she should be sure to care for his or her hands and feet. If the patient needs surgery, a doctor should be consulted about taking antibiotics. This is especially true if the patient needs intestinal surgery.

Rosalyn Carson-DeWitt, M.D.;
reviewed by David L. Horn, M.D., FACP

FURTHER READING

Anderson, D. J., et al. "Skin and Soft Tissue Infections in Older Adults." *Clinics in Geriatric Medicine* 23 (2007): 595.

Andreoli, Thomas E., et al., eds. *Andreoli and Carpenter's Cecil Essentials of Medicine.* 8th ed. Philadelphia: Saunders/Elsevier, 2010.

EBSCO Publishing. *DynaMed: Gas Gangrene.* Available through http://www.ebscohost.com/dynamed.

Folstad, Steven G. "Soft Tissue Infections." In *Emergency Medicine: A Comprehensive Study Guide*, edited by Judith E. Tintinalli. 6th ed. New York: McGraw-Hill, 2004.

Mandell, Gerald L., John E. Bennett, and Raphael Dolin, eds. *Mandell, Douglas, and Bennett's Principles and Practice of Infectious Diseases.* 7th ed. New York: Churchill Livingstone/Elsevier, 2010.

May, A. K. "Skin and Soft Tissue Infections." *Surgical Clinics of North America* 89 (2009): 403.

Meislin, H. W., et al. "Soft Tissue Infections." In *Rosen's Emergency Medicine: Concepts and Clinical Practice,* edited by J. A. Marx et al. 6th ed. St. Louis, Mo.: Mosby, 2006.

Wong, Jason K., et al. "Gas Gangrene." Available at http://www.emedicine.com/emerg/topic211.htm.

WEB SITES OF INTEREST

American Academy of Family Physicians
http://familydoctor.org

American Diabetes Association
http://www.diabetes.org

National Institutes of Health
http://www.nlm.nih.gov/medlineplus/diabeticfoot.html

Public Health Agency of Canada
http://www.phac-aspc.gc.ca

See also: Bacterial infections; Cellulitis; *Clostridium*; Disseminated intravascular coagulation; Fasciitis; Hyperbaric oxygen; Necrotizing fasciitis; Osteomyelitis; Wound infections.

Gastritis

CATEGORY: Diseases and conditions
ANATOMY OR SYSTEM AFFECTED: Digestive system, gastrointestinal system, intestines, stomach
ALSO KNOWN AS: Erosive or nonerosive gastritis, stress gastritis

DEFINITION

Gastritis is a condition in which the lining of the stomach, or mucosa, is inflamed. The lining of the stomach produces acid and enzymes to break down food and produces mucus to protect the stomach lining from the acid. Gastritis may be erosive or nonerosive. Erosive gastritis does not cause major inflammation but can cause the lining of the stomach to wear away, or erode.

CAUSES

Most cases of nonerosive gastritis are caused by infection with the bacterium *Helicobacter pylori.* Erosive gastritis may be caused by use of nonsteroidal anti-inflammatory drugs (NSAIDs) such as aspirin and ibuprofen. Drinking alcohol, using cocaine, and exposure to radiation may also cause erosive gastritis. Stresses such as trauma, major surgery, severe burns, or a critical illness may also cause erosive gastritis (in this case, often called stress gastritis). Less common causes of both erosive and nonerosive gastritis include autoimmune diseases, Crohn's disease, pernicious anemia, viruses, parasites, and bacteria other than *H. pylori.*

RISK FACTORS

Infection with *H. pylori* is a risk factor for gastritis. *H. pylori* may come from consuming contaminated water or food or from an infected person's saliva, vomit, or feces. Excessive use of NSAIDs, alcohol and drug abuse, exposure to radiation, and other gastrointestinal and autoimmune conditions increase the risk of gastritis. As persons age, the stomach lining thins, also increasing the risk.

SYMPTOMS

There may be no symptoms of gastritis. When symptoms do occur, they include dyspepsia (upper abdominal discomfort or pain), nausea, and vomiting. Bleeding may occur as a sign of erosive gastritis and could include blood in the vomit. Bowel movements may appear black and tarlike and may include blood.

SCREENING AND DIAGNOSIS

There is no screening test for gastritis. A biopsy through endoscopy, in which a thin, lighted tube with a camera is threaded down the throat and to the stomach to look at the stomach lining, is the most common diagnostic test. X rays of the upper gastrointestinal tract using barium may be ordered. Blood tests for anemia, tests for blood in the bowel movement, and breath and stool tests to determine if *H. pylori* is present are also part of the diagnosis.

TREATMENT AND THERAPY

The goal of therapy is to reduce the amount of acid in the stomach to promote healing. Medications such as antacids that neutralize acid and histamine 2 (H2) blockers and proton pump inhibitors (PPIs) that decrease acid production are commonly used. Prescription or over-the-counter medications may be ordered. If gastritis is caused by NSAIDs, the doctor may recommend the use of PPIs and stopping the use of NSAIDs, reducing the dose, or changing to another type of drug. If gastritis is caused by *H. pylori*, antibiotics may be prescribed for up to fourteen days. PPIs are also used to treat stress gastritis.

PREVENTION AND OUTCOMES

Although preventing gastritis may not be possible, there are steps that one can take to reduce symptoms. Eating small, frequent meals and avoiding spicy, fried, or fatty foods may help prevent indigestion and ease the effects of acid on the stomach. Limiting use of alcohol and quitting smoking may help. Also, one should take NSAIDs only when necessary and should consult a doctor about other options, such as acetaminophen.

Patricia Stanfill Edens, R.N., Ph.D., FACHE

FURTHER READING

Feldman, Mark, Lawrence S. Friedman, and Lawrence J. Brandt, eds. *Sleisenger and Fordtran's Gastrointestinal and Liver Disease: Pathophysiology, Diagnosis, Management.* New ed. 2 vols. Philadelphia: Saunders/Elsevier, 2010.

Kapadia, Cyrus R., James M. Crawford, and Caroline Taylor. *An Atlas of Gastroenterology: A Guide to Diagnosis and Differential Diagnosis.* Boca Raton, Fla.: Pantheon, 2003.

Kirschner, Barbara S., and Dennis D. Black. "The Gastrointestinal Tract." In *Nelson Essentials of Pediatrics*, edited by Karen J. Marcdante et al. 6th ed. Philadelphia: Saunders/Elsevier, 2011.

WEB SITES OF INTEREST

American Gastroenterological Association
http://www.gastro.org

National Digestive Diseases Information Clearinghouse
http://digestive.niddk.nih.gov

See also: Amebic dysentery; Antibiotic-associated colitis; Bacteria: Classification and types; Bacterial infections; *Escherichia coli* infection; *Helicobacter*; *Helicobacter pylori* infection; Infectious colitis; Inflammation; Intestinal and stomach infections; Peptic ulcer.

Genital herpes

CATEGORY: Diseases and conditions
ANATOMY OR SYSTEM AFFECTED: Genitalia, genitourinary tract, mouth, penis, peripheral nervous system, skin, vagina
ALSO KNOWN AS: Genital herpes simplex, herpes genitalis, herpes simplex 2, herpes simplex virus types 1 and 2

DEFINITION

Genital herpes is a highly contagious infection that is caused by a virus. Genital herpes causes fluid-filled blisters or sores on the skin of the genitals (areas on or around the vagina or penis). The infection can also cause blisters at the anal opening, on the buttocks or thighs, inside the vagina on the cervix, or in the urinary tract of women and men.

CAUSES

The infection is caused by the herpes simplex virus (HSV), of which there are two kinds: herpes simplex type 1 (HSV-1) and herpes simplex type 2 (HSV-2). HSV-2 is usually the cause of genital herpes, but the disease can also be caused by HSV-1, the virus that is associated with oral herpes (cold sores on the mouth).

Genital herpes is a common virus. In the United States, forty-five million people, or one of every five adolescents and adults, ages twelve years and older, are infected with HSV-2.

HSV is transmitted from skin-to-skin contact, especially in places that are warm and moist. The virus enters the body through a cut or opening in the skin or through mucous membranes, the moist inner lining of the urinary tract (in the vaginal area), or the digestive system that includes the mouth, esophagus, stomach, intestines, and anus. The virus stays in the nerve cells of the body, even if a person does not have symptoms or signs of genital herpes. Genital herpes is a chronic, lifelong infection with symptoms that will come and go (be active and inactive) throughout a person's life.

Speaking with a Healthcare Provider About Genital Herpes

SPECIFIC QUESTIONS TO ASK ABOUT GENITAL HERPES
What causes genital herpes?
How did I get infected?
What are the symptoms of a genital herpes outbreak?
Typically, how long will the outbreaks last?
What type of herpes simplex virus am I infected with?
How common is genital herpes?
How is genital herpes different than regular cold sores?
Are there any serious complications of genital herpes that I should be aware of?

SPECIFIC QUESTIONS ABOUT THE RISK OF DEVELOPING GENITAL HERPES
Based on my medical history, lifestyle, and family background, am I at risk for genital herpes?
How can I decrease my risk of contracting genital herpes?
How do I know if my partner has genital herpes? What physical signs or symptoms should I be looking for?
How do I recognize a genital herpes outbreak?
How should I prevent catching genital herpes?
How can I reduce the risk to my partner?

SPECIFIC QUESTIONS ABOUT TREATMENT OPTIONS
What type of medicine should I take to reduce the symptoms?
Can genital herpes be cured?
What medicine can I take to prevent outbreaks?
What are the benefits, side effects, and risks of the medications?
Will these medications interact with other medications, over-the-counter products, or dietary and herbal supplements?

How often is medicine taken or applied?
Are there any alternative or complementary therapies that will help me?
Are you aware of any ongoing research about genital herpes?
Is there any progress in research to find a cure or to prevent genital herpes entirely?
How can I stay abreast of the news about what's happening in genital herpes research?
Where can I find a support group about genital herpes?
Do you recommend any additional counseling?

SPECIFIC QUESTIONS ABOUT LIFESTYLE CHANGES
Is there anything else I can do to minimize any discomfort I may experience?
How do I tell my partner that I have genital herpes?
Do I have to tell my family about genital herpes?
How can I protect my partner?
Should my partner come in for a test and treatment?
Can I still have sex?
How will having genital herpes affect my relationship with my partner?
Are there any dietary changes I should make?
Will exercise affect genital herpes?

SPECIFIC QUESTIONS ABOUT OUTLOOK
How often will I have an outbreak?
How can I become pregnant if I have genital herpes?
How can I get my partner pregnant if I have genital herpes?
Can I take medication if I am pregnant? How can I protect my fetus?
Where can I get more information about genital herpes?

RISK FACTORS

Genital herpes is considered a sexually transmitted disease. One can spread the virus by touching, kissing, or having sexual contact, including vaginal, anal, and oral sex. Several factors lead to the spread of HSV, including having sexual contact with someone who does not have any obvious sores and with someone who has a clear outbreak of the virus. An outbreak means that the sexual partner has visible sores or blisters in the genital area. These sores give off (or shed) some of the virus that can infect the other partner. The virus is most contagious when the sores are visible and open and are producing a discharge.

SYMPTOMS

Once someone is infected, symptoms begin to appear within two to twenty days. The first outbreak is usually the most severe and lasts the longest. Early symptoms can last two to three weeks and can include discomfort (itching, burning, or pain) in the genital or anal area, discharge from the vagina, and a feeling of pressure in the abdomen.

RISK FACTORS

It is possible to develop genital herpes with or without the risk factors discussed here; however, the more risk factors one has, the greater the likelihood of becoming infected with genital herpes. Studies have found that cases of genital herpes have continued to increase. From the 1970's to the 1990's, the incidence of HSV-2, the virus that causes genital herpes, has increased by 30 percent.

Anyone who is sexually active (has vaginal, oral, or anal contact with others) can get genital herpes. If a person has oral herpes and performs oral sex, it is possible for that person's partner to develop genital herpes from that contact.

The following factors can increase the risk of becoming infected with genital herpes:

Behaviors. Having unprotected sex, becoming sexually active at a young age, having been sexually active for many years, having had several sexual partners, having a partner who is infected with genital herpes, and anal sex.

Gender. Women (one of every four women) are more likely than men (one of every five) to become infected with genital herpes.

Socioeconomics. The majority of new infections occur in adolescents and young adults (ages twenty to forty years). In young adults, HSV-1 infection is becoming a more common cause of genital herpes.

Health. Persons with a higher risk of genital herpes are those with human immunodeficiency virus infection, a history of other sexually transmitted infections, and a weak immune system.

Outside factors. Studies suggest there are several things that can trigger the virus and make it active, including stress, excessive sunlight, menstruation, and vigorous sexual activity.

Symptoms

Not all persons are aware they have genital herpes, mostly because they may not have symptoms. They may also not recognize the symptoms if they have them. When first infected, a person has the following symptoms, which appear within two to ten days:

Early symptoms that can last two to three weeks include itching, burning, and pain in the genital or anal area; discharge from the vagina; flulike symptoms, such as fever and swollen glands; and pressure in the abdomen (the area below the stomach).

As the infection progresses, symptoms of an outbreak include sores that start to form on the part of the body where the virus was contracted; sores that begin as small red bumps, develop into blisters, and then become painful open sores; sores or blisters that

appear and occur in clusters or small groupings; vaginal discharge; pain when urinating; and flulike symptoms, including fever, muscle aches, swollen glands, and headache.

The outbreak is coming to an end when, after a few days, the sores form a scablike outer layer and then fall off. The virus will recur and become active and inactive over time. The frequency of these recurrences varies from person to person. One may experience symptoms a number of times throughout a given year or may experience an outbreak only once or twice in a lifetime. Doctors and researchers do not yet know why these recurrences happen.

Every case of genital herpes is unique. The average number of outbreaks that a person experiences each year is about four or five. The first year of the virus is usually the worst. The first outbreak is usually the most severe and painful, with the second occurrence often happening only a few weeks later. As time goes on, the frequency of outbreaks lessens and the outbreaks become much less severe. Recurrences tend to become milder and last usually only a week.

Genital herpes also can result in no symptoms. One can still spread genital herpes even if he or she does not experience symptoms or if the symptoms are inactive.

Many people fail to recognize the symptoms of genital herpes. Women often confuse the discomfort with their menstrual period or with an itchy yeast infection. Men often confuse the symptoms with jock itch or friction burn. Symptoms of genital herpes have also been mistaken for insect bites or hemorrhoids.

Screening and Diagnosis

Sometimes genital herpes is easy to diagnose because the blisters or open sores around the genital area are easily visible, but oftentimes, for an adequate diagnosis, one will need more than an examination. Also, one can have genital herpes yet display no visible sores.

During an examination, laboratory tests will be done to determine if HSV is in the body. These tests will also determine whether the infection is caused by HSV-1 or by HSV-2.

The following tests are used to check for genital herpes:

Viral culture. If the infection is visible, the doctor will rub a swab over an open sore or blister to collect some cells. The cells are then tested to see if the virus is present in those cells. It is recommended that this culture test be taken within the first forty-eight hours after symptoms appear. The problem with this test is that if the body's immune system already killed the herpesvirus from that sore, the test may come back negative for genital herpes, leading to a false-negative diagnosis.

Blood tests. These blood tests are also called antibody tests because they measure HSV antibodies, the disease-fighting substances in the blood. If the blood tests show HSV antibodies, the affected person is most likely infected with HSV. Newer tests can even distinguish between HSV-1 and HSV-2. It is recommended that one wait a minimum of twelve to sixteen weeks from possible exposure to herpes so that the body has enough time to develop antibodies. This will ensure a more accurate blood test.

Specific blood tests include a point of care test, in which the physician gets a small blood sample from the patient (by pricking the skin). Results are available in less than ten minutes. This blood test checks for the presence of HSV-2 antibodies. The HerpeSelect ELISA (enzyme-linked immunoabsorbent assay), the HerpeSelect Immunoblot, and Captiva HSV IgG Type Specific ELISA all involve the patient going to a lab, where blood will be drawn from a vein for testing for HSV-1 or HSV-2 antibodies. Results are available in approximately one to two weeks. None of these tests, however, can pinpoint the site of the infection.

TREATMENT AND THERAPY

There is no cure for genital herpes and no surgical option for treatment. There are, however, medications that treat the symptoms and help prevent future outbreaks.

PREVENTION AND OUTCOMES

Because there is no cure, behavioral change is the best way to lower the risk of contracting the virus and spreading it to others. Abstaining or refraining from sex is the most certain way to avoid contracting genital herpes. Another preventive measure is to have a long-term mutually monogamous (only one exclusive sexual partner) with someone who does not have genital herpes. Persons should avoid sexual contact with others during a genital herpes outbreak, and one should always use a condom during sex. Persons with cold sores (a blister caused by HSV-1 infection) should avoid kissing other people and should avoid oral sex.

One should recognize when the disease is most contagious and know that the virus can be spread even if the person does not have visible sores or is not experiencing an outbreak. One should not touch any visible sores or blisters and should wash hands thoroughly with soap and warm water if a sore or blister is touched. One can ensure against spreading the virus to other parts of the body, such as the mouth or eyes, by not touching sores and then touching these uninfected areas.

One can also take medications, such as valacyclovir, that are approved by the U.S. Food and Drug Administration for use in preventing the spread of genital herpes. Taking valacyclovir only reduces the risk of transmission by 50 percent. A better way to protect oneself and one's partner is to take valacyclovir and use a condom.

Diane Safer, Ph.D.

FURTHER READING

American Academy of Dermatology. "Herpes Simplex." Available at http://www.aad.org. A brief but comprehensive discussion of the herpes simplex virus and its dermatological manifestations.

Drake, S., et al. "Improving the Care of Patients with Genital Herpes." *British Medical Journal* 321 (2000): 619-623. A clinician's guide to caring for persons with HSV genital infection.

Groves, M. J. "Transmission of Herpes Simplex Virus via Oral Sex." *American Family Physician* 73 (2006): 1153. Discusses how HSV infection, including cold sores, is transmissible through oral sex.

"Herpes Simplex." In *Ferri's Clinical Advisor 2011: Instant Diagnosis and Treatment*, edited by Fred F. Ferri. Philadelphia: Mosby/Elsevier, 2011. Provides recommendations on clinical treatments for HSV infections.

Langlais, Robert P., and Craig S. Miller. *Color Atlas of Common Oral Diseases.* 4th ed. Philadelphia: Lippincott Williams & Wilkins, 2009. Provides six hundred color photographs of the most commonly seen oral conditions, including HSV infections, and descriptive text for each condition.

WEB SITES OF INTEREST

American Social Health Association
http://www.ashastd.org

Centers for Disease Control and Prevention
http://www.cdc.gov/std/herpes

International Herpes Alliance
http://www.herpesalliance.org

National Institute of Allergy and Infectious Diseases
http://www.niaid.nih.gov

See also: Chancroid; Chlamydia; Cold sores; Contagious diseases; Genital warts; Gonorrhea; Herpes simplex infection; Herpesviridae; Herpesvirus infections; HIV; Human papillomavirus (HPV) infections; Human papillomavirus (HPV) vaccine; Men and infectious disease; Pelvic inflammatory disease; Sexually transmitted diseases (STDs); Trichomonas; Urethritis; Vaginal yeast infection; Viral infections; Warts; Women and infectious disease.

Genital warts

CATEGORY: Diseases and conditions
ANATOMY OR SYSTEM AFFECTED: Genitalia, mouth, skin, throat
ALSO KNOWN AS: Anogenital warts, condyloma acuminata, penile warts, venereal warts

DEFINITION

Genital warts are growths or bumps that appear on the vulva; in or around the vagina or anus; on the cervix, penis, scrotum, groin, or thigh; or, rarely, in the mouth or throat. The warts may be raised or flat, single or multiple, small or large. Some may cluster to form a cauliflower-like shape. This condition is one of the most common sexually transmitted diseases (STDs).

CAUSES

Genital warts are caused by the human papillomavirus (HPV). HPV is a family of more than eighty common viruses. Many types of HPV cause harmless skin warts that are often found on the fingers or feet. Only a few types are thought to cause genital warts.

HPV is easily spread during oral, genital, or anal sex with an infected partner. About two-thirds of people who have sex with a partner who has genital warts will also develop them. Warts can take several weeks or months to appear. Most people will be exposed to a form of HPV at some point in their lives, but not everyone will become infected or develop symptoms.

RISK FACTORS

Risk factors for HPV and genital warts include multiple sexual partners, women whose first male sexual partner has had two or more previous sexual partners, sex without condoms, sex at an early age, skin-to-skin contact with an infected partner, previous history of genital warts, pregnancy, smoking, and taking oral contraceptives. Persons age fifteen to thirty years are at higher risk.

SYMPTOMS

Genital warts often look like fleshy, raised growths. They have a cauliflower shape and often appear in clusters. In women, warts may be found in the area of the vulva, inside or around the vagina or anus, and on the cervix. In men, warts are less common. If present, they are usually found on the tip or shaft of the penis, on the scrotum, or around the anus. The following symptoms may also occur for women and for men: bleeding, itching, irritation, burning, and a secondary bacterial infection with redness, tenderness, or pus.

Complications of HPV include cancer. Most strains of HPV that produce genital warts do not cause cancer, but certain strains may cause cervical cancer. Less common are cancers of the vulva, anus, or penis. It is important for women to have yearly Pap tests, which can detect any HPV-related problems.

Genital warts may get larger during pregnancy and could make urination difficult. Warts in or near the vaginal opening may also block the birth canal during delivery.

SCREENING AND DIAGNOSIS

A doctor can diagnose genital warts by looking at them. If external warts are found on a woman, her cervix is usually also checked. In all patients, the doctor may use a special solution to help find lesions that do not have classic features.

An abnormal Pap test may indicate HPV, but the doctor will order more accurate tests, such as a colposcopy, to diagnose HPV. A colposcopy is a special device that allows the doctor to see if warts are in the cervix and vagina. The doctor may take a tissue sample (biopsy) and test it. During an HPV test, a swab of cells from the affected area can be checked for certain types of HPV.

TREATMENT AND THERAPY

Treatment, which depends on the size and location of the warts, helps the symptoms but does not cure the virus. The virus stays in the body, and warts or other problems may recur.

Treatments may include topical treatments. The doctor may recommend topical medications to be applied to the affected areas. They include imiquimod cream, podophyllum resin, podofilox solution, 5-fluorouracil cream, and trichloroacetic acid.

Other treatment options include cryosurgery (freezing the wart), electrocautery (burning the wart), and laser treatment, all of which destroy the warts. These methods are used on small warts and on large warts that have not responded to other treatment. A large wart can also be removed surgically. For warts that keep coming back, an antiviral drug, called alpha-interferon, can be injected into the wart.

PREVENTION AND OUTCOMES

The only way to completely prevent HPV from spreading is to avoid physical contact with an infected partner. Latex condoms may help reduce the spread of HPV infection and genital warts. Condoms are not 100 percent effective, however, because they do not cover the entire genital area. Other ways to prevent infection include abstaining from sex, having a monogamous relationship, and getting regular checkups for STDs. Women should get regular Pap tests, starting at age eighteen years or at the start of sexual activity.

The vaccine Gardasil protects against four types of HPV. Studies have shown that the vaccine reduced the number of precancerous cervical cell changes for up to three years after the shot. The vaccine is routinely given to girls ages eleven to twelve years, and a "catchup" vaccine is given to young women who have not been vaccinated. The U.S. Food and Drug Administration has also approved the use of Gardasil in males ages nine to twenty-six years.

Genital warts are rare in children. This diagnosis may indicate sexual abuse, which persons should report to authorities.

Michelle Badash, M.S.;
reviewed by David L. Horn, M.D., FACP

FURTHER READING

Behrman, Richard E., Robert M. Kliegman, and Hal B. Jenson, eds. *Nelson Textbook of Pediatrics.* 18th ed. Philadelphia: Saunders/Elsevier, 2007.

Centers for Disease Control and Prevention. "Genital Warts: Sexually Transmitted Diseases Treatment Guidelines 2010." Available at http://www.cdc.gov/std/treatment/2010/genital-warts.htm.

_____. "HPV Vaccines." Available at http://www.cdc.gov/hpv/vaccine.html.

Dunne, E. F., and L. E. Markowitz. "Genital Human Papillomavirus Infection." *Clinical Infectious Diseases* 43 (2006): 624.

EBSCO Publishing. *DynaMed: Condyloma acuminatum.* Available through http://www.ebscohost.com/dynamed.

Hanna, E., and G. Bachmann. "HPV Vaccination with Gardasil: A Breakthrough in Women's Health." *Expert Opinion on Biological Therapy* 6 (2006): 1223-1227.

Henderson, Gregory, and Batya Swift Yasgur. *Women at Risk: The HPV Epidemic and Your Cervical Health.* New York: Putnam, 2002.

Lowy, D. R., and J. T. Schiller. "Papillomaviruses and Cervical Cancer: Pathogenesis and Vaccine Development." *Journal of the National Cancer Institute Monographs* 23 (1998): 27-30.

McCance, Dennis J., ed. *Human Papilloma Viruses.* New York: Elsevier Science, 2002.

McLemore, M. R. "Gardasil: Introducing the New Human Papillomavirus Vaccine." *Clinical Journal of Oncology Nursing* 10 (2006): 559-560.

Markowitz, Lauri E., et al. "Quadrivalent Human Papillomavirus Vaccine: Recommendations of the Advisory Committee on Immunization Practices (ACIP)." *Morbidity and Mortality Weekly Report* 56 (March 23, 2007): 1-24.

"New Vaccine Prevents Cervical Cancer." *FDA Consumer* 40 (2006): 37.

"Quadrivalent Vaccine Against Human Papillomavirus to Prevent High-Grade Cervical Lesions." *New England Journal of Medicine* 356 (2007): 1915-1927.

U.S. Food and Drug Administration. "FDA Approves New Indication for Gardasil to Prevent Genital Warts in Men and Boys." Available at http://www.fda.gov.

Winer, R. L., et al. "Risk of Female Human Papillomavirus Acquisition Associated with First Male Sex Partner." *Journal of Infectious Diseases* 197 (2008): 279-282.

WEB SITES OF INTEREST

Centers for Disease Control and Prevention
http://www.cdc.gov/std

National Women's Health Information Center
http://www.womenshealth.gov

Planned Parenthood
http://www.plannedparenthood.org

Sex Information and Education Council of Canada
http://www.sieccan.org

See also: Acute cystitis; Bacterial vaginosis; Cervical cancer; Chancroid; Childbirth and infectious disease; Chlamydia; Genital herpes; Gonorrhea; Herpes simplex infection; Herpesviridae; Herpesvirus infections; HIV; Human papillomavirus (HPV) infections; Human papillomavirus (HPV) vaccine; Men and infectious disease; Pelvic inflammatory disease; Pregnancy and infectious disease; Sexually transmitted diseases (STDs); Trichomonas; Urethritis; Vaccines: Types; Vaginal yeast infection; Viral infections; Warts; Women and infectious disease.

German measles. *See* Rubella.

Germicides. *See* Chemical germicides.

Germs. *See* Bacteria; Pathogens; Viruses.

Gerstmann-Sträussler-Scheinker syndrome

CATEGORY: Diseases and conditions
ANATOMY OR SYSTEM AFFECTED: Brain, central nervous system
ALSO KNOWN AS: Genetic prion disease, transmissible spongiform encephalopathy

DEFINITION

Gerstmann-Sträussler-Scheinker (GSS) syndrome is a type of genetic prion disease. Prions are protein-aceous infectious particles that lack nucleic acid to replicate. Prion diseases may be sporadic or acquired, while a minority are inherited (10 to 15 percent). GSS syndrome is a rare, inherited, neurodegenerative disorder in which an abnormal prion causes the protein amyloid to be atypically deposited in the brain. Genetic prion diseases have an incidence of one case per million persons, translating into three hundred new cases per year worldwide.

CAUSES

GSS syndrome is caused by a mutation in the prion protein gene PRNP. The genetic mutation is inherited in an autosomal dominant manner, meaning each child has a 50 percent chance of inheriting GSS syndrome from an affected parent. However, some mutations originate in the affected person and are considered new in that person's family.

RISK FACTORS

A positive family history of GSS syndrome poses the greatest risk for inheritance of the disease. Although the disease may occur in persons of any ethnic background, prevalent mutations in those with European ancestry have been reported.

SYMPTOMS

Symptoms gradually appear during the third to sixth decade of life. Neurological findings include an unsteady walk, a lack of muscle coordination, and speech difficulties. This often progresses to cognitive dysfunction with slower thought processing and decreased concentration, increased muscle tone, swallowing difficulties, and diminished facial expressions. Vision and hearing loss may occur. GSS syndrome progresses slowly to the final stage, when an infected person is bedridden because of worsening symptoms. The disease lasts two to ten years and ultimately results in death from a secondary infection such as pneumonia or from a urinary infection.

SCREENING AND DIAGNOSIS

An electroencephalogram (EEG), magnetic resonance imaging (MRI), and analysis of cerebrospinal fluid may be performed, but none of these tests can independently establish the diagnosis. Sequencing of the PRNP gene is clinically available to establish that a genetic mutation is present, but sequencing is not 100 percent accurate. Prenatal diagnosis for a pregnancy by amniocentesis or chorionic villus sampling may be available if the mutation in PRNP has been identified in an affected parent. However, testing a pregnant woman for an adult-onset disorder is controversial.

Treatment and Therapy

No cure exists for GSS syndrome. Treatment is supportive only and entails medication for clinical symptoms or a feeding tube for swallowing difficulties. Antiviral therapies are not effective.

Prevention and Outcomes

Genetic prion diseases are not directly contagious; however, bodily fluid from a person with GSS syndrome is considered a biohazard and is disposed of appropriately. Preimplantation genetic diagnosis may be available for testing embryos for a mutation in the PRNP gene before implantation through in vitro fertilization.

Janet Ober Berman, M.S., CGC

Further Reading

Brown, David R., ed. *Neurodegeneration and Prion Disease.* New York: Springer, 2005.

Gambetti, P., et al. "Inherited Prion Diseases." In *Prion Biology and Diseases,* edited by Stanley B. Prusiner. 2d ed. Cold Spring Harbor, N.Y.: Cold Spring Harbor Laboratory Press, 2004.

Mastrianni, J. A. "The Genetics of Prion Diseases." *Genetics in Medicine* 4 (2010): 187-195.

Prusiner, Stanley B. "The Prion Diseases." *Scientific American* 272, no. 1 (January, 1995): 48-57.

Rowland, Lewis P., and Timothy A. Pedley, eds. *Merritt's Textbook of Neurology.* 12th ed. Philadelphia: Lippincott Williams & Wilkins, 2010.

Safar, J. R., et al. "Diagnosis of Human Prion Disease." *Proceedings of the National Academy of Science* 102 (2005): 3501-3506.

Web Sites of Interest

GeneTests
http://www.genetests.org

Genetic and Rare Diseases Information Center
http://rarediseases.info.nih.gov/gard

National Institute of Allergy and Infectious Diseases
http://www.niaid.nih.gov/topics/prion

National Institute of Neurological Disorders and Stroke: Transmissible Spongiform Encephalopathies Information Page
http://www.ninds.nih.gov/disorders/tse

National Organization for Rare Disorders
http://www.rarediseases.org

See also: Creutzfeldt-Jakob disease; Encephalitis; Fatal familial insomnia; Guillain-Barré syndrome; Kuru; Prion diseases; Prions; Subacute sclerosing panencephalitis; Variant Creutzfeldt-Jakob disease.

Giardia

Category: Pathogen
Transmission route: Ingestion

Definition

Giardia is a protozoan flagellate and the most common pathogen causing intestinal disease in humans worldwide. It is more common in developing countries but also found in developed countries. An estimated 280 million people worldwide have been infected with *Giardia*. *G. intestinalis* was first discovered in 1681 by Antoni van Leeuwenhoek, who examined his own diarrheal feces under a rudimentary microscope. *G. intestinalis* is also known as *G. lamblia* and *G. duodenalis*.

Natural Habitat and Features

The natural environment of *Giardia* is in rivers, lakes, and streams. Persons who hike or backpack may develop giardiasis by drinking water from these bodies of water. *Giardia* is a protozoan that, in its active disease-causing stage, resembles a pear that is cut in half, lengthwise. The parasite, once consumed, rapidly activates.

Giardia also can be transmitted in undercooked or raw foods, although waterborne contamination is believed far more common. When transmitted in food, it is most often transmitted through contaminated water used to prepare food or by an infected food handler. *Giardia* has also been reported in day-care centers where infant diapers are changed and where proper sanitation has not been practiced. Animal contamination of food may cause infection in humans,

Taxonomic Classification for *Giardia*

Kingdom: Protista
Subkingdom: Protozoa
Phylum: Sarcomastigophora
Subphylum: Mastigophora
Class: Zoomastigophora
Order: Diplomonadida
Family: Hexamitidae
Genus: *Giardia*
Species:
  G. intestinalis
  G. agilis
  G. muris
  G. ardeae
  G. psittaci
  G. microti

and some cross-species reports of *G. intestinalis* have been reported.

Giardia also infects amphibians, rodents, birds, voles, and muskrats. Ingestion of as few as ten cysts can trigger an active infection in the host. Note that in an average bowel movement of a person infected with giardiasis, three hundred million cysts could be deposited in the stool.

There are two key aspects to the life cycle of *Giardia*, including encystation and active infection. In the cyst stage, *Giardia* protects itself by creating a hard cyst, in which it can survive for long periods in damp, cool environments. The cyst comprises 40 percent protein and 60 percent carbohydrate; some studies have shown that the cyst is up to 0.5 micrometers (μm) in thickness. The cysts are oval-shaped and have outer and inner layers, comprising two protective membranes.

Once ingested, the parasite is activated by the gastric acid of the host, which triggers excystation (the end of the cyst stage) and the beginning of the second phase of the life cycle, in which the cyst is deactivated and activation of *Giardia* occurs. From two to four trophozoites (the active stage of the organism) may be excysted from each cyst. Each trophozoite reproduces itself at five to ten minute intervals. The reproduction stage is not completely understood, however, and experts disagree on whether, in these trophozoites, cell division leads to reproduction or if sexual reproduction (which has never been observed) leads to reproduction.

Excystation occurs in about fifteen minutes, starting with the flagella breaking through the cyst. The parasite uses its sucking disk like a suction cup to attach to the intestinal wall of the host. The trophozoite of *G. intestinalis* is up to 9 μm wide and 15 μm long. *G. intestinalis* consumes some of the nutrients eaten by the host before they can be used by the host. People who are most susceptible to infection are those whose immune systems are compromised.

There are two primary genetic groups of *G. intestinalis*, including assemblage A and B. Assemblage B appears to be more common in humans but B is the more studied form of the parasite.

G. intestinalis can survive a moderate level of chlorine, and according to the Centers for Disease Control and Prevention (CDC), *Giardia* can remain alive for up to one hour in chlorinated pools. Children and adults can become infected in pools that house the germ by swallowing the pool water.

G. intestinalis never enters the bloodstream of the infected host. Its actions are not entirely understood by experts, but it appears that the pathogen may release substances such as lectins or proteinases that can damage the epithelium of the host. *Giardia* may also trigger proteinase-activated receptors by the host, although *Giardia* itself never invades the skin. Some research also indicates that *Giardia* can cause a hypersecretion of chloride in infected humans and the malabsorption of sodium, glucose, and water, which together may be responsible for fluid accumulation of the host during infection.

According to the CDC, the number of all reported cases of giardiasis was 19,239 in 2006, 19,794 in 2007, and 19,140 in 2008.

PATHOGENICITY AND CLINICAL SIGNIFICANCE

Up to three stool specimens are needed to identify *Giardia,* and only sensitive immunoassays should be used to identify this pathogen. The enzyme-linked immunosorbent assay (ELISA) is one means of testing for *Giardia,* as is direct fluorescence testing (DFA). Cysts can be readily seen with the fluorescence method.

DRUG SUSCEPTIBILITY

The first-line treatment for *G. intestinalis* is metronidazole, given in a dosage of 250 milligrams three times per day for up to ten days. Resistance to metronidazole has been reported in about 20 percent of cases, and if such a resistance occurs, tinidazole may be given three times per day for seven days. If the pathogen is resistant to both metronidazole and tinidazole, then other drugs may be prescribed; these include albendazole, furazolidone, and quinacrine.

Christine Adamec, M.B.A.

FURTHER READING

Ankarklev, Johan, et al. "Behind the Smile: Cell Biology and Disease Mechanisms of *Giardia* Species." *Nature Reviews Microbiology* 8 (April, 2010): 413-422.

Buret, Andre G. "Mechanisms of Epithelial Dysfunction in Giardiasis." *Gut* 56 (2007): 316-317.

Espelage, Werner, et al. "Characteristics and Risk Factors for Symptomatic *Giardia lamblia* Infections in Germany." *BMC Public Health* 10 (2010). Available at http://www.biomedcentral.com/1471-2458/10/41.

Hill, David R., and Theodore E. Nash. "*Giardia lamblia.*" In *Mandell, Douglas, and Bennett's Principles and Practice of Infectious Diseases*, edited by Gerald L. Mandell, John F. Bennett, and Raphael Dolin. 7th ed. New York: Churchill Livingstone/Elsevier, 2010.

Kucik, Corry Jeb, Gary L. Martin, and Brett V. Sortor. "Common Intestinal Parasites." *American Family Physician* 69 (2004): 1161-1168.

Post, Robert E., and Barry L. Hainer. "Gastrointestinal Tract Infections." In *Management of Antimicrobials in Infectious Diseases: Impact of Antibiotic Resistance*, edited by Arch G. Mainous and Claire Pomeroy. 2d ed. Totowa, N.J.: Humana Press, 2010.

Schlossberg, David, ed. *Infections of Leisure.* 4th ed. Washington, D.C.: ASM Press, 2009.

Yoder, Jonathan S., Courtney Harral, and Michael J. Beach. "Giardiasis Surveillance—United States, 2006-2008." *Morbidity and Mortality Weekly Report* 59, no. SS-6 (June 11, 2010): 15-25.

WEB SITES OF INTEREST

American Academy of Family Physicians
http://familydoctor.org

American Gastroenterological Association
http://www.gastro.org

Canadian Association of Gastroenterology
http://www.cag-acg.org

Centers for Disease Control and Prevention
http://www.cdc.gov/parasites

See also: Amebic dysentery; Antibiotic-associated colitis; Antiparasitic drugs: Types; Ascariasis; Cholera; Cryptosporidiosis; Developing countries and infectious disease; Dracunculiasis; Giardiasis; Hookworms; Intestinal and stomach infections; Norovirus infection; Parasitic diseases; Travelers' diarrhea; Tropical medicine; Typhoid fever; Viral gastroenteritis; Waterborne illness and disease; Worm infections.

Giardiasis

CATEGORY: Diseases and conditions
ANATOMY OR SYSTEM AFFECTED: Abdomen, gastrointestinal system, intestines, stomach

DEFINITION

Giardiasis is a gastrointestinal infection caused by protozoa. It is one of the most common parasitic diseases and may be responsible for up to one billion cases annually worldwide.

CAUSES

Giardiasis is caused by a tiny parasite called *Giardia* lamblia. *Giardia* cysts are a resistant form of the parasite that can survive outside a human or animal body. These cysts cause the spread of this disease. For infection to occur, a person must ingest *Giardia* cysts by mouth. Once cysts are ingested, the parasites start growing and multiplying in the small intestine. Ingesting as few as ten parasitic cysts can cause an infection.

Giardiasis can be contracted by contact with feces containing the parasitic cysts. Infected feces can be human and animal (less often), including from beavers, cats, dogs, and cows. Giardiasis also can be contracted by eating food, drinking water, or swimming in water contaminated by the parasitic cysts, and by contact with a person's hands that are contaminated with parasite cyst-infected stool.

RISK FACTORS

Risk factors for giardiasis are unsanitary or crowded living conditions; drinking untreated water, such as well water or stream or lake water; low stomach acid,

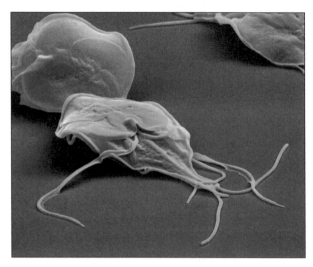

Giardia lamblia *is a parasitic organism that causes the gastrointestinal infection giardiasis.*

often found in elderly people and people on ulcer drugs; oral-anal sex; an impaired immune system; working or staying in a day-care center or nursing home; and international travel. Persons at higher risk are internationally adopted children, who may harbor more than one parasitic infection; hikers, campers, and swimmers; and young children and elderly adults.

SYMPTOMS

Symptoms usually start five to twenty-eight days after infection. Not all people who are infected have symptoms, but all people who are infected can transmit the disease. Symptoms may include diarrhea, acute or chronic; loose, greasy, foul-smelling stools; abdominal pain or cramps; bloating; gas; nausea or vomiting; weight loss; and, rarely, mild fever.

SCREENING AND DIAGNOSIS

A doctor will ask about symptoms and medical history and will perform a physical exam. Tests may include a laboratory exam of several (usually three) stool samples and stool testing (*Giardia* antigen test) for *Giardia* proteins. Some cases may require testing of a fluid or tissue sample from the intestine. If the patient is diagnosed with giardiasis, everyone living in that patient's household should be tested for infection.

TREATMENT AND THERAPY

Giardiasis is treated with a prescription antiparasitic drug. The medication is usually given for five to ten days and may include metronidazole, furazolidone, paromomycin, nitazoxanide, and tinidazole. This condition, however, may be resistant to any of these medications or to several others occasionally used. Resistance may complicate treatment and prolong illness.

PREVENTION AND OUTCOMES

To prevent getting or spreading giardiasis, one should take the following measures: Maintain good personal hygiene; wash hands several times a day, especially before eating or preparing food, after a bowel movement, and after changing a diaper; use bottled water for drinking, cooking, and brushing teeth when camping; purify untreated water before using (boil, filter, or otherwise sterilize); and thoroughly wash or peel raw fruits and vegetables before eating. When traveling overseas, one should use only bottled water for drinking, cooking, or brushing teeth and only should eat food that is adequately cooked and served steaming hot.

Children with diarrhea should not enter swimming pools, and swimming pools should be adequately chlorinated. Also, one should stay home from work and keep children home from school or day care until the infection disappears.

Rick Alan; reviewed by Daus Mahnke, M.D.

FURTHER READING

Adam, R. D. "Biology of *Giardia lamblia.*" *Clinical Microbiology Reviews* 14 (2001): 447.

Berger, Stephen A., and John S. Marr. *Human Parasitic Diseases Sourcebook.* Sudbury, Mass.: Jones and Bartlett, 2006.

Despommier, Dickson D., et al. *Parasitic Diseases.* 5th ed. New York: Apple Tree, 2006.

Hill, David R., and Theodore E. Nash. "*Giardia lamblia.*" In *Mandell, Douglas, and Bennett's Principles and Practice of Infectious Diseases*, edited by Gerald L. Mandell, John F. Bennett, and Raphael Dolin. 7th ed. New York: Churchill Livingstone/Elsevier, 2010.

Nash, T. E. "Surface Antigenic Variation in *Giardia lamblia.*" *Molecular Microbiology* 45 (2002): 585.

WEB SITES OF INTEREST

American Academy of Family Physicians
http://familydoctor.org

Canadian Association of Gastroenterology
http://www.cag-acg.org

Centers for Disease Control and Prevention
http://www.cdc.gov/parasites

See also: Amebic dysentery; Antiparasitic drugs: Types; Cryptosporidiosis; Diagnosis of protozoan diseases; Enteritis; Fecal-oral route of transmission; Food-borne illness and disease; *Giardia*; Intestinal and stomach infections; Norovirus infection; Parasitic diseases; Peritonitis; Prevention of protozoan diseases; Protozoa: Classification and types; Protozoan diseases; Sexually transmitted diseases (STDs); Soilborne illness and disease; Treatment of protozoan diseases; Waterborne illness and disease.

Gingivitis

CATEGORY: Diseases and conditions
ANATOMY OR SYSTEM AFFECTED: Gums, mouth, teeth, tissue
ALSO KNOWN AS: Gum disease

DEFINITION

Gingivitis is a mild, often reversible form of gum disease in which the gum tissue, which surrounds the teeth, is inflamed. If left untreated, gingivitis can progress to a serious condition called periodontitis (inflammation of the support tissue and bone).

CAUSES

Gingivitis is caused by a substance that forms on teeth called plaque. Plaque is a sticky material, composed of bacteria, mucus, food, and other substances. It hardens to form tartar or calculus. Plaque that is left on teeth for an extended time can cause gingivitis. Toxins produced by bacteria in dental plaque irritate the gum tissue and cause infection, inflammation, and pain.

RISK FACTORS

Risk factors for gingivitis include inadequate brushing and flossing; stress; clenching or grinding teeth; poor nutrition; diabetes; breathing through the mouth; human immunodeficiency virus infection; improper bite; advancing age; pregnancy; birth control pills; family members with gum disease; poorly fitting dentures; some medications taken for high blood pressure, heart disease, and depression; some seizure medications; drinking alcohol; smoking; and Down syndrome. Also, males are at higher risk for gingivitis.

SYMPTOMS

Gingivitis is often painless, with symptoms developing when the condition becomes worse. Symptoms may include swollen and puffy gums, tender gums, redness in the gums or around the teeth, bleeding gums during brushing or eating, gum tissue that recedes or changes shape, and persistent bad breath.

SCREENING AND DIAGNOSIS

A dentist will examine teeth and gums and assess them for swelling and areas where the tissue might be pulling away from the teeth and forming a pocket. Early diagnosis of the problem enables prompt treatment and the possibility of reversing the condition. One should see a dentist every six months for a cleaning because gingivitis may have no symptoms in its early stages.

TREATMENT AND THERAPY

Gingivitis therapy aims to remove the irritating plaque and prevent its return. Treatment includes regular dental checkups and good oral hygiene; careful and frequent brushing and flossing; a healthful diet that is low in saturated fat and rich in whole grains, fruits, and vegetables; and self-care brushing. One should thoroughly brush and floss teeth using a soft-bristled toothbrush held at a 45-degree angle to the line where the teeth and gums meet, and should move the brush in small circular movements along the gum line and chewing surfaces of the teeth. An electronic toothbrush may make brushing easier for people with physical limitations. One should replace the brush when the bristles become bent or frayed, or every three to four months.

Brushing removes bacteria from the teeth, but the brush cannot reach everywhere it is needed. Flossing helps rid food and bacteria from between the teeth. The best method for flossing includes holding the floss tight and then gently bringing it down between the teeth. One should avoid popping the floss against the gum. It is ideal to curve the floss around the tooth and rub up and down. Finally, it is best to adjust the floss so a fresh section is used for each tooth. A dentist may recommend additional self-care treatments, such as massaging the gums with a rubber tip. Rinses to fight bacteria and plaque buildup may help some persons.

Dental health professionals check for gingivitis and remove plaque that has built up on teeth. A visit every six months is usually considered adequate. Persons with gingivitis may need more frequent cleanings. If the disease progresses and plaque builds up below the gum line, the area should be scraped off and smoothed with dental tools. Accumulated plaque and tartar buildup make it easier for bacteria to grow.

If an area has progressed to periodontal disease, surgery or medication may be required. Treating an underlying medical problem may improve the health of the gums. In persons with recurring or persistent gingivitis, a dentist will evaluate whether some other condition may be contributing to the gum disease.

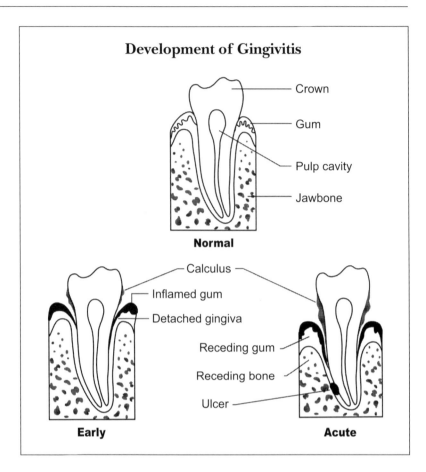

Development of Gingivitis

Crown
Gum
Pulp cavity
Jawbone
Normal

Calculus
Inflamed gum
Detached gingiva
Receding gum
Receding bone
Ulcer
Early
Acute

PREVENTION AND OUTCOMES

Strategies to prevent gingivitis include good dental habits, such as brushing teeth twice daily. There is some data that rotating oscillating electric toothbrushes are more effective in controlling gingivitis than is brushing by hand. Other strategies include flossing at least once a day, visiting a dentist's office for a cleaning every six months, eating balanced and nutritious meals, avoiding smoking, and avoiding alcohol.

Debra Wood, R.N.;
reviewed by Laura Morris-Olson, D.M.D.

FURTHER READING

Icon Health. *Gingivitis: A Medical Dictionary, Bibliography, and Annotated Research Guide to Internet References.* San Diego, Calif.: Author, 2004.

Lamont, R. J., and H. F. Jenkinson. "Life Below the Gum Line: Pathogenic Mechanism of Porphyromonas Gingivalis." *Microbiology and Molecular Biology Reviews* 62, no. 4 (1998): 1244-1263.

Langlais, Robert P., and Craig S. Miller. *Color Atlas of Common Oral Diseases.* 4th ed. Philadelphia: Lippincott Williams & Wilkins, 2009.

Newman, Michael G., Henry H. Takei, and Perry R. Klokkevold, eds. *Carranza's Clinical Periodontology.* 10th ed. St. Louis, Mo.: Saunders/Elsevier, 2006.

Parker, James N., and Philip M. Parker, eds. *The Official Patient's Sourcebook on Gingivitis.* San Diego, Calif.: Icon Health, 2002.

Sutton, Amy L., ed. *Dental Care and Oral Health Sourcebook.* 3d ed. Detroit: Omnigraphics, 2008.

WEB SITES OF INTEREST

American Academy of Periodontology
http://www.perio.org

American Dental Association
http://www.ada.org

Canadian Dental Association
http://www.cda-adc.ca

Canadian Dental Hygienists Association
http://www.cdha.ca

See also: Acute necrotizing ulcerative gingivitis; Cold sores; Herpes simplex infection; Herpesviridae; Herpesvirus infections; Inflammation; Mouth infections; Tooth abscess; Vincent's angina.

Glanders

CATEGORY: Diseases and conditions
ANATOMY OR SYSTEM AFFECTED: Blood, lungs, skin, upper respiratory tract

DEFINITION

Glanders is a highly infectious, life-threatening, disease caused by Burkholderia mallei, a potential biological warfare agent. It has been eradicated from most regions except Africa, Asia, the Middle East, Central America, and South America. Human infection occurs through the skin, lungs, or bloodstream.

CAUSES

B. mallei, classified as a category B priority pathogen by the National Institutes of Health and the Centers for Disease Control and Prevention (CDC), is highly infectious when aerosolized and is antibiotic resistant. It is a zoonotic agent because of its transmission between animals and humans. The bacteria exist in animal hosts (most often in horses, donkeys, and mules). Transmission of the disease in humans occurs through direct contact with tissue or bodily fluids of infected animals. The bacteria enter the body through minor cuts, through ingestion, or by inhalation of infected aerosols and then release toxins that interrupt cellular processes. Person-to-person transmission of the disease can occur.

RISK FACTORS

All ages can be affected by the disease. People in close contact with animals, such as veterinarians, and laboratory personnel working with B. mallei, are at greater risk of exposure.

SYMPTOMS

Clinical symptoms of glanders vary depending on the route of infection. A localized skin infection is characterized by rashes, bumps, and ulcerated lesions. An upper respiratory tract infection occurs when bacteria enter through mucous membranes (nose, eyes) and cause an increased nasal discharge and inflammation. Symptoms of pulmonary infection include cough, fever, difficulty breathing, and lung abscesses. Infection can disseminate to other areas and into the bloodstream (sepsis), causing fever, chills, muscle aches, chest pain, skin rash, diarrhea, liver and spleen enlargement, and multiorgan failure, followed by death. A chronic and progressive infection involves abscesses throughout the body.

SCREENING AND DIAGNOSIS

Glanders is a sporadic disease in humans, and any suspected cases should be reported to local health officials. Primary care physicians should consult with an infectious disease specialist and the CDC for diagnosis and treatment to prevent misdiagnosis. Diagnostic tests include sputum culture, chest X ray, radiography, and polymerase chain reaction assays. Definitive diagnosis of glanders requires isolating and confirming the presence of B. mallei from infected specimens.

TREATMENT AND THERAPY

Persons with glanders are treated with antibiotics based on the extent of the disease. The small number of human cases and clinical studies has limited the amount of information about effective antibiotic treatment. Some antibiotics, including sulfadiazine, have proven effective against glanders; however, extended multidrug therapy may be necessary. Glanders has a high mortality rate and, if left untreated, is quickly fatal.

PREVENTION AND OUTCOMES

Because there is no vaccine for glanders, preventive measures must be employed. In endemic areas, the identification and elimination of infected animals is essential in preventing human transmission. Within the health care, laboratory, and animal care settings, one should follow biosafety containment practices.

Rose Ciulla-Bohling, Ph.D.

FURTHER READING

Currie, Bart J. "*Burkholderia pseudomallei* and *Burkholderia mallei*: Melioidosis and Glanders." In *Mandell, Douglas, and Bennett's Principles and Practice of Infectious Diseases*, edited by Gerald L. Mandell, John F. Bennett, and Raphael Dolin. 7th ed. New York: Churchill Livingstone/Elsevier, 2010.

Larsen, Joseph C., and Nathan H. Johnson. "Pathogenesis of *Burkholderia pseudomallei* and *Burkholderia mallei*." *Military Medicine* 174 (2009): 647-651.

Rega, Paul P. "CBRNE—Glanders and Melioidosis." Available at http://emedicine.medscape.com/article/830235-overview.

WEB SITES OF INTEREST

Center for Biosecurity
http://www.upmc-biosecurity.org

Center for Food Security and Public Health
http://www.cfsph.iastate.edu/diseaseinfo

Centers for Disease Control and Prevention
http://www.cdc.gov

See also: Anthrax; Antibiotic resistance; Biological weapons; Bioterrorism; Botulinum toxin infection; Melioidosis; Respiratory route of transmission; SARS; Soilborne illness and disease; Zoonotic diseases.

Globalization and infectious disease

CATEGORY: Epidemiology

DEFINITION

The increased ease and frequency of international trade, travel, and migration have renewed concerns about the spread of infectious diseases. Infectious diseases such as cholera, yellow fever, and communicable meningococcal illnesses reemerged over the last quarter of the twentieth century, primarily because of the speed of international travel.

Twenty-first century outbreaks of H1N1 influenza and severe acute respiratory syndrome (SARS) have demonstrated the pace at which epidemics can be-

come globalized and the potential global economic impact. Newly identified infectious diseases must also be contained to prevent them from becoming pandemics. According to the World Health Organization (WHO), one new infectious disease is being identified each year (eleven hundred epidemics occurred between 2002 and 2007). Control of infectious diseases and prevention of pandemics require diligent monitoring of disease patterns, adherence to international regulations, reporting to world health authorities, and international response coordination when potential epidemics arise.

BACKGROUND

The spread of infectious diseases through travel and migration has presented a problem for public health as long as humans have been mobile. The best known of these diseases is perhaps the plague, caused by the bacterium Yersinia pestis. Outbreaks of plague occurred numerous times in history, and already in the fourteenth century it was recognized as an "imported" disease. Although germ theory and modes of disease transmission were as yet unknown, it was accepted that the disease was somehow transported by travelers and in goods arriving from plague-infected areas. This realization led to the establishment of a forty-day isolation period (or quarantine) to identify infected persons, which, however, did little to stop the spread of plague throughout Europe. In time, advances in medical knowledge, improvements in living conditions, and the development of vaccination programs helped reduce or eliminate some infectious diseases.

In modern times controlling the spread of infectious diseases has become much more complicated, and the speed of worldwide travel has made communication of potential disease events a high priority. Diseases considered regionally controlled or eradicated are being reintroduced into these areas; new infectious diseases such as viral hemorrhagic fevers have the potential to travel around the world in less than twenty-four hours.

MIGRATION

The extent of recent human migration has been a significant factor in the global spread of communicable diseases. In 2008, WHO estimated that there were 214 million international migrants, 740 million within-country migrants, and an unknown number of

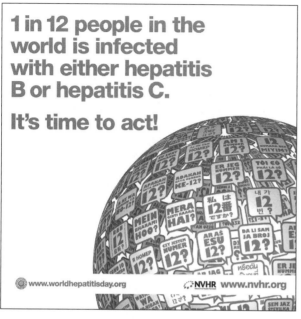

A World Health Assembly poster declares the widespread vulnerability of persons around the globe to hepatitis B and C. (AP/Wide World Photos)

undocumented migrants throughout the world. Migrant workers, refugees, and nomadic groups transport endemic diseases as they travel. Migration not only has spread infectious diseases (such as dengue fever) into areas where they were not previously seen but also has reintroduced diseases (such as tuberculosis) into areas where they had been controlled. Additionally, permanent migrants change the complexion of infectious disease patterns in the host country. Migration patterns are typically from developing nations to more prosperous areas, and residents of these poor regions generally lack adequate health care, nutrition, and sanitation, making them more susceptible to contracting infectious diseases and harboring pathogenic microorganisms.

Migrants who enter host countries through official means may be subjected to medical histories and physical screening to identify infectious and sexually transmitted diseases. Their movements may be tracked through travel documents and passports. Immigrants who have entered a country by unofficial (or illegal) means have not undergone such screening and may therefore be principal vectors for infectious diseases. Illegal (undocumented) immigrants are of particular concern because they are not screened, may fear seeking treatment for any diseases they already have, and may have contracted additional pathogens during their journey into the host country.

Chagas' disease, caused by Trypanosoma cruzi, provides an example of an infectious disease that has been globally spread to nonendemic areas. This organism is mainly transmitted by insects; however, it can also be spread through blood transfusions, organ transplants, contaminated food, and vertical transmission. Historically, Chagas' disease has been endemic to Mexico, Central America, and South America. From 2000 to 2007, however, it has been identified and documented in the United States, Canada, Europe, Australia, Japan, and regions of South America not previously affected. An estimated 2.9 percent and 2 percent, respectively, of documented Latin American immigrants to Europe and the United States were infected with T. cruzi, exemplifying a tropical disease that is now a global health concern.

The rate of tuberculosis (caused by Mycobacterium tuberculosis) cases among residents in the United Kingdom who are native born has been consistently controlled at a low rate. The number of tuberculosis cases among immigrants living in the United Kingdom, however, is high (from 2000 to 2008) because of migration. While the tuberculosis rate remained consistent at approximately 4 cases per 100,000 persons for the British-born population during this interval, the rate for migrants in the United Kingdom ranged from 80 to 102 cases per 100,000 persons (approximately 72 percent of total cases). A similar, though not as drastic, pattern was observed in the United States in 2008, in which the tuberculosis rates were 2 and 20 cases per 100,000 persons, respectively, for U.S.-born and foreign-born residents.

GLOBAL TRAVEL

Air travel has become the fastest and most efficient means of infectious disease movement across the globe. In 2009, 684 million passengers traveled internationally by air. A trip from New York City to either Beijing, China, or Mumbai, India, can be completed in about twenty-four hours. This is less time than the incubation periods of many communicable diseases. Many infectious diseases of concern are spread through airborne pathogens (such as influenza, SARS-associated coronavirus, and M. tuberculosis); therefore, they are ideally suited for transmission in a contained aircraft cabin.

The SARS epidemic provides a model of international airborne pathogen transmission within an aircraft cabin. Although it did not result in a catastrophic pandemic, this disease demonstrated how an outbreak can quickly spread to thirty-seven countries by international travelers. The disease itself has an incubation period of approximately seven days before symptoms appear, which allows it to unknowingly be transported anywhere around the world. The index case was a doctor from Guandong, China, who flew to Hong Kong in early 2003. The doctor had previously treated patients in Guandong with a respiratory illness that was, at the time, unidentified. While staying in Hong Kong, the doctor transmitted the disease to several other guests staying at the same hotel. One international business traveler subsequently transmitted the disease to twenty-two other passengers during air travel. All these transmissions occurred within days and before the onset of any symptoms of the disease in the persons who were infected.

Also of concern are diseases considered to be controlled or eradicated in a region that are imported back into the area. Measles was considered to be eliminated from the United States in 2000 because of a vaccination program that began in the 1960's; however, since this time, there have been periodic outbreaks of measles because of international travel. In the first six months of 2008, 131 cases of measles were reported to the U.S. Centers for Disease Control and Prevention (CDC), which is about twice the number reported on average per year from 2000 to 2007. Most (89 percent) of the cases during the outbreak in 2008 could be linked to international outbreaks.

Measles is still very common in China, Southeast Asia, and, to a lesser extent, Europe, where occasional outbreaks still occur. Travel to these areas or contact with foreign visitors accounted for only 17 of the 131 cases; association with these infected persons within the United States accounted for an additional 99 cases. The source of transmission for the remainder was unknown.

Most of the persons who contracted measles during this outbreak (91 percent) were either unvaccinated or had unknown vaccination statuses. In addition, 80 percent were less than twenty years of age, indicating that an increasing number of children are not being vaccinated because of religious objection or because of home schooling. (Children who are schooled at home are exempt from vaccination requirements.)

Measles is highly contagious. It quickly resurfaces in the United States when vaccination rates decline because it is still so prevalent in the rest of the world. The 2008 measles outbreak, with the highest rate of infection in the United States since 1996, illustrates the potential reemergence of an infectious disease that is considered controlled, particularly in areas with low vaccination rates.

INFECTIOUS DISEASE CONTROL

The spread of contagious diseases has been recognized as a threat to global health for several hundred years. Various health agencies recognized this and endeavored to engage international cooperation. The first cooperative effort to control cholera, plague, and yellow fever began in Europe in 1851, when the first International Sanitary Conference (ISC) was convened. By the mid-nineteenth century, the international shipping trade and the growth of transcontinental railroads had successfully swept the cholera epidemic throughout Europe. National regulations and quarantine were inconsistent and ineffective; cooperation among nations was the only method of monitoring and controlling disease propagation with minimal interference in international trade. Over the next century, these efforts resulted in international, legally binding regulations for international travel and transport. The ISC issued a series of regulations and gave rise to four international health agencies: the Pan American Sanitary Bureau (1902), the Office International de l'Hygiène Publique (1907), the Health Organisation of the League of Nations (1923), and WHO (1948). By 1951, these agencies had converged into WHO and issued the International Sanitary Regulations by the World Health Assembly. These international regulations expanded on the treaties issued by the ISCs.

Since the early 1950's, WHO has played a pivotal role in monitoring and controlling the spread of infectious diseases around the world. The goal of the International Sanitary Regulations was to control smallpox, typhoid fever, relapsing fever, yellow fever, cholera, and the plague, establishing standards for reporting international travelers and goods possibly carrying infectious diseases. WHO subsequently revised the regulations to include the eradication of smallpox and to focus on yellow fever, cholera, and plague. These regulations were replaced by the International Health Regulations in 2005 (revised 2007), which take a broader, more fundamental approach to protecting public health. The focal points are on preventing the global spread of infectious diseases with minimal interference in international travel and trade, and on stringent reporting policies regarding any health situation that poses a threat to public health. WHO also has programs to help member states track and respond to outbreaks that have the potential of developing into large-scale epidemics.

Developed countries, especially those successful in the eradication and control of various infectious diseases, have attempted to institute health regulations on international travelers, migrants, and imports. In response to health threats posed by human migration, some receiving countries have implemented restrictions on incoming migrants from areas with endemic infectious diseases of concern. These may include health screening, proof of vaccination, and potentially, quarantine. However, border control policies are rarely effective because of the sheer volume of persons who cross international borders over any period and because of the undetermined number of undocumented immigrants around the world. Even if it were possible to examine each person at a border crossing, diseases in the incubation stage could not be detected.

Noncatastrophic epidemics such as the SARS outbreak in early 2003 provide health care agencies with models of the global spread of infectious diseases. Using these models, the pattern of disease transmission can be predicted, allowing for the design of action plans in the event of a future infectious disease outbreak. SARS was the first example in the twenty-first century of an infectious disease outbreak that was tracked and contained by disease control measures. At the onset of the epidemic, little was known about the virus except that it could be spread by airborne transmission, that there was a fatality rate of about 10 percent, and that there were no vaccines or curative agents available. The release of public information and a global disease alert issued by WHO allowed potential travelers to be aware of the threat and to change their plans to avoid air travel or visiting areas in which SARS was identified. These actions had a substantial economic impact, but contact with infected persons could be minimized. Closely followed hygienic measures prevented the extensive spread of the disease among health care professionals. Further-

more, establishing the infectivity and incubation period of the virus facilitated tracking those persons who were infected and those who had been exposed.

In preparation for the Olympic Winter Games in Vancouver, Canada, in 2010, Canadian health authorities used known disease patterns from other mass human gatherings, such as the Hajj and the G-20 summit, to create a plan to identify and manage any potential infectious disease outbreaks. Before the Games, Canada had developed a Global Public Health Intelligence Network, a surveillance system that enabled them to acquire real-time information on potential disease threats (such as mumps, measles, and Norwalk-like virus) through the Internet. In conjunction with projected air-traffic patterns, health authorities developed models of potential patterns of infectious disease distribution. Had any infections be identified, alerts could have been issued to officials at the Games. Health officials in the native countries of visitors and athletes would also have been notified to prevent travelers from bringing any infectious diseases back from the Games to their home countries.

IMPACT

Migrants coming from poor countries require more health and social services and, therefore, place a tremendous burden on health services in host countries. In some receiving countries, migrants make up a majority of the population; in the United Arab Emirates, the country that receives more migrants than any other in the world, migrants are 71 percent of the population. WHO recognizes that migration is not a temporary phenomenon, and that high migration rates have a significant impact on the nature of diseases and health care systems of the host countries. Therefore, it urges receiving countries to make migrant health a high priority, stressing that the health of the native population is affected by the health of migrants and their children. However, migrants have specific medical, genetic, and cultural health care requirements, and the cost of providing this migrant-specific care cannot be estimated.

In addition to the impact of infectious diseases on the cost of health services, they also have a surprising impact on the global economy. This is particularly true for infections in which the modes of transmission are not definitively known. In the case of SARS, which was a relatively mild outbreak, the cost to the global economy was estimated at $30 billion to $100 billion. Most of this cost was borne by the travel, tourism, and other industries. Most of this deficit was absorbed by countries that continue to rely primarily on travel and tourism for their income. On a microlevel, however, persons lost their jobs, and their incomes. The long-term consequences of global disease outbreaks are often continued poverty and substandard living conditions.

To prevent a catastrophic pandemic, WHO has established regulations for the monitoring, reporting, and rapid response to any infectious disease events. The fundamental goal for WHO and other global health agencies is to provide access to health care for all, with the expectation that improved health in poor areas will result in less disease transmission and overall positive global health outcomes. The human population continues to grow, directing more focus on preventing the human-to-human transmission of communicable diseases.

Deborah A. Appello, M.S.

FURTHER READING

Fidler, David P. "The Globalization of Public Health: The First One Hundred Years of International Health Diplomacy." *Bulletin of the World Health Organization* 79 (2001): 842-849. A historical and political look at global public health since the start of the twentieth century.

Fricker, Manuel, and Robert Steffen. "Travel and Public Health." *Journal of Infection and Public Health* 1 (2008): 72-77. Public health examined through the lens of international travel.

International Air Transport Association. "Fact Sheet: Pandemic Preparedness." Available at http://www.iata.org/pressroom/facts_figures/fact_sheets. A guide to preparing for pandemics from an airline industry group.

Khan, Kamran, et al. "Preparing for Infectious Disease Threats at Mass Gatherings: The Case of the Vancouver 2010 Olympic Winter Games." *Canadian Medical Association Journal* 182, no. 6 (2010): 579-583. A case study of infectious disease preparedness.

Schmunis, Gabriel A., and Zaida E. Yadon. "Chagas' Disease: A Latin American Health Problem Becoming a World Health Problem." *Acta Tropica* 115 (2010): 14-21. A case study of one "local" disease that has begun to spread worldwide.

Smith, Richard D. "Responding to Global Infectious Disease Outbreaks: Lessons from SARS on the Role of Risk Perception, Communication, and Management." *Social Science and Medicine* 63 (2006): 3113-3123. A study of how global health agencies responded to the SARS crisis.

World Health Organization. *Health of Migrants: The Way Forward.* Geneva: Author, 2010. A focused study on the future of health in the context of world migration.

_____. *The World Health Report 2007: Global Public Health Security in the Twenty-First Century.* Geneva: Author, 2007. Examines the future of global health preparedness, response, and security for the twenty-first century.

WEB SITES OF INTEREST

Centers for Disease Control and Prevention
http://www.cdc.gov

Emerging and Reemerging Infectious Diseases Resource Center
http://www.medscape.com/resource/infections

Global Health Council
http://www.globalhealth.org

Health Protection Agency
http://www.hpa.org.uk

International Air Transport Association
http://www.iata.org

World Health Organization
http://www.who.int

See also: Biosurveillance; Centers for Disease Control and Prevention (CDC); Children and infectious disease; Developing countries and infectious disease; Disease eradication campaigns; Emerging and reemerging infectious diseases; Emerging Infections Network; Epidemics and pandemics: Causes and management; Epidemics and pandemics: History; Epidemiology; Outbreaks; Public health; Tropical medicine; Water treatment; World Health Organization (WHO).

Glycopeptide antibiotics

CATEGORY: Treatment

DEFINITION

Glycopeptide antibiotics are a class of antibiotics that contains glycosylated cyclic peptides and are used to treat infections. Glycopeptide antibiotics inhibit the synthesis of the cell walls of the gram-positive bacteria that cause many infections. Traditionally, this class of antibiotics has been used as a last line of defense to treat life-threatening infections after other treatments have failed.

CLASS MEMBERS

The first glycopeptide discovered was vancomycin in 1956, followed by U.S. Food and Drug Administration approval in 1958. Vancomycin has been the most widely used of this class, but more effective alternatives from this class have been developed. The most useful of these newer members is teicoplanin, which has a more effective ability to penetrate tissues; it also has a longer half-life. Others antibiotics in this class include bleomycin, brevianamide A and B, and oritavancin.

MODE OF ACTION

The members of this class of drugs bind tightly to the amino acid residue of acyl-D-alanyl-D-analine, located on the terminus of the pentapeptide peptidoglycan of several strains of gram-positive bacteria. This specific binding action of the drug prevents the bacteria from synthesizing their cell walls, thereby inhibiting their ability to cause an infection.

Ongoing research methods that include the sequencing and biosynthesis of gene clusters are part of the continued study of the mode of action of glycopeptides and part of the development of new members of the class. These research methods require the growth of bacterial cultures, isolation of their genomic deoxyribonucleic acid (DNA), cloning of the DNA fragments, identification of positive clones by using southern hybridization, and construction of libraries, which are screened using the polymerase chain reaction (PCR) technique. This analysis of gene clusters allows for identification of the specific genes that directly cause the binding of an antibiotic and for identification of the specific genes that can lead to drug resistance.

SIDE EFFECTS, COMPLICATIONS, AND LIMITATIONS

The glycopeptides cannot enter all tissues and, therefore, cannot treat infection in all tissues. Vancomycin is most effective when delivered intravenously, so pain and irritation can occur at the injection site and lead to what is known as red man syndrome; in turn, this can lead to blood disorders. Some bacterial strains can become resistant to the glycopeptide antibiotics.

IMPACT

Members of the glycopeptide antibiotic class of drugs have become indispensable in treating infectious diseases. The ability of glycopeptides to be effective even with only once-daily or twice-daily dosing has led to their application as an out-of-hospital therapy to treat infections that have been resistant to other classes of drugs. The glycopeptide antibiotic class is especially useful as an alternative to the beta-lactam antibiotic class for persons who are sensitive to that class of drugs.

Jeanne L. Kuhler, Ph.D.

FURTHER READING

Finch, Robert G., and George M. Eliopoulos. "Safety and Efficacy of Glycopeptide Antibiotics." *Journal of Antimicrobial Chemotherapy* 55 (2005): ii5-ii13.

Gould, Ian M., and Jos W. M. Van der Meer. *Antibiotic Policies: Fighting Resistance.* New York: Springer, 2007.

Nagarajan, Ramakris. *Glycopeptide Antibiotics.* West Palm Beach, Fla.: CRC Press, 1994.

Sanford, Jay P., et al. *The Sanford Guide to Antimicrobial Therapy.* 18th ed. Sperryville, Va.: Antimicrobial Therapy, 2010.

Uwe, Frank, and Evelina Tacconelli. *The Daschner Guide to In-Hospital Antibiotic Therapy.* New York: Springer, 2009.

Walsh, Christopher. *Antibiotics: Actions, Origins, Resistance.* Washington, D.C.: ASM Press, 2003. Examines such topics as how antibiotics block specific proteins, how the molecular structure of drugs enables such activity, the development of bacterial resistance, and the molecular logic of antibiotic biosynthesis.

WEB SITES OF INTEREST

eMedicineHealth: Antibiotics
http://www.emedicinehealth.com/antibiotics

National Institute of Allergy and Infectious Diseases
http://www.niaid.nih.gov/topics/
antimicrobialresistance

See also: Alliance for the Prudent Use of Antibiotics; Aminoglycoside antibiotics; Antibiotic resistance; Antibiotics: Types; Bacteria: Classification and types; Bacteria: Structure and growth; Bacterial infections; Cephalosporin antibiotics; Ketolide antibiotics; Lipopeptide antibiotics; Macrolide antibiotics; Microbiology; Oxazolidinone antibiotics; Penicillin antibiotics; Quinolone antibiotics; Superbacteria; Tetracycline antibiotics; Vancomycin-resistant enterococci infection.

Gonorrhea

CATEGORY: Diseases and conditions
ANATOMY OR SYSTEM AFFECTED: All

DEFINITION

Gonorrhea is an infection caused by bacteria. It is a common sexually transmitted disease (STD).

CAUSES

Gonorrhea is caused by the bacterium Neisseria gonorrhoeae. It is passed during vaginal, oral, or anal intercourse.

RISK FACTORS

Factors that increase the chance of gonorrhea include multiple sex partners, sexual intercourse with a partner who has a history of any STD, having sex without a condom, and a history of having a sexually transmitted disease. At higher risk are persons ages fifteen to twenty-nine years.

SYMPTOMS

Not all people who are infected will have symptoms. Some may have severe symptoms. If there are symptoms, they may appear two to ten days after contact with an infected partner. In some cases, they do not occur for up to one month.

People with gonorrhea may experience some, all, or none of the following symptoms: in men, discharge from the penis, a burning sensation while urinating, and tender or swollen testicles; in women, a burning sensation while urinating, abnormal vaginal discharge, abdominal pain, and unusual vaginal bleeding; and in men and women, anal itching, soreness, bleeding, painful bowel movements, eye infections, and blood infections.

SCREENING AND DIAGNOSIS

Three tests are commonly used to diagnose gonorrhea. These are the Gram's stain, in which a sample of the discharge from the penis or cervix is examined for the presence of bacteria (this test is more accurate for men than for women); the nucleic acid probe test, in which discharge or urine is tested for nucleic acids (these acids identify gonorrhea); and laboratory analysis, in which a smear of the discharge is sent to a lab and, after two days, checked for growth of bacteria.

TREATMENT AND THERAPY

The doctor may prescribe one of the following antibiotics for persons with gonorrhea: ceftriaxone, cefixime, ciprofloxacin, ofloxacin, and levofloxacin. One should take all the medication as prescribed, and all sexual partners should be tested and treated.

If gonorrhea is not treated, it can cause, in men, a painful condition of the testicles called epididymitis, which may lead to infertility. Untreated gonorrhea also can cause problems with the prostate and with the urethra, in which scarring inside the urethra can make it difficult to urinate.

In women, untreated gonorrhea can harm the reproductive organs through the onset of pelvic inflammatory disease (PID), a serious infection that can affect fertility.

PREVENTION AND OUTCOMES

The most effective way to prevent an STD is to abstain from sex. Other preventive measures are to always use latex condoms during sexual activity, to have only monogamous sex, and to have regular checkups for sexually transmitted diseases. Some other barrier methods of contraception may provide some protection.

Michelle Badash, M.S.;
reviewed by David L. Horn, M.D., FACP

FURTHER READING

Centers for Disease Control and Prevention. "Gonorrhea." Available at http://www.cdc.gov/std/gonorrhea/stdfact-gonorrhea.htm.

_____. "Sexually Transmitted Diseases Treatment

Guidelines 2010." Available at http://www.cdc.gov/std/treatment/2010.

"Gonococcal Infections." In *Harrison's Principles of Internal Medicine*, edited by Anthony Fauci et al. 17th ed. New York: McGraw-Hill, 2008.

Handsfield, H. H., et al. "*Neisseria gonorrhoeae*." In *Mandell, Douglas, and Bennett's Principles and Practice of Infectious Diseases*, edited by Gerald L. Mandell, John F. Bennett, and Raphael Dolin. 7th ed. New York: Churchill Livingstone/Elsevier, 2010.

Holmes, King K., et al., eds. *Sexually Transmitted Diseases*. 4th ed. New York: McGraw-Hill Medical, 2008.

Larsen, Laura. *Sexually Transmitted Diseases Sourcebook*. Detroit: Omnigraphics, 2009.

Workowski, K. A., et al. "Emerging Antimicrobial Resistance in *Neisseria gonorrhoeae*: Urgent Need to Strengthen Prevention Strategies." *Annals of Internal Medicine* 148 (2008): 606.

WEB SITES OF INTEREST

American Social Health Association
http://www.ashastd.org

Centers for Disease Control and Prevention
http://www.cdc.gov/std

Communicable Disease Control
http://www.gov.mb.ca/health/publichealth/cdc

National Institute of Allergy and Infectious Diseases
http://www.niaid.nih.gov

National Women's Health Information Center
http://www.womenshealth.gov

Sex Information and Education Council of Canada
http://www.sieccan.org

See also: Acute cystitis; Bacterial vaginosis; Chlamydia; Epididymitis; Herpes simplex infection; HIV; Men and infectious disease; *Neisseria*; Neisserial infections; Ophthalmia neonatorum; Pelvic inflammatory disease; Pregnancy and infectious disease; Prostatitis; Reiter's syndrome; Sexually transmitted diseases (STDs); Trichomonas; Urethritis; Vaginal yeast infection; Women and infectious disease.

Graft-versus-host disease

CATEGORY: Diseases and conditions
ANATOMY OR SYSTEM AFFECTED: Blood, bones, gastrointestinal system, immune system, liver, musculoskeletal system, skin, tissue

DEFINITION

Graft-versus-host disease (GVHD) occurs as a complication of a bone marrow or stem cell transplant when new cells are transplanted from a donor to a recipient. The tissue sample that is taken from the donor and inserted into the recipient is called a graft. The donor cells in the graft begin to create antibodies (proteins the immune system produces to fight infection). These foreign antibodies attack the recipient's healthy cells in the digestive system, skin, and liver.

Acute GVHD can occur soon after the transplantation, usually within the first one hundred days. Chronic GVHD can occur after the first one hundred days and can flare up at different times for several years after the transplantation. A person can experience both acute and chronic GVHD or just one of the syndromes.

CAUSES

GVHD is an immune response generated from the newly transplanted cells from an allogeneic donor, in which samples are taken from another person, either related or unrelated to the patient. Each person's chemical makeup is unique, and for transplantation to succeed, physicians must find donors who are similar to the recipient in chemical makeup.

Physicians look for certain proteins on blood cells called histocompatibility antigens (also known as HLA markers). These proteins are responsible for recognizing foreign invaders and for activating the immune system to eliminate any potential infections that are discovered. The HLA markers will be similar but will never be identical to the recipient's healthy cells, unless the donor and recipient are identical twins.

As the graft of cells begins to grow and integrate into the patient's body, the new cells recognize these slight differences and react by attacking other healthy cells within the patient's body, particularly cells found in the digestive tract, skin, and liver, just as a healthy immune system would attack bacteria or viruses. This process causes damage to these areas and complications for the patient.

Risk Factors

GVHD occurs only in persons who receive allogeneic grafts of peripherally collected stem cells, bone marrow, or umbilical cord blood to treat a variety of diseases, including certain cancers and sickle cell anemia. Umbilical cord blood grafts have less of a risk for GVHD than the other types of grafts, and grafts from unrelated donors have greater potential for causing GVHD than grafts from biological family members. Other risk factors include receiving a graft from a person of the opposite gender, older age of either the donor or the recipient, receiving a poorly matched graft, and having a cytomegalovirus (herpes) infection. Transplant recipients who have had their spleen removed are also at risk for GVHD. Men experience GVHD more often than do women.

People who have acute GVHD are at risk for developing chronic GVHD. Acute GVHD occurs in as many as 90 percent of allogeneic transplant recipients, with about 50 percent of occurrences considered to be clinically significant (that is, requiring medical intervention). Chronic GVHD affects as many as 80 percent of bone marrow transplant recipients.

Symptoms

Symptoms depend upon the area of the body that is affected. The skin is usually affected first, and the patient will usually experience burning, itching, and a rash. The skin will darken and have a reddish tone. The hands, feet, upper back, cheeks, neck, and ears are the most commonly affected areas. GVHD can progress to other areas of the body and include more serious skin complications, including blisters filled with a clear liquid. GVHD can resemble a severe burn. The most severe form can cause tissue necrosis (progressive skin-cell death).

When GVHD affects the liver, typical symptoms of liver disease occur, including jaundice (a yellowish tone to the skin and whites of the eyes), abdominal pain and cramping, weight gain, and an increase of fluid in the abdomen (ascites).

When GVHD includes the digestive tract, it affects the outer lining of the system (known as the mucosal lining). The most common symptom is diarrhea, which can be severe. The patient may also experience nausea and appetite loss.

The symptoms for each system can occur independently or at the same time. All three systems may be affected or only one or two. Symptoms can range from mild to life-threatening.

Screening and Diagnosis

To determine if a person has GVHD, physicians must rule out other diseases that have similar symptoms and that often occur in people who have bone marrow or stem cell transplants. These conditions include drug toxicity, reactions to radiation therapy or chemotherapy, bacterial or viral infections, or complications from total parental nutrition (tube feeding).

Diagnostic studies will depend on the part of the body that is affected. Because the risk is so high for GVHD in patients who receive an allogeneic stem cell or bone marrow transplant, they are often monitored for early signs of the disease through blood tests. Imaging scans and tissue biopsy of the affected system are often performed to rule out GVHD in persons who are experiencing symptoms. Endoscopy can be performed on persons who are experiencing digestive tract symptoms.

Treatment and Therapy

The first-line treatment for GVHD involves suppressing the immune system. Steroids are often prescribed for this. If this treatment does not work, a combination of methotrexate and mycophenolate is prescribed. In addition, therapies to alleviate digestive, skin, and liver symptoms also will be initiated.

Prevention and Outcomes

Suppressing the immune system is also used as an approach to GVHD prevention. In addition, finding the proper donor match is crucial to preventing GVHD. Taking steps to prevent acute GVHD will also help to prevent chronic GVHD.

Laura J. Pinchot, B.A.

Further Reading

Cancer Research U.K. "Graft Versus Host Disease." Available at http://www.cancerhelp.org.uk/coping-with-cancer/coping-physically/gvhd.

Eggert, Julie, ed. *Cancer Basics.* Pittsburgh, Pa.: Oncology Nursing Society, 2010. Describes skin, liver, and digestive problems associated with different types of cancer, including acute and chronic GVHD.

Latchford, Teresa. "Cutaneous Effects of Blood and

Marrow Transplantation" In *Principles of Skin Care and the Oncology Patient*. Pittsburgh, Pa.: Oncology Nursing Society, 2010. Provides a description and illustrations of GVHD and other skin problems associated with stem cell and marrow transplantation.

National Institutes of Health. "GVHD (Graft-Versus-Host-Disease): A Guide for Patients and Families After Stem Cell Transplant." Available at http://www.cc.nih.gov/ccc/patient_education/pepubs/gvh.pdf.

Ruiz, Phillip, Yaxia Zhang, and Shoib Sarwar. "Graft Versus Host Disease." Available at http://emedicine.medscape.com/article/886758-overview. A comprehensive overview of GVHD, including experimental treatments.

WEB SITES OF INTEREST

Leukemia and Lymphoma Society
http://www.leukemia-lymphoma.org

National Marrow Donor Program
http://www.marrow.org/patient

Patients Against Lymphoma
http://www.lymphomation.org

See also: Antibodies; Asplenia; Autoimmune disorders; Bloodstream infections; Immune response to bacterial infections; Immune response to viral infections; Immunity; Neutropenia; Osteomyelitis; Sepsis; T lymphocytes; Viral infections.

Gram staining

CATEGORY: Diagnosis
ALSO KNOWN AS: Gram's method, Gram's stain

DEFINITION

Gram staining is one of the most commonly used staining techniques in research and clinical laboratories. It is often the first test performed in inspecting bacterial morphology and in differentiating organisms into two broad classifications: gram-positive and gram-negative, which are based on the properties of an organism's cell walls. Danish scientist-inventor Hans

---

Key Terms: Gram Staining

- *Cell wall.* A structure outside the cell membrane of most bacteria, composed of varying amounts of carbohydrates, lipids, and amino acids

- *Gram-negative.* Referring to microorganisms that appear pink following the Gram-staining laboratory procedure

- *Gram-positive.* Referring to microorganisms that appear violet following the Gram-staining laboratory procedure

- *Gram's stain.* A laboratory method of staining bacteria as a primary means of differentiation and identification

- *Lipopolysaccharide (LPS).* A major component of the cell wall of gram-negative bacteria; the toxicity of LPS is associated with illnesses caused by gram-negative organisms

- *Mordant.* A chemical that acts to fix a stain within a physical structure; the role played by iodine in Gram's stain

- *Peptidoglycans.* Repeating units of sugar derivatives that make up a rigid layer of bacterial cell walls; found in both gram-positive and gram-negative cells

---

Christian Gram (1853-1938) developed the technique in 1882 to differentiate two bacterial species that exhibited similar clinical symptoms.

Gram staining involves four primary steps, after which gram-positive bacteria appear purple or blue under a light microscope and after which gram-negative bacteria are red or pinkish. This difference in appearance arises because of structural and biochemical differences in the cell walls of the two general classifications of bacteria, which also contribute to the physiological properties of the two groups. In particular, gram-positive bacteria have a thick cell wall made up largely of peptidoglycan, a substance that provides rigidity and strength to the wall. Gram-negative bacteria have significantly thinner cell walls with less peptidoglycan and have an additional outer membrane that contains lipids; this membrane is separated from the cell wall by the periplasmic space.

Of note, some bacteria fail to be definitively classified

using Gram's method and instead fall into gram-variable (in which bacteria may stain either gram-positive or gram-negative) or gram-indeterminate categories (in which bacteria are insusceptible to dyes and exhibit little or no stain).

METHOD

To prepare for Gram staining, bacteria are sampled (typically using an inoculation loop, a sterile toothpick, or a syringe), smeared into a thin layer on a microscope slide, allowed to dry briefly (to avoid cell lysis upon exposure to heat), and heat-fixed using a Bunsen burner or hot plate set to about 107° Fahrenheit (42° Celsius). The Gram's stain protocol itself consists of four primary steps. First, a small volume of the primary stain (crystal violet, methyl violet) is added to the smear, allowed to set for approximately twenty to sixty seconds depending on the size of the sample, and washed away with sterile water. Second, a small volume of trapping agent (Gram's iodine) is then added to the smear, allowed to set for twenty to sixty seconds, and washed away with sterile water. Third, a small volume of decolorizer (alcohol or acetone) is added to the smear briefly (for about five seconds or until color no longer runs off the slide) and then rinsed away with sterile water. Fourth, a small amount of counterstain (safranin or carbol fuchsin) is added to the smear, allowed to set for forty to sixty seconds, and then rinsed off with sterile water. After the specimens have been allowed to air dry completely, they can be observed using bright-field microscopy.

MECHANISM

Gram-negative and gram-positive bacteria appear reddish and bluish, respectively, after staining because of the elegant, complementary mechanisms of the reagents used in the Gram-staining procedure. Once dissolved into a water-based solution, the organic compound crystal violet (CV) dissociates into CV+ and chloride (Cl-) ions. Once bacteria have been submerged in CV solution, these ions penetrate through cell walls and membranes of both gram-positive and gram-negative bacteria; CV+ subsequently interacts with negatively charged components of bacterial cells and then stains cells purple.

Upon adding iodine solution (I- or I_3-) to already CV-stained bacterial smears, I- interacts with CV+ and forms large, insoluble CV-I complexes within the inner and outer layers of both gram-positive and gram-nega-

tive cells. In this context, iodine is said to act as a trapping agent, named so because it prevents the removal of CV-I complexes from gram-positive bacteria during the next decolorization step.

During the next step, alcohol, acetone, or another decolorizer readily penetrates and interacts with the lipid-rich cell membrane and thin peptidoglycan layer of gram-negative cells; this interaction strips these cells of their outer surfaces and leaves their inner cell-wall layers exposed. Consequently, CV-I complexes are washed from gram-negative cells during this step, leaving bacteria colorless or weakly stained. In contrast, decolorization causes peptidoglycan-rich, gram-positive cells to become dehydrated and their cell-wall pores to close, which prevents the large CV-I complexes from escaping, leaving cells purple or blue. It is critical to pay attention to the timing of the decolorization step, because CV (and its blue/purple color) may be removed from both gram-positive and gram-negative bacteria if the agent is left on too long; it can fail to be removed if not left on long enough. This step is the most likely source for introducing error or misinterpretation into Gram's stain results.

During the final step, the counterstain safranin gives colorless, gram-negative bacteria a red or pinkish color. Although this stain also permeates gram-positive bacteria, it typically has little influence on already darkly stained blue or purple cells.

IMPACT

Gram staining is arguably the most common research laboratory technique because it is often the first step in determining the identity of a bacterial sample and in appropriately deducing follow-up procedures. Advanced molecular techniques are available that are more reliable for precise and accurate identification of bacterial phylogeny.

In medicine, Gram staining is an invaluable resource for yielding fast results, because alternative laboratory-based culture methods can take several hours or days to reveal results. Gram staining can be performed on patients' body fluids or biopsies when bacterial infection is suspected (such as in cases of meningitis or sepsis). Gram staining can be helpful in deciding the appropriate treatment regimen, particularly because several antibiotics are active only against one of the two classifications of bacteria.

Gram staining is also used to monitor the quality and safety conditions in many other industries, including those that manufacture, process, and package water, foodstuffs, drugs, and medical devices.

Brandy Weidow, M.S.

FURTHER READING

Bergey, David H., et al., eds. *Bergey's Manual of Determinative Bacteriology.* 9th ed. Philadelphia: Lippincott Williams & Wilkins, 2000.

Beveridge, T. J., and L. L. Graham. "Surface Layers of Bacteria." *Microbiological Reviews* 55, no. 4 (1991): 684-705.

Black, Jacqueline G. *Microbiology: Principles and Explorations.* 7th ed. Hoboken, N.J.: John Wiley & Sons, 2008.

McClelland, R. "Gram's Stain: The Key to Microbiology." *Medical Laboratory Observer*, April, 2001, 20-31.

Madigan, Michael T., and John M. Martinko. *Brock Biology of Microorganisms.* 12th ed. Upper Saddle River, N.J.: Pearson/Prentice Hall, 2010.

Murray, Robert K., et al. *Harper's Illustrated Biochemistry.* 27th ed. Stamford, Conn.: Appleton & Lange, 2006.

Pagana, Kathleen Deska, and Timothy J. Pagana. *Mosby's Diagnostic and Laboratory Test Reference.* 9th ed. St. Louis, Mo.: Mosby/Elsevier, 2009.

Ryan, Kenneth J., and C. George Ray, eds. *Sherris Medical Microbiology: An Introduction to Infectious Diseases.* 5th ed. New York: McGraw-Hill, 2010.

Sutton, Scott. "The Gram Stain." *PMF Newsletter* 12, no. 2 (2006). Also available at http://microbiol. org/resources/monographswhite-papers/thegram-stain.

WEB SITES OF INTEREST

Biochemical Society
http://www.biochemistry.org

Protocolpedia
http://www.protocolpedia.com

Virtual Library of Biochemistry, Molecular Biology, and Cell Biology
http://www.biochemweb.org

See also: Acid-fastness; Bacterial infections; Bacteriology; Biochemical tests; Biostatistics; Diagnosis of bacterial infections; Immunoassay; Infection; Microbiology; Microscopy; Pathogens; Polymerase chain reaction (PCR) method; Pulsed-field gel electrophoresis; Serology; Virology.

Group A streptococcal infection

CATEGORY: Diseases and conditions
ANATOMY OR SYSTEM AFFECTED: Skin, throat, tissue, tonsils
ALSO KNOWN AS: Group A strep, *Streptococcus pyogenes* infection

DEFINITION

A group A streptococcal infection includes contagious illnesses caused by the bacterium *Streptococcus pyogenes.* The most common group A infection is strep throat. Other group A infections include impetigo (superficial skin infection) and serious deep tissue and blood infections. In rare cases, infection with group A strep can result in complications such as rheumatic fever and post-strep glomerulonephritis (kidney inflammation).

CAUSES

S. pyogenes bacteria are commonly found in the throat and on skin. During peak times between fall and spring, up to 20 percent of school-age children may carry the bacteria and may transmit it without becoming ill. The organism is spread person to person through respiratory droplets or through direct contact. Infected persons are contagious as long as they have symptoms. Infections that go untreated with antibiotics may be contagious beyond the symptomatic period.

While most cases of pharyngitis (strep throat) are viral, group A strep is the most common bacterial cause. Virulence factors of the bacterial cell influence the severity of the disease.

RISK FACTORS

Factors that increase the risk of developing localized group A strep infection, including strep throat and impetigo, are age (children of all ages), time of year (between fall and spring), and exposure to school-age children. Having a past history of group A strep infection may predispose one to future infection.

The risk of more severe invasive disease is increased by chickenpox infection, other infections of the skin, and immunosuppression of any cause. Infection with group A strep carries a risk of complications that include rheumatic fever and post-strep glomerulonephritis.

SYMPTOMS

Symptoms of strep throat include fever, sore throat, and swollen lymph nodes, sometimes accompanied by headache and vomiting. Redness, swelling, and pus may be present on the tonsils.

Symptoms of infection elsewhere depend on the area of the body, but usually include redness, inflammation, and swelling accompanied by fever. Symptoms of bacteremia (bacterial blood infection) often include fever and shaking chills.

SCREENING AND DIAGNOSIS

Diagnosis of strep throat may be made by laboratory test (rapid antigen test or throat culture) but often is made clinically if the signs and symptoms point to infection. The absence of typical viral symptoms, such as runny nose and cough, may indicate strep.

Group A strep infection is suspected when redness, inflammation, and swelling are present in an area that is a common location for that type of infection. A blood culture is required for diagnosis of strep bacteremia. Occasionally, a diagnosis is made following the appearance of one of the complications of strep infection, such as post-strep glomerulonephritis.

TREATMENT AND THERAPY

When a diagnosis of strep infection is confirmed or strongly suspected, antibiotic treatment is indicated to shorten the duration of symptoms, to shorten the time of contagiousness, and to prevent complications. Penicillin is effective when administered orally or by injection. Other antibiotics are used for persons allergic to penicillin.

PREVENTION AND OUTCOMES

Prevention involves minimizing the spread of bacteria. Frequent handwashing, careful personal hygiene, and avoiding the respiratory secretions of others help to prevent transmission.

Rachel Zahn, M.D.

FURTHER READING

Gerber, M. "*Streptococcus pyogenes* (Group A *Streptococcus*)." In *Principles and Practice of Pediatric Infectious Diseases*, edited by Sarah S. Long, Larry K. Pickering, and Charles G. Prober. 3d ed. Philadelphia: Churchill Livingstone/Elsevier, 2008.

Hahn, R. G., et al. "Evaluation of Poststreptococcal Illness." *American Family Physician* 71 (2005): 1949-1954.

Jaggi, P., and S. T. Shulman. "Group A Streptococcal Infections." *Pediatrics in Review* 27 (2006): 99-104.

Khan, Zartash Zafar, et al. "Streptococcus Group A Infections." Available at http://emedicine.medscape.com/article/228936-overview.

Landau, Elaine. *Strep Throat: Head-to-Toe Health*. Tarrytown, N.Y.: Benchmark Books, 2010.

WEB SITES OF INTEREST

Centers for Disease Control and Prevention
http://www.cdc.gov/ncidod/dbmd/diseaseinfo/groupastreptococcal_g.htm

KidsHealth
http://www.kidshealth.org

National Institutes of Health
http://www.nlm.nih.gov/medlineplus/streptococcalinfections.html

See also: Bacterial infections; Cellulitis; Contagious diseases; Impetigo; Necrotizing fasciitis; Penicillin antibiotics; Pharyngitis and tonsillopharyngitis; Rheumatic fever; Skin infections; Staphylococcal infections; *Staphylococcus*; Strep throat; Streptococcal infections; *Streptococcus*.

Group B streptococcal infection

CATEGORY: Diseases and conditions
ANATOMY OR SYSTEM AFFECTED: Gastrointestinal system, genitalia, genitourinary tract
ALSO KNOWN AS: Group B strep, *Streptococcus agalactiae* infection

DEFINITION

Group B streptococcal (GBS) disease is a bacterial infection. These bacteria live in the gastrointestinal and genitourinary tracts and are found in the vaginal or rectal areas of 10 to 35 percent of all healthy adult women.

GBS can cause illness in newborns, pregnant women, the elderly, and adults with other chronic medical conditions, such as diabetes or liver disease. In newborns, GBS is the most common cause of bacteremia or septicemia (blood infection) and meningitis (infection of the fluid and lining surrounding the brain). GBS in pregnant women and their fetuses and newborns are discussed here.

CAUSES

GBS is caused by the bacterium *Streptococcus agalactiae*. Not all fetuses and babies who are exposed to the bacterium will become infected, but those who have become infected with GBS got the infection in one of three ways: before birth, during delivery, and after birth. Before birth, bacteria in the vagina spread up the birth canal into the uterus and infect the amniotic fluid surrounding the fetus. The fetus becomes infected by ingesting the infected fluid. During delivery, the fetus can become infected by contact with bacteria in the birth canal; after birth, the newborn can be infected through physical contact with the mother.

RISK FACTORS

Factors that increase the risk of a baby contracting GBS are the mother having already had a baby with GBS disease, the presence of GBS bacteria in the current pregnancy, the mother having a urinary tract infection caused by GBS, going through labor or experiencing a rupture of the membranes before thirty-seven weeks gestation, experiencing a rupture of the membranes for eighteen hours or more before delivery, and the mother having a fever during labor.

SYMPTOMS

In pregnant women, GBS infections can cause endometritis, amnionitis, and septic abortion. In newborns, two forms of infection occur: early-onset and late-onset. Early-onset GBS disease usually causes illness within the first twenty-four hours of life. However, illness can occur up to six days after birth. Late-onset disease usually occurs at three to four weeks of age; it can occur any time from seven days to three months of age. Symptoms of both kinds of GBS include breathing problems, not eating well, irritability, extreme drowsi-

ness, unstable temperature (low or high), and weakness or listlessness (in late-onset disease).

SCREENING AND DIAGNOSIS

GBS can be diagnosed in a pregnant woman at a doctor's office. Testing for GBS should be done about one month before the baby is due. The doctor swabs the pregnant woman's vagina and rectum and sends these samples to a laboratory to test for GBS. Test results are available in twenty-four to forty-eight hours. The doctor may also order blood tests.

TREATMENT AND THERAPY

Women who test positive for GBS or who are at high risk may receive intravenous antibiotics during labor and delivery. Penicillin or ampicillin is usually used. Women who are allergic to penicillin or ampicillin may be given clindamycin or erythromycin instead. It is generally not recommended that women take antibiotics before labor to prevent GBS (unless GBS is identified in the urine). Studies have shown that antibiotics are not effective at earlier stages.

If the doctor suspects strep B infection in the newborn, the newborn might be kept in the hospital for observation by staff. If the baby is diagnosed with GBS, he or she will be treated with intravenous antibiotics for ten days. Even with the existence of screening tests and antibiotic treatment, some babies can still get GBS disease.

PREVENTION AND OUTCOMES

Methods to prevent GBS include screening pregnant women at thirty-five to thirty-seven weeks into the pregnancy and giving antibiotics during labor and delivery to women who are carriers of GBS bacteria, who have previously had an infant with invasive GBS disease, who have GBS bacterium in the present pregnancy, who go into labor or have a rupture of the membranes before the fetus has reached an estimated gestational age of thirty-seven weeks, who have a rupture of membranes for eighteen hours or more before delivery, who have a fever during labor, or who have a urinary tract infection with GBS. Another option is to give antibiotics (usually penicillin) to newborns who were exposed to the bacterium. No vaccine exists for the disease.

Skye Schulte, M.S., M.P.H.;
reviewed by David L. Horn, M.D., FACP

FURTHER READING

Centers for Disease Control and Prevention. "Provisional Recommendations for the Prevention of Perinatal Group B Streptococcal Disease." Available at http://www.cdc.gov/groupbstrep/guidelines/provisional-recs.htm.

Cunningham, F. Gary, et al., eds. *Williams Obstetrics.* 23d ed. New York: McGraw-Hill, 2010.

Martin, Richard J., Avroy A. Fanaroff, and Michele C. Walsh, eds. *Fanaroff and Martin's Neonatal-Perinatal Medicine: Diseases of the Fetus and Infant.* 2 vols. 8th ed. Philadelphia: Mosby/Elsevier, 2006.

Phares, C. R., et al. "Epidemiology of Invasive Group B Streptococcal Disease in the United States, 1999-2005." *Journal of the American Medical Association* 299, no. 17 (2008): 2056-2065.

Remington, Jack S., et al., eds. *Infectious Diseases of the Fetus and Newborn Infant.* 6th ed. Philadelphia: Saunders/Elsevier, 2006.

Wilson, Michael, Brian Henderson, and Rod McNab. *Bacterial Disease Mechanisms: An Introduction to Cellular Microbiology.* New York: Cambridge University Press, 2002.

WEB SITES OF INTEREST

American Congress of Obstetricians and Gynecologists
http://www.acog.org

Centers for Disease Control and Prevention
http://www.cdc.gov/groupbstrep

Group B Strep Association
http://www.groupbstrep.org

Society of Obstetricians and Gynaecologists of Canada
http://www.sogc.org

Women's Health Matters
http://www.womenshealthmatters.ca

See also: Bacterial infections; Bacterial meningitis; Bacterial vaginosis; Childbirth and infectious disease; Children and infectious disease; Endometritis; Genital herpes; Group A streptococcal infection; Neonatal sepsis; Ophthalmia neonatorum; Pregnancy and infectious disease; Sepsis; Streptococcal infections; *Streptococcus*; Women and infectious disease.

Guillain-Barré syndrome

CATEGORY: Diseases and conditions
ANATOMY OR SYSTEM AFFECTED: Brain, immune system, muscles, peripheral nervous system, spinal cord
ALSO KNOWN AS: Acute autoimmune neuropathy, acute idiopathic polyneuritis, acute inflammatory demyelinating polyneuropathy, acute inflammatory demyelinating polyradiculoneuropathy, acute inflammatory polyneuropathy, idiopathic polyneuritis

DEFINITION

Guillain-Barré syndrome is a rare condition that causes the immune system to attack the nerves outside the brain and the spinal cord. The syndrome is characterized by numbness, tingling, weakness, or paralysis in the legs, arms, breathing muscles, and face. It can affect all ages.

CAUSES

The exact cause of Guillain-Barré syndrome is unknown. However, in about 70 percent of persons, a recent infection or surgery is a trigger to an autoimmune response. This autoimmune response attacks the peripheral nerves, leading to weakness and a loss of sensation.

RISK FACTORS

Risk factors for Guillain-Barré syndrome may include recent gastrointestinal or respiratory infection by viruses or bacteria; recent surgery; a history of lymphoma, lupus, or acquired immunodeficiency syndrome; and a recent vaccination (especially influenza and meningococcal). The swine flu vaccine given in 1976-1977 was linked to many cases of Guillain-Barré syndrome. Since this time, influenza virus vaccines have been associated with only a marginally increased risk of Guillain-Barré syndrome. At higher risk for the syndrome are men and persons fifteen to thirty-five years of age and persons between sixty and seventy-five years of age.

SYMPTOMS

The first symptoms of Guillain-Barré syndrome include pain (lower back pain is the most common complaint); progressive muscle weakness on both sides of the legs, arms, and face; prickly, tingling sensations,

Key Terms: Guillain-Barré Syndrome (GBS)

- *Antibody.* A substance produced by plasma cells that usually binds to a foreign particle (antigen); in GBS, antibodies bind to myelin protein

- *Areflexia.* Loss of reflex

- *Autoimmune disorder.* A condition in which the immune system attacks the body's own tissue instead of foreign tissue

- *B cell.* A type of white blood cell that produces antibodies

- *CSF protein.* A protein in the cerebrospinal fluid whose level is usually very low

- *Demyelination.* A loss of the myelin coating of nerves

- *Macrophage.* A white blood cell that engulfs foreign protein; in Guillain-Barré syndrome, it also attacks myelin

- *Motor weakness.* Muscle weakness resulting from the failure of motor nerves

- *Myelin.* A soft material that forms a thick sheath around some nerve fibers

- *Nerve conduction velocity.* The speed at which a nerve impulse travels along a nerve

- *Neurogenic atrophy.* Shrinkage of muscle caused by a loss of nervous stimulation

- *Neuropathy.* A condition in which nerves are diseased, are inflamed, or show abnormal degeneration

- *Phagocytosis.* The process of engulfing particles

- *Polyneuropathy.* Neuropathy found in many areas

usually in the feet or hands; and a loss of normal reflexes.

Symptoms may develop over hours, days, or weeks. They will vary in severity from minimal to total paralysis, and they include respiratory weakness. The symptoms grow progressively worse. Most people experience the greatest weakness during the second or third week of illness. Related complications include facial weakness, blood pressure instability, heart rate changes, sweating abnormalities, cardiac arrhythmia, urinary and gastrointestinal dysfunctions, and breathing difficulty.

Most persons recover fully, but as many as 25 percent will have some residual symptoms. Five to ten percent have permanent, disabling deficits, and for 5 percent, the condition is fatal.

SCREENING AND DIAGNOSIS

A doctor will ask about symptoms and medical history and will perform a physical exam. Diagnosis is dependant on the physical exam and history, on cerebrospinal fluid findings, and on nerve conduction studies. The patient may also undergo a lumbar puncture, or spinal tap. For this test, a needle is inserted into the lower back to remove a sample of cerebrospinal fluid for testing. High levels of protein, and no infection in the patient, indicate the patient may have Guillain-Barré syndrome. Electrodiagnostic studies test the electrical conduction in the peripheral nerves and help differentiate Guillain-Barré from other disorders with similar symptoms.

TREATMENT AND THERAPY

Treatment aims to reduce the body's autoimmune response and decrease complications that result from immobility. Hospitalization is important because symptoms, including respiratory failure, cardiac arrhythmia, and blood pressure instability, may rapidly become more severe. Most affected persons need to be hospitalized for some time.

Common treatments for the syndrome include plasmapheresis, in which blood is removed from the body and passed through a machine that separates blood cells. The separated cells are then returned to the body with new plasma. This procedure may help shorten the course and severity of Guillain-Barré syndrome.

Another treatment option is high-dose immunoglobulin therapy. Intravenous infusion with immunoglobulins (antibodies) may help reduce the severity of a Guillain-Barré attack. Immunoglobulins are proteins that are naturally produced by the body's immune system.

Another treatment is mechanical ventilation. In 30 percent of cases, muscles necessary for breathing become paralyzed. This paralysis is treated with immediate emergency support from a mechanical ventilator. For pain control, the doctor may prescribe medications such as nonsteroidal anti-inflammatory drugs, gabapentin, carbamezepine, and narcotic analgesics.

PREVENTION AND OUTCOMES

There are no guidelines for the prevention of Guillain-Barré syndrome.

Michelle Badash, M.S.; reviewed by Rimas Lukas, M.D.

FURTHER READING

Abbas, Abul K., and Andrew H. Lichtman. *Basic Immunology: Functions and Disorders of the Immune System.* 2d ed. Philadelphia: Saunders/Elsevier, 2006.

Benatar. M., et al. "Guillain-Barré Syndrome." In *Ferri's Clinical Advisor 2011: Instant Diagnosis and Treatment,* edited by Fred F. Ferri. Philadelphia: Mosby/Elsevier, 2011.

Bradley, Walter G., et al., eds. *Neurology in Clinical Practice.* 5th ed. Philadelphia: Butterworth Heinemann/Elsevier, 2007.

Goetz, S. "Acute Inflammatory Demyelinating Polyradiculoneuropathy." In *Clinical Neurology*, edited by Michael J. Aminoff, David A. Greenberg, and Roger P. Simon. 7th ed. New York: McGraw-Hill Medical, 2009.

Parker, James N., and Philip M. Parker, eds. *The Official Patient's Sourcebook on Guillain-Barré Syndrome.* San Diego, Calif.: Icon Health, 2002.

Vucic, S., M. C. Kiernan, and D. R. Cornblath. "Guillain-Barré: An Update." *Journal of Clinical Neuroscience* 16, no. 6 (2009): 733-741.

WEB SITES OF INTEREST

Canadian Institute for Health Information
http://www.cihi.ca

Guillain-Barré Syndrome Foundation International
http://www.gbs-cidp.org

National Institute of Neurological Disorders and Stroke
http://www.ninds.nih.gov

Public Health Agency of Canada
http://www.phac-aspc.gc.ca

See also: Acute cerebellar ataxia; Autoimmune disorders; Bell's palsy; Creutzfeldt-Jakob disease; Gerstmann-Sträussler-Scheinker syndrome; Iatrogenic infections; Meningococcal meningitis; Myositis; Neisserial infections; Progressive multifocal leukoencephalopathy; Rabies; Viral meningitis.

H

H. pylori infection. *See Helicobacter pylori* infection.

Haemophilus

CATEGORY: Pathogen
TRANSMISSION ROUTE: Direct contact, inhalation

DEFINITION

Haemophilus is a gram-negative, nonmotile, non-spore-forming, pleiomorphic coccobacillus. Its name is derived from the Greek and means "blood lover." Most strains of *Haemophilus* require hemin (factor X) and NAD (factor V), both of which are naturally found in blood. Strains may be aerobes or facultative anaerobes. Many *Haemophilus* spp. are normal flora in the upper respiratory and urogenital tracts of humans and other animals.

Taxonomic Classification for *Haemophilus*

Kingdom: Bacteria
Phylum: Proteobacteria
Class: Gammaproteobacteria
Order: Pasteurellales
Family: Pasteurellaceae
Genus: *Haemophilus*
Species:
H. aegyptius
H. agni
H. avium
H. canis
H. ducreyi
H. haemolyticus
H. influenzae
H. paracuniculus
H. parahaemolyticus
H. parainfluenzae
H. parasuis

NATURAL HABITAT AND FEATURES

Although *Haemophilus* spp. are usually classified as coccobacilli, they are quite pleiomorphic and can take on various shapes in culture. Most are cultured on chocolate agar, a nutrient-dense agar with added denatured hemoglobin. Additional NAD is usually added to this agar when culturing *Haemophilus* spp. Incubation is best at 98.6° Fahrenheit (37° Celsius) and growth is enhanced in an incubator enriched with carbon dioxide. Most species are commensal in the upper respiratory tract and are opportunistic pathogens with relatively limited host ranges. The major pathogenic species in humans are *H. influenzae* and *H. ducreyi*.

PATHOGENICITY AND CLINICAL SIGNIFICANCE

H. influenzae was named when it was isolated in the 1890's from persons suffering from influenza. It was later shown to be a secondary bacterial infection and not the causative agent of that disease. It is similar to many other members of this genus. In fact, *H. aegyptius*, which causes conjunctivitis and Brazilian purpuric fever, has been reclassified as a subtype of *H. influenzae* rather than a separate species. Natural infections occur only in humans, although infection can be artificially induced in a few animal species.

Both encapsulated and nonencapsulated strains exist. The encapsulated strains show higher degrees of pathogenicity, most likely because the capsule offers some protection against the host's immune system and possibly increases the bacteria's virulence. Encapsulated strains are divided into six serotypes (a-f) with *H. influenzae* serotype B (Hib) being the most common pathogenic group. Before the widespread use of Hib vaccine, approximately 95 percent of all invasive *Haemophilus* infections in children, including 75 percent of meningitis cases, and 50 percent of *Haemophilus* infections in adults, were caused by Hib. Hib commonly causes meningitis, pneumonia, bacteremia, cellulitis, epiglottitis, and septic arthritis. It also can cause osteomyelitis and endocarditis. In developed countries, Hib infections in children have markedly decreased since the early 1990's, when the Hib vaccine became widely used. In the United States, for example, Hib infections in children decreased 99 percent between 1990 and 2000.

The percentage of infections caused by nonencapsulated *H. influenzae* (NTHi) has risen markedly since the introduction of the Hib vaccine. NTHi strains are present in the nasopharynx of 80 percent of the adult population and, because the strains lack capsules, are not affected by the vaccines that target capsular antigens. Migration of the NTHi bacteria from the nasopharynx can lead to otitis media (middle-ear infection), sinusitis, bronchitis, and pneumonia. Many of these infections are self-limiting because the immune system recognizes nonencapsulated strains more readily than those that are encapsulated. NTHi can also lead, more rarely, to disseminated systemic disease. Smoking, viral infections, chronic lung disease, and immunodeficiency can make NTHi infections much more likely. In 2006, NTHi accounted for almost two thirds of all *H. influenzae* infections in the United States.

Ampicillin has been the drug of choice for treating *H. influenzae*, but many strains have developed resistance to the penicillin family of antibiotics. Chloramphinicol has also been used, but chloramphenicol resistance is also on the rise. Second and third generation cephalosporins, fluoroquinolines, and clarithromycin are good alternatives. In severe cases, the cyclosporins cefotaxime and ceftriaxone can be administered intravenously.

H. ducreyi was first isolated in 1899. It is most commonly isolated from the urogenital mucosa of humans, the bacterium's only natural host. Like most members of its genus, *H. ducreyi* is a fastidious bacterium that requires enriched chocolate agar for growth. Genetic testing of *H. ducreyi* has shown it to be genetically related (albeit distantly) to other *Haemophilus* spp. and even to other members of Pasteurellaceae, although it has nutritional requirements similar to other members of this family. Some bacteriologists have suggested that *H. ducreyi* be placed as a monotypic genus in its own family.

H. ducreyi infection leads to chancroid (soft chancre), a common sexually transmitted disease in less developed countries in tropical and subtropical regions. The disease causes ulceration of the genitalia and is endemic to sub-Saharan Africa, especially among men who have sex with sex workers, who often are reservoirs for *H. ducreyi*. *H. ducreyi* infection in-

creases the likelihood of human immunodeficiency virus (HIV) transmission ten to one hundred times. Chancroid is uncommon in the United States, with the last major outbreak in the 1980's. Azythomycin is the drug of choice for treating *H. ducreyi* infections. Erythromycin, ciprofloxacin, and in severe cases, ceftriaxone are also used.

Other *Haemophilus* spp. that are commensal in humans only rarely cause opportunistic infections. *H. haemolyticus*, *H. parahaemolyticus*, and *H. parainfluenzae* are commonly found in the nasopharynx and oral cavities but are seen associated only with pharyngitis and other conditions in debilitated persons. It has been suggested that *H. avium* and *H. agni* be placed within other genera in the Pasteurellaceae family because they are genetically distant from all other *Haemophilus* spp. Other species, such as *H. paracuniculus* and *H. parasuis*, are somewhat genetically closer to the *Haemophilus* spp. that affect humans, but their taxonomy is under scientific review.

Richard W. Cheney, Jr., Ph.D.

FURTHER READING

Albritton, W. L. "Biology of *Haemophilus ducreyi*." *Microbiological Reviews* 53 (1989): 377-389.

Garrity, George M., ed. *The Proteobacteria*. Vol. 2 in *Bergey's Manual of Systematic Bacteriology*. 2d ed. New York: Springer, 2005.

Madigan, Michael T., and John M. Martinko. *Brock Biology of Microorganisms*. 12th ed. Upper Saddle River, N.J.: Pearson/Prentice Hall, 2010.

Spinola, Stanley M., Margaret E. Bauer, and Robert S. Munson, Jr. "Immunopathenogenesis of *Haemophilus ducreyi* Infection (Chancroid)." *Infection and Immunity* 70 (2002): 1667-1676.

WEB SITES OF INTEREST

American Academy of Pediatrics
http://www.healthychildren.org

National Institute of Allergy and Infectious Diseases
http://www.niaid.nih.gov

Todar's Online Textbook of Bacteriology
http://www.textbookofbacteriology.net

See also: Bacteria: Classification and types; Bacterial meningitis; Bronchitis; Cellulitis; Chancroid; Epiglottitis; *Haemophilus influenzae* infection; Hib vaccine; HIV; Influenza; Middle-ear infection; Pneumonia; Septic arthritis; Sinusitis.

Haemophilus influenzae infection

CATEGORY: Diseases and conditions
ANATOMY OR SYSTEM AFFECTED: Brain, ears, lungs, respiratory system

DEFINITION

Haemophilus influenzae is a small gram-negative bacterium that causes a variety of infections, primarily in young children. The species designation *influenzae* reflects the earlier misdiagnosis of this bacterium as the cause of influenza, which is a viral disease.

CAUSES

Strains of *H. influenzae* may be either encapsulated or nonencapsulated, and six distinct types of capsules are recognized. Most cases of serious invasive disease are caused by type B encapsulated strains (Hib), but bacteria of any subtype may be present as part of the normal respiratory tract flora in healthy persons. Humans are the only natural host of the organism, and disease is spread from person to person by inhalation of respiratory droplets or by direct contact with respiratory secretions.

RISK FACTORS

Young children who are not immunized are at high risk for contracting *H. influenzae* infections, particularly if contact has been established with a child with invasive Hib disease. Others at risk include people with human immunodeficiency virus (HIV) infection, sickle cell disease, asplenia (absent or nonfunctioning spleen), or malignant neoplasms.

SYMPTOMS

H. influenzae infections can result in a range of symptoms. Most are respiratory tract infections such as pneumonia, bronchitis, sinusitis, and otitis media and thus cause symptoms associated with those diseases, such as coughing, sneezing, and pain. Some strains cause invasive diseases and their accompanying symptoms, such as meningitis, epiglottitis, cellulitis, and septic arthritis.

SCREENING AND DIAGNOSIS

Persons with a suspected *H. influenzae* infection may have a sample taken for analysis. In the laboratory, *H. influenzae* cells are most easily cultured on chocolate agar, a rich growth medium containing essential growth factors from hemolyzed red blood cells. Colonies appear gray, with a diameter of 0.5 to 0.8 millimeters and usually with rough edges. Strains surrounded by a polysaccharide capsule usually produce larger colonies that are somewhat mucoid in appearance.

PREVENTION AND OUTCOMES

Until 1988, when the effective Hib conjugate vaccines were first introduced, Hib was the most common cause of bacterial meningitis in children in the United States. Acute epiglottitis caused by massive Hib colonization had a high mortality in children age two to four years. In the years since the widespread use of these vaccines, the incidence of invasive Hib disease in infants and young children has decreased by almost 99 percent.

Three different Hib conjugate vaccines are commercially available in the United States, and all show excellent effectiveness with minimal adverse reactions. Children as young as two months of age can be immunized. Either a two- or three-dose regimen is administered, depending on the vaccine prescribed, and a booster is recommended at age twelve to fifteen months.

TREATMENT AND THERAPY

Invasive Hib infections are most commonly treated with a third-generation cephalosporin antibiotic, such as cefotaxime or ceftriaxone. Meropenem or the combination of chloramphenicol and ampicillin have also been used effectively. For localized respiratory tract infections such as otitis media, oral amoxicillin is usually prescribed. Because as many as 5 to 50 percent of isolates from around the world are resistant to ampicillin, an oral cephalosporin may be required as well. Rifampin has proved to be successful as a chemoprophylaxis agent in households with a minimum of one contact younger than four years of age because it eliminates Hib from the pharynx in the vast majority of carriers.

Jeffrey A. Knight, Ph.D.

FURTHER READING

Brooks, George F., et al. *Jawetz, Melnick, and Adelberg's Medical Microbiology.* 25th ed. New York: McGraw-Hill Medical, 2010.

Madigan, Michael T., and John M. Martinko. *Brock Biology of Microorganisms.* 12th ed. Upper Saddle River, N.J.: Pearson/Prentice Hall, 2010.

Pan American Health Organization. World Health Organization. *Control of Diphtheria, Pertussis, Tetanus, "Haemophilus influenzae" Type B, and Hepatitis B Field Guide.* Washington, D.C.: Author, 2005.

Southwick, Frederick. *Infectious Diseases: A Clinical Short Course.* 2d ed. New York: McGraw-Hill, 2007.

WEB SITES OF INTEREST

American Academy of Otolaryngology—Head and Neck Surgery
http://www.entnet.org

Centers for Disease Control and Prevention
http://www.cdc.gov

National Institute of Allergy and Infectious Diseases
http://www.niaid.nih.gov

Pediatric Infectious Diseases Society
http://www.pids.org

See also: Bacteria: Classification and types; Bacterial infections; Bacterial meningitis; Bronchitis; Cellulitis; Children and infectious disease; Epiglottitis; *Haemophilus*; Hib vaccine; Influenza; Middle-ear infection; Pneumonia; Septic arthritis; Sinusitis.

Haemophilus influenzae vaccine. *See* Hib vaccine.

Hand, foot, and mouth disease

CATEGORY: Diseases and conditions
ANATOMY OR SYSTEM AFFECTED: Skin
ALSO KNOWN AS: Vesicular stomatitis with exanthem

DEFINITION

Hand, foot, and mouth disease is an enteroviral disease that usually affects children. It causes a vesicular eruption on the hands, feet, oral mucosa, and tongue.

CAUSES

The disease is usually caused by coxsackie virus A16 but may also be the result of infection with a number of other coxsackie viruses, echovirus 18, and enterovirus 71.

RISK FACTORS

Young children, age one to five years, are most commonly infected. The most common months for infection are those in the summer and early fall. Children may become infected when they come into contact with the oral secretions of infected children during nursery school or day-care outbreaks. Skin lesions and fecal material may also contribute to the spread of the disease. It is also common to spread infection to other family members. The incubation period is three to six days.

SYMPTOMS

The illness commences with a low-grade fever (100° to 101° Fahrenheit) and a sore mouth. Oral lesions begin as small red macules and rapidly evolve into fragile vesicles that rupture and leave painful ulcers. Any part of the mouth may be involved, but the hard palate buccal mucosa and tongue are mainly affected with an average of five to ten lesions. Similar lesions develop on the skin in the next one to two days and usually number twenty to thirty, but may be as many as one hundred. Discrete macular lesions, about 4 millimeters in diameter, appear on the hands and feet and sometimes the buttocks. These lesions often occur along skin lines and progress to become papules and white or gray flaccid vesicles containing infective virus. The lesions may be painful or tender, but there is no lymphadenopathy. The fever occurs during the first one to two days of the illness, which resolves in seven to ten days. Rarely, the viral infection is complicated by meningoencephalitis, carditis, or pneumonia.

SCREENING AND DIAGNOSIS

The diagnosis is usually made from the clinical signs and symptoms, but specimens from the mouth and skin lesions can be cultured for viruses or processed by polymerase chain reaction.

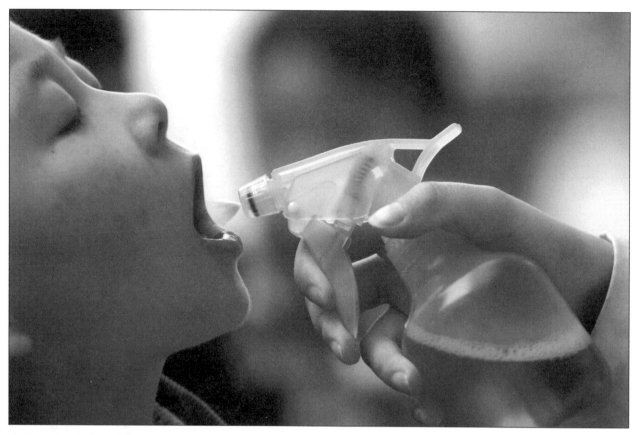

A doctor sprays disinfectant into the mouth of a child in China, hoping to prevent the spread of hand, foot, and mouth disease in 2009. (AP/Wide World Photos)

TREATMENT AND THERAPY

There is no specific treatment for hand, food, and mouth disease, which usually resolves without complications in about one week. Topical anesthetic agents, such as viscous lidocaine, may be used to soothe the discomfort of the mouth lesions.

PREVENTION AND OUTCOMES

Limiting one's contact with infected persons and handwashing after contact are the best preventive measures. Infected children's toys and other touched objects should be cleaned with a mild bleach solution.

H. Bradford Hawley, M.D.

FURTHER READING

Farrar, W. Edmund, et al. *Infectious Diseases: Text and Color Atlas.* 2d ed. New York: Gower Medical, 1992.

Hosoya, M., et al. "Diagnosis of Group A Coxsackievirus Infection Using Polymerase Chain Reaction." *Archives of Diseases of Childhood* 87 (2002): 316-319.

Long, Sarah S., Larry K. Pickering, and Charles G. Prober, eds. *Principles and Practice of Pediatric Infectious Diseases.* 3d ed. Philadelphia: Churchill Livingstone/Elsevier, 2008.

Modlin, John F. "Coxsackieviruses, Echoviruses, Newer Enteroviruses, and Parechoviruses." In *Mandell, Douglas, and Bennett's Principles and Practice of Infectious Diseases*, edited by Gerald L. Mandell, John F. Bennett, and Raphael Dolin. 7th ed. New York: Churchill Livingstone/Elsevier, 2010.

WEB SITES OF INTEREST

About Kids Health
http://www.aboutkidshealth.ca

American Academy of Family Physicians
http://familydoctor.org

American Academy of Pediatrics
http://www.healthychildren.org

Centers for Disease Control and Prevention
http://www.cdc.gov

See also: Coxsackie virus infections; Echovirus infections; Enterovirus infections; Fever; Mouth infections; Skin infections.

Hansen's disease. *See* Leprosy.

Hantavirus infection

CATEGORY: Diseases and conditions
ANATOMY OR SYSTEM AFFECTED: All
ALSO KNOWN AS: Hantavirus pulmonary syndrome

DEFINITION

Hantavirus infection is a deadly viral disease contracted from rodents. The infection results in flulike symptoms and serious breathing problems and often leads to death.

CAUSES

Hantavirus infection is caused when a person comes into contact with rodents that are infected with hantavirus, primarily when inhaling air containing hantaviruses from an infected rodent's urine or droppings. About 30 to 40 percent of people who contract hantavirus infection will die. In the United States, the deer mouse is the rodent most likely to carry hantavirus infection. Hantavirus infection cannot be passed between humans.

RISK FACTORS

Some factors thought to increase the risk of hantavirus infection include living near a forest, having rodents in the home, and having rodents in a work environment.

SYMPTOMS

Symptoms associated with hantavirus infection include fever, deep muscle aches, and a severe shortness of breath.

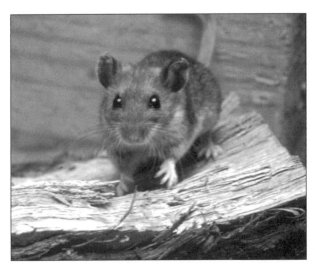

The deer mouse is a carrier of the hantavirus. (CDC)

SCREENING AND DIAGNOSIS

A doctor will ask about symptoms and medical history and will perform a physical exam. Other tests may include blood tests and a chest X ray.

TREATMENT AND THERAPY

There is no specific treatment for hantavirus infection. Treatment will focus on symptoms and on patient comfort.

PREVENTION AND OUTCOMES

The best way to prevent hantavirus infection is to control rodent infestation in and around the home. This involves sealing rodent entry holes or gaps with steel wool, lath metal, or caulk; trapping rodents using snap traps; and cleaning rodent food sources and nesting sites. In addition, when cleaning rodent-infested areas, one should wear rubber, latex, vinyl, or nitrile gloves; should not vacuum or sweep the area, because this may cause the virus to get into the air; and should wet contaminated areas with a bleach solution (such as 1.5 cups bleach in 1 gallon water) or household disinfectant. When everything is wet, contaminated materials should be removed with a damp towel before the area is mopped or sponged with the bleach solution or disinfectant, and dead rodents should be sprayed with disinfectant, double-bagged with all cleaning materials, and properly disposed of. Next, the local health department should be contacted for appropriate disposal methods.

Also, one should disinfect gloves with disinfectant or soap and water before taking them off, then thoroughly wash hands with soap and water or a waterless alcohol-based rub (such as a hand sanitizer) if soap is not available.

Krisha McCoy, M.S.;
reviewed by David L. Horn, M.D., FACP

FURTHER READING

Centers for Disease Control and Prevention. "Hantavirus Pulmonary Syndrome: What You Need to Know." Available at http://www.cdc.gov/ncidod/diseases/hanta/hps.

Cockrum, E. Lendell. *Rabies, Lyme Disease, Hanta Virus, and Other Animal-Borne Human Diseases in the United States and Canada.* Tucson, Ariz.: Fisher Books, 1997.

EBSCO Publishing. *DynaMed: Hantavirus Pulmonary Syndrome.* Available through http://www.ebscohost.com/dynamed.

Jonsson, C. B., L. T. Figueiredo, and O. Vapalahti. "A Global Perspective on Hantavirus Ecology, Epidemiology, and Disease." *Clinical Microbiology Reviews* 23, no. 2 (April, 2010): 412-441.

Meyer, Andrea S., and David R. Harper. *Of Mice, Men, and Microbes: Hantavirus.* San Diego, Calif.: Academic Press, 1999.

Murray, Patrick R., Ken S. Rosenthal, and Michael A. Pfaller. *Medical Microbiology.* 6th ed. Philadelphia: Mosby/Elsevier, 2009.

Shafts. C. "Hantavirus Pulmonary Syndrome." In *Ferri's Clinical Advisor 2011: Instant Diagnosis and Treatment,* edited by Fred F. Ferri. Philadelphia: Mosby/Elsevier, 2011.

Simpson, S. Q., et al. "Hantavirus Pulmonary Syndrome." *Infectious Disease Clinics of North America* 24, no. 1 (March, 2010): 159-173.

WEB SITES OF INTEREST

American Lung Association
http://www.lungusa.org

Canadian Centre for Occupational Health and Safety
http://www.ccohs.ca

Centers for Disease Control and Prevention
http://www.cdc.gov/ncidod/diseases/hanta/hps

Public Health Agency of Canada
http://www.phac-aspc.gc.ca

See also: Airborne illness and disease; Bubonic plague; Hemorrhagic fever viral infections; Histoplasmosis; Lassa fever; Monkeypox; Plague; Rabies; Rat-bite fever; Respiratory route of transmission; Rodents and infectious disease; Tularemia; Viral infections.

Head lice

CATEGORY: Diseases and conditions
ANATOMY OR SYSTEM AFFECTED: Hair, scalp, skin
ALSO KNOWN AS: Pediculosis

DEFINITION

Head lice are tiny, barely visible insectlike animals (arthropods) that may live on the scalp and cause itching. (The term "lice" is plural; the singular is "louse.") Head lice may also live in the eyebrows and eyelashes and in beards. Infestations in these areas sometimes are from a related species called pubic lice.

CAUSES

Head lice are spread by personal contact and by sharing combs, brushes, hats, and other contaminated personal items.

RISK FACTORS

Risk factors for head lice include sharing hair-grooming items, hats, and other personal items, and having personal contact with people who may have lice. Children are at higher risk for head lice.

SYMPTOMS

Symptoms for head lice include extreme itchiness, skin breaks and possible infection (caused by scratching), swollen lymph nodes, and bacterial infection (if scratching causes open areas on the scalp). Some persons with head lice do not have symptoms.

SCREENING AND DIAGNOSIS

A doctor will ask about symptoms and medical history and will perform a physical exam that includes looking at the head and scalp for lice and lice eggs (called nits). One should not self-diagnose or self-treat head lice. Some treatments can cause irritation and should be used only by people who have the infestation.

TREATMENT AND THERAPY

Treating head lice involves removing eggs and killing lice so that they cannot continue to lay eggs. Treatment may be difficult because in some regions lice have become resistant to many of the commonly used medications. Some experts recommend that treatment be given only when live adult lice are seen.

Treatment includes applying over-the-counter shampoo containing the insecticide permethrin. One should use medications as directed. Re-treatment at seven to ten days is usually required to kill any lice that hatch from remaining (unremoved) eggs.

Another treatment method is removing lice that are on the eyelashes, which may be difficult. Tweezers can be used to pick them off, and petroleum jelly (such as Vaseline) may be used to coat the eyelashes and kill the lice.

Unless instructed otherwise, one should remove eggs manually with specially designed combs. Eggs stick firmly to hair. Products such as Clear, which loosen the eggs, may assist in removal.

Most cases of head lice can be treated with over-the-counter preparations. However, there is increasing resistance to permethrin and pyrethrin in the United States. Malathion, which is available with a doctor's prescription, has become a first-line treatment because it kills both the lice and their eggs. In certain cases, a doctor may prescribe lindane, a neurotoxic that carries a U.S. Food and Drug Administration (FDA) warning. Malathion should be prescribed only to persons who are unable to take other medications or who have not responded to them. According to the FDA, lindane rarely causes serious side effects (such as seizure and death). Those especially susceptible are infants, the elderly, children and adults weighing less than 110 pounds, and persons with other skin conditions. Lindane is toxic and should not be overused.

PREVENTION AND OUTCOMES

Lice are common, especially in children. While no records are kept for accurate counts, some estimates show that as many as ten to fifteen million persons annually develop head lice in the United States. To prevent outbreaks of head lice, one should watch for signs of the disease, such as frequent head scratching. One should not share combs, brushes, hats, or other

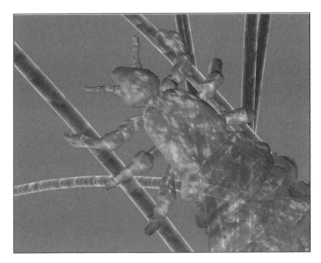

A micrograph image of a head louse. (AP/Wide World Photos)

personal items with people who may have lice, and should avoid close contact with people who may have lice.

All family members should be checked for lice and eggs a minimum of once each week. One should thoroughly wash and dry combs, brushes, hats, clothing, bedding, and stuffed animals in the home, and should vacuum carpeting and car seats. The parents or guardians of children with head lice should notify the child's school, camp, day-care provider, and friends' parents.

Jennifer Hellwig, M.S., RD;
reviewed by David L. Horn, M.D., FACP

FURTHER READING

Ashford, R. W., and W. Crewe. *The Parasites of "Homo sapiens": An Annotated Checklist of the Protozoa, Helminths, and Arthropods for Which We Are Home.* 2d ed. New York: Taylor & Francis, 2003.

Centers for Disease Control and Prevention. "Head Lice: Prevention and Control." Available at http://www.cdc.gov/lice/prevent.html.

Despommier, Dickson D., et al. *Parasitic Diseases.* 5th ed. New York: Apple Tree, 2006.

Diaz, J. H. "Lice (Pediculosis)." In *Mandell, Douglas, and Bennett's Principles and Practice of Infectious Diseases,* edited by Gerald L. Mandell, John E. Bennett, and Raphael Dolin. 7th ed. New York: Churchill Livingstone/Elsevier, 2010.

"Ectoparasites." In *Textbook of Family Medicine,* edited

by R. E. Rakel et al. 7th ed. Philadelphia: Saunders/ Elsevier, 2007.

Goddard, Jerome. *Physician's Guide to Arthropods of Medical Importance.* 4th ed. Boca Raton, Fla.: CRC Press, 2003.

Roberts, R. J. "Clinical Practice: Head Lice." *New England Journal of Medicine* 347, no. 17 (2002): 1381-1382.

U.S. Food and Drug Administration, Medication Guides. Available at http://www.fda.gov/drugs/drugsafety/ucm085729.htm.

WEB SITES OF INTEREST

American Academy of Dermatology
http://www.aad.org

Caring for Kids
http://www.caringforkids.cps.ca

Centers for Disease Control and Prevention
http://www.cdc.gov/parasites

KidsHealth
http://kidshealth.org

National Pediculosis Association
http://www.headlice.org

See also: Arthropod-borne illness and disease; Body lice; Crab lice; Fleas and infectious disease; Flies and infectious disease; Impetigo; Insecticides and topical repellants; Mites and chiggers and infectious disease; Parasitic diseases; Scabies; Skin infections.

Helicobacter

CATEGORY: Pathogen
TRANSMISSION ROUTE: Direct contact, ingestion

DEFINITION

Species of the bacterial genus *Helicobacter* cause a number of gastric and digestive accessory organ diseases in vertebrates. In humans, these diseases include gastroesophageal reflux disease (GERD) and stomach cancer.

Taxonomic Classification for *Helicobacter*

Kingdom: Bacteria
Phylum: Proteobacteria
Class: Epsilon Proteobacteria
Order: Campylobacterales
Family: Helicobacteraceae
Genus: *Helicobacter*
Species:
H. canis
H. cinaedi
H. fennelliae
H. hepaticus
H. heilmannii
H. pylori

NATURAL HABITAT AND FEATURES

Helicobacter was defined as a genus in 1989 and many of its species have since been discovered. *Helicobacter* spp. inhabit the gastric mucosa of many vertebrate animals, primarily birds and mammals. *H. pylori* was described by Robin Warren and Barry Marshall in 1983. It is the species most often found in humans and has been extensively studied; most other *Helicobacter* spp. are like it in characteristics and growth patterns.

H. pylori is a gram-negative, *S*-shaped, or curved-rod bacterium. The bacterium is a microaerophile, requiring small amounts of oxygen and growing best in the presence of 5 to 10 percent oxygen and 5 to 10 percent carbon dioxide. Specimens range from 0.5 to 0.9 micrometers (μm) wide and 2 to 4 μm long. Occasionally, *V*-shaped, *U*-shaped, straight, or spherical forms of *H. pylori* are found either in culture or within the human host.

Members of this genus are characterized by possessing sheathed flagella (usually seven in *H. pylori*), which have a covering continuous with the outer membranes of the body wall, an external glycocalyx, the presence of menoquinone-6, and G+C content of chromosomal DNA (deoxyribonucleic acid) of 35 to 40 mol percent. Cultured colonies of *H. pylori* grow within about three to five days, and are convex, circular, and translucent in appearance.

In addition to *pylori*, human infections have been caused by *canis, cinaedi, fennelliae, hepaticus,* and *heilmannii.* Some researchers have suggested a link between *hepaticus* and gallbladder cancer in humans; this bacterium is primarily found in rodents. *Heilmannii*, usually restricted to cats and dogs, may infect humans and cause chronic gastritis.

PATHOGENICITY AND CLINICAL SIGNIFICANCE

H. pylori is the causative factor of stomach ulcers and of many cases of GERD, chronic gastritis, and stomach cancer, particularly gastric mucosa-associated lymphoid tissue (MALT) lymphoma (MALToma). The bacterium also is associated with cases of iron deficiency anemia.

Approximately 50 percent of the world's population is infected with *H. pylori*. Most people have no ill effects, but for those who do, the outcome without treatment can be painful, debilitating, and even fatal. About one in six persons with *H. pylori* infection will develop an ulcer or stomach cancer.

Research indicates that most infections are acquired during childhood by person-to-person contact, primarily through direct contact with the saliva or fecal material of an infected person, often a family member. There is some evidence that *H. pylori* also can be transmitted through untreated water. Living in crowded conditions, living in areas where there is no reliable source of hot water, and living with someone who is already infected with *H. pylori* are all important risk factors influencing the spread of this bacterial disease. Among the persons who seek treatment for *H. pylori* infections, 29 percent are white, 60 percent are Hispanic, and 54 percent are of African descent.

Symptoms of an *H. pylori* infection include an ache or burning sensation in the stomach or abdomen, nausea, vomiting, frequent burping, a bloated feeling, and unexplained weight loss. Physicians test for the presence of *H. pylori* by blood tests, urea breath tests, stool sample tests, and endoscopy. The blood test for this bacterium has some inaccuracy because if a person has had *H. pylori* in the past and has been treated for it, antibodies for the bacterium may remain in the blood. The urea breath test is considered to be a more accurate indicator of an infection. It is based upon the ability of the bacteria to break down urea into carbon dioxide. The patient swallows a capsule containing a tiny amount of radioactive urea, and ten to twenty minutes later, a breath sample is collected and analyzed. If radioactive carbon dioxide is present, this indicates an active *H. pylori* infection.

Endoscopy can also be used to check for ulcers and stomach cancer, as gastric tissue can be removed for biopsy during the procedure.

DRUG SUSCEPTIBILITY

A combination of antibiotic drugs and either proton pump inhibitors (PPIs) or histamine (H-2) blockers generally provide an effective treatment for *H. pylori* infections. Usually, amoxicillin and clarithromycin are prescribed together, or a combination of metronidazole, tetracycline, and bismuth subsalicylate may be given to the patient. PPIs, including omeprazole, lansoprazole, pantoprazole, rabeprozole, or esomeprazole, are prescribed to control the production of stomach acid. Histamine blockers such as ranitidine, famotidine, cimetidine, and nizatidine may also be effective in suppressing acid production.

Antibiotic treatment should be closely supervised because some strains of *H. pylori* have become resistant to metronidazole and clarithromycin. Treatment protocols are usually of two weeks' duration; however, longer-term treatment, especially of acid reduction medicines, may be needed for some patients.

Lenela Glass-Godwin, M.S.

FURTHER READING

Feldman, Mark, Lawrence S. Friedman, and Lawrence J. Brandt, eds. *Sleisenger and Fordtran's Gastrointestinal and Liver Disease: Pathophysiology, Diagnosis, Management.* New ed. 2 vols. Philadelphia: Saunders/Elsevier, 2010. A comprehensive textbook of gastrointestinal diseases and physiology. Contains excellent endoscopic photographs.

Fox, James G., et al. "Hepatic *Helicobacter* Species Identified in Bile and Gallbladder Tissue from Chileans with Chronic Cholecystitis." *Gastroenterology* 114, no. 4 (1998): 755-763. Reports on a study of bile-resistant *Helicobacter* species associated with gallbladder disease.

Owen, R. J. "*Helicobacter*: Species Classification and Identification." *British Medical Bulletin* 54, no. 1 (1998): 17-30. Provides information on the molecular structure of the type species and discussion of other *Helicobacter* species associated with vertebrate disease.

Verijola, Lea, et al. "Detection of *Helicobacter* Species in Chronic Liver Disease and Chronic Inflammatory Bowel Disease." *Annals of Medicine* 39. no. 7 (2007): 554-560. A report on the role of *Helicobacter* in diseases other than those of the stomach.

WEB SITES OF INTEREST

American Gastroenterological Association
http://www.gastro.org

Helicobacter Foundation
http://www.helico.com

National Digestive Diseases Information Clearinghouse
http://digestive.niddk.gov/ddiseases

Todar's Online Textbook of Bacteriology
http://www.textbookofbacteriology.net

See also: Bacterial infections; Gastritis; *Helicobacter pylori* infection; Intestinal and stomach infections; Microbiology; Peptic ulcer.

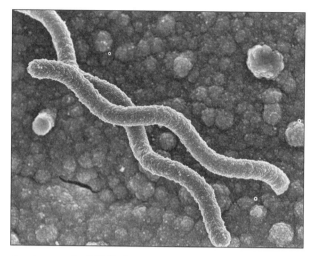

A micrograph of Helicobacter pylori bacteria.

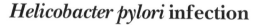

Helicobacter pylori infection

CATEGORY: Diseases and conditions
ANATOMY OR SYSTEM AFFECTED: Gastrointestinal system, intestines, stomach

DEFINITION

Helicobacter pylori is a gram-negative bacillus that causes an infection of the inner mucus lining of the stomach. It is the primary cause of gastric ulcers. The prevalence of *H. pylori* infection worldwide is more than 50 percent of the population and is much higher in developing countries.

CAUSES

H. pylori infections can result from the ingestion of food or liquids contaminated with the bacterium *H. pylori*, a spiral-shaped organism with multiple flagella that allow the organism to readily attach to the stomach mucosa. The organism survives by using the enzyme urease to break urea down to ammonia and bicarbonate, which neutralizes the strong gastric acidity. The bacterial secretions stimulate the formation of inflammatory cytokines, leading to chronic gastritis. The mucus layer is damaged and thinned by *H. pylori* secretions of cytotoxins and by enzymes such as proteases and phospholipases. With the loss of the protective mucus layer, the strong acids of the stomach attack and damage the stomach lining, resulting in peptic ulcers. The majority of peptic ulcer cases in the United States are associated with *H. pylori* infections.

RISK FACTORS

There is a much greater risk of contracting *H. pylori* infection in developing countries because of unsanitary conditions. Contaminated food and water are primary sources, but other sources include contact with the stool, vomit, or saliva of an infected person.

SYMPTOMS

The majority of *H. pylori* infections do not cause symptoms. When the infection causes inflammation and ulcers, symptoms can include abdominal pain, nausea, frequent burping, bloating, and weight loss. Immediate medical help is needed if severe abdominal pain, difficulty swallowing, or bloody stools or vomit are experienced.

SCREENING AND DIAGNOSIS

There are three primary ways to diagnosis *H. pylori* infection. In endoscopy, a physician threads a flexible tube into the stomach to remove and examine a tissue sample for the presence of the bacterium. A breath test involves a patient ingesting a test meal containing radioactively labeled urea. *H. pylori* breaks down the urea, forming radioactive carbon dioxide, which is detected. Finally, a blood test detects the presence of antibodies against *H. pylori*, which could indicate a current or prior infection.

TREATMENT AND THERAPY

Treatment usually consists of the administration of three drugs simultaneously for seven to fourteen days. One of the drugs, omeprazole (Prilosec), is a proton pump inhibitor (PPI). The other two drugs are antibiotics, typically clarithromycin and andamoxicillin. The PPIs are necessary to suppress gastric acid production, which improves the effectiveness of the antibiotics.

PREVENTION AND OUTCOMES

Although the mode of transmission of *H. pylori* is not fully understood, what is known is that improved sanitation is an essential preventive measure. A vaccine against the bacillus is under development.

David A. Olle, M.S.

FURTHER READING

Chey, William D., and Benjamin C. Y. Wong. "American College of Gastroenterology Guidelines on the Management of *Helicobacter pylori* Infection." *American Journal of Gastroenterology* 102 (2007): 1808-1825.

McCoil, Kenneth E. L. "*Helicobacter pylori* Infection." *New England Journal of Medicine* 362 (2010): 1597-1604.

Rosenberg, J. J. "*Helicobacter pylori.*" *Pediatrics in Review* 31, no. 2 (February, 2010): 85-86.

Sultan, Mutaz I., et al. "*Helicobacter pylori* Infection." Available at http://emedicine.medscape.com/article/929452-overview.

WEB SITES OF INTEREST

American Gastroenterological Association
http://www.gastro.org

Helicobacter Foundation
http://www.helico.com

National Digestive Diseases Information Clearinghouse
http://digestive.niddk.gov/ddiseases

See also: Bacterial infections; Gastritis; *Helicobacter*; Intestinal and stomach infections; Microbiology; Peptic ulcer.

Hemorrhagic fever viral infections

CATEGORY: Diseases and conditions
ANATOMY OR SYSTEM AFFECTED: All
ALSO KNOWN AS: Viral hemorrhagic fever

DEFINITION

Hemorrhagic fever viral infections (HFVIs) are caused by four distinct families of viruses: arenavirus, bunyavirus, filovirus, and flavivirus. These viruses are round structures with an average diameter of 110 to 130 nanometers (1 billionth of a meter). They are covered with a lipid (fat) membrane. A cross-section view of the viruses shows grainy particles.

HFVIs are characterized by fever and bleeding disorders, which can progress to shock and death. However, these viruses can also produce a mild infection with little or no symptoms. The viruses are present throughout the globe, and most of them are totally dependent on a host organism, such as a rodent or insect, for replication and survival. This host organism is known as a vector.

CAUSES

Arenavirus, bunyavirus, filovirus, and flavivirus are all ribonucleic acid (RNA) viruses (RNA is a long chain of nucleotide units). Humans contract one of these viruses through contact with the urine, saliva, or feces of infected rodents. For viruses that have an insect vector, the disease occurs from a bite. Some arenaviruses, such as Machupo and Lassa, can be spread by person-to-person contact. For example, hospital workers caring for infected persons can acquire the infection. Other viruses can enter the body through inhaled airborne particles or by direct contact with broken or abraded (chafed) skin.

Each virus is usually associated with a specific rodent or insect host species, or with a closely related species. These host species (vectors) maintain the virus within their bodies and are not known to exhibit any symptoms of viral illness. Rodents, mosquitoes, and ticks are found in most areas on Earth.

Arenaviruses. These arenaviruses are divided into two groups: the New World or Tacaribe complex and the Old World or Lassa complex. Both groups produce infections in humans. In Africa (Old World), Lassa virus causes Lassa fever; in South America (New

World), arenavirus infections are caused by the Machupo virus, which leads to Bolivian hemorrhagic fever; the Guanarito virus, which causes Venezuelan hemorrhagic fever; the Junin virus, which causes Argentine hemorrhagic fever; and the Sabia virus, which causes Brazilian hemorrhagic fever. Infections with the lymphocytic choriomeningitis virus, which causes lymphocytic choriomeningitis, have been reported in the Americas, Australia, Europe, and Japan.

Approximately 400,000 Lassa fever infections occur annually, with a mortality rate of about 20 percent; the disease's vector is a rat, *Mastomys natalensis*. Bolivian hemorrhagic fever has a mortality of about 30 percent; its vector is the vesper mouse, *Calomys callosus*. Venezuelan hemorrhagic fever also has a mortality rate of about 30 percent; its vectors are the short-tailed cane mouse (*Zygodontomys brevicauda*) and Alston's cotton rat (*Sigmodon alstoni*).

Bunyaviruses. These viruses commonly infect insects and rodents, and some infect humans. Others cause plant diseases. Bunyavirus vectors are mosquitoes, ticks, and sandflies. The only exception is the hantavirus, which is spread through contact with deer mice feces. Transmission of these viruses is usually seasonal. For example, viruses transmitted by mosquitoes are more common in summer. Some of these viruses cause serious illness and death. Two examples are the Crimean-Congo hemorrhagic fever virus and the hantavirus, which causes hantavirus hemorrhagic fever. Crimean-Congo hemorrhagic fever is a tick-borne viral infection with a mortality rate of about 30 percent. Hantavirus causes high fever, pulmonary edema (fluid in the lungs), pulmonary failure, and hypotension (dangerously low blood pressure); it has a mortality rate of approximately 55 percent.

Filoviruses. These viruses are the Ebola virus and the Marburg virus. Despite sometimes causing mild illness, they are two of the most virulent (deadly) viruses on the planet. Filoviruses cause a severe viral hemorrhagic fever disease, mainly in sub-Saharan Africa. The vector for the Ebola virus is unknown. However, researchers theorize that a human infection first occurs through contact with an infected animal. This infected human then transmits the infection through contact with blood or secretions from another infected person; thus, family members and health care workers are at increased risk. Mortality rates range from 50 to 90 percent, depending on the particular viral strain.

The Marburg virus is also spread through body

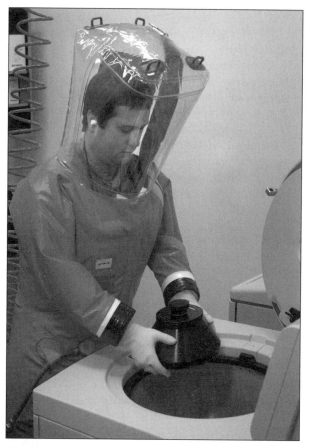

Hemorrhagic fever viral infections are the main foci of the CDC's Special Pathogens Branch. Here, a branch microbiologist wears air-tight protective clothing during testing. (CDC)

fluids. A suspected vector is the Egyptian fruit bat, *Rousettus aegyptiacus*. Marburg virus infections have a mortality rate of about 25 percent. Recovery may be prolonged in some persons and is complicated by hepatitis (liver inflammation), myelitis (muscle inflammation), orchitis (testicular inflammation), or uveitis (eye inflammation).

Flaviviruses. These viruses cause dengue fever, Kyasanur forest disease, Omsk hemorrhagic fever, and yellow fever. Yellow fever is endemic to tropical regions of Africa and the Americas. The virus primarily affects humans and nonhuman primates (such as monkeys) and is transmitted through the bite of infected *Aedes aegypti* mosquitoes. It can cause devastating epidemics, which can result in many fatalities. Both in Africa and South America, despite large-scale vaccination campaigns to prevent and control these outbreaks, the risk of major yellow fever epidemics exists, particularly in densely populated, poor, urban settings. Yellow fever is considered to be an emerging, or reemerging, disease of significant importance.

An even greater threat is dengue fever. It is the most prevalent insect-borne virus affecting humans. It is present in more than one hundred countries, and 50 million to 100 million cases occur each year. Dengue fever is transmitted through the bite of an infected *A. aegypti* or *A. albopictus* mosquito. Breeding sites for the mosquitoes that transmit dengue virus have increased, partly because of population growth and uncontrolled urbanization in tropical and subtropical countries.

RISK FACTORS

Taken together, viruses that cause HFVIs are present throughout the globe; however, the overall risk of contracting an infection is low. Furthermore, because each virus is often associated with a specific host, it is usually present only in the area where that host lives. Some viruses are present only in isolated regions; thus, the risk of transmission is extremely low. However, some infections, such as dengue, Lassa, and yellow fevers, are common in certain regions, mainly South America and sub-Saharan Africa. These areas are known as endemic areas for those diseases.

Some infections, such as dengue fever, flare with periodic outbreaks; thus, travel to a region during an epidemic increases the risk of infection. The risk of infection in an endemic area is greater if one hikes or camps in the countryside rather than staying in a hotel and taking guided tours. Infection from a virus outside the endemic area is possible because of air travel or because of bioterrorism.

The risk of a rodent-borne infection increases in rodent-infested buildings, by living in the country, or by living near an area where rodents congregate (such as trash storage areas). The risk of insect-borne infection increases by being outdoors with exposed areas of skin, particularly at night.

The following persons are at increased risk: hospital workers ranging from health care professionals to janitorial staff, laboratory workers, and researchers studying these viruses. For example, hospital personnel in Africa caring for patients with Ebola frequently contract the disease.

SYMPTOMS

Infected humans may remain healthy and exhibit no symptoms. If symptoms occur, they often begin with a gradual onset of flulike symptoms (fever, muscular aches, and cough). If the disease progresses during the next few days, infected persons often experience a sore throat, headache, chest pain, abdominal pain, vomiting, and diarrhea. Further progression leads to bleeding from the gums, the intestinal tract, and other internal organs; next occurs facial swelling and conjunctivitis (inflammation and swelling of the eyelids and portions of the eyeballs). At this stage, hematuria (blood in the urine) commonly occurs. With further progression comes temporary or permanent hearing loss, pulmonary edema (fluid in the lungs), and encephalitis (brain inflammation). Late stages of the disease can lead to shock, seizures, coma, and death.

Severe multisystem disease occurs in about 20 percent of cases. Hemorrhage and tissue damage occurs in the liver, spleen, and kidneys. The mortality rate for these cases ranges from 15 to 100 percent.

SCREENING AND DIAGNOSIS

In the early stages of infection, the symptoms are similar to those of many other viral infections: fever, muscular aches, and cough. Early diagnosis is essential for treatment; however, the similarity of the symptoms to a much less virulent viral infection hampers an early diagnosis. Despite this, researchers are developing and evaluating accurate and uncomplicated diagnostic tests for hemorrhagic fever infections. A definite diagnosis can be made in a highly specialized laboratory only, one that can detect the presence of a virus or antibodies to it. Antibodies are gammaglobulin proteins that are present in blood or other bodily fluids; they are used by the immune system to identify and inactivate foreign organisms, such as bacteria and viruses. A test known as an enzyme-linked immunosorbent assay (ELISA) test is used; this biochemical technique can detect the presence of an antibody or an antigen in a sample. Specific ELISA tests are required for each virus.

TREATMENT AND THERAPY

No established drug treatments or cures exist for most HFVIs. The antiviral drug ribavirin is effective for Lassa fever if given early in the course of the disease. However, it might cause birth defects, so women taking the medication should avoid pregnancy at that time.

Treatment for HFVIs consists mainly of supportive care, such as the replacement of fluid loss, blood and blood product (platelet) transfusions, and the maintenance of blood pressure. This supportive care keeps the infected person in a reasonable state of health, which allows the body time to develop antibodies to the virus. These antibodies attack and inactivate the virus. If this occurs, the infected person regains his or her health and is immune to further attacks from the virus.

Complicating the immune response to these viruses is their ability to mutate (evolve) into different, and sometimes more virulent, strains of the virus. If a significant difference exists between the original and mutated strains, the immune system will not recognize the virus and repeat illness is possible. For example, dengue viruses have evolved rapidly as they have spread worldwide; more virulent strains have spread across Asia and the Americas.

Research into HFVIs is focused on vector (rodents and mosquitoes) control and on developing vaccines and antiviral medications. Researchers are looking for an appropriate animal model for vaccine testing. Nonhuman primate models can most reliably mimic human disease; however, less costly and more readily available rodent models are also being studied. Genetic inhibitors of these viruses are being identified in genetics laboratories. The antiviral activity of the natural human hormones, dehydroepiandrosterone and epiandrosterone, and sixteen synthetic derivatives are under investigation.

PREVENTION AND OUTCOMES

Vaccines are present for yellow fever and Argentine hemorrhagic fever. These vaccines are about 96 percent effective in preventing infection; however, they have a significant level (30 to 35 percent) of adverse effects. Essentially, these vaccines produce a mild case of the viral disease. The side effects of the vaccines include headache, fever, nausea and vomiting, weakness, myalgia (muscle pain), retroocular pain (pain behind the eyeballs), dizziness, low back pain, exanthema (widespread rash), mildly decreased blood cell and platelet counts, and microhematuria (blood in the urine that is visible microscopically).

The best prevention is to avoid contact with the rodent and insect vectors. For rodent control, garbage should be placed in rodent-proof containers. As a further precaution, these containers should be placed as far from a home as possible. Placement of traps and

pesticides in attics and other areas can control the rodent population. The risk of mosquito bites can be reduced by staying indoors at night, applying insect repellants, and wearing full-length clothing. Window screens should be placed to prevent entrance of mosquitoes into a home. If entrance cannot be completely prevented, sleeping nets should be placed over beds. Spraying with pesticides will also reduce the insect population. Prevention includes avoiding mosquito bites and promoting a clean community environment to discourage rodents from entering homes. In recent years, vector control programs have been eliminated, often because of lack of government funding. This increases the risk of infection.

For those hemorrhagic fever viruses that can be transmitted from one person to another, avoiding close physical contact with infected people and their body fluids is the most important way of controlling the spread of disease. Infection control techniques include isolating infected persons and wearing protective clothing. Other infection control recommendations include proper use, disinfection, and disposal of instruments and equipment (such as needles and thermometers) used in treating or caring for persons with these infections.

Researchers are focused on developing strategies for these diseases in the following areas: containment, treatment, and vaccines. Furthermore, they are attempting to develop methods for earlier diagnosis of these diseases.

Robin Wulffson, M.D., FACOG

FURTHER READING

Berger, Stephan A., Charles H. Calisher, and Jay S. Keystone. *Exotic Viral Diseases: A Global Guide.* Lewiston, N.Y.: B. C. Dekker, 2003. A guide to viral diseases written primarily, but not solely, for the clinician. Examines the epidemiology, signs, symptoms, and treatments of all unusual viral infections of humans.

Centers for Disease Control and Prevention. "What Are Viral Hemorrhagic Fevers?" Available at http://www. cdc.gov/ncidod/dvrd/spb/mnpages/dispages/ vhf.htm. A look at HFVIs, provided by the CDC's special pathogens branch.

Grady, D. *Deadly Invaders: Virus Outbreaks Around the World, from Marburg Fever to Avian Flu.* Boston: Kingfisher, 2006. A readable introductory student text covering viral epidemics. The book begins with an account of the author's trip to Angola to cover an outbreak of Marburg fever. Other viral diseases are covered in subsequent chapters and include avian flu, human immunodeficiency virus infection, SARS, and West Nile virus.

Howard, Colin R., ed. *Viral Haemorrhagic Fevers.* Boston: Elsevier, 2005. Part of the Perspectives in Medical Virology series, this book is an informative introductory guide to hemorrhagic fevers for students and general readers.

Parker, J., and P. Parker. *The Official Patient's Sourcebook on Viral Hemorrhagic Fevers.* San Diego, Calif.: Icon Health, 2003. Although this book is mostly useful to doctors, caregivers, and other health professionals, it also provides guidance for general readers on finding information on viral hemorrhagic fevers, from the essentials to the most advanced areas of research.

WEB SITES OF INTEREST

American Society of Tropical Medicine and Hygiene
http://www.astmh.org

Centers for Disease Control and Prevention
http://www.cdc.gov

National Center for Emerging and Zoonotic Infectious Diseases
http://www.cdc.gov/ncezid

Universal Virus Database
http://www.ictvdb.org

World Health Organization
http://www.who.int

See also: Antiviral drugs: types; Arenaviridae; Dengue fever; Ebola hemorrhagic fever; Fever; Filoviridae; Marburg hemorrhagic fever; Mosquito-borne viral encephalitis; Mosquitoes and infectious disease; Rodents and infectious disease; Viral infections; Yellow fever.

Hepadnaviridiae

CATEGORY: Pathogen
TRANSMISSION ROUTE: Direct contact

DEFINITION

The hepadnaviruses are a family of viruses that causes infection of the hepatocytes, often resulting life-threatening conditions such as liver cancer in humans and animals. Hepadnavirus is specifically responsible for hepatitis B (hepatitis A, C, and D are caused by other viruses), which is a significant public health problem.

Taxonomic Classification for Hepadnaviridiae

Order: Unassigned
Family: Hepadnaviridiae
Genus: *Orthohepadnavirus*
Species: Hepatitis B virus

NATURAL HABITAT AND FEATURES

The hepadnavirus is made up of two very small genomes of partially double-stranded and partially single-stranded circular DNA (deoxyribonucleic acid), one being positive-sense and the other negative-sense. The virions are small and spherical, and enveloped, and they are 40 to 48 nanometers (nm) in diameter. Reverse transcriptase is used for virus replication in the host during infection.

Most strains of the virus replicate only in specific hosts, making in vitro laboratory experiments extremely difficult. However, the duck hepatitis virus, which shares several fundamental features with human hepatitis B, serves as an excellent in vitro and in vivo study model.

PATHOGENICITY AND CLINICAL SIGNIFICANCE

Approximately 1.2 million people have chronic hepatitis B in the United States, and many do not know they are infected. It is most commonly spread through sexual contact and is fifty to one hundred times more infectious than human immunodeficiency virus (HIV). Ninety percent of children infected with the hepatitis B virus (HBV) are infected as infants. Each year, three thousand people will die from hepatitis B-related liver disease.

After a person is first infected, he or she can develop what is known as acute stage hepatitis B, which can range from a severe infection to a mild illness with few or no symptoms. Acute hepatitis usually occurs the first six months after exposure to the virus. Many people are able to fight the infection, clear the virus from their body, and never show signs of hepatitis infection. However, if the infection remains in the body, the virus progresses to the chronic stage, in which it cannot be cleared from the body. This stage requires treatment and management to prevent the potential life-threatening complications of the disease, including liver failure, cirrhosis, and liver cancer.

Symptoms for both acute and chronic hepatitis are similar, although in some people, chronic hepatitis symptoms can take several years or even decades to appear. Acute hepatitis will usually appear forty days to six months after exposure, except in children, who are usually asymptomatic. Some of the most common symptoms are fever, arthritis, abdominal pain, thrombocytopenia, dark urine, joint pain, gray stools, and jaundice.

DRUG SUSCEPTIBILITY

Several options are available for drug treatment for HBV; however, the drugs should be used in concert with the unique biochemistry of HBV. As the acute stage of the virus progresses into several stages, drugs are either very effective at reducing the viral load, completely ineffective, or harmful to the patient. A chronic patient may remain on antiviral therapy throughout his or her life.

Careful monitoring of both the acute and chronic patient should occur during drug therapy. Patients without other medical comorbidities have the best treatment success, but even patients with common comorbidities such as HBV and HIV can keep both viruses under control and lead healthy lives with careful monitoring of antiviral therapy.

Most therapies involve a combination of interferon and several antivirals. Interferon is the preferred drug for younger patients. There are many antivirals in use; however, resistance is an ongoing issue. New drugs that stimulate B cell and T cell responses to achieve suppression of the viral replication have been studied as options to the conventionally used drugs.

Safe hepatitis B vaccines are available for persons of all ages and are recommended as part of an infant's vaccine schedule. It is especially important also to immunize high-risk groups, including intravenous-drug users, infants born to women with HBV, health care workers who come in contact with blood as part of the job, persons who engage in unprotected sex with multiple partners, persons from countries where HBV is endemic, persons on dialysis, and inmates in jails and prisons. Persons with kidney or liver disease also are at risk.

S. M. Willis, M.S., M.A.

FURTHER READING

American Liver Foundation. "Hepatitis B." Available at http://www.liverfoundation.org/abouttheliver/info/hepatitisb.

"Hepatitis B." In *Red Book: 2009 Report of the Committee on Infectious Diseases*, edited by Larry K. Pickering et al. 28th ed. Elk Grove Village, Ill.: American Academy of Pediatrics, 2009.

Jafri, Syed-Mohammed R., and Anna Suk-Fong Lok. "Antiviral Therapy for Chronic Hepatitis B." *Clinical Liver Disease* 14 (2010): 425-438.

Roggendorf, M., D. Yang, and M. Lu. "The Woodchuck: A Model for Therapeutic Vaccination Against Hepadnaviral Infection." *Pathologie Biologie* 58 (2010): 308-314.

WEB SITES OF INTEREST

Hepatitis B Foundation
http://www.hepb.org

Virus Pathogen Database and Analysis Resource
http://www.viprbrc.org/brc

See also: Contagious diseases; Hepatitis A; Hepatitis C; Hepatitis D; Hepatitis E; Hepatitis vaccines; HIV; Vaccines: Types; Viral hepatitis; Viral infections; Viruses: Structure and life cycle; Viruses: Types.

Hepatitis A

CATEGORY: Diseases and conditions
ANATOMY OR SYSTEM AFFECTED: Abdomen, gastrointestinal system, liver
ALSO KNOWN AS: Hep A, infectious hepatitis

DEFINITION

Hepatitis A is an infection of the liver that is caused by the hepatitis A virus. The infection was formerly called infectious hepatitis.

CAUSES

The hepatitis A virus is usually found in the stool (feces) of people who have the infection. It is spread by putting something in one's mouth that has been infected with the hepatitis A virus; by drinking water contaminated by raw sewage; by eating hepatitis-contaminated food, especially if it has not been properly cooked; by eating raw or partially cooked shellfish contaminated by raw sewage; and by having sexual contact (particularly anal sex) with a person who is infected with the hepatitis A virus.

RISK FACTORS

Risk factors for hepatitis A include close contact with an infected person (although the virus is generally not spread by casual contact); using household items that were used by an infected person but were not properly cleaned; having sex with multiple partners; having sex with a partner who has hepatitis A; traveling to or spending long periods of time in a country where hepatitis A is common or where sanitation is poor; injecting drugs, especially if sharing needles; changing diapers or toilet training young children; being in day-care centers or other similar facilities; and receiving plasma products (as do people with hemophilia).

SYMPTOMS

Hepatitis A does not always cause symptoms. Adults are more likely to have them than children. Symptoms include tiredness, loss of appetite, fever, nausea, abdominal pain or discomfort, jaundice (yellowing of the eyes and skin), darker colored urine, light or chalky colored stools, rash, itching, and muscle pain.

SCREENING AND DIAGNOSIS

A doctor will ask about symptoms and medical history and will perform a physical exam. Tests may include a blood test to look for hepatitis A antibodies (proteins that the body has made to fight the hepatitis A virus), liver function studies, and, in severe cases, a liver biopsy (removing a sample of liver tissue to be examined).

TREATMENT AND THERAPY

There are no specific treatments. The goals of hepatitis A treatments are to keep the patient as comfortable as possible, to prevent the infection from being passed to others, and to prevent more liver damage by

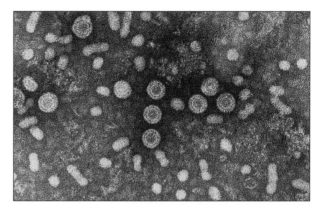

The hepatitis A virus in infected liver tissue. (AP/Wide World Photos)

helping the patient avoid substances such as medications and alcohol that might stress the liver while it is healing.

The disease will usually go away without treatment within two to five weeks. About 15 percent of people who are infected by hepatitis A will have relapsing symptoms. This can happen for up to nine months. In almost all cases, once a person recovers, there are no lasting effects and the person will be immune to the virus. In rare cases, the infection is severe, necessitating a liver transplant.

PREVENTION AND OUTCOMES

Prevention includes proper sanitary habits, such as washing one's hands with soap and water (important after using the toilet or changing a diaper); washing one's hands with soap and water before eating or preparing food; avoiding using household utensils that a person with hepatitis A may touch; ensuring that all household utensils are carefully cleaned; avoiding sexual contact with a person with hepatitis A; avoiding the use of injectable drugs and especially avoiding sharing needles. If one travels to a high-risk region, he or she should take the following precautions: drink bottled water, avoid ice chips, wash fruits well before eating, and eat well-cooked food.

Another preventive measure is to have an immunoglobulin (Ig) injection, which contains antibodies that provides temporary protection from hepatitis A. The Ig injection can last about one to three months and must be given before exposure to the virus or within two weeks after exposure.

Getting a hepatitis A vaccine is another measure. This vaccine is made from inactive hepatitis A virus and is highly effective in preventing infection. It provides full protection four weeks after the first injection. A second injection provides protection lasting up to twenty years. The vaccine is also used after exposure. If given within two weeks, it can prevent infection.

The hepatitis A vaccine is recommended for all children who are twelve months of age, children ages twelve months or older living in high-risk areas, people traveling to areas where hepatitis A is prevalent, people who have anal sex, drug users, people with chronic liver disease, people with blood-clotting disorders such as hemophilia, children who live in areas where hepatitis A is prevalent, and people who will have close contact with an adopted child from a medium- or high-risk area. One should consult a doctor before getting the vaccine.

Rick Alan; reviewed by David L. Horn, M.D., FACP

FURTHER READING

Boyer, Thomas D., Teresa L. Wright, and Michael P. Manns, eds. *Zakim and Boyer's Hepatology: A Textbook of Liver Disease.* 5th ed. Philadelphia: Saunders/Elsevier, 2006.

Centers for Disease Control and Prevention. "Hepatitis A: Questions and Answers." Available at http://www.cdc.gov.

EBSCO Publishing. *Health Library: Hepatitis A Vaccine.* Available through http://www.ebscohost.com.

_____. *Health Library: Hepatitis Prevention for Travelers.* Available through http://www.ebscohost.com.

Feldman, Mark, Lawrence S. Friedman, and Lawrence J. Brandt, eds. *Sleisenger and Fordtran's Gastrointestinal and Liver Disease: Pathophysiology, Diagnosis, Management.* New ed. 2 vols. Philadelphia: Saunders/Elsevier, 2010.

Frank, Steven A. *Immunology and Evolution of Infectious Disease.* Princeton, N.J.: Princeton University Press, 2002.

Palmer, Melissa. *Dr. Melissa Palmer's Guide to Hepatitis and Liver Disease.* Rev. ed. Garden City Park, N.Y.: Avery, 2004.

Ronco, Claudio, and Rinaldo Bellomo, eds. *Critical Care Nephrology.* 2d ed. Philadelphia: Saunders/Elsevier, 2009.

"An Updated Recommendation from the Advisory Committee on Immunization Practices (ACIP) for Use of Hepatitis A Vaccine in Close Contact of Newly Arriving International Adoptees." *Morbidity and Mortality Weekly Report* 58 (2009): 1006.

WEB SITES OF INTEREST

American Liver Foundation
http://www.liverfoundation.org

Canadian Institute for Health Information
http://www.cihi.ca

Hepatitis Foundation International
http://www.hepfi.org

Immunization Action Coalition
http://www.immunize.org

See also: Cancer and infectious disease; Contagious diseases; Fecal-oral route of transmission; Food-borne illness and disease; Hepatitis B; Hepatitis C; Hepatitis D; Hepatitis E; Hepatitis vaccines; HIV; Sexually transmitted diseases (STDs); Viral hepatitis; Viral infections; Waterborne illness and disease.

Hepatitis B

CATEGORY: Diseases and conditions
ANATOMY OR SYSTEM AFFECTED: Abdomen, gastrointestinal system, liver
ALSO KNOWN AS: Hep B

DEFINITION

Hepatitis B is a liver disease caused by the hepatitis B virus (HBV). Most hepatitis B infections clear up within one to two months without treatment. When the infection lasts more than six months, it can develop into chronic hepatitis B, which can lead to chronic inflammation of the liver, cirrhosis (scarring of the liver), liver cancer, liver failure, or death.

CAUSES

HBV is spread through contact with the body fluids of an infected person. These fluids include blood, semen, vaginal fluids, and saliva. A woman with hepatitis can pass the virus to the fetus during birth. HBV is not spread through food or water.

RISK FACTORS

The following factors may increase one's risk of getting hepatitis B: having sex with someone infected with hepatitis B or who is a carrier of hepatitis B; injecting illicit drugs, especially with shared needles; having more than one sexual partner; being a man who has sex with men; and living in the same home with someone who is infected with hepatitis B.

Another risk factor is employment as someone who has contact with human body fluids. These workers include first aid or emergency workers, funeral directors, medical personnel, rescue workers, firefighters, police personnel, dentists, and dental assistants.

Other risk factors are having a sexually transmitted disease when having contact with hepatitis B; traveling to areas of the world where hepatitis B is common, such as China, southeast Asia, and sub-Saharan Africa; receiving a blood transfusion before 1992 (the year a more reliable test to screen blood was developed); receiving multiple transfusions of blood or blood products, as do hemophiliacs (a risk that has been greatly reduced with modern blood screening techniques); working or being a patient in a hospital or long-term care facility; working or being incarcerated in a jail or prison; being bitten so that the skin is broken by someone whose saliva contains the virus; and receiving hemodialysis treatment.

SYMPTOMS

Symptoms may appear about 25 to 180 days after one is exposed to the virus. The most common symptoms are yellowing skin and eyes (jaundice), fatigue that lasts for weeks or even months, abdominal pain in the area of the liver (upper right side of the abdomen), loss of appetite, nausea, vomiting, joint pain, low-grade fever, dark urine and light-colored stool, widespread itching, and rash.

SCREENING AND DIAGNOSIS

A doctor will ask about symptoms and medical history and will perform a physical exam. Hepatitis B is diagnosed with blood tests. These blood tests are also used to monitor the virus's effect on the liver. For chronic cases, the patient may need a liver biopsy (the removal of a sample of liver tissue for testing).

TREATMENT AND THERAPY

If the patient has an uncomplicated case, he or she can expect to recover completely. Persons with chronic hepatitis B may be treated with medication to help reduce the activity of the virus and also to prevent liver failure. These medications include interferon alfa-2b (Intron A) injection, lamivudine (Epivir-HBV) oral medication, adefovir (Hepsera) oral medication, and entecavir (Baraclude) oral medication.

Persons who have chronic hepatitis B should avoid further injury to the liver by avoiding alcohol and certain medications, dietary supplements, and herbs. One should discuss these supplements and herbs with a doctor before taking.

One can prevent spreading the infection to others by notifying one's own doctors, dentists, and sexual partner or partners; by avoiding donating blood or organs for transplant; and by discussing one's hepatitis B status with a doctor during pregnancy or before becoming pregnant to ensure the baby receives treatment.

PREVENTION AND OUTCOMES

Hepatitis B can be prevented with a vaccination. It consists of three injections that are given over a period of six months. Protection is not complete without all three injections. Persons at increased risk for hepatitis B should be vaccinated.

In addition, to prevent the transmission of hepatitis B, one should use condoms during sexual intercourse or should abstain from sex, limit the number of sexual partners, avoid injecting drugs and avoid sharing needles or syringes, and avoid sharing personal items that might have blood on them (such as razors, toothbrushes, manicuring tools, and pierced earrings). Persons who get a tattoo or a body piercing should ensure that the artist or piercer properly sterilizes the equipment. Infection can occur if the tools have another person's blood on them.

Health care and public safety workers should get vaccinated against hepatitis B; should always follow routine barrier precautions and safely handle needles and other sharp instruments; should wear gloves when touching or cleaning up body fluids on bandages, tampons or sanitary pads, and linens; and should cover open cuts or wounds.

Pregnant women should have a blood test for hepatitis B. Infants born to women with hepatitis B should be treated within twelve hours of birth.

Karen Schroeder Kassel, M.S., RD, M.Ed.;
reviewed by David L. Horn, M.D., FACP

FURTHER READING

American Liver Foundation. "Hepatitis B." Available at http://www.liverfoundation.org/abouttheliver/info/hepatitisb.

Boyer, Thomas D., Teresa L. Wright, and Michael P. Manns, eds. *Zakim and Boyer's Hepatology: A Textbook of Liver Disease.* 5th ed. Philadelphia: Saunders/Elsevier, 2006.

Centers for Disease Control and Prevention. "Hepatitis B." Available at http://www.cdc.gov/hepatitis/hbv.

Feldman, Mark, Lawrence S. Friedman, and Lawrence J. Brandt, eds. *Sleisenger and Fordtran's Gastrointestinal and Liver Disease: Pathophysiology, Diagnosis, Management.* New ed. 2 vols. Philadelphia: Saunders/Elsevier, 2010.

Frank, Steven A. *Immunology and Evolution of Infectious Disease.* Princeton, N.J.: Princeton University Press, 2002.

Palmer, Melissa. *Dr. Melissa Palmer's Guide to Hepatitis and Liver Disease.* Rev. ed. Garden City Park, N.Y.: Avery, 2004.

Pan American Health Organization. World Health Organization. *Control of Diphtheria, Pertussis, Tetanus, "Haemophilus influenzae" Type B, and Hepatitis B Field Guide.* Washington, D.C.: Author, 2005.

WEB SITES OF INTEREST

American Liver Foundation
http://www.liverfoundation.org

Canadian Institute for Health Information
http://www.cihi.ca

Canadian Liver Foundation
http://www.liver.ca

Hepatitis B Foundation
http://www.hepb.org

Hepatitis Foundation International
http://www.hepfi.org

See also: Blood-borne illness and disease; Cancer and infectious disease; Childbirth and infectious disease; Contagious diseases; Hepatitis A; Hepatitis C; Hepatitis D; Hepatitis E; Hepatitis vaccines; HIV; Liver cancer; Saliva and infectious disease; Sexually transmitted diseases (STDs); Viral hepatitis; Viral infections.

Hepatitis C

CATEGORY: Diseases and conditions
ANATOMY OR SYSTEM AFFECTED: Abdomen, gastrointestinal system, liver
ALSO KNOWN AS: Hep C

DEFINITION

Hepatitis C is an infection of the liver caused by the hepatitis C virus (HCV).

CAUSES

The hepatitis C virus (HCV), which is carried in the blood of an infected person, is most often spread through contact with infected blood, such as through injecting illicit drugs with shared needles; receiving HCV-infected blood transfusions (before 1992) or blood clotting products (before 1987); receiving an HCV-infected organ through transplantation; receiving long-term kidney dialysis treatment (the machine might be tainted with HCV-infected blood); sharing toothbrushes, razors, nail clippers, or other personal hygiene items contaminated with HCV-infected blood; being accidentally stuck by an HCV-infected needle (a special concern for health care workers); frequent contact with HCV-infected people (a special concern for health care workers); and receiving a tattoo, body piercing, or acupuncture with unsterilized or improperly sterilized equipment.

Hepatitis C can also spread through an HCV-infected woman to her fetus at the time of birth, through sexual contact with someone infected with HCV, through sharing a straw or inhalation tube when inhaling drugs with someone infected by HCV, and through receiving a blood transfusion. HCV cannot spread through the air, unbroken skin, casual social contact, or breast-feeding.

RISK FACTORS

Factors that increase the chance of HCV infection include having received a blood transfusion before 1992, having received blood clotting products before 1987, having long-term kidney dialysis treatment, getting a tattoo or body piercing, injecting illicit drugs (especially with shared needles), and having sex with partners who have hepatitis C or other sexually transmitted diseases.

In-Home Medical Testing for Hepatitis C

In-home medical testing has become increasingly popular as a result of its convenience, privacy, and affordability. Home tests can help determine the potential risk for developing a health problem, such as an infectious disease, even when no immediate signs or symptoms exist. Home tests also can enable persons to follow a specific medical condition more accurately.

Several home tests are available for over-the-counter purchase, including those that test for hepatitis C. One should not use home test kits as stand-alone measures to determine the need for medical care. Rather, one should use the results in conjunction with proper medical advice to confirm the test results.

Most reports state that the test kits approved by the U.S. Food and Drug Administration (FDA) are either "about as accurate" or "fairly accurate," when compared to those that a doctor would use, provided that the instructions are carefully followed. No test is 100 percent accurate; test accuracy is improved when the test instructions are read, understand, and followed carefully. A home test kit will require accurate timing, specific collection materials, and typically a body fluid sample. Failure to comply with any of these factors could result in an inaccurate reading. If a product is not approved by the FDA, then the test's safety and efficacy is in question. Purchasing diagnostic test kits on the Web can be particularly problematic, because not all test kits available as a Web purchase are FDA-approved and some are illegal to sell online.

A search of the Clinical Laboratory Improvement Amendments (CLIA) database will inform persons if a home test has FDA approval. To use this search engine, one must know if the test is considered a "test kit" (a person takes a sample, performs the test, and analyzes it) or a "collection kit" (a person takes a sample but sends it to a laboratory for analysis). Collection kits are not listed on the CLIA database, although one can contact the FDA directly to find out if a kit is FDA-approved.

The FDA maintains another database called Manufacturer and User Facility Device Experience (MAUDE), which lists reports on problems with kits and testing devices. *Consumer Reports* magazine and its Web site also provide additional product comparison information for a handful of home tests.

Bonita L. Marks, Ph.D.

SYMPTOMS

Eighty percent of people with hepatitis C have no symptoms. Over time, the disease can cause serious liver damage. Symptoms may include fatigue, loss of appetite, jaundice (yellowing of the eyes and skin), darker colored urine, chalky and light-colored stools, loose and light-colored stools, abdominal pain, aches and pains, itching, hives, joint pain, nausea, and vomiting. Also, cigarette smokers may suddenly dislike the taste of cigarettes.

Chronic hepatitis C infection may cause some of the foregoing symptoms and also weakness, severe fatigue, and loss of appetite. Serious complications of hepatitis C infection include a chronic infection that will lead to cirrhosis (scarring) and progressive liver failure and an increased risk of liver cancer.

SCREENING AND DIAGNOSIS

A doctor will ask about symptoms and medical history and will perform a physical exam. Tests may include blood tests to look for hepatitis C antibodies (proteins that the body has made to fight the hepatitis C virus) or genetic material from the virus, liver function studies to initially determine and follow how well a person's liver is functioning, an ultrasound of the liver to assess liver damage, and a liver biopsy (removal of a sample of liver tissue to be examined).

TREATMENT AND THERAPY

Hepatitis C is usually treated with combined therapy, consisting of interferon (given by injection) and ribavirin (given orally). These medications can cause difficult side effects and they also have limited success rates. In unsuccessful cases, chronic hepatitis C can cause cirrhosis (scarring) and serious liver damage. A liver transplant may be needed.

PREVENTION AND OUTCOMES

To prevent becoming infected with hepatitis C, one should not inject illicit drugs (using shared needles has the highest risk), should avoid sex with partners who have sexually transmitted diseases (STDs), should practice safer sex (by using, for example, latex condoms) or abstain from sex, should limit the number of sexual partners, should not share personal items that might have blood on them (such as razors, toothbrushes, manicuring tools, and pierced earrings), and should avoid handling items that may be contaminated by HCV-infected blood. One also should donate his or her own blood before elective surgery so that this blood can be used if a blood transfusion is required during that surgery.

To prevent spreading hepatitis C to others if one is infected, one should notify his or her dentist and physician before receiving checkups or treatment, should get hepatitis A and B vaccinations, and should not donate blood or organs for transplant.

Rick Alan; reviewed by David L. Horn, M.D., FACP

FURTHER READING

American Liver Foundation. "Hepatitis C." Available at http://www.liverfoundation.org/abouttheliver/info/hepatitisc.

Boyer, Thomas D., Teresa L. Wright, and Michael P. Manns, eds. *Zakim and Boyer's Hepatology: A Textbook of Liver Disease.* 5th ed. Philadelphia: Saunders/Elsevier, 2006.

Centers for Disease Control and Prevention. "Hepatitis C." Available at http://www.cdc.gov/hepatitis/hcv.

Everson, Gregory T., and Hedy Weinberg. *Living with Hepatitis C: A Survivor's Guide.* 5th ed. New York: Hatherleigh Press, 2009.

Feldman, Mark, Lawrence S. Friedman, and Lawrence J. Brandt, eds. *Sleisenger and Fordtran's Gastrointestinal and Liver Disease: Pathophysiology, Diagnosis, Management.* New ed. 2 vols. Philadelphia: Saunders/Elsevier, 2010.

Frank, Steven A. *Immunology and Evolution of Infectious Disease.* Princeton, N.J.: Princeton University Press, 2002.

National Digestive Diseases Information Clearinghouse. "What I Need to Know About Hepatitis C." Available at http://digestive.niddk.nih.gov/ddiseases/pubs/hepc_ez.

Palmer, Melissa. *Dr. Melissa Palmer's Guide to Hepatitis and Liver Disease.* Rev. ed. Garden City Park, N.Y.: Avery, 2004.

Ronco, Claudio, and Rinaldo Bellomo, eds. *Critical Care Nephrology.* 2d ed. Philadelphia: Saunders/Elsevier, 2009.

WEB SITES OF INTEREST

American Liver Foundation
http://www.liverfoundation.org

Canadian Institute for Health Information
http://www.cihi.ca

Canadian Liver Foundation
http://www.liver.ca

Hepatitis Foundation International
http://www.hepfi.org

See also: Blood-borne illness and disease; Cancer and infectious disease; Childbirth and infectious disease; Contagious diseases; Hepatitis A; Hepatitis B; Hepatitis D; Hepatitis E; Hepatitis vaccines; HIV; Liver cancer; Sexually transmitted diseases (STDs); Viral hepatitis; Viral infections.

Hepatitis D

CATEGORY: Diseases and conditions
ANATOMY OR SYSTEM AFFECTED: Liver
ALSO KNOWN AS: Delta agent, delta hepatitis, hepatitis D virus

DEFINITION

Hepatitis D is a viral infection of the liver caused by the hepatitis D virus. The hepatitis D virus is infective only in persons who are also infected with active hepatitis B. Hepatitis D can initiate an infection at the same time as the initial hepatitis B infection (coinfection), or it can infect a person with lifelong (chronic) hepatitis B infection (superinfection). There are two types of hepatitis D: acute and chronic. Chronic infection can cause serious liver damage, or cirrhosis, and death.

CAUSES

Hepatitis D is caused by the hepatitis delta virus (HDV), which is a small, circular, enveloped ribonucleic acid (RNA) virus. HDV requires the help of a Hepadnavirus (hepatitis B virus, or HBV) for its own replication. The delta virus is an incomplete viral particle. Its companion virus, HBV, actually forms a covering over the HDV particle.

RISK FACTORS

Hepatitis B infection may occur simultaneously when HDV is spread, or the person may already have hepatitis B. In either case, transmission of HDV can occur in one of several ways: when blood from an infected person enters the body of a person who is not infected; through contact with other body fluids, such as semen, vaginal fluids, or saliva; and through contact with shared needles or through needle-sticks or other sharp exposures on the job. Rarely, transmission can occur from an infected woman to her fetus during childbirth.

SYMPTOMS

The symptoms of hepatitis D may include fatigue, loss of appetite, diarrhea, dark urine, abdominal pain, muscle pain, joint pain, sore throat, nausea, and vomiting. These early symptoms may be confused with symptoms common to the stomach flu.

SCREENING AND DIAGNOSIS

A doctor can test for hepatitis D through a series of blood tests that identify HDV antigen. Diagnostic tests may include liver enzyme tests, which look at certain levels of liver enzymes in the blood. Other tests will look for antibodies that the body has made against the hepatitis D virus.

TREATMENT AND THERAPY

Each type (acute and chronic) of hepatitis D is treated differently. There are no specific medicines that can cure hepatitis D, so treatment for acute hepatitis D is focused on dealing with symptoms or complications. Even without specialized treatment for acute hepatitis D, most people recover completely within a few weeks.

Although there are some indications that certain medicines used to treat hepatitis B may be effective against hepatitis D, there are no drugs that are approved to treat a chronic hepatitis D infection. These medicines include alpha interferon and pegylated alpha interferon. There is no consent, however, on how much of these medicines should be used or on a time line for use.

PREVENTION AND OUTCOMES

The best prevention against hepatitis D infection is to obtain a vaccination against hepatitis B. Persons who are not infected with hepatitis B cannot contract hepatitis D.

Camillia King, M.P.H.

FURTHER READING

Boyer, Thomas D., Teresa L. Wright, and Michael P. Manns, eds. *Zakim and Boyer's Hepatology: A Textbook of Liver Disease.* 5th ed. Philadelphia: Saunders/Elsevier, 2006.

Feldman, Mark, Lawrence S. Friedman, and Lawrence J. Brandt, eds. *Sleisenger and Fordtran's Gastrointestinal and Liver Disease: Pathophysiology, Diagnosis, Management.* New ed. 2 vols. Philadelphia: Saunders/Elsevier, 2010.

Taylor, J. M. "Hepatitis Delta Virus." *Virology* 344 (January, 2006): 71-76.

WEB SITES OF INTEREST

American Liver Foundation
http://www.liverfoundation.org

Centers for Disease Control and Prevention
http://www.cdc.gov/hepatitis

Hepatitis Foundation International
http://www.hepfi.org

World Health Organization
http://www.who.int/csr/disease/hepatitis/whocdscsrncs20011

See also: Blood-borne illness and disease; Childbirth and infectious disease; Contagious diseases; Hepatitis B; Hepatitis vaccines; HIV; Liver cancer; Saliva and infectious disease; Secondary infection; Sexually transmitted diseases (STDs); Treatment of viral infections; Viral hepatitis; Viral infections.

Hepatitis E

CATEGORY: Diseases and conditions
ANATOMY OR SYSTEM AFFECTED: Gastrointestinal system, intestines, liver
ALSO KNOWN AS: Hepatitis E virus

DEFINITION

Hepatitis E is a viral liver infection transmitted through the intestinal tract. Hepatitis E, which is an acute, short-lived illness that can sometimes cause liver failure, is more common in regions of the world that lack clean water and environmentally safe sanitation.

CAUSES

Hepatitis E is primarily spread by fecal-oral transmission. It is commonly found in countries where human waste contaminates the water sources. Large outbreaks have occurred in Asia and South America that have poor sanitation. In the United States and Canada, no outbreaks have been reported, but persons traveling to an endemic region may return infected with the hepatitis E virus (HEV).

RISK FACTORS

Risk factors for hepatitis E are factors that do not seem to be a direct cause of the disease. Hepatitis E occurs in both epidemic and sporadic-endemic forms usually associated with contaminated drinking water. Because this disease is primarily a result of a lack of water filtration in underdeveloped countries, there are no specific risks associated with it. Water filtration systems are prevalent in most developed countries, such as the United States, Canada, and China, and in the countries of Europe. Historically, the only major waterborne epidemics have occurred in Asia and North and West Africa.

SYMPTOMS

The symptoms of hepatitis E include flulike symptoms, fever, fatigue, nausea, vomiting, loss of appetite, abdominal pain, diarrhea, and jaundice.

SCREENING AND DIAGNOSIS

Cases of hepatitis E are not clinically evident from other types of acute viral hepatitis. Diagnoses are usually made by blood tests that detect elevated levels of specific antibodies to hepatitis E in the body or by reverse transcriptase polymerase chain reaction. However, these tests are not yet widely available.

When waterborne hepatitis occurs in developing countries, especially if the disease is more severe in pregnant women, hepatitis E should be suspected if hepatitis A has been excluded. If laboratory tests are not available, epidemiologic evidence can help in establishing a diagnosis.

TREATMENT AND THERAPY

Hepatitis E is classified as a viral disease, so there is no effective treatment of acute hepatitis. Consequently, antibiotics are of no significance in the treatment of the viral infection. Hepatitis E infections usually remain in the intestinal tract, and hospitalization is gen-

erally not required. However, there are reports of HEV damaging and destroying liver cells, so much so that the liver cannot function. This is called fulminant liver failure, a condition that can lead to death. Pregnant women are at a higher risk of dying from fulminant liver failure. This increased risk is not constant with any other type of viral hepatitis.

The majority of persons who recover from acute infection do not continue to carry HEV and, thus, cannot pass the infection to others. No available therapy can alter the course of acute infection. Also, there are no vaccines for hepatitis E that have been approved by the U.S. Food and Drug Administration.

PREVENTION AND OUTCOMES

Prevention is the most effective approach against hepatitis E. The most effective way to prevent hepatitis E is to provide and consume safe drinking water and to take precautions to use sterilized water and beverages when traveling to an endemic region.

Camillia King, M.P.H.

FURTHER READING

Feldman, Mark, Lawrence S. Friedman, and Lawrence J. Brandt, eds. *Sleisenger and Fordtran's Gastrointestinal and Liver Disease: Pathophysiology, Diagnosis, Management.* New ed. 2 vols. Philadelphia: Saunders/Elsevier, 2010.

Kamar, N., et al. "Hepatitis E Virus and Chronic Hepatitis in Organ-Transplant Recipients." *New England Journal of Medicine* 358 (2008): 811-817.

Shrestha, M. P., et al. "Safety and Efficacy of a Recombinant Hepatitis E Vaccine." *New England Journal of Medicine* 356 (2007): 895-903.

WEB SITES OF INTEREST

American Liver Foundation
http://www.liverfoundation.org

Centers for Disease Control and Prevention
http://www.cdc.gov/hepatitis

Hepatitis Foundation International
http://www.hepfi.org

World Health Organization
http://www.who.int/csr/disease/hepatitis/whocdscsredc200112

See also: Developing countries and infectious disease; Emerging and reemerging infectious diseases; Endemic infections; Fecal-oral route of transmission; Hepatitis D; Hepatitis vaccines; Treatment of viral infections; Viral hepatitis; Viral infections; Waterborne illness and disease.

Hepatitis vaccines

CATEGORY: Prevention

DEFINITION

Hepatitis is inflammation of the liver caused by a viral infection. There are five types of hepatitis infection: A, B, C, D, and E. Not all of these types of hepatitis, however, can be prevented by vaccination.

PREVENTION

The types of viral hepatitis that can be prevented by a vaccine are hepatitis A and hepatitis B. Hepatitis A can be prevented by the use of Havrix or Vaqta. Hepatitis B can be prevented by the use of Engerix-B or Recombivax HB. Both A and B can be prevented by the use of Comvax, Pediarix, and Twinrix. A vaccine for hepatitis E is being tested but has not been approved by the U.S. Food and Drug Administration.

Hepatitis A vaccine is available for people in high-risk groups, such as day-care and nursing-home staff, laboratory staff, and those traveling to parts of the world where hepatitis is common. Routine childhood immunization against hepatitis A is also recommended.

Hepatitis B vaccine is given to all infants and unvaccinated children. The vaccine is available for adults at high risk, such as health care professionals, intravenous-drug users, and those who do not practice safer sex.

REQUISITE DOSAGES

Dosages are administered at intervals. No vaccine series should be restarted. Licensed combination vaccines may be used when any component of the combination is indicated and when its other component (or components) is not contraindicated. The use of licensed combination vaccines is preferred over separate injection of their equivalent component vaccines.

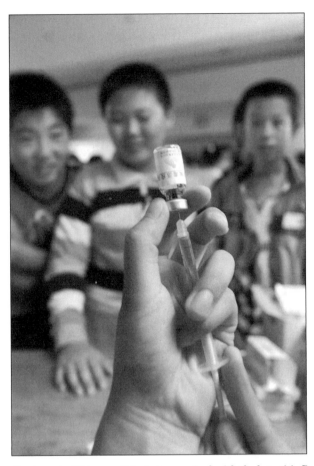

Students in China wait to be immunized with the hepatitis B vaccine in 2009. (AP/Wide World Photos)

Engerix-B or Recombivax HB should be used for the hepatitis B vaccine birth dose.

IMPACT

Hepatitis A and B are highly contagious. Hepatitis A is spread readily in locations with poor sanitary conditions and hepatitis B is spread through contact with the blood or body fluids of infected persons. However, hepatitis A, along with hepatitis E, are typically caused by the ingestion of contaminated food or water. Of the many persons at risk of being infected with these diseases, those who are at higher risk include people who work or travel in areas with high rates of infection and all children older than age one year.

Margaret Ring Gillock, M.S.

Further Reading

Centers for Disease Control and Prevention. "Global Routine Vaccination Coverage, 2009." *MMWR: Morbidity and Mortality Weekly Report* 59 (2010): 1367-1371.

Dienstag, J. L. "Hepatitis B Virus Infection." *New England Journal of Medicine* 359 (2008): 1486-1500.

Jou, J. H., and A. J. Muir. "In the Clinic: Hepatitis C." *Annals of Internal Medicine* 148 (2008): ITC6-1-ITC6-16.

Plotkin, Stanley A., and Walter A. Orenstein, eds. *Vaccines.* 5th ed. Philadelphia: Saunders/Elsevier, 2008.

Sjogren, M. H. "Hepatitis A." In *Sleisenger and Fordtran's Gastrointestinal and Liver Disease: Pathophysiology, Diagnosis, Management,* edited by Mark Feldman, Lawrence S. Friedman, and Lawrence J. Brandt. New ed. 2 vols. Philadelphia: Saunders/Elsevier, 2010.

Web Sites of Interest

Centers for Disease Control and Prevention
http://www.cdc.gov/hepatitis

Hepatitis Foundation International
http://www.hepfi.org

Vaccine Research Center
http://www.niaid.nih.gov/about/organization/vrc

World Health Organization
http://www.who.int/immunization

See also: Asplenia; Childbirth and infectious disease; Developing countries and infectious disease; Emerging and reemerging infectious diseases; Endemic infections; Fecal-oral route of transmission; Hepatitis A; Hepatitis B; Hepatitis C; Hepatitis D; Hepatitis E; Inflammation; Sexually transmitted diseases (STDs); Vaccines: History; Vaccines: Types; Viral hepatitis; Viral infections; Virology; Waterborne illness and disease.

Herpes simplex infection

Category: Diseases and conditions
Anatomy or system affected: Genitalia, mouth, skin
Also known as: Cold sore, fever blister, genital herpes

Definition

Herpes simplex infection is a sore or blister caused by the herpes simplex virus (HSV) that can occur on the face or the genital area. The blisters contain fluid that harbors the virus.

Causes

Herpes simplex infection is caused when the virus is transmitted by person-to-person contact or by contact with contaminated items. HSV type 1 usually causes cold sores or blisters on the lips, while HSV type 2 is usually the cause of genital herpes. Kissing, oral sex, or other sexual acts may transmit the virus. Sharing infected items (fomites), such as lipstick, dishes, and towels, may also cause infection. Pregnant women may infect their fetuses during a vaginal birth.

Risk Factors

Exposure to someone with an active infection and contact with contaminated items are risk factors for infection with HSV. Newborns and persons who are stressed or who have a weak immune system are more at risk. Previous infection with herpes simplex is a risk factor in future infections. Unprotected sex is a risk factor for genital herpes.

Symptoms

The presence of small, painful blisters that are filled with fluid is the primary symptom of infection with HSV. A tingling or painful sensation may occur before blister development. Blister development may take a few weeks after exposure to the virus.

Screening and Diagnosis

There is no recommended routine screening test for the HSV. For cold sores, diagnosis is usually made based on symptoms. A physician will ask about previous cold sores, current stress levels, tingling or pain before the blister developed, and exposure to others with cold sores. For genital herpes, a herpes viral culture of the fluid in the blister may be used in addition to the physician's examination. A herpesvirus antigen test involves the use of a microscope to find markers on cells that indicate infection. A polymerase chain reaction test can be used with fluids from sores, blood, or spinal fluid to look for genetic material and can determine if the virus is type 1 or type 2.

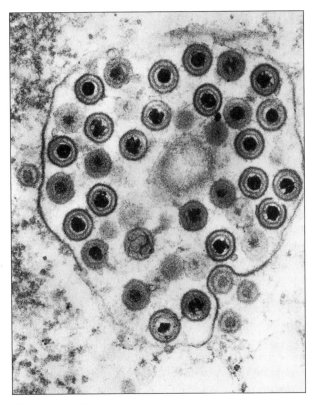

A herpes simplex virus.

TREATMENT AND THERAPY

Outbreaks of herpes simplex infection may occur several times a year. Cold sores usually will clear up on their own or with over-the-counter treatments. Persons who have frequent cold sores, an impaired immune system, a cold sore that does not heal, or severe symptoms including pain, should contact a doctor. Oral antiviral drugs may be prescribed by the doctor if outbreaks are severe. Cold or warm cloths applied to the blister may ease the pain.

Genital herpes requires a visit to a physician. There is no treatment that can cure genital herpes, but medication is available to treat outbreaks and to suppress the virus.

PREVENTION AND OUTCOMES

One should not share personal items with persons who have visible cold sores, should refrain from eating and drinking from shared plates and cups, and should use good handwashing technique. Genital herpes can be transmitted even when blisters are not present, so one should abstain from sexual contact when blisters

are visible. Latex condoms, when correctly used, may reduce the risk of herpes simplex infection, but they cannot eliminate infection.

Patricia Stanfill Edens, R.N., Ph.D., FACHE

FURTHER READING

Gordon, Sara C., et al. "Viral Infections of the Mouth." Available at http://emedicine.medscape.com/article/1079920-overview.

James, S. H., and R. J. Whitley. "Treatment of Herpes Simplex Virus Infections in Pediatric Patients: Current Status and Future Needs." *Clinical Pharmacology and Therapeutics* 88 (2010): 720-724.

Kane, Melissa, and Tatyana Gotovkina. "Common Threads in Persistent Viral Infections." *Journal of Virology* 84 (2010): 4116-4123.

Khare, Manjiri. "Infectious Disease in Pregnancy." *Current Obstetrics and Gynaecology* 15 (2005): 149-156.

WEB SITES OF INTEREST

American Social Health Association
http://www.ashastd.org

Centers for Disease Control and Prevention
http://www.cdc.gov/std

HerpesGuide.ca
http://www.herpesguide.ca

See also: Childbirth and infectious disease; Cold sores; Genital herpes; Herpesviridae; Herpesvirus infections; Mouth infections; Oral transmission; Pregnancy and infectious disease; Saliva and infectious disease; Sexually transmitted diseases (STDs); Viral infections.

Herpes zoster infection

CATEGORY: Diseases and conditions
ANATOMY OR SYSTEM AFFECTED: Abdomen, muscles, peripheral nervous system, skin
ALSO KNOWN AS: Ramsay Hunt syndrome, shingles

DEFINITION

Herpes zoster infection, or shingles, is a painful skin rash with blisters that usually occurs in a band around one side of the abdomen. Shingles occurs after a previous episode of chickenpox, a childhood disease that was especially common before the availability of a vaccination. In rare cases, shingles can affect the facial nerve and cause muscle weakness or facial paralysis; this condition is called Ramsay Hunt syndrome.

CAUSES

Shingles is caused by the varicella zoster virus. After infecting a person with chickenpox, the virus stays in some nerves of the body but remains dormant or inactive. There is no known reason why the virus becomes active and causes shingles.

RISK FACTORS

Persons who have had chickenpox may develop shingles. The risk for developing shingles, which is most common in older adults, increases with age. A weakened immune system may create a higher risk for shingles too. A weakened immune system can be caused by human immunodeficiency virus (HIV) infection, acquired immunodeficiency syndrome (AIDS), long-term steroid use, and cancer treatments.

SYMPTOMS

The first symptoms of shingles include pain, burning, or tingling on one side of the body from the middle of the back to the breastbone in the front. Red patches that develop into fluid-filled blisters on the skin occur in most people. The blisters eventually break and form small ulcers that dry and become crusty. These crusts fall off in two to three weeks, and scarring rarely occurs. The rash may occur on the face, ears, and mouth, and around the eyes. Additional symptoms include pain, chills, fever, difficulty moving facial muscles, headache, a general uncomfortable feeling, joint pain, swollen glands, and hearing, vision, and taste problems.

SCREENING AND DIAGNOSIS

There is no screening test for shingles. Diagnosis is made based on symptoms and a history of chickenpox infection. Pain on one side of the body and the telltale rash usually indicate shingles, but the examining physician may also take fluid or tissue samples from the blisters and send them to a laboratory for testing. A blood test may show an increase in white blood cells and antibodies to the varicella zoster virus, but this test does not confirm that the rash is caused by shingles.

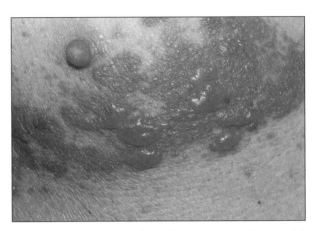

Rash and blisters on the chest of a ninety-year-old man with shingles, or herpes zoster infection.

TREATMENT AND THERAPY

Antiviral medicines in pill form or given intravenously may be prescribed to reduce pain, decrease the risk of complications, and shorten the course of the disease. Corticosteroids, such as prednisone, may be used to decrease swelling and pain. Pain medicines and antihistamines in pill or cream form may be used to reduce pain and itching. A cream containing an extract of pepper called capsaicin may be used to prevent postherpetic neuralgia, a condition in which pain and irritation persists after the blisters disappear. Soothing baths with oatmeal, calamine lotion, and cool cloths or compresses may also relieve discomfort. One should keep the rash area clean and should disinfect items used for treatment.

PREVENTION AND OUTCOMES

Persons who have not had chickenpox or the chickenpox vaccine should avoid coming in contact with the rash and blisters of a person with shingles or chickenpox. For persons age sixty years and older, a herpes zoster vaccine is available that may reduce complications from shingles. The person with shingles is contagious until the blisters dry out.

Patricia Stanfill Edens, R.N., Ph.D., FACHE

FURTHER READING

Ward, Mark A. "Varicella." In *Conn's Current Therapy 2011*, edited by Robert E. Rakel, Edward T. Bope, and Rick D. Kellerman. Philadelphia: Saunders/ Elsevier, 2010.

Weaver, Bethany A. "Herpes Zoster Overview: Natural

History and Incidence." *Journal of the American Osteo-pathic Association* 109 (2009): S2-S6.

Whitley, Richard J. "Varicella-Zoster Virus." In *Mandell, Douglas, and Bennett's Principles and Practice of Infectious Diseases*, edited by Gerald L. Mandell, John F. Bennett, and Raphael Dolin. 7th ed. New York: Churchill Livingstone/Elsevier, 2010.

WEB SITES OF INTEREST

American Academy of Dermatology
http://www.aad.org

National Immunization Program
http://www.cdc.gov/nip

National Institute of Neurological Disorders and Stroke
http://www.ninds.nih.gov/disorders/shingles

National Shingles Foundation
http://www.vzvfoundation.org

See also: Aging and infectious disease; Bell's palsy; Chickenpox; Herpes simplex infection; Herpesviridae; Herpesvirus infections; Immunity; Immunization; Postherpetic neuralgia; Reinfection; Scabies; Shingles; Skin infections; Stress and infectious disease; Viral infections.

Herpesviridae

CATEGORY: Pathogen
TRANSMISSION ROUTE: Direct contact

DEFINITION

The herpesviridae family comprises more than one hundred viruses that infect mammals, primarily. Eight of the viruses are associated with human infections. All known herpesviruses consist of a large double-stranded deoxyribonucleic acid (DNA) genome enclosed within an icosahedral capsid. This capsid ranges in size from 100 to 300 nanometers and is surrounded by a membranous envelope.

NATURAL HABITAT AND FEATURES

Most members of the herpesviridae are found naturally in humans. Initial infection generally results in

---

Taxonomic Classification for Herpesviridae
Kingdom: Unassigned
Order: Herpesvirales
Family: Herpesviridae
Subfamily: Alphaherpesvirinae
Genera: *Simplexvirus, Varicellovirus*
Order: Herpesvirales
Family: Herpesviridae
Subfamily: Betaherpesvirinae
Genera: *Cytomegalovirus, Roseolovirus*
Order: Herpesvirales
Family: Herpesviridae
Subfamily: Gammaherpesvirinae
Genera: *Lymphocryptovirus, Rhadinovirus*

pclinical disease that can take different forms depending upon the cells infected. All herpesviruses can undergo latency, in which a virus is retained within a proportion of infected cells but is not undergoing active replication. The virus may be reactivated at any time, resulting in recurrence of clinical symptoms and in the shedding of the virus.

The herpesviruses are largely species-specific. Humans are the sole reservoir for the viruses, though a minimum of one simian virus, *H. simiae*, also known as monkey B virus and now called cercopithecine herpesvirus-1, can pass from rhesus monkeys to humans.

PATHOGENICITY AND CLINICAL SIGNIFICANCE

The diversity of the human herpesviruses coupled with the types of cells they infect result in a variety of diseases with which they are associated. The specific clinical appearance following infection depends upon the site and form of exposure.

Human herpesvirus-1 (HHV-1) and human herpesvirus-2 (HHV-2). HHV-1 and HHV-2, formerly called herpes simplex-1,2, initially infect surface epithelial cells, resulting in cold sores or fever blisters. The virus then establishes latency in nerve ganglia associated with the site of infection. HHV-1 is primarily a childhood infection that leads to sores around the mouth; it is generally transmitted by children who, by touching herpes lesions, pass the virus to others. HHV-2 historically was a sexually transmitted virus that led to genital sores.

Human herpesvirus-1 (HHV-3). Initial exposure to

HHV-3, formerly called the varicella zoster virus, leads to the childhood disease chickenpox. The virus is generally passed through respiratory secretions. As a childhood disease, chickenpox is usually mild; if the first infection is in an adult, however, the disease may be more severe and potentially life-threatening. The virus remains in a latent state within nerve ganglia. Reactivation of the virus produces a rash, usually in the trunk region, called shingles.

Human herpesvirus-4 (HHV-4). Also called the Epstein-Barr virus, HHV-4 is a respiratory virus, infecting the glands of the nasopharynx region. Initial exposure may result in the so-called kissing disease known as infectious mononucleosis. The virus establishes latency in lymphocytes. The same virus is associated with two forms of cancer: Burkitt's lymphoma and nasopharyngeal carcinoma, and has been linked to Hodgkin's disease.

Human herpesvirus-5 (HHV-5). Also known as cytomegalovirus, HHV-5 is passed with respiratory secretions and establishes latency in lymphocytes. The virus is generally harmless in otherwise healthy persons. However, the virus can cross the placenta, so infection in a pregnant woman can lead to severe birth defects and disorders to her child.

Human herpesvirus-6 (HHV-6) and Human herpesvirus-7 (HHV-7). Associated with roseola in infants, HHV-6 is sometimes referred to as sixth disease, in which children may develop a rashlike illness. It is latent in lymphocytes and is likely passed in respiratory secretions. Also latent in lymphocytes, HHV-7 is not, however, associated with any known disease.

Human herpesvirus-8 (HHV-8). The site of latency for HHV-8 is unknown. In healthy persons, the virus appears harmless, but in immunosuppressed persons, such as those who have human immunodeficiency virus infection, the reactivation of HHV-8 may result in Kaposi's sarcoma.

DRUG SUSCEPTIBILITY

All of the human herpesviruses establish latency in cells specific to that virus and all are maintained for the life of the infected person. Antiviral treatment is often useful in suppressing viral growth, limiting the pathological effects of the disease, and reducing the ability of the virus to pass from one person to another. However, the virus is never completely eliminated from the infected person, and recurrence of the infection may sporadically take place.

All of the antiviral drugs proven effective in treatment of Herpesviridae infections have been DNA analogs, molecules that structurally resemble those used in synthesis of DNA during viral replication but that actually inhibit the process. The principle underlying the use of these drugs takes advantage of the fact that these viruses encode their own unique DNA polymerase, which preferentially incorporates the analogs in place of the correct nucleotides during DNA synthesis. The equivalent cell polymerase, used in replicating cell DNA, is less likely to use these same analogs. Consequently, normal cell replication is unaffected.

The earliest developed of these analogs was acyclovir, a molecule similar in structure to the thymdine normally used in DNA. Incorporation of the drug into replicating DNA inhibits the elongation of the growing strand, blocking viral replication.

Similar analogs, including valacyclovir, vidarabine, and ganciclovir, were developed for the treatment of herpes simplex and other herpesviruses. All of these analogs act either by directly inhibiting the viral polymerase or by blocking the chain growth of replicating DNA.

Richard Adler, Ph.D.

FURTHER READING

Brooks, George, et al. *Jawetz, Melnick, and Adelberg's Medical Microbiology*. 25th ed. New York: McGraw-Hill, 2010. Among the most useful of the medical microbiology texts. Chapters provide useful overviews without overwhelming the reader with minutiae. Several chapters address the herpesviruses and antiviral therapy.

Knipe, David M., and Peter M. Howley, eds. *Fields' Virology*. 5th ed. Philadelphia: Wolters Kluwer Health/Lippincott Williams & Wilkins, 2007. Arguably one of the most complete compendia on animal viruses. Several chapters deal with the human herpesviruses.

Strauss, James, and Ellen Strauss. *Viruses and Human Disease*. 2d ed. Boston: Academic Press/Elsevier, 2008. Extensive summary of the most important human pathogens. Chapters are arranged on the basis of types of genomes and include sections on newly emerging diseases.

Wagner, Edward K., and Martinez J. Hewlett. *Basic Virology*. 3d ed. Malden, Mass.: Blackwell Science, 2008. Summary of viral replication and pathogenesis.

Several portions of chapters deal specifically with the herpesviruses.

WEB SITES OF INTEREST

HerpesGuide.ca
http://www.herpesguide.ca

International Committee on Taxonomy of Viruses
http://www.ictvonline.org

Universal Virus Database
http://www.ictvdb.org

Viral Zone
http://www.expasy.org/viralzone

See also: Antiviral drugs: Types; Chickenpox; Childbirth and infectious disease; Cold sores; Cytomegalovirus infection; Epstein-Barr virus infection; Herpes simplex infection; Herpes zoster infection; Herpesvirus infections; HIV; Pregnancy and infectious disease; Sexually transmitted diseases (STDs); Shingles; Viral infections; Viruses: Structure and life cycle; Viruses: Types.

Herpesvirus infections

CATEGORY: Diseases and conditions
ANATOMY OR SYSTEM AFFECTED: All

DEFINITION

Herpesviruses are large, complex viruses composed of double-stranded DNA (deoxyribonucleic acid). More than one hundred herpesviruses are known, but only eight infect humans. The human herpesvirus (HHV) family is divided into three subfamilies based on the duration of viral reproductive cycle, ability to grow in cell culture, and location of the latent virus in the body. Alphaherpesvirinae contains the simplexviruses (HSV-1 and HSV-2) and varicellovirus (VZV), while Betaherpesvirinae includes cytomegalovirus (HCMV) and roseolovirus (HHV-6 and HHV-7). Gammaherpesvirinae is composed of lymphocryptovirus (Epstein-Barr virus, or EBV) and Kaposi's sarcoma-associated herpesvirus (HHV-8).

CAUSES

Herpesvirus infections are highly contagious and spread by direct personal contact through sharing saliva or secretions or by contact with skin that is shedding the virus. After primary infection, the herpesvirus remains latent in the body in an inactive phase. However, under stressors, the virus enters a lytic cycle, whereby it replicates, travels to the skin surface, and reactivates the infection.

RISK FACTORS

Persons who are immunocompromised, such as those with human immunodeficiency virus (HIV) infection or cancer or those who have had an organ transplant, have the greatest risk for contracting herpesvirus infections. Unprotected sex increases transmission risk too.

Predisposing factors for reactivation of a latent virus include colds or fevers, exposure to ultraviolet radiation, hormonal fluctuations, stress, and trauma. Some infections occur more frequently in the winter and spring seasons.

Young children are at greater risk for certain herpesvirus infections, such as cytomegalovirus (CMV) and chickenpox, while increasing age is associated with more severe symptoms when VZV is reactivated. Risk factors for vertical transmission of herpesviruses include primary infection within the pregnancy, prolonged rupture of the amniotic sac before delivery, and vaginal delivery.

SYMPTOMS

An incubation period exists from initial herpesvirus contact to the appearance of clinical symptoms. Primary exposure may be asymptomatic or symptomatic.

Clinical findings associated with HSV-1 and, less commonly, HSV-2 include cold sores, otherwise known as fever blisters. These painful fluid-filled blisters occur on the mouth, lips, and nose and may be accompanied by swelling of the gums and lips. Recurrences typically occur in the same location.

Genital herpes are more common with an HSV-2 rather than an HSV-1 infection. Herpetic lesions appear as open sores or as red bumps on the genitalia, anus, thighs, or buttocks and may be associated with painful urination or abnormal discharge. Primary genital herpes takes longer to heal than recurrent outbreaks because of a lack of immune resistance.

HSV-2 is also the primary virus implicated with neonatal herpes, which may cause skin lesions and central nervous system abnormalities of the neonate when contracted through the vaginal birth canal.

Primary VZV infection causes chickenpox and subsequently confers lifelong immunity to varicella. VZV reactivation results in herpes zoster, or shingles. Herpes zoster is characterized by a vesicular rash on the specific segment of the body where the varicella infection previously occurred and by pain that may persist for some time after the rash is treated. Fetal varicella syndrome occurs with primary maternal varicella exposure in the first and second trimester of pregnancy, causing mental retardation, seizures, and underdeveloped limbs.

Children and adults with CMV infection are often asymptomatic, but the virus causes the most common congenital infection in the United States. Severely affected newborns may have hearing loss, vision loss, mental retardation, cerebral palsy, seizures, and liver disease. Roseolovirus is often seen in children and causes roseola infantum, characterized by a fever and a faint pink rash that begins on the body trunk and spreads to the extremities. Symptoms generally spontaneously resolve, but seizures may occur during the febrile period.

Infants become susceptible to EBV when maternal antibody protection disappears following birth. Infected children may be asymptomatic or have mild flulike symptoms, but infections in adulthood lead to mononucleosis, hepatitis, and encephalitis. Symptoms last for several months after initial onset. When reactivated, EBV increases the risk for cancers including Hodgkin's and Burkitt's lymphoma.

HHV-8 has little consequence in a healthy person but manifests with flulike symptoms. In an immunosuppressed person, a primary infection is more severe and possibly fatal. HHV-8 causes Kaposi's sarcoma, an aggressive tumor and the most common malignancy found with acquired immunodeficiency syndrome. HHV-8 has also been implicated with diseases such as sarcoidosis and multiple myeloma.

Screening and Diagnosis

Often, laboratory tests are not needed to diagnose a herpesvirus infection, as symptoms are clinically recognizable. Serology and polymerase chain reaction studies are available to confirm many infections, although the tests are not always accurate or useful for treatment. Prenatal tests, such as an amniocentesis, are diagnostic for cytomegalovirus and varicella, as they confer a risk to the pregnancy if vertically transmitted during pregnancy. Physical examinations are also performed in pregnancy and labor to detect active genital herpes outbreaks.

Treatment and Therapy

Treatment for most herpesvirus infections remains supportive because many infections spontaneously resolve. Topical creams, ointments, and lotions are available for pain, and acetaminophen can be taken to reduce fevers. Antiviral medications are prescribed for some but not all herpesviruses to shorten the duration of symptoms; these are most effective when taken at the first sign of illness. Steroids are controversial for mononucleosis from EBV as a means to reduce swelling of the throat and tonsils.

Prevention and Outcomes

Although people are most contagious during an active outbreak of herpesvirus, the virus is shed in saliva, feces, or skin after an infection has apparently resolved. Therefore, proper hygienic practices, such as frequent handwashing, sterilizing of household items, and avoiding the sharing of toiletries, are all recommended. Safe sexual practices, such as abstinence or the use of condoms, are encouraged.

Despite myriad recommendations, herpesvirus infections are lifelong and have no efficacious method of prevention or cure. The exception is the VZV vaccines that are routinely administered to children and immunocompetent adults. Other vaccines for CMV infections are in clinical trials.

Janet Ober Berman, M.S., CGC

Further Reading

Edelman, Daniel C. "Human Herpesvirus 8: A Novel Human Pathogen." *Virology Journal* 2 (2005): 1-32. Description of the most recent discovery of HHV-8 and its implication in herpesvirus disease.

James, S. H., and R. J. Whitley. "Treatment of Herpes Simplex Virus Infections in Pediatric Patients: Current Status and Future Needs." *Clinical Pharmacology and Therapeutics* 88 (2010): 720-724. Review of HSV-1 and HSV-2 infections and symptomatology in newborn and pediatric patients.

Oxman, Michael N. "Zoster Vaccine: Current Status and Future Prospects." *Vaccines* 51 (2010): 197-213.

Article compares and contrasts HSV to VZV when discussing the possibility of future herpesvirus vaccines.

WEB SITES OF INTEREST

HerpesGuide.ca
http://www.herpesguide.ca

International Herpes Alliance
http://www.herpesalliance.org

See also: Chickenpox; Childbirth and infectious disease; Cold sores; Cytomegalovirus vaccine; Epstein-Barr virus infection; Herpes simplex infection; Herpes zoster infection; Herpesviridae; HIV; Kaposi's sarcoma; Pregnancy and infectious disease; Saliva and infectious disease; Sarcoidosis; Sexually transmitted diseases (STDs); Shingles; Treatment of viral infections; Viral infections; Viruses: Structure and life cycle; Viruses: Types.

Hib vaccine

CATEGORY: Prevention
ALSO KNOWN AS: *Haemophilus influenzae* type B vaccine

DEFINITION

The Hib vaccine protects against disease caused by the bacterium *Haemophilus influenzae* type B. This bacterium (also called Hib) can lead to infection of the coverings of the spinal cord and brain (meningitis) and infections of the epiglottis (epiglottitis) and blood (sepsis), among other areas of the body. These infections are dangerous and can be fatal, even with adequate treatment.

Other strains of *H. influenzae* exist and are commonly referred to as nontypeable *H. influenzae*. These strains can cause infection, though these diseases are much less virulent than those caused by *H. influenzae*. These infections, which are common in the ear, sinuses, and lower respiratory tract, rarely spread to the bloodstream and rarely cause meningitis

MECHANISM

The Hib vaccine is made by taking the shell (the polysaccharide coating) of the Hib bacterium and linking it to another protein. Injection of this safe combination incites the body to produce an immune response against this Hib bacteria coating without actually causing the disease, thus protecting against future infection.

HISTORY

The first version of the Hib vaccine was released in 1985 and was placed on the recommended pediatric immunization schedule starting in 1989. The vaccine eventually was combined with the DTaP (diphtheria, tetanus, and pertussis) vaccine in 1996 as TriHIBit (diphtheria, tetanus, pertussis, and *Haemophilus influenzae* type B) and later with the DTaP and inactivated poliovirus vaccines as Pentacel.

ADMINISTRATION

Children should receive the Hib vaccine at two, four, six, and twelve to fifteen months of age. The vaccine is commonly administered in combination with DTaP and poliovirus in the combination vaccine Pentacel.

IMPACT

The Hib vaccine is highly effective at preventing the diseases commonly caused by the bacterium *H. influenzae*. Before the development of this vaccine, Hib was the leading cause of meningitis in children. It is estimated that the mortality rate among infants and children who contracted this illness was 5 percent, with an even greater incidence of permanent brain damage or hearing loss, or both, among survivors. It is important to note that other bacterial causes of meningitis still exist, but the incidence of meningitis overall has dramatically declined since the Hib vaccine was added to the immunization schedule.

Epiglottitis, a serious disease that was most commonly caused by Hib, was widespread before Hib vaccination became standard. Epiglottitis has virtually disappeared as a disease, and many pediatricians have learned of this illness only by anecdote.

Jennifer Birkhauser, M.D.

FURTHER READING

Behrman, Richard E., Robert M. Kliegman, and Hal B. Jenson, eds. *Nelson Textbook of Pediatrics.* 18th ed. Philadelphia: Saunders/Elsevier, 2007.
Harvey, Richard A., Pamela C. Champe, and Bruce D. Fisher. *Lippincott's Illustrated Reviews: Microbiology.*

2d ed. Philadelphia: Lippincott Williams & Wilkins, 2006.

Loehr, Jamie. *The Vaccine Answer Book: Two Hundred Essential Answers to Help You Make the Right Decisions for Your Child.* Naperville, Ill.: Sourcebooks, 2010.

Plotkin, Stanley A., Walter A. Orenstein, and Paul A. Offit. *Vaccines.* 5th ed. Philadelphia: Saunders/Elsevier, 2008.

WEB SITES OF INTEREST

Centers for Disease Control and Prevention
http://www.cdc.gov/vaccines

Children's Hospital of Philadelphia, Vaccine Education Center
http://www.chop.edu/service/vaccine-education-center

See also: Bacterial meningitis; Epiglottitis; *Haemophilus*; *Haemophilus influenzae* infection; Sepsis; Vaccines: Types.

Histoplasma

CATEGORY: Pathogen
TRANSMISSION ROUTE: Inhalation

DEFINITION

Histoplasma is a genus of fungi containing a single species that is the causative agent of the disease histoplasmosis.

**Taxonomic Classification
for *Histoplasma***

Kingdom: Fungi
Phylum: Ascomycota
Subphylum: Ascomycotina
Class: Ascomycetes
Order: Onygenales
Family: Onygenaceae
Genus: *Histoplasma* (*Ajellomyces*)
Species: *H. capsulatum*

NATURAL HABITAT AND FEATURES

The species *H. capsulatum* includes two varieties, *H. capsulatum* var. *capsulatum* and *H. capsulatum* var. *duboisii*. *H. c.* var. *capsulatum* is a New World variety that causes histoplasmosis involving primarily the pulmonary and reticuloendothelial systems, whereas *H. c.* var. *duboisii*, the cause of African histoplasmosis, usually involves infections of the bones and skin.

Histoplasma is a naturally occurring fungus that is generally found in soil contaminated with either bird or bat droppings. It is endemic to the Ohio, Tennessee, Missouri, and Mississippi river basins of the United States. The fungus is also found in tropical areas of Central America, South America, eastern Asia, Australia, and eastern and central Africa, often in caves that contain bat guano (feces).

Histoplasma is a thermally dimorphic fungus, which means that it has two morphs, or forms, depending upon the temperature at which it grows. At temperatures of approximately 77° Fahrenheit (25° Celsius), an average soil temperature, it grows in mold form. Colonies at this temperature grow slowly and have a granular to cottony texture and a whitish color that turns buff brown as the fungus ages. Once within a human host, growing at normal body temperature of 98.6° F (37° C), ovoid, cream-colored budding yeast cells are formed. While within soil, the hyphae, or fungal strands, are septate and hyaline. Conidiophores, the spore-bearing portions of the fungus, grow at right angles to the parent colony, and both macroconida and microconidia are present. The macroconidia are unicellular, large, tuberculate, thick-walled structures. These macroconidia are also called tuberculo-chlamydospores or macroaleurioconidia. *Histoplasma* microconidia are unicellular and round and possess either rough or smooth walls.

Histoplasma grows best in moist, acidic soil conditions such as those found in caves, poultry houses, and silos serving as bird roosts. The fungus can contaminate soil for years and spores can be inhaled when the soil is disturbed.

PATHOGENICITY AND CLINICAL SIGNIFICANCE

When spores of *H. capsulatum* from contaminated soil are inhaled, they lodge in the lungs. In the alveoli of the lungs, macrophages of the immune system attack the fungal spores and transport them to the lymph nodes of the chest. Inflammation, scarring, and calcification can then occur in the lungs. The majority of people who contract histoplasmosis, however, have no symptoms, but for some, an acute pulmonary phase of the disease occurs. Symptoms of acute pulmonary symptomatic histoplasmosis infection start within three to seventeen days of initial exposure. This phase is characterized by cold or flulike symptoms and may last two weeks or longer. Fever, periodic sweats, muscle aches, a dry cough, chest pain, and loss of appetite often occur.

Rare but serious complications of acute phase infection include enlargement of the lymph nodes of the chest, causing esophageal or airway obstruction and making swallowing and breathing extremely difficult. Fibrosing mediastinitis, severe scarring of the lymph nodes in the chest, may also cause chest pain and breathlessness and can be life-threatening. Pericarditis (inflammation of the pericardial sac around the heart), meningitis (inflammation of the meninges and cerebrospinal fluid of the brain and spinal cord), and arthritis are all severe complications of acute histoplasmosis cases. Adrenal insufficiency may also occur if adrenal glands are destroyed by the fungus.

Chronic pulmonary cases of histoplasmosis symptomatically mimic tuberculosis. These cases usually occur in patients who already have a lung disease, such as emphysema. Disseminated or systemic cases of histoplasmosis affect multiple organ systems and can prove fatal to elderly or immunocompromised persons. Liver and spleen enlargement, Addison's disease, meningitis, pericarditis, and pneumonia may all result from disseminated histoplasmosis.

Ocular histoplasmosis damages the retina, resulting in scar tissue that can lead to leakage and subsequent vision loss. In cases of African histoplasmosis, skin lesions and osteolytic lesions, particularly in the skull, ribs, and vertebrae, frequently develop. Also common is fever and lymph node enlargement.

Fungal samples from sputum, blood, and infected organs can be cultured in the laboratory for definitive diagnosis of histoplasmosis. However, this process may take as long as four weeks, so it is not the diagnostic tool of choice for suspected cases of disseminated histoplasmosis. Blood samples may reveal antigens or antibodies against *Histoplasma*; antigens may also be present in the urine of infected persons. If a person has been infected in the past with *Histoplasma*, blood tests can give false-positive results, which may mask a different type of infection.

Fungal stain tests can be conducted on tissue samples, but because other fungi resemble *H. capsulatum*, a misdiagnosis is possible with this technique. Chest X rays, computed tomography (CT) scans, and bronchoscopies may also be useful in assisting with a definitive diagnosis.

DRUG SUSCEPTIBILITY

Treatment with amphotericin B for one to two weeks is standard for severe cases of acute pulmonary symptomatic histoplasmosis. Steroid treatment with drugs such as methylprednisone may follow amphotericin B once patients are stabilized. Treatment with itraconazole may continue for one year following serious cases. Other antifungal drugs such as fluconazole and ketoconazole may occasionally be used.

For chronic pulmonary histoplasmosis cases that involve cavitary lesions within the lungs, treatment includes long-term itraconazole use and surgical intervention. Ocular histoplasmosis treatment requires steroids. Antifungal treatment is of little use for the rare, severe complications of pericarditis and fibrosing mediastinitis.

Lenela Glass-Godwin, M.S.

FURTHER READING

Hage, C. A., et al. "Histoplasmosis." In *Harrison's Principles of Internal Medicine*, edited by Joan Butterton. 17th ed. New York: McGraw-Hill, 2008.

Hospenthal, D. R., and H. J. Becker. "Update on Therapy for Histoplasmosis." *Infectious Medicine* 26 (2009): 121-124. Discusses the current drug and surgery protocols for various types of histoplasmosis.

Kauffman, C. A. "Histoplasmosis: A Clinical and Laboratory Update." *Clinical Microbiology Reviews* 20, no. 1 (2007): 115-132. Provides a recent review of testing and treatment for histoplasmosis.

Ryan, Kenneth J., and C. George Ray, eds. *Sherris Medical Microbiology: An Introduction to Infectious Diseases.* 5th ed. New York: McGraw-Hill, 2010. A textbook presentation of histoplasmosis culture and diagnostic techniques.

WEB SITES OF INTEREST

American Lung Association
http://www.lungusa.org

Centers for Disease Control and Prevention
http://www.cdc.gov

DoctorFungus
http://doctorfungus.org

Systematic Mycology and Microbiology Laboratory
http://www.ars.usda.gov

See also: Airborne illness and disease; *Aspergillus*; Blastomycosis; Bronchiolitis; Bronchitis; Chromoblastomycosis; Coccidiosis; Cryptococcosis; Fungi: Classification and types; Histoplasmosis; Legionnaires' disease; Mucormycosis; Paracoccidioidomycosis; Pneumocystis pneumonia; Psittacosis; Soilborne illness and disease; Tuberculosis (TB); Whooping cough.

Histoplasmosis

CATEGORY: Diseases and conditions
ANATOMY OR SYSTEM AFFECTED: Lungs, respiratory system

DEFINITION

Histoplasmosis is a fungal infection that often causes a respiratory illness.

CAUSES

Histoplasmosis is caused by a fungal infection of the lungs. Humans become infected by exposure to bird and bat droppings.

RISK FACTORS

Risk factors for histoplasmosis includes work that involves contact with bird or bat droppings (such as in an aviary); activities that put one in contact with bird or bat droppings (such as in cave exploration); keeping birds as pets; living along river valleys; living in the states of Mississippi, Ohio, Kentucky, Illinois, Indiana, Missouri, or Tennessee; living in eastern Canada, Mexico, Central or South America, southeast Asia, or Africa; recent travel to a location where histoplasmosis is common; and having a medical condition, such as human immunodeficiency virus (HIV) infection, that weakens the immune system.

SYMPTOMS

Many persons do not have symptoms, but those who do have symptoms have symptoms such as weakness, headache, achy muscles, joint pain, fever, chills, malaise (a feeling of discomfort or uneasiness), hemoptysis (coughing up blood), chest pain, cough, shortness of breath, weight loss, mouth sores, enlarged liver and spleen, skin rashes, and loss of vision.

SCREENING AND DIAGNOSIS

A doctor will ask about symptoms and medical history and will perform a physical exam. Tests may include blood tests, a blood culture, a sputum culture, a pulmonary function test, skin testing, urine antigen testing, X rays of chest or abdomen (or both), and bone marrow tests.

TREATMENT AND THERAPY

Treatment includes the use of antifungal medications, which may include amphotericin B or itraconazole. Persons with acquired immunodeficiency syndrome may require treatment with an antifungal medication for the rest of their lives to prevent further attacks of histoplasmosis.

PREVENTION AND OUTCOMES

Persons who anticipate being exposed to bird or bat droppings should wear face masks, and persons with weakened immune systems should completely avoid bird and bat droppings.

Rosalyn Carson-DeWitt, M.D.

FURTHER READING

"Clinical Practice Guidelines for the Management of Patients with Histoplasmosis: 2007 Update by the Infectious Diseases Society of America." *Clinical Infectious Diseases* 45 (2007): 807.

Hage, C. A., et al. "Histoplasmosis." In *Harrison's Principles of Internal Medicine,* edited by Anthony Fauci et al. 17th ed. New York: McGraw-Hill, 2008.

Kaufman, C. A. "Histoplasmosis." *Clinics in Chest Medicine* 30 (2009): 217.

McPhee, Stephen J., and Maxine A. Papadakis, eds. *Current Medical Diagnosis and Treatment 2011.* 50th ed. New York: McGraw-Hill, 2011.

Mason, Robert J., et al., eds. *Murray and Nadel's Textbook of Respiratory Medicine.* 5th ed. Philadelphia: Saunders/Elsevier, 2010.

Myers, Adam. *Respiratory System.* Philadelphia: Mosby/Elsevier, 2006.

WEB SITES OF INTEREST

Centers for Disease Control and Prevention
http://www.cdc.gov

National Institute of Allergy and Infectious Diseases
http://www.niaid.nih.gov

Public Health Agency of Canada
http://www.phac-aspc.gc.ca

See also: Airborne illness and disease; Allergic bronchopulmonary aspergillosis; Antifungal drugs: Types; Aspergillosis; Bats and infectious disease; Birds and infectious disease; Blastomycosis; Chromoblastomycosis; Cryptococcosis; Diagnosis of fungal infections; Fecal-oral route of transmission; Fungal infections; Fungi: Classification and types; *Histoplasma*; Immune response to fungal infections; Mucormycosis; Psittacosis; Soilborne illness and disease; Tuberculosis (TB).

HIV

CATEGORY: Diseases and conditions
ANATOMY OR SYSTEM AFFECTED: All
ALSO KNOWN AS: Human immunodeficiency virus

DEFINITION

HIV is a virus that attacks white blood cells called helper T cells (CD4). These cells are part of the immune system, and they fight infections and disease. An HIV infection can leave a person vulnerable to many illnesses.

Acquired immunodeficiency syndrome (AIDS) is a late stage of HIV. It reflects severe damage to the immune system. An opportunistic infection, a type of infection that occurs only in people with compromised immune systems, will also exist in persons with HIV infection.

CAUSES

HIV is spread through contact with HIV-infected blood or other body fluids, including semen, vaginal fluid, and breast milk. AIDS is caused by the destruction of T cells (whose destruction is caused by HIV infections).

HIV is spread through sexual contact with an HIV-infected person, especially through vaginal or anal intercourse; through transfer of HIV from a woman to her fetus during pregnancy and from a woman to her child at birth; through breast-feeding; through a break in the skin with an HIV-contaminated needle; and through a blood transfusion with HIV-infected blood (now rare because all donated blood is tested for HIV, a practice that began in 1985).

Rarely, HIV can be spread through blood from an HIV-infected person getting into an open wound of another person, being bitten by someone infected with HIV, and sharing personal hygiene items (such as razors or toothbrushes) with an HIV-infected person.

RISK FACTORS

Factors that increase the chance of getting HIV include having multiple sexual partners; sharing needles to inject drugs; being regularly exposed to HIV-contaminated blood or other body fluids (a concern for health care workers); receiving donor blood products, tissue, or organs, or having been artificially inseminated; and having a sexual relationship with a person already infected with HIV. Persons who are at increased risk include those who were born to an HIV-infected woman and immigrants from geographic regions with high numbers of persons with AIDS (such as east-central Africa and Haiti). The risk factor for developing AIDS is having an HIV infection.

SYMPTOMS

HIV may not cause symptoms for a number of years, but early symptoms may appear one or two months after a person is infected and may last a couple of weeks. The symptoms include rapid weight loss; a dry cough; a sore throat; recurring fever; night sweats; extreme, unexplained fatigue; swollen lymph nodes in armpits, neck, or groin; white spots on the tongue or in the mouth or throat; a headache; discomfort from light; a rash; depression; an irritable mood; and memory loss or other neurological disorder.

After these initial symptoms pass, there may be no symptoms for months to years. The following symptoms may occur over the course of one to three years: swollen lymph glands all over the body; fungal infections of the mouth, fingernails, and toes; repeated vaginal infections (such as yeast infection and trichomoniasis); development of many warts; exacerbations of prior conditions such as eczema, psoriasis, and herpes infection; shingles; night sweats; weight loss; and chronic diarrhea.

Ten years or more can pass before HIV progresses to AIDS. This happens when levels of helper T cells fall below certain levels and opportunistic infections arise. Examples of opportunistic infections and other complications of AIDS include thrush (an overgrowth of yeast); pneumonia (particularly pneumocystis pneumonia); invasive fungal infections (resulting in brain or lung infections, or both); toxoplasmosis infection; tuberculosis; viral brain infection; Kaposi's sarcoma; lymphoma; cervical cancer; eye disease caused by cytomegalovirus infection; intestinal infections, especially from *Shigella, Salmonella,* and *Campylobacter;* severe weight loss (wasting syndrome); severe skin rashes; reactions to medications; and psychiatric problems, including depression and dementia.

SCREENING AND DIAGNOSIS

A doctor will ask about symptoms, medical history, and risk factors, and will perform a physical exam. Blood tests may be ordered, including an ELISA (enzyme-linked immunoabsorbent assay) test and a Western blot test. An ELISA test is used to detect HIV infection (95 percent of persons tested will have a positive test within three months of infection and 99 percent will have a positive test within six months of infection). If an ELISA test is negative but the patient still thinks he or she may have HIV, a retest should be requested for one to three months following the initial test. The Western blot test is usually administered to confirm the diagnosis of HIV infection if the ELISA test was positive.

TREATMENT AND THERAPY

Medications can prevent, delay, or control the development of AIDS in many people infected with HIV. Drugs that fight HIV are often given in combination (highly active antiretroviral therapy, or HAART) and are often referred to as an AIDS cocktail. These drugs include nucleoside reverse transcriptase inhibitors, such as AZT (zidovudine or ZDV), ddC (zalcitabine), ddI (dideoxyinosine), d4T (stavudine), 3TC (lamivudine), emtricitabine (Emtriva), and abacavir (Ziagen). In some patients, abacavir can cause a hypersensitivity reaction, which can be life-threatening. Researchers have found that screening for a particular gene can help prevent this reaction.

Other drugs include nucleotide reverse transcrip-

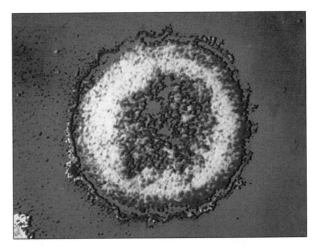

The human immunodeficiency virus. (PhotoDisc)

tase inhibitors, such as delavirdine (Rescriptor), nevirapine (Viramune), efavirenz (Sustiva), and etravirine (Intelence); protease inhibitors, such as ritonavir (Norvir), saquinavir (Invirase), indinavir (Crixivan), amprenavir (Agenerase), fosamprenavir (Lexiva), nelfinavir (Viracept), lopinavir (Kaletra), atazanavir (Reyataz), tipranavir (Aptivus), and darunavir (Prezista); and a combination pill called atripla (Efavirenz, Tenofovir, and Emtricitabine). Still others include the HIV fusion inhibitors enfuvirtide (Fuzeon) and maraviroc (Selzentry), and the integrase inhibitor raltegravir (Isentress). Drugs that fight AIDS-related infections include those that treat pneumonia, thrush, repeated herpes infections, and *Toxoplasma* brain infections.

PREVENTION AND OUTCOMES

The best way to prevent HIV infection is to abstain from sex. Persons who do have sex (any sexual act that results in the exchange of bodily fluids) should insist on the use of a latex condom.

Other preventive measures include not sharing needles for drug injection; limiting the number of sexual partners; avoiding sexual partners who are HIV-positive or who inject drugs; and avoiding receiving transfusion of unscreened blood products. Health care workers should wear appropriate latex gloves and facial masks during all procedures, carefully handle and properly dispose of needles, and carefully follow universal precautions.

Persons who live with an HIV-infected person should wear appropriate latex gloves if handling HIV-infected

In Her Own Words: Living with HIV

Forty-six-year-old Beverly tested positive for HIV infection. The health educator tried to stay abreast of the latest research and was optimistic about the future. Here is her story:

What was your first sign that something was wrong? What symptoms did you experience?

I didn't have any symptoms but knew I had put myself at risk. I had been an IV [intravenous] drug user for sixteen years and had unprotected sex with someone who tested positive for HIV. I knew in my heart I could be infected but was afraid to be tested. But I knew people who were HIV positive and knew if they could deal with it, so could I. Finally in 1993, I went for testing. I didn't start to show symptoms of a faltering immune system until 1996, when I developed vaginitis, colds, and sinus infections that were more severe than ever before.

What was the diagnosis experience like?

My doctor had tried to convince me to be tested, but I didn't want my insurance company to know if I was HIV positive. I went to a clinic that provided anonymous testing. My name was not identified with the results. The woman who gave me the results looked more scared than I was. She gave me the name of a doctor, but I didn't go. At the time, I was dead set against starting on drugs to treat HIV. My instincts served me well. Now they do not recommend that early treatment.

What was your initial and then longer-term reaction to the diagnosis?

I was in shock. The positive result didn't hit me until the next day. I worked as a counselor in a drug-recovery program when I learned the result. A month or two later, I changed jobs and began working as a chemical dependency counselor with HIV-positive men. Now I work with an agency that advocates for and trains women and children who are affected by HIV. I like helping people. It's spiritually uplifting to know that I am making a difference in someone's health. I stay on the cutting edge. I read everything I can get my hands on. There's an ever-changing landscape of treatments. I want to avail myself to them and survive as long as possible.

How is your disease treated?

I receive medications through a clinical trial. I recently took a break from the drugs. The drugs have side effects, including a shifting of fat tissue, high blood fats, and cholesterol. But the side effects are mild. I recently developed high blood pressure, probably from the drugs. I also see a primary care physician for routine health needs and an acupuncturist, who offers a holistic approach. It's important to remain mindful of other health issues.

Did you have to make any lifestyle or dietary changes in response to your illness?

I try to make sure I get enough rest. I'm not as good about making opportunities to regularly exercise, but I try. I take nutritional supplements and eat a healthful diet. I watch my sugar intake. The medications can cause insulin resistance, so I have to be careful. I don't smoke, drink alcohol, or take recreational drugs.

Did you seek any type of emotional support?

After I tested positive, I went to a 12-step AA [Alcoholics Anonymous] meeting for people with HIV. It was a cornerstone of support. I now work in a supportive environment.

Did or does your condition have any impact on your family?

My immediate family has been supportive. Just as I had to go through the process from denial to acceptance, my loved ones had to as well. I say let people who love you know your status. If you don't have loved ones, find people to care about.

An area that's still difficult for me is dating. During the four years from my drug recovery to HIV diagnosis, I didn't date. I knew if I were dating, I would have to deal with it. Once I was tested, I started dating immediately. The last person I was involved with was HIV positive. If I don't know the man's status or do know that he is negative, it's hard to tell him.

What advice would you give to anyone living with this disease?

If you are at risk and don't know your HIV status, seek support and get tested. There are treatments that can make a huge difference in your quality of life and survival, and there will be more in the future. But you can't avail yourself, if you don't know your status.

Be honest with yourself and educate yourself. If you are living with HIV or anything serious, the more you accept the situation, the more you will make the best of what happens.

As told to Debra Wood, R.N.

bodily fluids; cover with bandages any cuts and sores of all persons in that residence; avoid sharing personal hygiene items, such as razors and toothbrushes; and carefully handle and properly dispose of needles that have been used for medication.

One should inform former or potential sexual partners of one's HIV status, avoid donating blood or organs, and consult a doctor or other health care provider about contraception.

Studies have found that circumcised men are significantly less likely to develop HIV infection compared with uncircumcised men. HIV-infected women who want to become pregnant should consult a doctor to discuss ways to lower the chance their child will be born with HIV infection. Infected women with newborns should not breast-feed.

Rick Alan; reviewed by David L. Horn, M.D., FACP

FURTHER READING

Bailey, R. C., et al. "Male Circumcision for HIV Prevention in Young Men in Kisumu, Kenya: A Randomised Controlled Trial." *The Lancet* 369 (February 24, 2007): 643-656.

Centers for Disease Control and Prevention. "HIV/AIDS A-Z Index." Available at http://www.cdc.gov/hiv/az.htm.

Clark, Rebecca A., Robert T. Maupin, Jr., and Jill Hayes Hammer. *A Woman's Guide to Living with HIV Infection.* Baltimore: Johns Hopkins University Press, 2004.

Fan, Hung Y., Ross F. Conner, and Luis P. Villarreal. *AIDS: Science and Society.* 5th ed. Sudbury, Mass.: Jones and Bartlett, 2007.

Fehervari, Zoltan, and Shiman Sakaguchi. "Peacekeepers of the Immune System." *Scientific American,* October, 2006, 56-63.

Friedman-Kien, Alvin, and Clay J. Cockerell. *Color Atlas of AIDS.* 2d ed. Philadelphia: Elsevier Health Sciences, 1996.

Mallal, S., et al. "HLA-B5701 Screening for Hypersensitivity to Abacavir." *New England Journal of Medicine* 358 (2008): 568-579.

Matthews, Dawn D., ed. *AIDS Sourcebook.* 3d ed. Detroit: Omnigraphics, 2003.

Rey, D., et al. "Virologic Response of Zidovudine, Lamivudine, and Tenofovir Disoproxil Fumarate Combination in Antiretroviral-Naive HIV-1-Infected Patients." *Journal of Acquired Immune Deficiency Syndrome* 43 (2006): 530-534.

St. Georgiev, Vassil. *Opportunistic Infections: Treatment and Prophylaxis.* Totowa, N.J.: Humana Press, 2003.

Stine, Gerald J. *AIDS Update 2010.* New York: McGraw-Hill Higher Education, 2010.

WEB SITES OF INTEREST

AIDSgov
http://www.aids.gov

AIDSinfo
http://aidsinfo.nih.gov

Canadian AIDS Treatment Information Exchange
http://www.catie.ca

Centers for Disease Control and Prevention, National Center for HIV/AIDS, Viral Hepatitis, STD, and TB Prevention
http://www.cdc.gov/nchhstp

Foundation for AIDS Research
http://www.amfar.org

See also: AIDS; Antibodies; Antiviral drugs: Mechanisms of action; Antiviral drugs: types; Autoimmune disorders; Blood-borne illness and disease; Breast milk and infectious disease; Cancer and infectious disease; Contagious diseases; HIV vaccine; Immunity; Immunoassay; Incubation period; Kaposi's sarcoma; Maturation inhibitors; Men and infectious disease; Opportunistic infections; Oral transmission; Penicilliosis; Pneumocystis pneumonia; Pregnancy and infectious disease; Protease inhibitors; Reverse transcriptase inhibitors; Saliva and infectious disease; Seroconversion; Sexually transmitted diseases (STDs); Social effects of infectious disease; T lymphocytes; Thrush; Viral infections.

HIV vaccine

CATEGORY: Prevention
ALSO KNOWN AS: Human immunodeficiency virus vaccine

DEFINITION

A vaccine prevents disease by enabling the body's immune response to an infectious agent. Vaccines

Experimental HIV Vaccine

Close to thirty years of intensive research, and a global expenditure of more than $6 billion, has yielded no vaccine to prevent HIV infection. Indeed, one notorious trial was halted early when vaccinated persons actually suffered an increased risk of HIV infection.

There are a number of complex reasons that candidate (experimental) vaccines have proven ineffective. One reason is that the molecules on the surface of the virus to which the immune system's antibodies can bind are much more variable than in typical pathogens. The HIV genome, composed of ribonucleic acid, can accumulate mutations at frequencies up to one hundred times higher than genomes composed of deoxyribonucleic acid like the human genome. Thus, selection pressure because of an immune response against one set of HIV surface molecules will rapidly lead to the evolution of resistant strains displaying distinct sets of surface molecules. Indeed, multiple highly divergent strains are found in persons with HIV infection in different regions of the globe.

In September, 2009, a U.S.-Thai team of investigators announced the first demonstration of reduced risk of HIV infection after immunization. The study employed a combination of two vaccines that had individually failed to be effective in previous experiments. Low-to-moderate-risk HIV-negative volunteers age eighteen to thirty years were given injections of vaccine or placebo and subsequently tested for infection every six months for three years. In the control group, 74 of 8,198 subjects were infected by the end of the study; in the vaccinated group, 51 of 8,197 subjects became infected. Those figures reflect a statistically significant 31.2 percent reduction of probability of infection after vaccination.

Although the observed effect was encouraging, the results include a number of caveats. The vaccine combination targets the HIV strain encountered most frequently in Thailand and therefore would not be expected to provide immunity to the strains responsible for most infections in Africa, Europe, North America, and elsewhere. Vaccination had no apparent effect on the severity of infection in subjects who contracted HIV during the study. Lastly, the vaccine's efficacy is far below the 80 percent threshold required for approval for public distribution.

Carina Endres Howell, Ph.D.

contain elements of the infectious agent in preparations not meant to cause disease, but to stimulate production of antibodies against the infectious agent. These antibodies prevent disease development. Although rare cases of persons with immunity to the human immunodeficiency virus (HIV) have been reported, mostly, natural immunity to HIV infection has not been effectively isolated or studied.

DEVELOPMENT CHALLENGES

Typical vaccine development procedures look at how the body naturally protects itself from reinfection with a disease causing agent. If someone has mumps or measles as a child, that person will not suffer a second bout with the disease because his or her body has built up a natural immune antibody response to the viruses causing these diseases. Scientists look at antibodies produced by immune people and try to reproduce the same response with a vaccine. Researchers developing HIV vaccines are challenged because they lack this natural immune response model.

HIV infection is not a disease until the infection reduces a certain type of white blood cell (CD4+ T cells) to a very low level. Once this CD4 count lowers enough, the HIV infected person will have acquired immunodeficiency syndrome (AIDS). Vaccines prevent disease, not infection. People can carry HIV infections for years without developing AIDS. HIV vaccine development aims to immunize against the infection, and not only against the disease. This is another significant challenge for HIV vaccine development.

IMPACT

HIV vaccination provides hope for AIDS disease prevention and protection against the transmission of HIV infection. Experiments with three main vaccine approaches involve deoxyribonucleic acid (DNA) vaccines, recombinant vector vaccines, and component vaccines. All three approaches aim to produce antibodies against HIV.

DNA vaccines use parts of the HIV genetic code, a tiny ring of HIV DNA called a plasmid. Needle-free injection technology pushes DNA plasmids directly into the skin cells and immune cells. Electroporation devices increase skin cell plasmid uptake by using electrical pulses that open cell pores, admitting the plasmids. Once inside skin immune cells, the HIV genes produce HIV proteins (antigens). These antigens would provoke an immune antibody response and provide protection against HIV infection.

Recombinant vector vaccines use a carrier to bring HIV genes into the body. A part of the HIV genetic code is combined with the genetic code of another virus, a virus that typically does not cause human disease. This recombinant DNA, after introduction to the body, becomes a vector for the HIV genes. As with DNA vaccines, the newly introduced HIV genes would produce HIV antigens, resulting in host antibody production and HIV immunity.

Both of the foregoing techniques involve modern genetic manipulations. Component or protein vaccines, also known as subunit vaccines, use portions of HIV to stimulate an immune response. This is the classic type of vaccine, but even this classic approach now uses modern gene technology. Genetic engineering is used to produce HIV portions used in these component vaccines.

HIV vaccine development must overcome intricate challenges. Modern technologies provide hope and promise with this important disease prevention endeavor.

Richard P. Capriccioso, M.D.

FURTHER READING

Grandi, Guido, ed. *Genomics, Proteomics, and Vaccines.* Hoboken, N.J.: John Wiley & Sons, 2004.

Morrow, Matthew P., and David B. Weiner. "DNA Drugs Come of Age." *Scientific American* 303, no. 1 (July, 2010) 48-53.

Plotkin, Stanley A., Walter A. Orenstein, and Paul A. Offit. *Vaccines.* 5th ed. Philadelphia: Saunders/Elsevier, 2008.

U.S. Department of Health and Human Services. "Preventive HIV Vaccines." Available at http://aidsinfo.nih.gov.

Watkins, David I. "Basic HIV Vaccine Development." *Topics in HIV Medicine* 16, no. 1 (March/April, 2008): 7-8. Available at http://www.iasusa.org/pub/topics/2008/issue1/7.pdf.

WEB SITES OF INTEREST

AIDSinfo
http://aidsinfo.nih.gov

Foundation for AIDS Research
http://www.amfar.org

HIV Vaccine Trials Network
http://www.hvtn.org

International AIDS Society-USA
http://www.iasusa.org

See also: AIDS; Antibodies; Autoimmune disorders; Blood-borne illness and disease; HIV; Immunity; Immunoassay; Maturation inhibitors; Men and infectious disease; Opportunistic infections; Protease inhibitors; Reverse transcriptase inhibitors; Seroconversion; Sexually transmitted diseases (STDs); Social effects of infectious disease; T lymphocytes; Vaccines: Types; Viral infections.

Home remedies

CATEGORY: Treatment
ALSO KNOWN AS: Herbal remedies, home treatments, natural cures, natural remedies

DEFINITION

Home remedies are forms of treatment or cures for illnesses and diseases. These remedies are made from common, usually inexpensive ingredients found in the home or garden.

HISTORY

Western medicine depends primarily on prescribed or over-the-counter medications to treat or cure disease. Historically, however, women (especially) in the home employed various herbs or foods to treat illness. By trial and error, some remedies worked effectively, while others did not. Those that successfully cured illnesses were passed through generations as accepted treatments for common ailments.

Some home remedies, such as chicken soup for an upper respiratory illness or the common cold, have become traditions, and studies have demonstrated a scientific basis to explain their success. For example, researchers published findings in the October, 2000 issue of *Chest,* the journal of the American College of Chest Physicians. They detailed how eating chicken soup stopped neutrophil migration, providing a mild

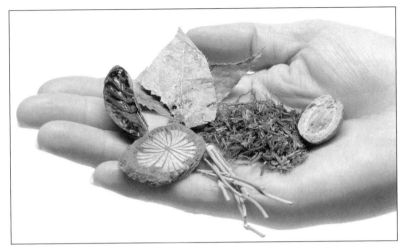

A variety of herbs have been associated with preventing and treating infectious diseases and conditions. (PhotoDisc)

anti-inflammatory response that suppressed cold symptoms. Other home remedies also have scientific rationale and include willow bark powder for headache. Willow bark contains salicin, a substance later compounded into acetylsalicylic acid or aspirin, which inhibits the production of prostaglandins, providing analgesic relief of pain and fever.

GENERAL TYPES

One type of home remedy comes from the use of herbs grown in kitchen gardens or in containers in small living spaces. These herbs can be harvested as medicinals, flavorings, insect repellant, or room deodorants. Herbs that might be grown for medicinal use include lavender, yarrow, sage, bee balm, and flowering thyme.

Herbs can be processed in different ways to make them useful home remedies. They may be used to make infusions, decoctions, or tinctures for illnesses. Various teas, for example, can be steeped for ten to twenty minutes to become an infusion for the relief of indigestion or nausea, to use as an antiseptic foot soak, or to perfume a bath or pillow to manage insomnia. Drinking tea has historically been a preventive measure and a restorative option for health. The intense level of polyphenols or catechins in green tea acts as an antioxidant to promote health and support the immune system against disease. Other forms of home remedies include poultices, ointments, salves, elixirs, tonics, and aromatics. Food in whole form, dried, or juiced can offer treatment to specific ailments.

HOME REMEDIES AND INFECTIONS

Some home remedies seem to make common sense. For example, garlic has been used for more than three thousand years as a home remedy for various ailments. Allicin, one of about one hundred chemicals found in garlic, provides natural antibiotic, antiviral, and antifungal benefits. Garlic powder can be used in a foot soak to kill the fungus of athlete's foot, can be used to treat oral thrush, and can be included in many recipes to add flavor yet also to destroy harmful bacteria in the stomach.

Salt water, a safe and inexpensive home remedy, can be used as an effective antibiotic because many types of bacteria cannot live in a salty environment. Gargling with salt water to relieve a sore throat or toothache can be a valuable approach at home. Salt water can also be used as a topical treatment.

Echinacea has long been considered an effective home remedy for colds, earache, sore throats, and flu. The action of echinacea is antibiotic, antifungal, and antiviral and is believed to boost the immune system. Research in 2005 by the National Center for Complementary and Alternative Medicine did not confirm the effectiveness of echinacea at a low dose, but studies continue about this popular herbal remedy.

The use of camphor, eucalyptus, and menthol, such as in vapor rubs, has been found to display antifungal properties. A study at Michigan State College of Nursing concluded that nail bed fungus can be treated effectively by application of a vapor rub compound used twice daily. Thyme oil is also touted as an effective home remedy for fungal infections of the nails.

Other home remedies for infections include *Melaleuca alternifolia* or Austrian tea tree oil, goldenseal, *pau d'arco* bark made into tea, oil of oregano, and manuka honey. Future studies of home remedies may prove them useful in treating infections.

IMPACT

At a time when medications are too expensive for most budgets and which come with undesired side effects, home remedies are becoming more and more attractive to many in mainstream society. Consumers are seeking less costly, safe alternatives to treat illnesses and to manage diseases. Many people are uninsured, have high deductibles on their health insurance policies, or have experienced adverse reactions to traditional pharmaceuticals. People from all walks of life have returned to time-tested approaches to disease treatment and health promotion. They have decided that the home and garden remedy approach to treating illness makes sense, and the price is right. Many health care providers, too, support the use of safe home remedies.

One should be cautious, however, before using home remedies, especially if one has a complicated illness or is taking medicines (prescribed or over the counter) that might interact with a home remedy. One should always consult with a health care provider before using home remedies to determine their usefulness and safeness in treatment.

Marylane Wade Koch, M.S.N., R.N.

FURTHER READING

Freeman, Lyn. *Mosby's Complementary and Alternative Medicine: A Research-Based Approach.* 2d ed. St. Louis, Mo.: Mosby, 2004.

Micozzi, Marc S., ed. *Fundamentals of Complementary and Integrative Medicine.* 3d ed. St. Louis, Mo.: Saunders/Elsevier, 2006.

Rennard, Barbara O., et al. "Chicken Soup Inhibits Neutrophil Chemotaxis in Vitro" *Chest* 118, no. 4 (2000): 1150-1157. Also available at http://chest-journal.chestpubs.org/content/118/4/1150.full.pdf+html.

Trivieri, Larry, Jr., and John W. Anderson, eds. *Alternative Medicine: The Definitive Guide.* 2d ed. Berkeley, Calif.: Ten Speed Press, 2002.

White, Martha, et al. *Traditional Home Remedies.* Dublin, N.H.: Yankee, 1997.

WEB SITES OF INTEREST

National Center for Complementary and Alternative Medicine
http://nccam.nih.gov

Natural Antiseptics, Antibiotics, and Antifungals
http://www.mostlyherbs.com/antiseptics.html

See also: Alternative therapies; Bacterial infections; Cold sores; Common cold; Fungal infections; Infection; Influenza; Over-the-counter (OTC) drugs; Strep throat; Treatment of bacterial infections; Treatment of fungal infections; Treatment of viral infections; Viral infections.

H1N1 influenza

CATEGORY: Diseases and conditions
ANATOMY OR SYSTEM AFFECTED: Lungs, respiratory system
ALSO KNOWN AS: Global swine flu, H1N1 infection, human swine flu, influenza A (H1N1), new H1N1 flu, novel H1N1 flu, pig flu, swine flu, swine influenza, type A (H1N1) flu

DEFINITION

The H1N1 flu, originally called swine flu, is a respiratory infection. The H1N1 flu, which spread to humans and reached the level of a pandemic, or worldwide outbreak, in 2009, can cause mild to severe symptoms.

CAUSES

There are two main types of influenza virus: type A and type B. The 2009 outbreak was caused by a new mixture of different kinds of influenza type A. This strain passes from human to human, so it may spread rapidly. The H1N1 flu spreads in the same way as the seasonal flu, that is, by breathing in droplets after an infected person coughs or sneezes and by touching a contaminated surface and then touching one's eyes, nose, or mouth. The virus can survive on surfaces and infect a person for two to eight hours after that person has touched the contaminated surface.

RISK FACTORS

The main risk factor for getting the H1N1 flu is contact with an infected person. Also, having a chronic health condition (such as cardiovascular disease, respiratory disease, diabetes, or cancer) may increase the risk of a more severe form of the infection. Eating pork or pork products or drinking tap water are not risk factors for the H1N1 flu.

People younger than the age of twenty-five years are more likely to be affected by the virus. The H1N1 flu is less likely to affect the elderly because older people may have developed immunity against the virus. At highest risk are children younger than two years old and teenagers younger than nineteen years old who are on long-term aspirin regimens.

Factors that increase the risk of developing complications from the H1N1 flu include pregnancy; recent (within two weeks) childbirth; diabetes; a weakened immune system, such as human immunodeficiency virus infection; immunosuppressive drugs; disorders that may affect breathing; chronic lung, heart, kidney, liver, nerve, or blood conditions; chronic care facilities; and, according to some reports, obesity.

SYMPTOMS

The following symptoms may be caused by the H1N1 flu, but they may also be caused by other conditions: fever and chills, sore throat, cough, severe muscle aches, severe fatigue, headache, runny nose, nasal congestion, sneezing, watery eyes, and gastrointestinal symptoms such as nausea, diarrhea, and vomiting. Persons should consult a doctor if having both a fever of 100° Fahrenheit (37.8° Celsius) or higher and either a stuffy nose (that makes it difficult to breathe through the nose), a runny nose (that causes one to wipe often), a cough, or a sore throat.

Exposure to the H1N1 flu can occur when a person is within six feet of someone known to have or someone suspected of having the H1N1 flu. Exposure also can occur when living, traveling, or having traveled to a place with confirmed cases of H1N1 flu.

Severe cases of H1N1 flu can cause pneumonia. Deaths have occurred, but this has been rare. The H1N1 flu can also worsen existing medical conditions.

One should seek urgent medical care if experiencing any of the following emergency warning signs: In adults, the signs include a fever of 100° F (37.8° C) or higher for more than three days, trouble breathing or shortness of breath, bloody or colored sputum, pain or pressure in chest or belly, sudden dizziness, confusion, severe vomiting or vomiting that does not stop, or flulike symptoms that get better then come back with a fever and a worse cough.

Emergency warning signs in children include fast breathing or trouble breathing, blue or gray skin, not drinking enough fluids, severe vomiting or vomiting that does not stop, difficulty waking up, being too irritable to be held, having little or no desire to play or

interact, lacking alertness, having flulike symptoms that get better then come back with a fever and a worse cough, and having a fever with a rash.

SCREENING AND DIAGNOSIS

A doctor will ask the patient about his or her symptoms and medical history. Diagnosis of the flu is usually based on symptoms. In some cases, the doctor may take samples from the patient's nose or throat to confirm the diagnosis.

TREATMENT AND THERAPY

Most people with the flu do not need antiviral medicine, but one should check with a doctor to see if antiviral medicine is needed. One also should consult a doctor before buying or using products sold through the Web that claim to treat H1N1 flu.

Persons in a high-risk group or who have a severe illness (such as breathing problems) will need antiviral medicine. Antiviral medicines do not cure the flu, but they may help relieve symptoms and shorten the time one is sick, especially if taken within forty-eight hours of the first symptoms.

Antiviral medicines used to treat the H1N1 flu include the following prescription drugs: oseltamivir (Tamiflu); zanamivir (Relenza), which may worsen a person's asthma or chronic obstructive pulmonary disease (COPD); peramivir, an investigational intravenous medicine that the U.S. Food and Drug Administration has allowed doctors to use for hospitalized patients if other antiviral medicines do not work; and oseltamivir (and perhaps zanamivir), which may increase the risk of self-injury and confusion shortly after taking, especially in children (who should be closely monitored for signs of unusual behavior). Other antiviral medications (such as amantadine or rimantadine) that are sometimes used to treat some kinds of seasonal flu do not work against the H1N1 flu.

There are other measures patients can take, such as getting extra rest; drinking increased amounts of liquids, including water, juice, and decaffeinated tea; and taking over-the-counter (OTC) pain relievers such as acetaminophen, ibuprofen, or (in adults) aspirin. Aspirin is not recommended for children or teenagers with a current or recent viral infection because of the risk of Reye's syndrome. One should consult the doctor about medicines that are safe for children (including other OTC products, such as decongestants, saline nasal sprays, and cough medicines).

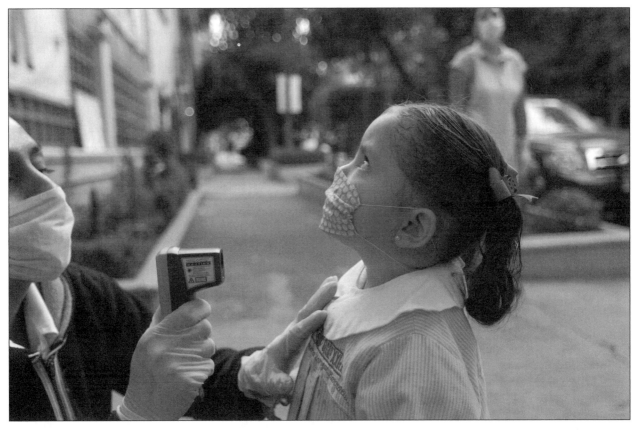

A schoolteacher checks a girl for fever in Mexico City in 2009. Students were kept from school during the H1N1 influenza, or swine flu, outbreak. (AP/Wide World Photos)

Cough and cold products can cause serious side effects in young children.

One alternative therapy may be a helpful form of treatment too. Researchers found that products (such as Sambucol and ViraBLOC) containing an herb called elderberry decreased flu symptoms in some studies. One should be aware, however, that herbal remedies are not regulated by the U.S. government. The herbal supplements purchased by consumers may not have the same ingredients as the supplements studied; they also may contain impurities.

PREVENTION AND OUTCOMES

An H1N1 flu vaccine is available. The vaccine comes in two forms: as a nasal spray and as a shot. The nasal spray is given in two doses (one month apart) for children ages two to nine years and in one dose for persons ages ten to forty-nine years. The shot will be given in two doses (one month apart) to children ages six months to nine years and in one dose for people ages ten years and older. One should consult a health care provider about the appropriate vaccine.

To avoid getting the H1N1 flu, one should wash his or her hands with soap and water often, especially after contacting someone who is sick; use rubbing-alcohol-based hand cleaners when water is not available; avoid close contact with persons who have respiratory infections, because the flu can spread starting one day before and ending seven days after symptoms appear; and avoid crowded gatherings, especially if one is at high risk for complications from H1N1 flu. (A disposable face mask could be used if one is unable to avoid crowded areas where H1N1 flu has been confirmed.)

Other preventive measures are to cover one's mouth and nose with a tissue when coughing or sneezing, and then throwing away the tissue after use (coughing or sneezing into one's elbow or upper sleeve is also helpful); avoid spitting; avoid sharing drinks or personal items; avoid biting one's nails; and avoid putting one's hands near one's eyes, mouth, or nose. Another measure is to keep surfaces clean by wiping them with a household disinfectant, but to avoid using cleaning products sold through the Web that claim to prevent the H1N1 flu. One should consult a doctor before using such products.

If caring for someone who has the H1N1 flu, one should follow the following steps: To prevent areas from being contaminated, one should try to keep the person who is sick in one room and should wash his or her hands after having contact with the sick person. If one is unable to avoid close contact with a sick person, it is helpful to cover one's mouth and nose with a face mask (or a respirator, if available). Also, one should limit contact with other members of the sick person's household or community while taking care of the person.

The person who is sick should have little contact with others and stay home from school or work. Going to school or work is possible if one feels well, but one should remember to keep track of his or her health and to take precautions (such as washing one's hands).

To prevent getting the H1N1 flu, one could take medications such as zanamivir (Relenza) or oseltamivir (Tamiflu). These drugs may be considered for people who have close contact with an infected person (who has a confirmed or suspected infection) and for those who have conditions that put them at high risk for complications. These persons include those with a chronic health condition or with an suppressed immune system and persons who are younger than the age of nineteen years and are on a long-term aspirin regimen; sixty-five years of age or older; younger than five years of age; those who are pregnant; those who are living in a nursing home; and those who are employed as a health care or public health worker who has contact with persons with confirmed or suspected infections.

Rebecca J. Stahl, M.A., and
Brian S. Alper, M.D., M.S.P.H.;
reviewed by Brian S. Alper

FURTHER READING

Centers for Disease Control and Prevention. "Key Facts About Swine Influenza (Swine Flu)." Available at http://www.cdc.gov/swineflu/key_facts.htm.

EBSCO Publishing. *DynaMed: Influenza.* Available through http://www.ebscohost.com/dynamed.
_____. *DynaMed: Pandemic (H1N1) 2009.* Available through http://www.ebscohost.com/dynamed.
_____. *Health Library: Flu.* Available through http://www.ebscohost.com.
Jamieson, Denise J., et al. "H1N1 2009 Influenza Virus Infection During Pregnancy in the USA." *The Lancet* 374 (2009): 451-458.
Myers, Kendall P., Christopher W. Olsen, and Gregory C. Gray. "Cases of Swine Influenza in Humans: A Review of the Literature." *Clinical Infectious Diseases* 44 (2007): 1084-1088.
U.S. Food and Drug Administration. "FDA Warns Web Sites Against Marketing Fraudulent H1N1 Flu-Virus Claims." Available at http://www.fda.gov.
Zakay-Rones, Z., et al. "Inhibition of Several Strains of Influenza Virus In Vitro and Reduction of Symptoms by an Elderberry Extract (*Sambucus nigra l.*) During an Outbreak of Influenza B Panama." *Journal of Alternative and Complementary Medicine* 1 (1995): 361-369.
_____. "Randomized Study of the Efficacy and Safety of Oral Elderberry Extract in the Treatment of Influenza A and B Virus Infections." *Journal of International Medical Research* 32, no. 2 (2004): 132-140.

WEB SITES OF INTEREST

Centers for Disease Control and Prevention
http://www.cdc.gov/flu

Flu.gov
http://www.flu.gov

Public Health Agency of Canada
http://www.phac-aspc.gc.ca

World Health Organization
http://www.who.int

See also: Airborne illness and disease; Avian influenza; Contagious diseases; Epidemics and pandemics: Causes and management; Hygiene; Infection; Influenza; Influenza vaccine; Respiratory route of transmission; Seasonal influenza; Viral infections; Viral upper respiratory infections.

Hookworms

CATEGORY: Pathogens
TRANSMISSION ROUTE: Direct contact, ingestion

DEFINITION

Hookworms are parasitic, threadlike roundworms (nematodes) that infect the small intestines of their host. Two species of hookworm are known to infect humans: *Ancylostoma duodenale*, also known as old world hookworm, and *Necator americanus*, also known as new world or American hookworm. Listed as one of the neglected tropical diseases (NDT) by the World Health Organization, hookworm infection is estimated to affect about one-quarter of the world's population.

Taxonomic Classification for Hookworms

Kingdom: Animalia
Phylum: Nematoda
Order: Strongylida
Family: Ancylostomatidae, Uncinariidae
Genera: *Ancylostoma, Necator*
Species:
A. duodenale
N. americanus

NATURAL HABITAT AND FEATURES

Hookworms are most often found in rural areas of tropical and subtropical countries such as those in Asia, East Africa, South America, and the southeastern United States. The eggs are deposited in the soil from human feces because of poor sanitation or because of the use of human feces as fertilizer. For the eggs to develop into larvae, the soil must be warm, shaded, sandy, or loamy, and must have sufficient moisture. The eggs hatch in one to two days into larvae that are able to penetrate skin and enter their human host. Ingestion of larvae from contaminated food is also possible.

Once inside the host, the larvae migrate through the body through the circulatory system and then through the lungs to the small intestines, where they adhere to the intestinal lining with their teeth or cutting plates. The worms will feed on their host's blood and proteins.

Six weeks after initial host penetration, the worm will have reached the adult reproductive stage. The oval eggs exit the body with the passage of stools. Depending on the species, each female can generate thousands of eggs per day. Hookworm life spans average one to two years, and some live up to ten years.

N. americanus ranges from six to twelve millimeters (mm) long and has a round body. Males are typically smaller than females. *A. duodenale* is slightly larger at eight to thirteen mm long and has an *S* shape at its front end.

PATHOGENICITY AND CLINICAL SIGNIFICANCE

The penetration of the skin by larvae causes an allergic reaction around the site of entry that is known as ground itch. Larvae migration through the body may also cause mild pulmonary distress such as asthma, bronchitis, or coughing.

Minor hookworm infections are typically asymptomatic. When many worms are present, the most critical pathology is human blood loss, which leads to iron deficiency anemia. Heavy infestation may also result in extreme fatigue and lethargy, fever, malnutrition, and digestive disruptions such as nausea, abdominal pain, diarrhea, and discolored stools. Severe infection in children can cause developmental delays.

Hookworm infections may be prevented through sanitary disposal of human feces and by wearing shoes in areas where hookworm larvae are likely to be found. Despite efforts to control and eradicate hookworms, they remain a worldwide public health concern. The U.S. Centers for Disease Control and Prevention lists hookworm as the second most common parasitic worm infection. In the face of hookworm's prevalence and its disruption to daily life, and because of concern over building resistance to drugs, the Human Hookworm Vaccine Initiative, composed of educational and research institutions from around the world, is working to develop a vaccine against hookworm infection.

DRUG SUSCEPTIBILITY

Hookworm infections may be treated with albendazole, mebendazole, and pyrantel pamoate. Reexamination of stools should occur two weeks after initial drug therapy to ensure the parasites have been eradicated. In addition to drug therapy, iron supplements may be necessary.

Susan E. Thomas, M.L.S.

FURTHER READING

Brooker, Sam, and Donal A. P. Bundy. "Soil-Transmitted Helminths (Geohelminths)." In *Manson's Tropical Diseases*, edited by Gordon C. Cook and Alimuddin I. Zumla. 22d ed. Philadelphia: Saunders/Elsevier, 2009.

Diemert, D. J., J. M. Bethony, and P. J. Hotez. "Hookworm Vaccines." *Clinical Infectious Diseases* 46 (2006): 282-288.

Fetouh, Nagla. "*Ancylostoma duodenale.*" University of Michigan, Museum of Zoology. Available at http://animaldiversity.ummz.umich.edu.

Hays, Harlan. "*Necator americanus.*" University of Michigan, Museum of Zoology. Available at http://animaldiversity.ummz.umich.edu.

Hotez, Peter J. "Neglected Tropical Disease Control in the 'Post-American World.'" *PLoS Neglected Tropical Diseases* 4, no. 8 (August, 2010). Available at http://www.plosntds.org.

"Intestinal Nematodes." In *Diagnostic Medical Parasitology*, edited by Lynne Shore Garcia. 5th ed. Washington, D.C.: ASM Press, 2007.

Kucik, Corry Jeb, et al. "Common Intestinal Parasites." *American Family Physician* 69 (2004): 1161-1168.

WEB SITES OF INTEREST

Centers for Disease Control and Prevention
http://www.cdc.gov/ncidod/dpd/parasites/hookworm

Neglected Tropical Diseases Coalition
http://www.neglectedtropicaldiseases.org

Sabin Vaccine Institute: Human Hookworm Vaccine Initiative
http://www.sabin.org/vaccine-development/vaccines/hookworm

See also: Ascariasis; Cholera; Developing countries and infectious disease; Fecal-oral route of transmission; Food-borne illness and disease; Giardiasis; Intestinal and stomach infections; Parasites: Classification and types; Parasitic diseases; Shigellosis; Travelers' diarrhea; Tropical medicine; *Vibrio*; Water treatment; Waterborne illness and disease; Worm infections.

Hordeola

CATEGORY: Diseases and conditions
ANATOMY OR SYSTEM AFFECTED: Eyes, tissue, vision
ALSO KNOWN AS: Sty

DEFINITION

A hordeolum is a small infection of the glands in the eye, located in the eyelids. The infection causes a red bump on the eyelid that may look like a pimple. This type of infection, also known as a sty, is usually quite painful. There are two types of hordeola: external, which occurs when the infection is external to the eyelash line, and internal, which occurs when the infection is inside the eyelash line. Hordeola are often easily diagnosed, and prompt treatment often prevents progression of the infection.

CAUSES

A hordeolum is caused by a blockage in the small glands located along the eyelid margin. These glands produce oil, and the blockage prevents normal drainage of the gland. If bacteria are trapped in the gland, an infection can develop. Fluid and pus cause the area to become red and inflamed. In 90 to 95 percent of cases, the resulting infection is caused by the bacterium *Staphylococcus aureus* (also known as staph). It is possible to have more than one hordeolum at a time, and it is common for them to recur.

RISK FACTORS

Hordeolum infection is a common condition, although the exact incidence in the United States is not known. Some conditions may increase the risk of developing a hordeolum; these conditions include poor eyelid hygiene, chronic illness, and a previous hordeolum (hordeola often recur in the same eyelid).

SYMPTOMS

A hordeolum usually begins as a red and swollen area on or in the eyelid. Often, the area is tender and painful. In addition to the red, painful bump, other symptoms include tearing of the eye and blurred vision or a sensation of a foreign body or scratchiness in the eye. Sometimes the swollen area has a point or yellowish spot. This area is where the discharge of pus will occur when the hordeolum drains.

Internal hordeola are usually more painful and are less likely to come to a point without the assistance of a doctor. If a person experiences redness and painful swelling in the eye, or any change in vision, he or she should consult an eye doctor immediately because these symptoms may be caused by other health conditions.

SCREENING AND DIAGNOSIS

In most cases, a simple eye exam is all that is necessary to confirm the diagnosis of a hordeolum. Other than looking at the person's eye, special tests are not usually necessary for diagnosis.

TREATMENT AND THERAPY

Often, hordeola resolve spontaneously on their own. In these cases, only hot compresses to assist the drainage are needed. Warm compresses can be applied four to six times a day for several minutes a session. However, if they do not drain on their own, hordeola often respond quickly to simple treatment from a doctor. If left untreated, the infection may continue to grow or may lead to other conditions. Chalazia occurs when the gland is blocked but no infection is present. Cellulitis occurs when the infection spreads to the tissue of the eyelid or beyond.

Drainage of the lesion is the first step in treating the hordeolum. If the hordeolum does not drain on its own, a doctor may assist by lancing the hordeolum. The pus and contents of the swollen area can then be drained. One should not lance the hordeolum without the assistance of a doctor; permanent damage to the eye or eyelid can occur.

In some cases, antibiotics are also given to ensure that the entire infection is eliminated. Antibiotics may be given in oral form, or as eye drops or eye ointment. In many cases, antibiotics alone are ineffective.

PREVENTION AND OUTCOMES

The best prevention against developing a hordeolum is to keep the area around the eye as clean as possible. One should always wash his or her hands thoroughly before touching one's eyes and should refrain from rubbing the eyes.

Although it may not be possible to prevent the development of every hordeolum, obtaining prompt treatment when one occurs is the best way to prevent recurrences. One should not attempt to drain the hordeolum. Any squeezing or poking at the hordeolum may cause more damage. The infection may be spread inadvertently, or damage to the eye could result.

Finally, one should contact a doctor immediately if experiencing vision problems, if there is a blister or crusting on the eyelid, if the white of the eye becomes red, if the hordeolum bleeds, or if experiencing pain.

Maria Borowski, M.A.;
reviewed by Christopher Cheyer, M.D.

FURTHER READING

Cassel, Gary H., Michael D. Billig, and Harry G. Randall. *The Eye Book: A Complete Guide to Eye Disorders and Health.* Baltimore: Johns Hopkins University Press, 2001.

"Chalazion/Hordeolum." In *The Wills Eye Manual: Office and Emergency Room Diagnosis and Treatment of Eye Disease,* edited by J. P. Ehler et al. 5th ed. Baltimore: Lippincott Williams & Wilkins, 2008.

Fort, G. G., et al. "Hordeolum (Stye)." In *Ferri's Clinical Advisor 2011: Instant Diagnosis and Treatment,* edited by Fred F. Ferri. Philadelphia: Mosby/Elsevier, 2011.

Mueller, J. B., et al. "Ocular Infection and Inflammation." *Emergency Medicine Clinics of North America* 26 (2008): 57.

Pasternak, A., and B. Irish. "Ophthalmologic Infections in Primary Care." *Clinics in Family Practice* 6 (2004): 19-33.

Riordan-Eva, Paul, and John P. Whitcher. *Vaughan and Asbury's General Ophthalmology.* 17th ed. New York: Lange Medical Books/McGraw-Hill, 2007.

Sutton, Amy L., ed. *Eye Care Sourcebook: Basic Consumer Health Information About Eye Care and Eye Disorders.* 3d ed. Detroit: Omnigraphics, 2008.

WEB SITES OF INTEREST

American Academy of Ophthalmology
http://www.aao.org

American Optometric Association
http://www.aoa.org

Canadian Association of Optometrists
http://www.opto.ca

Canadian Ophthalmological Society
http://www.eyesite.ca

See also: Abscesses; Bacterial infections; Boils; Conjunctivitis; Eye infections; Keratitis; Ophthalmia neonatorum; Pilonidal cyst; Staphylococcal infections; *Staphylococcus;* Trachoma.

Horizontal disease transmission

CATEGORY: Transmission

DEFINITION

Horizontal disease transmission refers to the passing of a disease or pathogen from one person to another who are in the same generation. The disease is not passed from woman to fetus in the perinatal period; this is done through vertical disease transmission. Symptoms depend on the specific type of acquired infection. Horizontal disease transmission occurs by direct or indirect pathogenic contact.

ROUTES OF TRANSMISSION

Horizontal transmission arises by direct contact through touching or sharing of saliva and secretions. For example, if one sexual partner has an infection, that infection may be transmitted to another partner through genital, anal, or oral contact. More than twenty-five sexually transmitted diseases (STDs) exist, including human immunodeficiency virus (HIV) infection, chlamydia, gonorrhea, and herpes. The respiratory route is another common pathway for direct contact, whereby an infected person coughs or sneezes droplets onto a susceptible person. The pathogen enters the body through the nose, mouth, or eye and causes infections such as influenza, chickenpox, and strep throat.

Indirect transmission occurs when a person has contact with an object (fomite) or host that carries the pathogen, allowing transmission without physical contact. Infections that are spread by contact with inanimate contaminated objects are warts, syphilis, and impetigo. Risk factors include improper handwashing technique, inadequate sterilization of objects, and living in close quarters, especially under unsanitary conditions. Indirect contact with insects or animals acting as disease vectors will also lead to horizontal disease transmission. Mosquitoes transfer malaria and ticks transfer Lyme disease to humans.

TESTING AND PREVENTION

Laboratory blood work or a physical exam, or both, will diagnose a horizontally transmitted disease. Antibiotics, antiviral medications, and vaccinations are available for some infections. In the case of STDs, precautions such as abstinence or condom use help prevent future horizontal transmission. One should also clean soiled laundry and bath towels and should avoid sharing personal toiletries.

IMPACT

Prevention of horizontal disease transmission is of paramount importance from a public health perspective. One study estimated there are 333 million new cases of syphilis, gonorrhea, trichomoniasis, and chlamydia in one year worldwide, with HIV remaining prevalent in both developed and developing countries. If not adequately controlled, some infections can cause global pandemics, such as the H1N1 influenza outbreak. In addition, the financial impact of any pandemic is extremely high.

Janet Ober Berman, M.S., CGC

FURTHER READING

Martinson, Francis E., et al. "Risk Factors for Horizontal Transmission of Hepatitis B Virus in a Rural District in Ghana." *American Journal of Epidemiology* 147 (1997): 478-487.

Okinyi, M., et al. "Horizontally-Acquired HIV Infection in Kenyan and Swazi Children." *International Journal of STD and AIDS Online* 20 (2009): 852-857.

Wilkinson, D., and G. Rutherford. "Population-Based Interventions for Reducing Sexually Transmitted Infections, Including HIV Infection." *Cochrane Database of Systematic Reviews* (2001): CD001220. Available through *EBSCO DynaMed Systematic Literature Surveillance* at http://www.ebscohost.com/dynamed.

WEB SITES OF INTEREST

American Social Health Association
http://www.ashastd.org

Centers for Disease Control and Prevention
http://www.cdc.gov/std

See also: Bacterial infections; Chlamydia; Gonorrhea; Herpes simplex infection; Herpesvirus infections; HIV; Mouth infections; Oral transmission; Pathogens; Primary infection; Saliva and infectious disease; Sexually transmitted diseases (STDs); Transmission routes; Trichomonas; Vertical disease transmission; Viral infections.

Hospitals and infectious disease

CATEGORY: Epidemiology

ALSO KNOWN AS: Health-care-associated infections, nosocomial infections

DEFINITION

Infections acquired in hospitals and health care facilities involve approximately 5 to 10 percent of persons admitted to acute-care or long-term-care facilities, according to the Centers for Disease Control and Prevention (CDC). These percentages mean that about ninety thousand persons per year get care-facility infections, also called nosocomial infections, making nosocomial infection the fourth leading cause of death in the United States. To be diagnosed as nosocomial, the infection must not be associated with the admitting diagnosis and must occur because of a patient's exposure to the surrounding pool of infectious agents. The infection usually becomes clinically evident after forty-eight hours (and during hospitalization) or within thirty days of discharge. These infectious agents can colonize a person's skin, respiratory tract, genitourinary tract, gastrointestinal tract, and bloodstream.

Hospital-Acquired Infections

According to the U.S. Department of Health and Human Services, the following four conditions account for 78 percent of all hospital-acquired infections:

- Urinary tract infections (34 percent)
- Surgical site infections (17 percent)
- Bloodstream infections (14 percent)
- Pneumonia (13 percent)

CAUSES

Most hospital acquired infections are caused by bacteria, viruses, or parasites. The causative organisms can be introduced through endotracheal (ET) intubation, catheterization, gastric drainage tubes, and intravenous procedures for medication delivery, blood transfusions, or nutrition supplementation. Infection also occurs through surgical procedures and by health care workers' failing to wash their hands before procedures and between encountering patients. Other causes of hospital acquired infections include prolonged hospitalization, the severity of the patient's underlying illness, the prevalence of antibiotic-resistant bacteria from the prolonged use or overuse of antibiotics, contaminated air-conditioning systems, contaminated water systems, lack of an appropriate ratio of nurses to patients, and overcrowding of beds. Later studies suggested that the uniforms and laboratory coats of hospital personnel may also help transfer pathogens. Also, it has been suggested that the shedding of epithelial tissues from the patients onto their hospital clothing may contribute to infections. Other reservoirs of contamination include stethoscopes, blood pressure cuffs, bed pans, water pitchers, telephones, and other objects. Airborne infections in hospitals may contribute to infections that include tuberculosis and herpes varicella.

The most common hospital acquired infection is that of the urinary tract, accounting for about 40 percent of cases. Placing a catheter into the bladder for delivery of medication, for measuring urinary output, for the relief of pressure, or for other medical reasons creates a port of entry for infectious agents. The healthy bladder is normally sterile; it contains no harmful bacteria or other organisms. The catheter can pick up bacteria or organisms from the urethra, providing an easy route to the bladder. This infection can occur because of improper sterilization techniques, which creates a mechanical entry for infection through, for example, multiple tries to insert the catheter; even the composition of the catheter can lead to infection of the bladder. It is now recognized that a major cause of nosocomial infection is the picking up of bacteria, such as *Escherichia coli* (*E. coli*), or other organisms from the intestinal tract and transferring them to the bladder. Irritation from the catheter's insertion and prolonged use of the catheter can transfer bacteria (and a fungus called *Candida*). An infection caused by an indwelling catheter will need long-term treatment with antibiotics; this long-term treatment can compromise the patient's immune system, thereby causing further harm.

Nosocomial pneumonia is the second leading hospital-acquired infection, accounting for about 20 percent of cases. Bacteria and other microorganisms enter the respiratory system through procedures treating respiratory illnesses. The placement of ET tubes for mechanical ventilation is of primary concern. If ET tubes are inserted (such as by a paramedic) while the patient is outside a hospital or even in an emergency room, the risk of infection is greater. The introduction of aids for ensuring adequate ventilation often lead to infection. Aspiration from the nose, throat, and lungs is a direct pathway for introduction of microorganisms.

Accounting for about 17 percent of cases of hospital acquired infection is surgery. Agents of infection include contaminated surgical equipment, the contaminated hands of health care providers, contaminated dressings, trauma wounds, burn wounds, and pressure sores from prolonged bed rest or wheel chair use. The continuous delivery of medications, transfusions, antibiotics, or nutrients through the bloodstream by intravenous (IV) routes is a common cause of infection. Improper technique causes bacteria to enter the body at the placement of IVs and increases the risk of infection the longer the IVs are in place. Infections in the blood are of special concern because they can produce disseminating infections. Gastrointestinal procedures, such as colonoscopy; obstetric procedures; and kidney dialysis can also lead to major infections.

Antibiotic resistance has led to an increase in several other nosocomial infections, including superinfections. Generally, the major causative pathogens for hospital acquired infections relate to the location of the involved body system or systems, except for the bloodstream, which when infected can cause dissemination of the infection to all major organs. By classifying major pathogens according to the organ systems they affect, one can differentiate among these varying pathogens. The major pathogens for the genitourinary system are gram-negative enterics, fungi, and enterococci. Bloodstream infectious agents are usually coagulase-negative staphylococci, enterococci, fungi, *Staphylococcus aureus*, *Enterobacter* species, *Pseudomonas*, and *Acinetobacter baumannii* (which causes substantial antimicrobial resistance). Surgical-site infections include *S. aureus*, *Pseudomonas*, coagulase-negative staphylococci, and (rarely) enterococci, fungi, *Enterobacter* species, and *E. coli*.

Ventilator-associated pneumonia is designated as either early or late onset. Early onset begins within the first three to four days of mechanical ventilation. The infections are usually antibiotic-sensitive and are most often caused by *S. pneumoniae*, *H. influenza*, or *S. aureus*. Late-onset infections that are antibiotic-resistant

and are main causative agents are those caused by *Ps. aeruginosa*, *Actinobacter* spp., and *Enterobacter* spp. Other pneumonias caused by gram-negative bacterium are *Klebsiella pneumoniae*, *Legionella*, or methicillin-resistant *Staphyloccocus aureus* (MRSA), known as the superbug.

The newest hospital-acquired infection is colitis, caused by the organism *Clostridium difficile*. This gram-positive, anaerobic, spore-forming bacillus is responsible for antibiotic-associated diarrhea and colitis. The infection is caused by a disturbance of the normal bacterial flora in the colon, precipitated by antibiotic therapy. The colonization of *C. difficile* releases two toxins: toxin A, an endotoxin, and toxin B, a cytotoxin, leading to mucosal inflammation and damage of the colon.

RISK FACTORS

Although all hospital patients are susceptible to nosocomial infections, young children, especially those in the neonatal intensive care unit (ICU); adult ICU patients; the elderly; and patients with compromised immune systems are more likely to acquire these infections. Other risk factors include having underlying diseases such as chronic lung disease, diabetes, or cardiac disease; being obese; being malnourished; having a malignancy; having a remote infection; using prophylactic antibiotics; and hospitalization before surgery (especially for twelve hours or longer), which increases the patient's exposure to the reservoir of infectious agents.

SYMPTOMS

The primary sign of infection is fever. A person's admission temperature and those temperatures recorded at the time of hospitalization and after hospitalization are paramount for recognizing a developing infection. Other symptoms of infection include an increased respiratory rate; increased pulse rate; sweating, especially at night; chest pain; productive phlegm with coughing or an inability to cough; pain and discharge from the nose or mouth; fatigue; difficulty and pain with swallowing; nausea; vomiting; excessive diarrhea; pain with urination or blood present in urine; reduced urine output; redness and swelling with pustular discharge around surgical wounds or openings in sutures from skin closures with exposure to subcutaneous tissues; and the development of skin rashes.

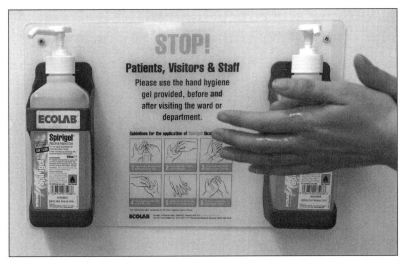

Resistant pathogens easily spread in hospitals and other health care facilities. Hand sanitizers for staff and visitors are now commonly used to stop the spread of disease. (AP/Wide World Photos)

SCREENING AND DIAGNOSIS

The foregoing signs and symptoms suggest infection. One should consult a doctor immediately if any of these symptoms are present during or after hospitalization. The first diagnostic tool is a complete physical examination, which includes laboratory studies and X rays. Other tests include extensive blood testing, with a complete blood count that looks for an increase in infection-fighting white blood cells; a complete urinalysis that includes culture and checks for a sensitivity to antibiotics; two blood samples drawn twenty minutes apart for culture and sensitivity; sputum for culture and sensitivity; and wound cultures for culture and sensitivity. Ancillary tests include abdominal X rays or computed tomography (CT) scans (a detailed X ray that identifies abnormalities of fine tissue structure); kidney X rays; kidney, liver, and pancreas function tests; blood gas tests; and tests for fungus infective agents.

TREATMENT AND THERAPY

While waiting for the laboratory culture and sensitivity results, which may take up to forty-eight hours to complete, one should begin broad-spectrum antibiotic therapy. This usually includes penicillin, cephalosporins, tetracycline, or erythromycin, and supplemental oxygen if needed. The doctor will need to know if the patient is allergic to certain antibiotics or if the patient has been on prolonged antibiotic therapy. It is usual to combine antibiotics for therapy, so, for best results, the doctor must determine if the infecting organism is gram-positive or gram-negative or whether it is anaerobic bacteria, resistant bacteria, or fungi. Once the causative agent for infection has been identified, aggressive therapy begins. Recommended treatments include vancomycin, imipenem plus cilastatin, meropenem, azteonam, piperacillin plus tazobactam, ceftazidme, and cefepime. If MRSA is suspected, limezoid can be used.

Other treatments that can be used to supplement antibiotic therapy include pulmonary hygiene and respiratory treatments, aggressive wound care, fever control until the antibiotics show evidence of effectiveness, body cleansing, changing of hospital garments, and extreme sterile techniques when treating the patient (which may include putting the patient in reverse isolation for protection of further exposure to infections). Close monitoring of cardiac status, urine output, and pulmonary functions is recommended. The changing of catheters, IV lines, gastrointestinal (GI) tubes, and other invasive forms of exposure may also be ordered by the doctor. The hospital's medical team and infectious disease control team will monitor the patient's status and present complete documentation of the case.

PREVENTION AND OUTCOMES

The recommendations for the prevention of infections acquired in hospitals and other health care facilities cover a broad geographic, demographic, cultural, and ecological spectrum. The recommendations are based on the type of causative agents as precursors for disease in the associated populations. Requirements, although based on sound science, can sometimes be misinterpreted or even ignored. A good foundation for practice is to bring together basic infection-control measures and the history of epidemiology. Historically, this practice could have begun in the nineteenth century with Florence Nightingale, who believed respiratory secretions could be dangerous, and with Ignaz Semmelweis, a nineteenth century obstetrician who demonstrated that routine handwashing could prevent the spread of puerperal fever. Joseph Lister, a nineteenth century professor of surgery, was the first to realize the connection between the suppuration of wounds and the discoveries of the fermentation process (by chemist and microbiologist Louis Pasteur) in the mid-nineteenth century. Lister published his findings in 1867 and was credited with helping to start the practice sterilizing operating rooms with carbolic acid.

The CDC began hospital surveillance in the United States in the 1960's. The 1970's saw the introduction of training courses in disease prevention and the establishment of the CDC's Division of Healthcare Quality and Promotion for hospital infection programs and the National Nosocomial Infections Surveillance System. The Study on the Efficacy of Nosocomial Infection Control was conducted in the early 1970's. The Healthcare Infection Control Practices Advisory Committee was formed in 1991 and, in 2005, hospitals began contributing surveillance to the National Healthcare Safety Network, which was reworked with a comparison study in 2007. The initiatives created by these agencies and programs provide guidelines for improvement in the prevention of hospital acquired infections.

These guidelines include adopting infection control programs in accordance with the CDC to track trends in infection rates, ensuring that one practitioner is available for every two hundred beds in hospitals and other health care facilities, identifying high-risk medical procedures, strict adherence by medical staff and visitors to handwashing policies, and other sterilization techniques. These include using sterile gowns, gloves, masks, and barriers; sterilizing reusable equipment, including ventilators, humidifiers, or other respiratory equipment that comes in contact with a patient's respiratory tract; frequently changing wound dressings and using antimicrobial ointments; removing nasalgastric and endotracheal tubes as soon as possible; using antibacterial-coated venous catheters; preventing infection by airborne microbes through wearing masks (by hospital personnel and patients); limiting the use of high-risk procedures such as urinary catheterization; isolating patients with known infections; and reducing the general use of antibiotics.

M. Barbara Klyde, PA

FURTHER READING

Clancy, Carolyn. "Simple Steps Can Reduce Health Care-Associated Infections: Navigating the Health Care System." Rockville, Md.: Agency for Healthcare Research and Quality, 2008. Available at http://www.ahrq.gov/consumer/cc/cc070108.htm.

Helms, Brenda, et al. "Improving Hand Hygiene Compliance: A Multidisciplinary Approach." *American Journal of Infection Control* 38, no. 7 (2010): 572-574.

Heymann, David L., ed. *Control of Communicable Diseases Manual.* 19th ed. Washington, D.C.: American Public Health Association, 2008.

Kuehnert, Matthew J., et al. "Methicillin-Resistant *Staphylococcus aureus* Hospitalizations, United States." *Emerging Infectious Diseases* 11, no. 6 (2005).

Kushner, Thomasine Kimbrough. *Surviving Healthcare: A Manual for Patients and Their Families.* New York: Cambridge University Press, 2010.

Peleg, Anton Y., and David C. Hooper. "Hospital-Acquired Infections Due to Gram-Negative Bacteria." *New England Journal of Medicine* 362, no. 19 (2010): 1804-1813.

Turnock, Bernard, J. *Public Health: What It Is and How It Works.* 3d ed. Sudbury, Mass.: Jones and Bartlett, 2004.

Weber, David J., et al. "Role of Hospital Surfaces in the Transmission of Emerging Health Care-Associated Pathogens: Norovirus, *Clostridium difficile*, and *Acinetobacter* Species." *American Journal of Infection Control* 38, no. 5, suppl. (2010): S25-S33.

WEB SITES OF INTEREST

Agency for Healthcare Research and Quality
http://www.ahrq.gov

Association for Professionals in Infection Control and Epidemiology
http://www.knowledgeisinfectious.org

Clean Hands Coalition
http://www.cleanhandscoalition.org

National Institute of Allergy and Infectious Diseases
http://www.niaid.nih.gov

Public Health Agency of Canada
http://www.phac-aspc.gc.ca

See also: Airborne illness and disease; Antibiotic resistance; Antibiotic-associated colitis; Antibiotics: Types; Bacterial infections; Bloodstream infections; Chemical germicides; Contagious diseases; Drug resistance; Emerging and reemerging infectious diseases; Epidemiology; Fever; Fever of unknown origin; Iatrogenic infections; Methicillin-resistant staph infection; Necrotizing fasciitis; Opportunistic infections; Osteomyelitis; Primary infection; Prosthetic joint infections; Public health; Puerperal infection; Respiratory route of transmission; Secondary infection; Superbacteria; Transmission routes; Vancomycin-resistant enterococci infection; Viral infections; Wound infections.

Hosts

CATEGORY: Transmissionn

DEFINITION

A host is a living thing upon which another organism, a parasite, depends for survival. A parasite lives on or in the body of the host. To live, the parasite relies on the host to provide food, water, warmth, protection, and conditions for reproduction. The parasite does not provide anything beneficial in return and may cause the host to become ill.

PARASITIC INFECTION

Parasites target a specific species of host for optimum survival. They are much smaller than their hosts and reproduce at a faster rate, so they are able to survive and procreate without killing the host.

Skin parasites attach themselves to a host and feed on the host's blood. They typically lay their eggs on the skin surface, where their offspring may also feed on the host or be released into the environment to find other hosts.

Other parasites may be found in uncooked or undercooked meat, raw vegetables, and contaminated, dirty drinking water. They may also be carried on hands that have not been washed after handling animals, soil, or feces. Thus, parasites may be inadvertently ingested. The eggs and offspring of ingested parasites are shed into the environment in the host's feces. Some parasites are deposited into hosts through insect bites. For example, mosquitoes are carriers of the protozoa that cause malaria.

ADVERSE EFFECTS ON THE HOST

If the host were to die, the parasite would lose its life support, so the parasite does not deliberately kill its host. However, its presence affects the host's health. Parasites in the intestinal tract may prevent the host from absorbing nutrients. Parasites traveling in the bloodstream may clog blood vessels, lymph vessels, and bile ducts. Parasites residing in tissues and organs may cause damage by producing toxins that destroy the cells.

PREVENTION

One can prevent a parasitic infection through adequate handwashing technique, including the use of soap and water, after handling animals and raw meats, after working in soil, and before handling food. Cooking raw meats to sufficiently high temperatures also helps prevent infection. In addition, one can use insect repellent to ward off parasites.

IMPACT

The Centers for Disease Control and Prevention tracks the incidence of reportable parasitic diseases in the United States. About 7.4 million cases of trichomoniasis, a sexually transmitted parasitic disease, are reported every year, followed in frequency by giardiasis (2 million cases) and cryptosporidiosis (300,000 cases). Toxoplasmosis, caused by a food-borne parasite, leads to the death of more than 375 persons annually.

Diagnostic tests for parasitic diseases include direct examination of fecal samples for parasites and their eggs (ova), endoscopy or colonoscopy to directly observe parasites in the gastrointestinal tract, and examination of blood samples under a microscope. Treatments include antibiotics such as metronidazole and antimalarial drugs such as chloroquine.

Bethany Thivierge, M.P.H.

FURTHER READING

Marquardt, William C., ed. *Biology of Disease Vectors.* 2d ed. New York: Academic Press/Elsevier, 2005.

Reidl, Joachim, et al. "*Vibrio cholerae* and Cholera: Out of the Water and Into the Host." *FEMS Microbiological Reviews* 26 (June, 2002): 125-139.

Sasse, Amber. "A Lousy Reason for Asthma and Allergies: Parasites May Reduce Their Hosts' Risk of Developing Immune Dysfunctions." *Popular Science,* April 22, 2009.

Tolan, Robert W., Jr. "Infections in the Immunocompromised Host." Available at http://emedicine.
medscape.com/article/973120-overview.

WEB SITE OF INTEREST

Centers for Disease Control and Prevention
http://www.cdc.gov/parasites

See also: Arthropod-borne illness and disease; Blood-
borne illness and disease; Carriers; Food-borne illness and disease; Insect-borne illness and disease;
Parasites: Classification and types; Parasitic diseases;
Pathogenicity; Pathogens; Transmission routes; Vectors and vector control; Virulence; Waterborne illness
and disease.

Human immunodeficiency virus. *See* HIV.

Human papillomavirus (HPV) infections

CATEGORY: Diseases and conditions
ANATOMY OR SYSTEM AFFECTED: Anus, cervix, genitalia, penis skin, vagina

DEFINITION

Human papillomaviruses (HPVs) are members of
the Papillomaviridae family that selectively infect the
epithelium of skin and mucous membranes. These infections may produce no symptoms or may produce
several types of common warts, or they may be associated with a number of both benign and cancerous
tissue growths. More than one hundred different HPV
genotypes have been identified, and more than forty
of these infect the genital epithelium. Low-risk types
cause benign lesions such as common warts and genital warts, while high-risk types can cause invasive cervical cancer. It is estimated that the annual incidence
of genital HPV infections in the United States is 5.5
million, making this the most commonly acquired
viral sexually transmitted disease.

CAUSES

Genital HPV is a double-stranded deoxyribonucleic

acid (DNA) virus that is transmitted by skin-to-skin
contact with an infected partner, regardless of the partner's gender. Sexually transmitted HPV can spread
through vaginal, anal, or oral sex. Individual strains of
HPV are associated with specific clinical symptoms and
are classified by their risk of causing cervical cancer.
HPV-6 and HPV-11, which are identified with most of
the more benign lesions, such as genital warts, are the
two most common low-risk types. HPV types 16 and 18,
which can cause abnormal cellular development in
the cervix, leading to invasive cervical cancer, are the
two most common high-risk types. Scientists have established that persistent infection with high-risk genital HPV is necessary for the development of cervical
cancer.

RISK FACTORS

One of the most significant risk factors for acquiring HPV, both among men and women, is having
many sex partners over the course of one's life. The
risk for genital HPV infection in women is increased
the earlier a woman began having sex. In men, the
number of lifetime and recent sex partners, and the
frequency of sex, are significant risk factors. Recent
studies have concluded that males who are not circumcised are at a greater risk than circumcised men
for contracting HPV-related penile cancer, and that
circumcision may reduce the risk of infection. Men
and women who participate in receptive anal intercourse are at risk for anal HPV infection, which may
result in anal warts or anal cancer.

SYMPTOMS

Clinical manifestations of genital HPV include genital warts, dysplasia (abnormal growth or development
of cells), and cancer of the cervix, vulva, vagina, anus,
and penis. In women, HPV-related disease occurs
more often at the cervix. HPV infection is the principal cause of all cervical cancers and is responsible for
5.2 percent of all cancers. Cervical cancer is the second
leading cancer among women worldwide. Nearly ten
million women in the United States have HPV infection without clinically detectable symptoms.

Exposure to genital HPV usually occurs soon after
starting sexual activity. In most affected women, HPV
infections are temporary and present no symptoms;
often, neither genital warts nor cervical dysplasia will
develop. About 70 percent of new infections resolve
spontaneously within one year and 90 percent do so

within two years. Only a minority of these cases progress to cervical cancer.

Following an incubation period of several months after exposure, however, a lesion such as cervical dysplasia or a genital wart may appear in some women. During this period of active growth, a sustained immune response to the HPV virus is generated. Following this immune response, there is a period of host containment, after which either remission continues or cancer develops.

SCREENING AND DIAGNOSIS

Cervical cancer develops over a long period of time, during which HPV causes cells on or around the cervix to develop abnormally; this change is known as cervical intraepithelial neoplasia, which could progress to precancer (changes in the cells that can become cancer). Most often, however, abnormal cells disappear without treatment.

A Pap test (Pap smear), sometimes called cervical cytology screening, is the best way to detect abnormal or potentially abnormal cell changes in the vagina and uterine cervix; the existence of these cell changes might be an early sign of precancer of the cervix. With the Pap test, cells are collected from the cervical area and examined under a microscope. If a Pap test shows the presence of abnormal cells, a physician will suggest follow-up care, which may include repeat Pap testing or HPV DNA testing. The HPV DNA test detects the genetic material of high-risk types of HPV that are associated with cancer, including specific subtypes such as HPV-16 and HPV-18. The American Congress of Obstetricians and Gynecologists recommends that women should have their first Pap test within three years of becoming sexually active or by age twenty-one years.

TREATMENT AND THERAPY

There is no known cure for HPV infection; the HPV virus itself cannot be treated. Several options exist for the treatment of common warts. HPV infection is not always eliminated by removing warts; if the virus is still present in the body, it can reappear following treatment.

Common skin warts can be removed at home with over-the-counter medications such as salicylic acid. A doctor can use cryotherapy to freeze, and, thus, remove the wart with liquid nitrogen. Genital warts can be treated with medications such as imiquimod, podo-

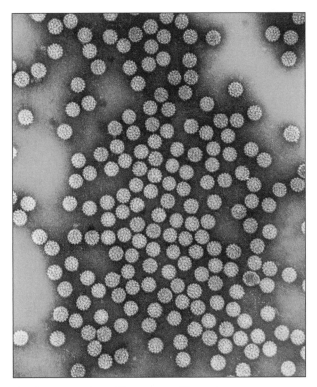

A microscopic view of human papillomaviruses.

phyllotoxin, podophyllum, and trichloroacetic acid, or they may be physically removed with laser therapy or minor surgery.

If the infection has resulted in cell changes that might potentially progress to cervical cancer, four treatment options are available. One approach is to watch and wait; most of the time these cell changes will heal by themselves. If they do not, cryotherapy may be applied. Conization, or cone biopsy, removes the abnormal areas. In a process known as LEEP (loop electrosurgical excision procedure), the abnormal cells are removed with a painless electrical current.

PREVENTION AND OUTCOMES

The only effective way to prevent HPV infection is to avoid contact with infectious lesions. One of the most significant risk factors for acquiring HPV is having many lifetime sex partners, therefore limiting the number of sex partners can limit the number of potential infections. Condoms reduce the risk of infection in vaginal, anal, and oral sex and protect against genital warts, cervical dysplasia, and invasive cervical cancer.

The Pap test and HPV DNA test are essential tools for the screening and prevention of cervical cancer. Two vaccines are available that protect against the types of HPV that cause most cases of genital warts and cervical cancer. Gardasil protects against HPV types 6, 11, 16, and 18, while Cervarix protects against types 16 and 18. The vaccines are most effective if given before a girl or woman is exposed to HPV.

Gerald W. Keister, M.A.

FURTHER READING

Bonnez, William, and Richard C. Reichman. "Papillomaviruses." In *Mandell, Douglas, and Bennett's Principles and Practice of Infectious Diseases*, edited by Gerald L. Mandell, John E. Bennett, and Raphael Dolin. 7th ed. New York: Churchill Livingstone/Elsevier, 2010.

Bosch, F. X., et al. "The Causal Relation Between Human Papillomavirus and Cervical Cancer." *Journal of Clinical Pathology* 55 (2002): 244-265.

Munoz, N., et al. "Epidemiologic Classification of Human Papillomavirus Types Associated with Cervical Cancer." *New England Journal of Medicine* 348 (2003): 518-527.

Reichman, Richard C. "Human Papillomavirus Infections." In *Harrison's Principles of Internal Medicine*, edited by Joan Butterton. 17th ed. New York: McGraw-Hill, 2008.

Steben, Marc, and Eliane Duarte-Franco. "Human Papillomavirus Infection: Epidemiology and Pathophysiology." *Gynecologic Oncology* 107 (2007): S2-S5.

Trottier, H., and E. L. Franco. "The Epidemiology of Genital Human Papillomavirus Infection." *Vaccine* 24, suppl. 1 (March 30, 2006): S1-S15.

Weaver, Bethany A. "Epidemiology and Natural History of Genital Human Papillomavirus Infection." *Journal of the American Osteopathic Association* 106, no. 3, suppl. 1 (March, 2006): S2-S8.

WEB SITES OF INTEREST

American Cancer Society
http://www.cancer.org

American Social Health Association
http://www.ashastd.org

Centers for Disease Control and Prevention, National Center for HIV, STD, and TB Prevention
http://www.cdc.gov/std

Gynecologic Cancer Foundation
http://www.thegcf.org

National Cancer Institute
http://www.cancer.gov/cancertopics/hpv-vaccines

See also: Cancer and infectious disease; Cancer vaccines; Cervical cancer; Children and infectious disease; Chlamydia; Contagious diseases; Genital herpes; Genital warts; Gonorrhea; Herpes simplex infection; HIV; Human papillomavirus (HPV) vaccine; Pelvic inflammatory disease; Prevention of viral infections; Sexually transmitted diseases (STDs); Syphilis; Trichomonas; Urethritis; Warts.

Human papillomavirus (HPV) vaccine

CATEGORY: Prevention

DEFINITION

Two brands of the human papillomavirus (HPV) vaccine, Cervarix and Gardasil, have been approved by the U.S. Food and Drug Administration. Both brands can prevent most cases of cervical cancer in girls and women if the vaccine is given before exposure to HPV. Gardasil can also prevent genital warts in both females and males.

More than forty types of HPV can infect the genital areas of both males and females. Most HPV types cause no symptoms and resolve on their own. Some types of HPV, however, cause cervical cancer in girls and women and other, less common, genital cancers (of the anus, vagina, and vulva). Some types of HPV can cause genital warts in males and females. Because the HPV vaccine does not prevent all kinds of cervical cancer, females who receive the HPV vaccine still need to have regular Pap tests.

CANDIDATES FOR VACCINATION

The HPV vaccine should be given before beginning sexual activity with another person. The vaccine is most effective in persons who have not been exposed to HPV.

The vaccine is recommended for girls age eleven and twelve. However, the vaccines can be adminis-

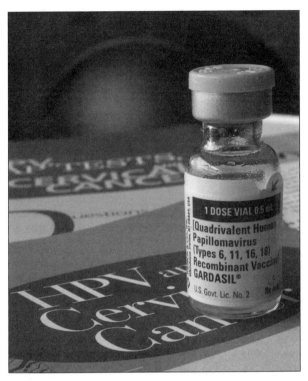

One dose of the vaccine Gardasil, used to prevent human papillomavirus infections. (AP/Wide World Photos)

tered in girls as young as nine years of age. Also, girls and women through age twenty-six years can receive the vaccine if they had not received any or all of the shots when they were younger. Males age nine through twenty-six years can receive the HPV vaccine to help prevent genital warts.

DOSAGE

The HPV vaccine is given as a three-dose series. Each dose is 0.5 milliliters, administered intramuscularly, preferably in a deltoid muscle. It is best to use the same vaccine brand for all three doses. The minimum time between dose one and dose two of the vaccine is four weeks; between does two and dose three is twelve weeks. The minimum time between dose one and dose three is twenty-four weeks. Doses that were received after a shorter-than-recommended time interval should be given again.

RISKS

Generally, the HPV vaccine is very safe, but mild to moderate reactions have been reported. Reactions in-

clude pain, redness, itching, bruising, or swelling at the injection site; mild to moderate fever; headache; nausea; vomiting; dizziness; and fainting. Persons who are allergic to the ingredients of the vaccines, including yeast, should not receive the vaccine, nor should pregnant girls or women.

IMPACT

The HPV vaccine is the first preventive cancer vaccine. Initially, the vaccine was controversial because some parents and religious groups claimed it would make casual sex more acceptable, especially among girls. Lawmakers are debating whether to make this vaccine mandatory.

Claudia Daileader Ruland, M.A.

FURTHER READING

Boston Women's Health Collective. *Our Bodies, Ourselves: A New Edition for a New Era.* 35th anniversary ed. New York: Simon & Schuster, 2005.

Centers for Disease Control and Prevention. "FDA Licensure of Bivalent Human Papillomavirus Vaccine (HPV2, Cervarix) for Use in Females: Recommendations of the Advisory Committee on Immunization Practices (ACIP)." *Morbidity and Mortality Weekly Report*, May 28, 2010, 626-629.

_____. "FDA Licensure of Quadrivalent Human Papillomavirus Vaccine (HPV4, Gardasil) for Use in Males: Recommendations of the Advisory Committee on Immunization Practices (ACIP)." *Morbidity and Mortality Weekly Report*, May 28, 2010, 630-632.

_____. "HPV Vaccine Information for Young Women." Available at http://www.cdc.gov/std/hpv/stdfact-hpv-vaccine-young-women.htm.

Dunne, E. F., and L. E. Markowitz. "Genital Human Papillomavirus Infection." *Clinical Infectious Diseases* 43 (2006): 624.

Larsen, Laura. *Sexually Transmitted Diseases Sourcebook.* Detroit: Omnigraphics, 2009.

McCance, Dennis J., ed. *Human Papilloma Viruses.* New York: Elsevier Science, 2002.

Plotkin, Stanley A., Walter A. Orenstein, and Paul A. Offit. *Vaccines.* 5th ed. Philadelphia: Saunders/Elsevier, 2008.

"Quadrivalent Vaccine Against Human Papillomavirus to Prevent High-Grade Cervical Lesions." *New England Journal of Medicine* 356 (2007): 1915-1927.

Trottier, H., and E. L. Franco. "The Epidemiology of

Genital Human Papillomavirus Infection." *Vaccine* 24, suppl. 1 (March 30, 2006): S1-S15.

Web Sites of Interest

American Cancer Society
http://www.cancer.org

American Social Health Association
http://www.ashastd.org

GirlsHealth.gov
http://www.girlshealth.gov

Gynecologic Cancer Foundation
http://www.thegcf.org

National Cancer Institute
http://www.cancer.gov/cancertopics/hpv-vaccines

WomensHealth.gov
http://www.womenshealth.gov

See also: Cancer and infectious disease; Cancer vaccines; Cervical cancer; Children and infectious disease; Chlamydia; Contagious diseases; Genital herpes; Genital warts; Gonorrhea; Herpes simplex infection; HIV; Human papillomavirus (HPV) infections; Pelvic inflammatory disease; Prevention of viral infections; Sexually transmitted diseases (STDs); Syphilis; Trichomonas; Urethritis; Warts.

Hygiene

Category: Prevention
Also known as: Body hygiene, personal hygiene

Definition

Hygiene involves more than cleanliness; it encompasses the habits humans practice to reduce the risk of receiving and transmitting infectious diseases.

Types of Hygienic Practice

Handwashing. Studies have shown that handwashing is the single most effective way to protect oneself from illness and to avoid passing microorganisms to others. Hands should be washed often, particularly before preparing food; after handling uncooked meat; before eating; after using the toilet; after changing a diaper; after sneezing, coughing, or blowing one's nose; before inserting and removing contact lenses; after gardening or working in dirt or soil; and after touching animals or cleaning up after them.

One should wash hands in clean, preferably warm, running water with a lathering liquid or bar soap. Hands should be rubbed together, making sure the soap contacts all skin surfaces, for a minimum of fifteen to twenty seconds. The soap should then be rinsed off with running water. Hands may be dried with a clean cloth towel, paper towel, or air dryer.

If soap and water are not available, one can use an alcohol-based hand sanitizer. Hands should be rubbed together until the alcohol evaporates and the hands are dry.

Showering and bathing. Bathing or showering with comfortably hot, clean water and liquid or bar soap that lathers removes dirt and sweat that contain microorganisms and also moisturizes the skin to create a more efficient barrier. Clean and moisturized skin also promotes the healing of cuts, abrasions, burns, and rashes.

Oral hygiene. Brushing and flossing one's teeth after meals protect the teeth and gums from dental caries, or cavities, and periodontal disease. Regular visits to a dentist and dental hygienist keep the oral cavity clean and allow for the early detection and treatment of tooth, gum, and mouth diseases.

Covering coughs and sneezes. When a person sneezes or coughs, saliva and other mucus containing bacteria and viruses are released as droplets into the air. To limit transmission, sneezes and coughs should be covered using a disposable tissue, a handkerchief, one's sleeve, or one's hand, which should be washed as soon as possible after coughing or sneezing into it.

Environmental hygiene. Housekeeping is important because disinfecting surfaces, especially in the kitchen and bathroom, kills disease-causing bacteria. All cloth towels should be washed in hot water with detergent. Dishes should be washed with dish soap and hot water.

Impact

Hygiene practices, especially handwashing, reduce the incidence of illness, lower the cost of medical care associated with illness, decrease the number of lost days from work and school, and potentially save lives.

Bethany Thivierge, M.P.H.

Handwashing and Bacterial Resistance

Antibacterial soaps contain antibacterials, a subclass of antimicrobials, which kill or inhibit the growth of bacteria and other microorganisms. Antiseptics are antimicrobial agents that are sufficiently nontoxic to be applied to human tissue. Antibiotics are chemicals that inhibit a specific pathway or enzyme in a bacterium and are critical to the treatment of a bacterial infection. When bacteria are exposed to sublethal concentrations of an antibiotic, resistance can develop through the elimination of normal bacteria, allowing the resistant bacteria to survive and reproduce. The question has been whether exposure to antibacterial products can promote antibiotic resistance. The answer is that the use of antibacterial products may actually increase the prevalence of antibiotic-resistant bacteria.

Antibiotic resistance is irreversible and unavoidable because of the selective pressure on bacteria to become resistant. This selection is in large part a result of the widespread use of antibiotics to increase growth rates in livestock and a result of unnecessary and improper use of antibiotics to restore and maintain human health. The indiscriminate use or overuse of antibiotics has been widely blamed for the appearance of superbacteria, bacteria that are unaffected by more than one antibiotic. In addition, a widely used antibacterial agent used in toothpaste, kitchen utensils and appliances, clothing, cat litter, and toys could lead to the development of resistant strains of bacteria.

Triclosan is a good example of the potent antibacterial and antifungal agents that are increasingly used to produce "germ-free" consumer products. Triclosan used to be considered a broad-spectrum antiseptic rather than a true antibiotic. As a general biocide, triclosan was not expected to have a specific target in the bacterial cell. However, researchers at Tufts University School of Medicine determined that triclosan specifically interferes with an enzyme important in the synthesis of plasma membrane lipids. As triclosan kills off normal bacteria, it could make way for the growth of strains with triclosan-insensitive enzymes. More troubling, one of the front-line antibiotics commonly used to treat tuberculosis, isoniazid, targets the same enzyme, raising the possibility that the use of triclosan will lead to new drug-resistant strains of *Mycobacterium tuberculosis*.

Consumers are convinced that the use of products with antimicrobial chemicals will lower the risk of infection. This has not been demonstrated scientifically, but effective handwashing has been demonstrated to prevent illness. However, the key to effective handwashing is the length of time (15 to 30 seconds) spent scrubbing, not the inclusion of antibacterials in the soap. Regular soap, combined with scrubbing action, physically dislodges and removes microorganisms. The constant exposure of bacteria to sublethal concentrations of triclosan promotes the development of resistance; the substitution of antibacterial soap for proper handwashing techniques will eventually render triclosan ineffective.

Laurie F. Caslake, Ph.D.

FURTHER READING

American Medical Association. "Hand Washing, Alcohol-Based Rubs Help Curb Influenza Outbreaks." *American Medical News* 52, no. 6 (2009).

Centers for Disease Control and Prevention. *An Ounce of Prevention Keeps the Germs Away: Seven Keys to a Safer, Healthier Home.* Atlanta: Author, 2002.

Heymann, David L., ed. *Control of Communicable Diseases Manual.* 18th ed. Washington, D.C.: American Public Health Association, 2004.

Marriot, Norman G., and Robert B. Gravani. *Principles of Food Sanitation.* 5th ed. New York: Springer, 2006.

Wallace, Robert B., ed. *Maxcy-Rosenau-Last Public Health and Preventive Medicine.* 15th ed. New York: McGraw-Hill, 2007.

WEB SITES OF INTEREST

American Dental Hygienists' Association
http://www.adha.org/oralhealth/brushing.htm

Centers for Disease Control and Prevention
http://www.cdc.gov/cleanhands

Clean Hands Coalition
http://www.cleanhandscoalition.org

See also: Bacterial infections; Centers for Disease Control and Prevention (CDC); Chemical germicides; Decontamination; Disinfectants and sanitizers; Hospitals and infectious disease; Iatrogenic infections; Infection;

Prevention of bacterial infections; Prevention of fungal infections; Prevention of parasitic diseases; Prevention of protozoan diseases; Prevention of viral infections; Public health; Schools and infectious disease; Viral infections; Viruses: Types; Water treatment.

Hyperbaric oxygen

CATEGORY: Treatment
ALSO KNOWN AS: Hyperbaric medicine, hyperbaric oxygen therapy, hyperbaric oxygenation, hyperbarics

DEFINITION

Hyperbaric oxygen therapy (HBOT) involves the delivery of 100 percent oxygen to a person in a pressurized chamber. The elevated pressure markedly increases the amount of dissolved oxygen in the bloodstream, thereby substantially augmenting tissue oxygenation. Potential infectious disease applications of HBOT include treatment of clostridial myositis and myonecrosis (gas gangrene), necrotizing soft-tissue infections (such as necrotizing fasciitis), chronic osteomyelitis, and intracranial abscesses.

PHYSIOLOGY

At normal atmospheric pressure, most oxygen in the blood is bound to hemoglobin; a small amount exists in solution. During a hyperbaric oxygen treatment session, pressure within the chamber is raised to 1.5 to 3.0 atmospheres absolute (ATA), forcing a high concentration of oxygen into solution. When breathing 100 percent oxygen at 3.0 ATA, the partial pressure of oxygen in the arterial circulation increases from the normobaric level of roughly 100 millimeters of mercury (mmHg) to approximately 2,000 mmHg. The steep partial pressure gradient in oxygen tension between the hyperoxic blood and the tissues leads to diffusion of oxygen into the cells. With 100 percent

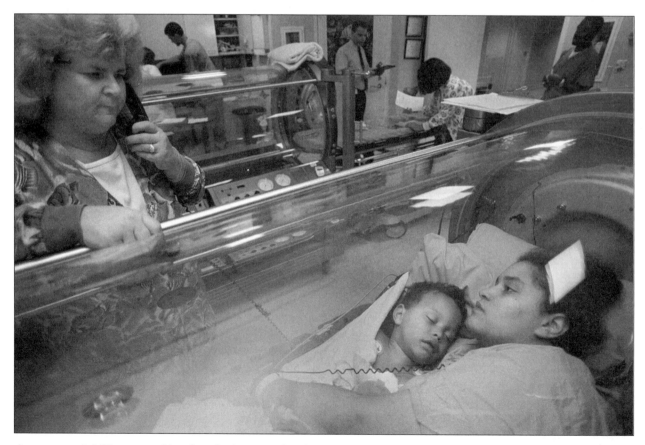

A woman and child are treated in a hyperbaric oxygen chamber following exposure to a toxic agent. (AP/Wide World Photos)

oxygen at 3.0 ATA, tissue oxygen tension increases roughly tenfold, from 55 mmHg to approximately 500 mmHg.

INHIBITORY AND BACTERICIDAL EFFECTS

HBOT for infectious disease indications may be included as part of a multimodality treatment approach, typically in combination with surgical debridement and intravenous antimicrobial therapy. Hyperoxia may combat bacterial infections through a variety of complementary mechanisms. High tissue oxygen tension during HBOT markedly increases the production of reactive oxygen species, or free radicals, which may oxidize and denature structural bacterial proteins and exotoxins. Sufficiently elevated tissue oxygen tension may also inhibit replication and metabolism of anaerobic bacteria. During periods of metabolic inactivity, toxin production temporarily slows or stops, potentially limiting further spread of the infection to surrounding tissues.

ENHANCED PHAGOCYTIC AND ANTIMICROBIAL FUNCTIONS

Increased tissue oxygen tension during hyperbaric therapy may augment the antimicrobial and phagocytic functions of polymorphonuclear leukocytes and tissue macrophages. These phagocytes lose effectiveness at the low oxygen tensions that commonly occur in infected body sites. Certain antibiotics that lose efficacy in low oxygen environments may also become more effective with an HBOT-induced increase in tissue oxygen tension at the site of infection.

IMPACT

The infectious conditions for which HBOT may be indicated are associated with a significant risk of disfigurement, morbidity, and mortality. Research indicates a trend toward a potential role for HBOT in improving outcomes with these conditions. Large-scale, randomized-controlled clinical trials will help determine the most appropriate settings and treatment protocols for the adjuvant use of HBOT for potentially catastrophic bacterial infections.

Tina M. St. John, M.D.

FURTHER READING

Bitterman, Haim. "Bench-to-Bedside Review: Oxygen as a Drug." *Critical Care* 13 (2009): 205.

Gill, Adrian L., and Chris N. A. Bell. "Hyperbaric Oxygen: Its Uses, Mechanisms of Action, and Outcomes." *QJM: An International Journal of Medicine* 97 (2004): 385-395.

Goldman, Robert J. "Hyperbaric Oxygen Therapy for Wound Healing and Limb Salvage: A Systematic Review." *PM&R* 1 (2009): 471-489.

Jain, Kewal K. *Textbook of Hyperbaric Medicine*. 5th ed. Cambridge, Mass.: Hoegrefe, 2009.

Rabinowitz, R. P., and E. S. Caplan. "Hyperbaric Oxygen." In *Mandell, Douglas, and Bennett's Principles and Practice of Infectious Diseases*, edited by Gerald L. Mandell, John F. Bennett, and Raphael Dolin. 7th ed. New York: Churchill Livingstone/Elsevier, 2010.

WEB SITE OF INTEREST

Undersea and Hyperbaric Medical Society
http://www.uhms.org

See also: Gangrene; Infection; Myositis; Necrotizing fasciitis; Osteomyelitis; Treatment of bacterial infections; Wound infections.

I

Iatrogenic infections

CATEGORY: Diseases and conditions
ANATOMY OR SYSTEM AFFECTED: All

DEFINITION

Iatrogenic infections are those infections transmitted during medical treatment and care. A study published by the *Journal of the American Medical Association* reported that iatrogenic infection contributes to about 225,000 deaths in the United States each year. After heart disease and cancer, iatrogenic illness is the third leading cause of death in the United States.

CAUSES

Iatrogenic infection is complex because it has so many causes, including chance, negligence, medical error, and interactions of prescription drugs. Nosocomial infections, another leading cause of iatrogenic illness, are those that occur during hospitalization or through treatment in another health care setting. Pathogens for infection in these facilities include vomit, blood, urine, and feces. Some microorganisms can be spread through the air. Postsurgical patients are particularly vulnerable to hospital acquired infection. Illnesses can be transmitted by health care providers who neglect proper methods of sanitation.

RISK FACTORS

The risks associated with adverse drug reactions typically occur when health care providers lack understanding and education about the prescribed drug. One of the most significant issues in drug-drug interactions resulting in iatrogenic illness is a change in the gastrointestinal tract and liver that leads to metabolic problems. Alcohol intake and smoking can also affect the way drugs are metabolized.

One study of hospitalized patients showed that up to one-half of drug-related problems occur because of errors in prescribing, administering, dispensing, and transcribing records of drugs. Inadequate monitoring of patients was cited in another study, meaning that the appropriate laboratory tests were either not ordered or were incorrectly interpreted.

Also, a lack of sanitation frequently leads to iatrogenic illness. This could happen in a wide range of settings, from food waste and dirty restrooms to devices, such as surgical equipment, catheters, and wound dressings, that are supposed to be sterile.

Rare diseases can be transmitted during corneal transplants, by contaminated dura matter (the layers surrounding the brain and spinal cord), through blood transfusion, and by dental pulp, which has been implicated in the spread of the incurable Creutzfeldt-Jakob disease.

SYMPTOMS

Affected persons experience a wide range of symptoms, illnesses, disorders, and conditions. Some of the most frequently studied include autistic spectrum disorder, ovarian hyperstimulation syndrome, fat intolerance after cholecystectomy, rupture of the tracheobronchial tree, colitis, hypoglycemia, back pain, neuropathy after hysterectomy, rectourethral fistula, acute estrogen deficiency, temporomandibular joint symptoms, and small perforations of the colon during colonoscopy.

SCREENING AND DIAGNOSIS

By applying rigorous methodology, researchers can study, for example, the epidemiology of drug-induced illnesses. Such research includes a consideration of the frequency of a drug-induced disease, nonmedical contributing factors, the dose and route of administration of all drugs taken by the patient, the time and place of drug-induced diseases, and the specific characteristics of each patient. Other kinds of iatrogenic illness, such as nosocomial infections, are often monitored by the medical provider's risk-management or quality-assurance departments.

TREATMENT AND THERAPY

Measures for the treatment of iatrogenic illness include antiseptics, antibiotics, and better surgical techniques. Anesthesia may be used to control pain.

Because there are hundreds of varieties of iatrogenic illness, each requiring individualized treatment, this section will outline the therapeutic course for a patient who is at high risk for developing a common type of iatrogenic, adverse drug reaction: dyspepsia caused by treatment with ibuprofen.

Patients with dyspepsia, or indigestion, have symptoms such as upper abdominal pain, belching, nausea, vomiting, abdominal bloating, and satiety. For patients taking ibuprofen, there is also a risk of internal bleeding, and the medical team will have to screen for this. The patient may also experience warning signs such as weight loss, blood in the stool, fever, and vomiting. The medical team also needs to check on the patient's diet, and it needs to screen for depression and anxiety. Other factors under consideration should include the patient's age, medical history, concurrent drug use, use of herbal medicines, and use of food supplements. Treatment cannot safely begin until all differential diagnoses have been excluded.

If the dyspepsia is caused by abnormal function of the gastrointestinal muscles, a smooth muscle relaxant will increase motility and improve symptoms. Dyspepsia with the production of stomach acid may be treated with a proton pump inhibitor or misoprostol. After weighing the risks and benefits, the physician may ask the patient to reduce or stop the ibuprofen.

PREVENTION AND OUTCOMES

Nosocomial infection can be addressed by decontamination measures such as cleaning, disinfection, sterilization, and ventilation. Vulnerable patients with wounds can be protected with sterile dressings and isolation precautions. Adequate air flow and moisture control help to keep microorganisms such as bacteria and fungi in check. Health care providers can limit the risk of iatrogenic illness by containing or removing infectious materials, instituting single-use devices, and standardizing drug equipment. Some hospitals are experimenting with financial incentives for handwashing, as studies have shown that medical staff fail to wash their hands more than half of the time.

Many quality improvement approaches to iatrogenic illness focus on the design of systems for control of hospital infections and adverse drug reactions. Targeting people has been less effective. In a system-focused environment, mechanisms such as medical audit, peer review, and risk management offer valuable feedback to every member of the health care team, making it easier to implement evidence-based preventive measures. The evidence-based environment also fosters meta-analysis to improve clinical practice.

Merrill Evans, M.A.

FURTHER READING

Ayliffe, Graham A. J., et al. *Hospital-Acquired Infection: Principles and Prevention.* Oxford, England: Butterworth-Heinemann, 1999. Administrative aspects, risk assessment, cleaning, disinfection, and sterilization for infection control in hospitals.

Merry, Alan, and Alexander McCall Smith. *Errors, Medicine, and the Law.* New York: Cambridge University Press, 2003. Argues that many medical accidents are linked to the complexity of modern health care and calls for a more informed alternative to the "blaming culture" in medicine.

Morath, Julianne M., and Joanne E. Turnbull. *To Do No Harm: Ensuring Patient Safety in Health Care Organizations.* San Francisco: Jossey-Bass, 2005. A manual on patient safety for health care personnel.

Preger, Leslie, ed. *Iatrogenic Diseases.* 2 vols. Boca Raton, Fla.: CRC Press, 1986. Offers helpful advice on diagnosing iatrogenic diseases. Includes bibliographical references and an index.

Sharpe, Virginia A., and Alan I. Faden. *Medical Harm: Historical, Conceptual, and Ethical Dimensions of Iatrogenic Illness.* New York: Cambridge University Press, 1998. A discussion about nosocomial infection, the adverse effects of drug treatment, and recommendations for limiting iatrogenic harm.

Starfield, Barbara. "Is U.S. Health Really the Best in the World?" *Journal of the American Medical Association* 284, no. 4 (2000): 483-485. A landmark article that includes statistics showing the effects of doctors' medical errors.

Steele, K. "Iatrogenic Illness on a General Medicine Service at a University Hospital." *Quality and Safety in Health Care* 13 (2004): 76-81. This article considers the circumstances under which the benefit of hospitalization exceeds the risk to the patient.

Tisdale, James E., et al., eds. *Drug-Induced Diseases: Prevention, Detection, and Management.* Bethesda, Md.: American Society of Health-System Pharmacists, 2005. Discusses the magnitude and significance of drug-induced diseases, including the impact on the health care system.

WEB SITES OF INTEREST

Agency for Healthcare Research and Quality
http://www.ahrq.gov

Clean Hands Coalition
http://www.cleanhandscoalition.org

National Institute of Allergy and Infectious Diseases
http://www.niaid.nih.gov

Public Health Agency of Canada
http://www.phac-aspc.gc.ca

See also: Bacterial infections; Bloodstream infections; Decontamination; Disinfectants and sanitizers; Drug resistance; Emerging and reemerging infectious diseases; Fever of unknown origin; Fungal infections; Hospitals and infectious disease; Hygiene; Infection; Opportunistic infections; Outbreaks; Prevention of bacterial infections; Prevention of fungal infections; Prevention of viral infections; Public health; Viral infections; Wound infections.

Idiopathic thrombocytopenic purpura

CATEGORY: Diseases and conditions
ANATOMY OR SYSTEM AFFECTED: Blood, immune system, spleen
ALSO KNOWN AS: Immune thrombocytopenic purpura

DEFINITION

Idiopathic thrombocytopenic purpura (ITP) is a treatable blood disorder. Antibodies that are produced in the spleen attack and destroy the body's own blood-clotting cells (platelets), which help stop bleeding. Normally, platelets move to damaged areas of the body and stick together, forming a sort of barrier against germs. If there are not enough platelets in the body, bleeding injuries are difficult to stop. Although people with ITP have a lower than normal number of platelets in their blood, all other blood cell counts are normal.

There are two types of ITP. Acute ITP, which lasts less than six months and usually occurs in children, is the most common. Chronic ITP lasts more than six months and usually occurs in adults.

CAUSES

The cause of most cases of ITP is unknown. In children, the disorder has been linked to viral infections. It is believed that in these cases the immune system becomes confused and begins attacking healthy platelet cells. When too many platelets are destroyed, ITP can result. The disorder in adults has not been linked to viral infections. Some cases of ITP are thought to be caused by drugs, infection, or other immune disorders. Pregnant women too sometimes develop the disorder.

RISK FACTORS

Persons with an increased chance of developing ITP include children who have had a recent viral infection or have had a live-virus vaccination (which may sometimes put a child at a higher risk); women, usually younger than age forty years; and women in general, who are two to three times more likely to get ITP than are men.

SYMPTOMS

Both adults and children may notice the following symptoms of ITP: easy bruising, dark urine or stools, bleeding for longer than normal following an injury, unexplained nosebleeds, bleeding from the gums, heavier-than-normal menstrual periods (in adult women), red dots called petechiae on the skin (petechiae may occur in groups and resemble a rash), and, in rare cases, bleeding within the intestinal tract or brain.

SCREENING AND DIAGNOSIS

A doctor will ask about symptoms and medical history and will perform a physical exam. Tests may include a complete blood count (CBC), in which a blood sample is tested to see if the numbers of different blood cells are normal; and a bone marrow test, in which a needle is inserted into the skin and into the bone and a small amount of bone marrow is removed. The sample is tested to ensure the marrow contains normal numbers of platelet-producing cells. This test is done to rule out other disorders. Another test is a computed tomography (CT) scan (in rare cases). The CT scan is done if there is a concern about bleeding in the brain.

TREATMENT AND THERAPY

Treatment for ITP is different for children and for adults. Most children recover from ITP without any treatment. However, a doctor may recommend the following: medications to increase platelet counts in the blood, such as steroids (for example, prednisone), which lowers the activity of the immune system and keeps it from destroying platelets; and gamma globulin infusions (an antibody-containing protein that slows down platelet destruction). An infusion means that the injection is given by IV (intravenously) or through a shot. It usually works more quickly than steroids. Both of these treatments work but both can have side effects. Eighty-five percent of children who have ITP recover within a year and do not experience the problem again.

Two newer drugs stimulate platelet production: eltrombopag (Promacta) and romiplostim (Nplate). Using these drugs and also using the targeted monoclonal antibody rituximab (Rituxan) may prevent the need for a splenectomy. A splenectomy is the surgical removal of the spleen. This procedure stops the destruction of platelets because the antibodies are made in the spleen. In adults, if drug intervention does not do enough to raise platelet counts, the doctor may recommend a splenectomy.

A splenectomy leaves the body more vulnerable to infection from other sources. This surgery is usually not performed until medications have proven ineffective. Doctors also sometimes recommend lifestyle changes when platelet counts are low, including avoiding contact sports; patients also are recommended to wear a helmet during sports activities.

PREVENTION AND OUTCOMES

Because the cause of ITP is unknown, there are no specific ways to prevent the disease. However, because bleeding and injury can be serious for people with ITP, one should take precautions to avoid injury, such as using padding on an infant's crib or around a play area and ensuring that older children wear helmets and protective gear when playing sports (to help reduce bruising injuries). Persons with low platelet counts should stop playing contact sports.

People who have ITP should also avoid medications that contain aspirin or ibuprofen. These medicines can reduce platelet function. To help stay healthy, one should eat a healthful diet, low in saturated fat and rich in whole grains, fruits, and vegetables; get regular exercise; lose weight if overweight; stop smoking; and drink alcohol, if desired, only in moderation (two drinks per day for men and one drink per day for women).

Amanda Dameron, M.A.;
reviewed by Igor Puzanov, M.D.

FURTHER READING

Bick, Roger L. *Disorders of Thrombosis and Hemostasis: Clinical and Laboratory Practice.* 3d ed. Philadelphia: Lippincott Williams & Wilkins, 2002.

Bussel, J. B., et al. "Eltrombopag for the Treatment of Chronic Idiopathic Thrombocytopenic Purpura." *New England Journal of Medicine* 357, no. 22 (November 29, 2007): 2237-2247.

George, J. N. "Platelets." *The Lancet* 355 (April 29, 2000): 1531-1539.

George, J. N., et al. "Update on Idiopathic Thrombocytopenic Purpura." Available at http://www.hematology.org/publications/hematologist/2010/4965.aspx.

Karpatkin, S. "Autoimmune (Idiopathic) Thrombocytopenic Purpura." *The Lancet* 349 (1997): 1531-1536.

Lichtman, Marshall A., et al., eds. *Williams Hematology.* 7th ed. New York: McGraw-Hill, 2006.

McCrae, Keith R., ed. *Thrombocytopenia.* New York: Taylor & Francis, 2006.

Newland, A., et al. "An Open-Label, Unit Dose-Finding Study of AMG 531, a Novel Thrombopoiesis-Stimulating Peptibody, in Patients with Immune Thrombocytopenic Purpura." *British Journal of Haematology* 135, no. 4 (2006): 547-553.

WEB SITES OF INTEREST

American Academy of Family Physicians
http://familydoctor.org

National Heart, Lung, and Blood Institute
http://www.nhlbi.nih.gov

National Institute of Diabetes and Digestive and Kidney Diseases
http://www2.niddk.nih.gov

Public Health Agency of Canada
http://www.phac-aspc.gc.ca

See also: AIDS; Antibodies; Asplenia; Autoimmune disorders; Disseminated intravascular coagulation; HIV; Sepsis.

Imidazole antifungals

CATEGORY: Treatment

DEFINITION

Imidazole antifungals belong to the azole family, which also includes triazole and thiazole. An imidazole functional group, which is a five-membered ring containing two nitrogens, differentiates these drugs from other members of the azole family. Thiazole groups are similar rings with one nitrogen and one sulfur, while triazoles contain three nitrogens.

Imidazoles are used primarily to treat two types of yeast infection: oral thrush and vaginal candidiasis. They are as effective as polyene antifungals such as nystatin for oral thrush and somewhat more effective for vaginal candidiasis.

MECHANISM OF ACTION

Imidazole antifungals act similarly to triazole and thiazole antifungals. They work by inhibiting cytochrome P450 demethylase, an enzyme responsible for converting lanosterol to ergosterol. Because ergosterol is a major component of fungal cell membranes, blocking this conversion leads to buildup of lanosterol. Lanosterol contains a 14 alpha-methyl group not present in ergosterol. Because of the different shape and physical properties of this sterol, the fungal cell membrane exhibits permeability changes and becomes leaky. Key cellular components can leak, and cell death results.

DRUGS IN THIS CLASS

Ketoconazole is the only drug in this category that is approved for topical and systemic use. Oral absorption is erratic and dependent on an acidic pH. Ketoconazole effectiveness will be dramatically lowered if taken with antacids or other drugs that lower gastric pH. It also is less effective if taken with drugs that are inducers of the CYP3A4 pathway and can lead to an increase in blood levels of other drugs metabolized by this pathway. Ketoconazole is now used mainly as a topical drug because of these drug interactions and the availability of more effective agents. Ketoconazole is available as a cream, lotion, suppository, and shampoo.

Other drugs in this class are topical agents used to treat superficial fungal and yeast infections. In some cases, the drugs are too toxic for systemic use. In others, they are so extensively and quickly degraded by first-pass metabolism in the liver that an insufficient amount of the drug would remain in the bloodstream to treat systemic infections.

Clotrimazole (Lotrimin, Gyne-Lotrimin, Mycelex) and miconazole (Monistat, Desenex) are the most commonly used of these agents and are effective against *Candida*, some other yeasts, and some gram-positive bacteria. Powders, creams, and topical sprays may be used to treat ringworm and athlete's foot. Vaginal infections are best treated with vaginal creams (to be inserted internally) and suppositories. Oral thrush is treated with oral suspensions and troches. Rash is among the more common adverse effects associated with these products.

IMPACT

Approximately 75 percent of women experience at least one instance of vaginal candidiasis in their lifetime, and antifungal drugs represent a necessary treatment option for many. Antibiotic use is one of the primary predisposing factors for *Candida* infections; it is likely that the need for drugs to treat these infections will continue to remain high based on antibiotic prescription frequency. Over-the-counter imidazole products are available and are best used by persons with recurring infections who can accurately diagnose symptoms. Initial infections should be diagnosed by a health care professional.

Karen M. Nagel, Ph.D.

FURTHER READING

Griffith, R. K. "Antifungal Drugs." In *Foye's Principles of Medicinal Chemistry*, edited by Thomas L. Lemke and William O. Foye. 6th ed. Philadelphia: Wolters Kluwer, 2008.

Gullo, Antonio. "Invasive Fungal Infections." *Drugs* 69 (2009): 65-73.

Murray, Patrick R., Ken S. Rosenthal, and Michael A. Pfaller. *Medical Microbiology*. 6th ed. Philadelphia: Mosby/Elsevier, 2009.

Ryan, Kenneth J. "Pathogenesis of Fungal Infection." In *Sherris Medical Microbiology*, edited by Kenneth J. Ryan and C. George Ray. 5th ed. New York: McGraw-Hill, 2010.

WEB SITES OF INTEREST

Centers for Disease Control and Prevention, Division of Foodborne, Bacterial, and Mycotic Diseases
http://www.cdc.gov/nczved/divisions/dfbmd

Microbiology and Immunology On-line: Mycology
http://pathmicro.med.sc.edu/book/mycol-sta.htm

U.S. Food and Drug Administration
http://www.fda.gov

See also: Antifungal drugs: Mechanisms of action; Antifungal drugs: Types; Fungal infections; Fungi: Classification and types; Mold infections; Treatment of fungal infections; Vaginal yeast infection.

Immune response to bacterial infections

CATEGORY: Immune response

DEFINITION

The immune system defends itself against infectious organisms (pathogens) such as bacteria by utilizing physical barriers that prevent bacteria from entering the body and by detecting and eliminating bacteria after they enter the body. Cells, proteins, tissues, and organs work together in a coordinated response, the immune response, to defend against microorganisms.

When a bacterial infection develops, the immune system responds through a series of steps by activating certain cells and by producing substances that recognize and react to invading microorganisms, or antigens. Bacterial antigens are generally proteins present on the surface of a bacterium.

TYPES OF IMMUNITY

Physical barriers are the immune system's first line of defense. They comprise the skin, mucous membranes, mucus, and tears. Unless damaged through injury or other means, the skin generally protects against invasion by microorganisms. Mucous membranes (that is, the linings of the mouth, nose, and eyelids) are effective barriers and are generally coated with secretions, such as lysozyme, that fight microorganisms. Organisms that penetrate physical barriers are identified and eliminated by white blood cells and antibodies. Adaptive immunity, comprised of cell-mediated and antibody-mediated immunity, is an important component of defense against bacterial infection. In antibody-mediated, or humoral, immunity, the immune response is mediated by antibodies (immunoglobulins), which are specific proteins produced in response to antigens. Cell-mediated immunity is mediated by effector T cells (T lymphocytes).

CELLS INVOLVED IN AN IMMUNE RESPONSE

The immune system is made up of a coordinated network of cells, tissues, and organs. White blood cells, or leukocytes, circulate and detect and destroy microbes. Two basic types of leukocytes are phagocytes and lymphocytes. Phagocytes ingest invading organisms and lymphocytes help recognize invaders and eliminate them. The neutrophil is the most common type of phagocyte and is primarily involved in fighting bacteria; an increase in neutrophil numbers generally is triggered by infection. Leukocytes circulate in the bloodstream to provide a coordinated effort for the immune system to monitor and protect against bacterial infection.

B and T lymphocytes (B and T cells) have separate functions: B cells seek targets and send defenses and T cells, in various forms, destroy the invading organism. With stimulation by antigens, T cells comprise several forms, or classes, of effector T cells: killer (cytotoxic), helper, and suppressor.

Killer T cells destroy specific target cells. Helper T cells help other cells, such as B cells, produce antibodies; they also help activated killer T cells destroy foreign cells (macrophages), which enables the killer T cells to ingest foreign cells efficiently. T cells also produce cytokines that activate other cells. B cells have receptors on their surface, where antigens attach stimulate cells to become antibody-secreting cells.

PRIMARY AND SECONDARY IMMUNE RESPONSE

A primary immune response occurs the first time antigens are encountered. At subsequent encounter with the same antigens, a secondary immune response occurs. Before an infection, precursor T or B cells are present as resting cells, but during the course of an adaptive immune response, the immune system activates T cells or triggers B lymphocytes to produce

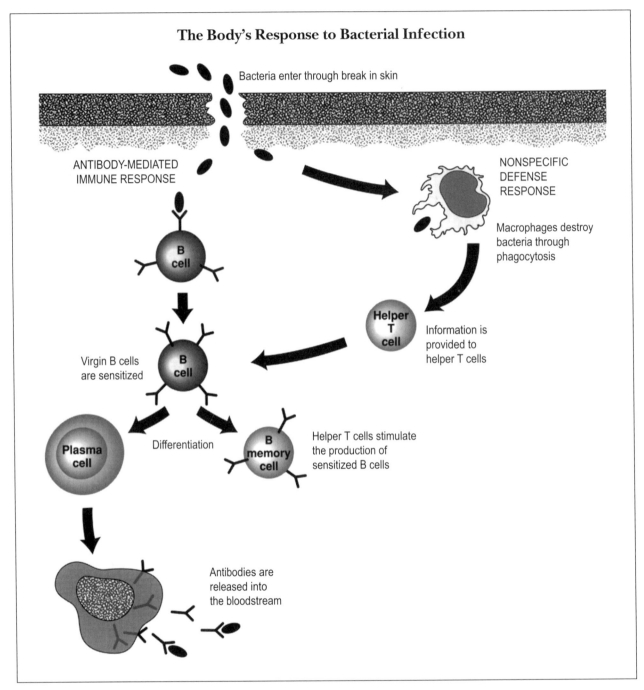

The Body's Response to Bacterial Infection

The immune system responds to a bacterial infection by producing antibodies directly or through phagocytosis, in which a macrophage, a type of white blood cell, engulfs a bacterium and further stimulates antibody production.

antibodies. After initially encountering an antigen, sufficient amounts of antibody take several days to produce, with only small amounts formed during the first few days; circulating antibodies are undetectable until about one week after initial encounter. The primary immune response is relatively slow, with antigens first needing to be recognized, processed, and presented by antigen-presenting cells. Antibody levels need to reach sufficient levels for the host to develop resistance (which may take several days or weeks).

A second encounter with microbial antigens leads to an accelerated immune response, called the secondary or memory response. During the secondary response, memory B cells "remember" and rapidly recognize antigens. Memory B cells then multiply and change into plasma cells; large amounts of antibodies are generated in only one to two days. Similarly, memory T cells rapidly develop into effector cells. The secondary immune response is very quick, efficient, and effective. This specific immune response prevents people from contracting certain diseases more than once.

Antigen-Presenting Cells

The primary immune response is initiated when an antigen penetrates epithelial surfaces and comes into contact with macrophages or other antigen-presenting cells. An antigen-presenting cell is usually either a macrophage or a dendritic cell and, in combination with either a B or T cell, is required for an immune response. Antigens, such as bacterial cells, are ingested and processed by antigen-presenting cells and then presented to lymphocytes to initiate the immune response.

Processing by a macrophage results in antigen fragments being attached in combination with cell surface molecules known as MHC. The antigen-MHC complex is presented to helper T cells, which recognize processed antigen and develop into effector T cells. When a macrophage presents antigen to a B cell, the B cell is signaled to generate antibodies specific for that antigen.

Cell Signaling

Helper T cells provide signals, such as interleukins or cytokines, that stimulate cells to proliferate and function more efficiently. The interaction between an antigen-presenting macrophage and a helper T cell results in secretion of interleukin-1 from macrophages that, in turn, stimulate helper T cells to mature and produce other cytokines, including interleukin-2 and -4. Interleukin-2 stimulates proliferation of other T cells and interleukin-4 causes B cells to develop into antibody-secreting plasma cells. Interleukin-2 also activates killer T cells to destroy cells with antigen on

their surfaces. When a B cell is stimulated by interleukin-4, the B cell grows and divides to form an army of identical B cells, each capable of producing large amounts of identical antibody molecules.

Impact

The immune system prevents and defends against bacterial infections. Antibody-mediated and cell-mediated immune responses are generated during almost all infections, but the magnitude and importance of each response varies, depending on the host and the infectious agent. As people age, they usually become immune to more microorganisms, as the immune system comes into contact with increasing numbers of antigens through a person's life. In general, adults and teenagers tend to get fewer bacterial infections than younger children because their bodies have learned to recognize and immediately attack antigens to which they are exposed.

C. J. Walsh, Ph.D.

Further Reading

Coico, Richard, and Geoffrey Sunshine. *Immunology: A Short Course.* 6th ed. Hoboken, N.J.: Wiley-Blackwell, 2009. A clear and comprehensive introduction to essential topics in modern immunology.

DeFranco, Anthony L., Richard M. Locksley, and Miranda Robertson. *Immunity: The Immune Response in Infectious and Inflammatory Disease.* New York: Oxford University Press, 2007. An introduction for undergraduates and medical students to the immune response to infection. Includes chapters on the immune response to specific microorganisms.

Mak, Tak W., and Mary E. Saunders. *Primer to the Immune Response.* Maryland Heights, Mo.: Academic Press/Elsevier, 2008. Provides an understandable introduction to immunology. A resource for college students, students studying medicine, and those in health professions.

Web Sites of Interest

Microbiology and Immunology On-line: Immunology
http://pathmicro.med.sc.edu/book/immunol-sta.htm

Todar's Online Textbook of Bacteriology
http://www.textbookofbacteriology.net

See also: Antibodies; Bacteria: Classification and types; Bacteria: Structure and growth; Bacterial infections; Bacteriology; Immune response to viral infections; Immunity; Immunodeficiency; Infection; Inflammation; Mutation of pathogens; Pathogenicity; Primary infection; Reinfection; Secondary infection; Seroconversion; Superbacteria; T lymphocytes; Virulence.

Immune response to fungal infections

CATEGORY: Immune response
ALSO KNOWN AS: Mycoses

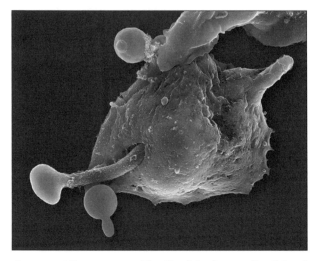

A neutrophil, center, engulfs cells of the fungus Candida albicans.

DEFINITION

The immune response is the mechanism by which the body recognizes and defends itself against invading microbes, including fungi. The more effective the body's immune response, the more successfully it combats the development and severity of infection. A breakdown of the immune response can have dire consequences.

BASIC IMMUNE SYSTEM COMPONENTS

Skin and mucous membranes are the first line of defense against microbes. If these are penetrated, the body's immune response becomes active. Lymphocytes, specialized white blood cells, react to the presence of substances called antigens on the surface of invading fungal spores or molds. The two major types of lymphocytes are T cells (T lymphocytes) and B cells (B lymphocytes). T cells attack antigens directly. B cells produce antibodies, circulating proteins that bind to specific antigens and make it easier for immune cells to destroy the antigens.

Other contributors to the immune response to fungal infections include macrophages and other phagocytes, which are blood cells that surround and digest foreign bodies; complement, which are specialized proteins in the blood that act in sequence to mediate inflammation and the immune response; and neutrophils, which are circulating white blood cells that play a major role in destroying fungal pathogens.

Lymphocytes may develop a "memory" of invading antigens they encounter. This allows the immune system to respond faster and more efficiently on future exposure to the same antigens. For superficial, noninvasive infections, this memory is not long lasting, so a recurrence of infection often occurs after treatment has been discontinued.

IMMUNE RESPONSE TO FUNGI IN HEALTHY PERSONS

Humans inhale or ingest thousands of fungal spores every day. Of the more than 200,000 species of fungi, fewer than 100 are associated with human infection. In healthy persons, most potentially pathogenic fungi produce mild, even subclinical, transitory infection, if any infection. In these situations, the body's immune system has responded quickly and effectively to the pathogens.

Some fungal pathogens, however, challenge the body's immune response, even in healthy persons. *Histoplasma capsulatum*, in its yeast form, can be resistant to killing by macrophages. *H. capsulatum* can actually multiply within macrophages. Progressive pulmonary infection or disseminated disease may result. *Candida albicans* may bind to complement, and by so doing can short-circuit the immune response. *Coccidioides immitis* contains a substance in its wall that resists its destruction, a critical step in the immune response. *Cryptococcus neoformans*, unlike other pathogenic fungi, is an encapsulated yeast. The capsule helps to impair destruction of the fungus by phagocytes. Despite setbacks by such challenges, in most healthy persons the immune response recoups, with T-cell-mediated responses and a proliferation of neutrophils playing a major role.

With most fungal pathogens, antibodies do not contribute significantly to the immune response. C. neoformans is an exception, so much so that rising titers of antibodies against C. neoformans are evidence of recovery from illness. In contrast, high titers of C. immitis-specific antibodies are associated with dissemination and a worsening clinical course.

IMMUNE RESPONSE TO FUNGI IN IMMUNOCOMPROMISED PERSONS.

Invasive fungal infections are a major threat to immunocompromised persons. Both underlying disease and therapy can compromise the immune response and cause it to malfunction, resulting in an increased risk for severe and systemic fungal infections. Leukemia, diabetes ketoacidosis, sarcoidosis, chronicgranulomatous disease, and acquired immunodeficiency syndrome (AIDS) are examples of diseases that have a direct impact on the functioning of the immune response. Leukemia can severely deplete neutrophils, resulting in neutropenia, a low level of circulating neutrophils. Diabetes ketoacidosis has a negative impact on lymphocytes by increasing serum acidity. The lesions caused by sarcoidosis and chronic granulomatous disease interfere with the functioning of macrophages. Human immunodeficiency virus (HIV), the virus that causes AIDS, attacks and destroys helper T cells. Consequently, T-cell-mediated immunity is compromised.

Agents used to treat cancer and AIDS or to suppress rejection of solid or stem-cell transplants and high-dose, long-term therapy with corticosteroids increase the risk for severe and systemic fungal infections by suppressing the immune response. In particular, they cause neutropenia and depression of the T-cell-mediated immune response. Neutropenia is a major contributor to the emergence of disseminated candidiasis and severe aspergillosis, zygomycosis, and hyalophomycosis (caused by *Fusarium* species). High-dose, long-term use of corticosteroids impairs both macrophage and neutrophil function. This contributes to the development of severe aspergillosis, cryptococcosis, and zygomycosis (also called mucormycosis).

IMPACT

As the number of immunocompromised persons increases, both from disease (such as AIDS) and from treatment (such as immunosuppressive chemotherapy), fungal infections are emerging as a major cause of morbidity and mortality. These infections include particularly virulent strains and fungi rarely observed as pathogenic in the past. Greater understanding of the factors contributing to the breakdown of the immune response in these situations has become critical to controlling these opportunistic infections.

Ernest Kohlmetz, M.A.

FURTHER READING

Kavanaugh, Kevin, ed. *New Insights in Medical Mycology.* New York: Springer, 2007.

Ryan, Kenneth J., and George Ray. *Sherris Medical Microbiology: An Introduction to Infectious Diseases.* 5th ed. New York: McGraw-Hill Medical, 2010.

Shoman, Shmuel, and Stuart M. Levitz. "The Immune Response to Fungal Infections." *British Journal of Haematology* 129 (2005): 569-582.

WEB SITES OF INTEREST

Microbiology and Immunology On-line: Immunology
http://pathmicro.med.sc.edu/book/immunol-sta.htm

Systematic Mycology and Microbiology Laboratory
http://www.ars.usda.gov

See also: Airborne illness and disease; Antibodies; Antifungal drugs: Types; Diagnosis of fungal infections; Fever; Fungal infections; Fungi: Classification and types; *Fusarium*; *Histoplasma*; Immunity; Mycoses; Polyene antifungals; Prevention of fungal infections; Respiratory route of transmission; Soilborne illness and disease; T lymphocytes; Treatment of fungal infections.

Immune response to parasitic diseases

CATEGORY: Immune response

DEFINITION

Parasites are large multicellular organisms that undergo multiple stages of development, inhabit a variety of biological niches, and produce a range of antigens and metabolic secretions; thus, the human body's immune response to these organisms is necessarily complex.

IMMUNE RESPONSE

Information on the human immune system's reaction to parasites is based largely on laboratory models. In general, once parasites (such as helminths, or worms) are identified, the immune system works to expel or isolate the organisms and to minimize their harmful effects. Although the response varies by invading species, it typically involves binding and inactivation of antigens, the release of cytotoxic agents, regulated hypersensitivity reactions, and tissue repair.

In mucosal areas (such as the gastrointestinal tract), a strong helper T cell (T lymphocyte) type 2 (T_H2) response is common, although the exact route has not been identified and likely depends on the invading organism. In many cases, helminth antigens are recognized by T cells in the human gut's lymphoid tissues, a recognition that sparks the production of cytokines (interleukins), mucus-producing cells, and immunoglobulin E (IgE). IgE antibodies then react with parasite antigens, leading to the release of mediators from mast cells and of eosinophils and basophils; inflammation soon follows. The gastrointestinal environment becomes toxic, and the smooth muscles contract, causing diarrhea and inducing the worms to leave or be expelled. The larval stages of some nematodes are damaged by toxic proteins released by eosinophils only after they leave the gut and migrate through the body.

Tissue-dwelling trematodes and filarial nematodes also trigger a T_H2 response that includes the destruction of larvae by eosinophils, the formation of granulomas around *Schistosoma* eggs, and the production of nodules around the adult *Onchocerca volvulus*. Mast cells may play a larger role in expelling nematodes from tissue, possibly by making blood vessels more permeable. Neutrophils also work with eosinophils and macrophages to destroy parasites lodged in tissues. Nevertheless, the T_H2 response appears to be less protective in these areas, in which chronic infections are the norm. The T_H1 response (such as the secretion of interferon and activation of macrophages that destroy organisms) may be more important here, especially in early infections.

Although antigen-specific T cell responses are stimulated during the initial stages of an infestation, as the body is exposed to parasite antigens over time, the immune response often becomes muted, or down-regulated. This modified T_H2 response has been noted in chronic infections with filarial worms, *Schistosoma*, and gastrointestinal tract nematodes, and it features an anti-inflammatory component that inhibits allergic responses. The actual mechanism behind the dampened response is unknown, but it appears that host macrophages may somehow be alternatively activated and recruited to the site of infection by parasites, creating an environment that favors the organisms' survival. Interleukin 10, which is produced by regulatory T cells and helps to regulate the strength of T_H1 and T_H2 responses, also is likely involved. In addition to aiding in the suppression of inflammation, alternatively activated macrophages promote wound healing and damage repair (such as from hookworm bites).

PARASITE EVASION

The persistence of parasites across species is a testament to their ability to successfully elude or neutralize host defense mechanisms. In many cases, the adult worm's large size and motility make it difficult to eradicate through phagocytosis (ingestion). Some parasites also disguise themselves by adopting host antigens or by continually changing or turning down the expression of their own antigens. Other parasites evade destruction by shedding their outer coat, modulating their numbers to avoid detection, and accelerating growth and production of offspring when encountering hosts with potent immune systems.

Helminths also can interfere directly with the host's immune response, doing so, for example, by secreting products that suppress T cell and B cell function, that interfere with the work of macrophages, that bind to immunoglobulins, and that dampen mast-cell signals. Some parasites also establish a relationship with the host known as premunition, in which an existing infection is allowed to continue, but new infestations by the same species are destroyed. This condition benefits both the host and the parasite because it avoids superinfection in the host and controls "overcrowding" by parasites.

IMMUNOPATHOLOGY

Occasionally, the body's reaction to parasites causes self-injury or otherwise impairs functioning. Hypersensitivity reactions such as hives and swelling can be by-products of the immune response to worm antigens. During chronic infection, circulating antibodies and parasite antigens can coat cells or lodge in vessels or tissues and cause damage or blockages.

Immune responses to larval and egg stages of parasite development also can lead to pathology. For example, immune system attacks on migrating larvae can damage tissue inadvertently. In addition, many of the symptoms associated with onchocerciasis (such as rashes, lesions, severe visual impairment, and epilepsy) are attributed to antibody- and cell-mediated responses to dead or dying larvae. Similar cell-mediated pathologies can occur with granuloma formation in schistosomiasis. Over time, as the eggs die and the granulomas resolve, fibrosis can develop and obstruct blood flow to the liver or bladder. This scarring also can inhibit the liver's ability to purify blood and can cause excessive bleeding.

IMPACT

According to the World Health Organization, soil-dwelling roundworms and flatworms affect 2 billion people worldwide, and waterborne helminths affect another 500 to 600 million. Although parasitic infections are generally not fatal, they are associated with multiple disease states, delayed child development, and human suffering.

Continued research on helminth biology and the body's immune responses to the organisms can spur the development of effective vaccines. In addition, studies of the T_H2 response and the parasite's ability to suppress immunity may one day provide cures for infectious diseases and provide critical information about autoimmune and allergic disorders. The use of worms, eggs, and purified proteins of nematode parasites to promote protection from allergy and autoimmunity also has been investigated in preclinical and clinical trials.

Judy Majewski, M.S.

FURTHER READING

Anthony, Robert M., et al. "Protective Immune Mechanisms in Helminth Infection." *Nature Reviews Immunology* 7 (2007): 975-987. A thorough review of the T_H2 immune response to helminth infections.

Dunne, David W., and Anne Cooke. "A Worm's Eye View of the Immune System: Consequences for Evolution of Human Autoimmune Disease." *Nature Reviews* 5 (May, 2005): 420-426. An overview of how imbalance between parasite and host can lead to immunopathology.

Maizels, R. M. "Exploring the Immunology of Parasitism: From Surface Antigens to the Hygiene Hypothesis." *Parasitology* 136 (2009): 1549-1564. A review of research on helminth immunology.

Noble, Elmer R., and Glenn A. Noble. *Parasitology: The Biology of Animal Parasites.* Philadelphia: Lea & Febiger, 1982. Background reading on parasites by phylum that is written for undergraduate students.

Roberts, Larry S., and John Janovy, Jr. *Gerald D. Schmidt and Larry S. Roberts' Foundations of Parasitology.* 8th ed. Boston: McGraw-Hill, 2009. A classic work focusing on the parasites of humans.

WEB SITES OF INTEREST

Microbiology and Immunology On-line: Immunology
http://pathmicro.med.sc.edu/book/immunol-sta.htm

National Institutes of Health
http://health.nih.gov/topic/parasiticdiseases

Neglected Tropical Disease Program
http://www.neglecteddiseases.gov

See also: Antiparasitic drugs: Mechanisms of action; Antiparasitic drugs: Types; Diagnosis of parasitic diseases; Immunity; Infection; Inflammation; Parasites: Classification and types; Parasitic diseases; Parasitology; Pathogens; Prevention of parasitic diseases; T lymphocytes; Treatment of parasitic diseases; Worm infections.

Immune response to prion diseases

CATEGORY: Immune response

DEFINITION

Prion diseases are rare and fatal degenerative brain disorders caused by mutated proteins in the brain that aggregate and form visible "holes" that show a spongy appearance seen through a microscope, hence the name "spongiform encephalopathies." Certain prion diseases, such as scrapie (a disease of sheep and goats), and two human diseases, Creutzfeldt-Jacob disease (CJD) and kuru, are transmitted by an infectious agent, namely a prion. Variant CJD and Gerstmann-Sträussler-Scheinker syndrome are two familial forms of prion diseases and are considered genetically inherited neurodegenerative disorders.

The causative agent of prion diseases is the cell surface prion protein (PrPc). PrPc is expressed on the surface of almost all cells in the body but are in extremely high concentrations on neurons in the peripheral and central nervous systems. However, no evidence has been found of an immune response or antibody detection against prions.

IMMUNE SYSTEM

Controversy surrounds the role of the immune system in prion disease. On one hand, a potential exists for immunization as a form of treatment; on the other hand, the involvement of the immune system may actually play a role in promoting disease in lymphoid organs and may be a detrimental factor in establishing a disease state. Prion diseases are unusual because they lack any nucleic acid, which is the chemical building block of deoxyribonucleic acid (DNA), which makes up the genes that generally code for proteins. Therefore, the pathogenic potential of prions lies in their protein conformation, which can induce the transformation of the host cellular protein (PrPc) to the disease state (PrPsc).

Prions use the immune system and lymphoreticular cells to gain access to the brain. It has been shown that a humoral immune response to the prion protein (PrPc) may inhibit prion infection. Reports in the literature using the mouse as a model have shown that anti-PrPc antibodies can possibly prevent prion disease. This suggests that immunization can possibly help to prevent prion infection and manifestation of disease. However, data demonstrates that there is a lack of immune response against prions, and that the immune system may actually help, rather than hinder, the propagation of prions.

PrPc AND THE LACK OF IMMUNE RESPONSE IN SCRAPIE DISEASE

Scrapie is a prion disease of rodents, sheep, and goats, and it expresses a modified cellular form of the prion protein (PrPsc). Scientists have shown that scrapie infection fails to elicit an immune response. There are no antibodies detected against prions be-cause the PrPsc is a modified version of a host cellular prion protein (PrPc). Therefore, organisms will not see the modified scrapie version as foreign. Thus, host organisms of prion infection are tolerant of both PrPc and PrPsc and cannot consequently induce an immune response by either scrapie infections or immunization with scrapie prions injected to elicit a response. Because the cell surface prion protein is found in most cells, including lymphocytes of the immune system, a prion infection—which is not seen as foreign by T-lymphocytes—will not generate an immune response.

LYMPHOID TISSUES

There is evidence suggesting that the lymphoid system, including the spleen, lymph nodes, bone marrow, and peripheral blood, may influence the course of prion diseases. Data suggest a number of possibilities for prion disease: The susceptibility of prion infection correlates with the maturation of the immune system during the growth and development of an organism; corticosteroids, made by the lymphoid system, reduce the susceptibility to scrapie in experimental animal studies; stimulated white blood cells increase the susceptibility of scrapie; removal of the spleen delays the onset of clinical symptoms of mice that were infected with prions; and studies with immunodeficient mice have shown more precision in the role of the immune system in prion disease.

The lymphoid organs have also been shown to replicate prions. The immune system is able to propagate PrPsc proteins even while the brain remains unaffected. The involvement of the lymphoid system in prion infection may involve a specific factor in lymphoid cells that aid in prion replication. These may involve chaperone proteins, which help to enhance production of other proteins.

IMPACT

One interesting fact regarding the involvement of the immune system in prion disease is that no significant pathologic lesion occurs, whereas infection of the brain is always accompanied by vascular degeneration, astrocytosis, neuronal loss, and possibly amyloid deposition. Future studies on the mechanism by which prion diseases interact with the immune system, and particularly the lymphoid cells, may lead to a better design of drugs that could impair the peripheral steps in prion disease.

The involvement of the immune system in prion diseases remains debatable. More scientific information is needed to determine if the immune system plays a large role and, if it does, whether that role has a generally positive or negative affect on prion disease states.

Susan M. Zneimer, Ph.D., FACMG

FURTHER READING

Aucouturier, P., et al. "Short Analytic Review: Prion Diseases and the Immune System." *Clinical Immunology* 96, no. 2 (2000): 79-85.

Berg, L. J. "Insights into the Role of the Immune System in Prion Diseases." *Proceedings of the National Academy of Science* 91 (1994): 429-432.

Murphy, Kenneth, Paul Travers, and Mark Walport. *Janeway's Immunobiology.* 7th ed. New York: Garland Science, 2008.

Polymenidou, M., et al. "Humoral Immune Response to Native Eukaryotic Prion Protein Correlates with Anti-Prion Protection." *Proceedings of the National Academy of Science* 101 (2004): 14670-14676.

Prusiner, Stanley B. "The Prion Diseases." *Scientific American* 272, no. 1 (January, 1995): 48-57.

_____, ed. *Prion Biology and Diseases.* 2d ed. Cold Spring Harbor, N.Y.: Cold Spring Harbor Laboratory Press, 2004.

WEB SITES OF INTEREST

Centers for Disease Control and Prevention
http://www.cdc.gov/ncidod/dvrd/prions

Creutzfeldt-Jakob Disease Foundation
http://www.cjdfoundation.org

Genetic and Rare Diseases Information Center
http://rarediseases.info.nih.gov/gard

National Institute of Allergy and Infectious Diseases
http://www.niaid.nih.gov/topics/prion

National Institute of Neurological Disorders and Stroke, Transmissible Spongiform Encephalopathies Information Page
http://www.ninds.nih.gov/disorders/tse

National Organization for Rare Disorders
http://www.rarediseases.org

National Prion Disease Pathology Surveillance Center
http://www.cjdsurveillance.com

See also: Creutzfeldt-Jakob disease; Encephalitis; Fatal familial insomnia; Gerstmann-Sträussler-Scheinker syndrome; Immunity; Kuru; Prion diseases; Prions; Subacute sclerosing panencephalitis; Variant Creutzfeldt-Jakob disease.

Immune response to protozoan diseases

CATEGORY: Immune response

DEFINITION

Protozoa are simple single-celled organisms that are part of the animal kingdom. A number of protozoan species infect humans by inhabiting the body as parasites. The parasitic protozoans of importance are species of amebas, flagellates, and sporozoan. The most recognized ameba is *Entamoeba histolytica*.

IMMUNE RESPONSE

The host's immune system interacts with the infectious organism in a vigorous way, as the host aims to eliminate the organism. Protozoa cause persistent and chronic infections, mainly because the host's natural immunity cannot fight all protozoa. Many types of protozoa have evolved to evade specific types of immunity. Indeed, protozoa can activate dissimilar, specific immune responses, different from those of bacteria, viruses, and fungi.

Trypanosoma cruzi is an obligate intracellular parasite that invades different types of cells in vertebrate hosts, and *Toxoplasma gondii* can disseminate in the host because it can change and infect many nucleated cells in its path. Research indicates that cell-mediated immunity against protozoan infection is promoted by CD40-CD40L interaction. CD40-CD40L interaction is critical to the outcome of infection in a number of parasite models.

Some vital information on the paradigms of the T_H (helper T cell, or T lymphocyte) immune response came from a study on immunity to *Leishmania* infection. Host resistance to *Leishmania* leads to the protozoan's multiplication as an amastigote. This multiplication occurs within macrophages that are contingent on the polarization of the immune response to T_H1. The CD40-CD40L interaction is important for promoting T_H1 immune response. Numerous studies have focused on the impact of these types of interaction on the outcome of infection.

The studies on *Leishmania* point to a major role of CD40-CD40L interaction in distorting the immune response of T_H1 for the antiparasite to defend. This interaction is crucial for a positive outcome of infection from a number of parasite models. The stimulation of CD40 proved to be useful in expanding the T_H1-type response.

Protozoan parasites possess a strong ability to adapt into different host environments. They have developed many ways to corrupt the immune system's response.

PARASITE EVASION

Parasites have a variety of mechanisms to break through the immune system's defenses. For example, complement proteins are activated when an infection is recognized. Complements are specialized proteins in the blood that act in sequence to mediate inflammation and the immune response; complements, which include cell membrane receptors and serum proteins, work to destroy infection. In leishmaniasis, the parasite would inhibit the serum proteins and cell membrane receptors by degrading the host's vital proteins. The parasite would continue to interfere with the complement by attacking its nature to bind with the parasite membrane.

Studies have shown that immune evasion does not always lead to an increase in pathogenicity. For example, a decline of the inflammatory response, and a decrease in its severity, can occur when helminths (worms) evade the immune system.

IMMUNOPATHOLOGY

The body reacts strongly to parasites, but parasites have mechanisms of escape; sometimes they can injure the organs of the body and the immune system. These protozoan infections lead to tissue damage and disease. Chronic infection often is caused by the immune system itself, as it responds to the parasite, to antigens, and to changes to the cytokines. Some parasites can acquire a coating of what are called antigen-antibody complexes, or noncytotoxic antibodies that block the binding of certain antibody to the parasite surface. Also, the parasitic protozoan infection can produce host immunosuppression, which will limit the host's ability to kill the parasite. Over time, these parasites can cause lesions and organ damage. Lesions can appear on the mouth, nose, and other areas of the body. In other forms, protozoa can travel in the bloodstream and enlarge the liver, spleen, lymph nodes, and bone marrow.

IMPACT

Leishmaniasis is the most significant protozoan disease worldwide. Infection with the parasitic species, of which there are several found worldwide, can, in its severe form, disfigure a person and can cause death. The World Health Organization (WHO) estimates that there are more than 12 million cases around the world at any given time, with an annual mortality of 60,000 persons. WHO further estimates that 350 million people are at risk for infection worldwide. The impact of leishmaniasis over the years has been underestimated and under-reported. No effective medicine or vaccine exists for leishmaniasis.

Marvin L. Morris, M.P.A.

FURTHER READING

Cohen, Jonathan, William G. Powderly, and Steven E. Opal. *Infectious Diseases*. 3d ed. St. Louis, Mo.: Mosby/Elsevier, 2010. Discusses infectious disease challenges, newer strains of swine influenza, HIV/AIDS, and SARS.

Katsambas, Andreas, and Clio Dessinioti. "Diseases Caused by Protozoa." In *Conn's Current Therapy 2011*, edited by Robert E. Rakel, Edward T. Bope, and Rick D. Kellerman. Philadelphia: Saunders/Elsevier, 2010. Provides treatment recommendations for protozoan diseases found worldwide.

Lupi, O., et al. "Tropical Dermatology: Tropical Diseases Caused by Protozoa." *Journal of the American Academy of Dermatology* 60, no. 6 (2009): 897-925. Examines the different types of protozoa found in tropical regions and the impact these diseases have on public health.

Maizels, R. M. "Exploring the Immunology of Parasitism: From Surface Antigens to the Hygiene Hypothesis." *Parasitology* 136 (2009): 1549-1564. A review of research on parasite immunology.

See also: Developing countries and infectious disease; Diagnosis of protozoan diseases; Leishmaniasis; Parasites: Classification and types; Parasitic diseases; Prevention of protozoan diseases; Protozoa: Structure and growth; Protozoan diseases; Toxoplasmosis; Treatment of protozoan diseases; *Trichomonas*; Tropical medicine; *Trypanosoma*.

Immune response to viral infections

CATEGORY: Immune response

DEFINITION

Viral infections are caused by viral particles that replicate in the host cell. These viral particles then produce more genetic material for new particles and also incorporate their own genetic material into the host cell's genome. As part of its immune response, the human immune system attacks these viral particles to undermine their effect on the body.

Viruses are fought with specific and nonspecific mechanisms, involving either a humoral or cellular response. These two immune responses involve the formation of specific antibodies that are generated to kill viral antigens, the production of interferon by host cells to inhibit viral function, and the production of natural killer cells that recognize and kill the virus.

SPECIFIC TYPES

Humoral immune response. A humoral (body fluid) response to viral infection blocks or neutralizes the viral particles' ability to infect a host cell. The immu-

noglobulin genes in the human immune system are integrally involved in this process. When viruses infect a human host cell, they are considered foreign antigens. The human host cell will then generate antibodies that recognize the specific antigen. Once an antibody is formed, it will then continue to replicate and attack the antigen, thereby neutralizing the viral impact on the host cell.

Cellular immune response. A cellular response to viral infection kills the virus by attacking proteins that reside on viral cell surfaces, such as glycoproteins, or by attacking core proteins of the virus. This attack is made by T cell lymphocytes that will recognize the cell surface proteins of a virus. The killer T cells will destroy the cell and the virus in the cell. Another cellular response is the production of interferons, which are hormones produced by the body when viruses are present.

SPECIFIC METHODS

Interferons. Interferons (IFNs) are proteins made by lymphocytes produced in the human immune system that are released in response to a viral infection. IFNs are part of a group of cytokines that "interfere" with viral replication within the host human cell. They also activate other immune cells, such as natural killer cells and macrophages, and increase the recognition of viral infections for other immune cells to respond. Before a human cell is killed by a virus, it first produces and releases IFNs. These IFNs will then communicate with neighboring host cells to set off a chain reaction to produce and release protein factors called interferon-stimulated genes, which will fight the virus.

Cytotoxic T-cell lymphocytes. Cytotoxic T-cell lymphocytes (CTLs) are virus-specific cells that recognize specific viral antigens that have been synthesized or produced within a human cell. These cells are located on the cell surface on virtually all somatic cells in the human body, so they can respond to practically all the viral antigens it recognizes. CTLs can destroy these viral particles. However, CTLs, in the process of destroying viral particles, also can destroy the involved human cell, which could lead to more damage and injury to the human body. Liver damage, for example, is caused by the virus-specific CTL rather than by the virus itself in the case of hepatitis B infection.

Natural killer cells. Antidependent cell-mediated cytotoxicity (ADCC) is a mechanism in the human immune system and part of cell-mediated immunity that involves effector cells to lyse, or kill, a pathogen (such as a virus) that has been bound by antibodies. Thus, as part of the humoral immune response, antibodies are released to bind to a viral particle, thereby allowing other cells in the immune system to attach to the antibody-antigen complex and destroy it directly.

One ADCC method is the activation of natural killer (NK) cells, which will recognize part of the antibody that is attached to the virus. NK cells are large granular lymphocytes produced by the immune system that make up approximately 2 to 5 percent of peripheral blood lymphocytes. These NK cells, once attached to the viral-antibody complex, will release cytokines, such as interferons and cytotoxic granules, that enter the target cell and promote cell death by triggering the apoptosis (regulated cell death) process. This process is similar, but independent of, responses by CTLs.

IMPACT

All living organisms, including humans, have to develop protective mechanisms against infectious organisms, including viruses, if they are to survive. The complexity of the many infectious particles found on Earth has forced the human body to develop numerous and complicated methods to fight these foreign substances. These methods, which include producing and releasing vast amounts of specific and nonspecific proteins to fight infection, define the immune response.

Susan M. Zneimer, Ph.D., FACMG

FURTHER READING

Coffin, J. M., S. H. Hughes, and H. E. Varmus, eds. *Retroviruses.* Cold Spring Harbor, N.Y.: Cold Spring Harbor Laboratory Press, 2002. Also available at http://www.ncbi.nlm.nih.gov/books/nbk19403. This volume is a major source of information on retroviruses, their classification, production, and replication; also examines how retroviruses infect host cells.

Koyoma, Shohei, et al. "Innate Immune Response to Viral Infection." *Cytokine* 43, no. 3 (2008): 336-341. A review of the different types of immune response to virus infections, including the involvement of immune receptors, the recognition of viruses, sig-naling pathways and communication for immune response, and the factors inhibiting host immune response.

Lane, Thomas, ed. *Chemokines and Viral infection.* New York: Springer, 2006. This book examines the functional roles of chemokines and their receptors in the immune response against well-known viral pathogens.

Murphy, Kenneth, Paul Travers, and Mark Walport. *Janeway's Immunobiology.* 7th ed. New York: Garland Science, 2008. The standard textbook in graduate and medical-school immunology courses because of its clear writing style, organization, and scientific accuracy. Includes color illustrations.

Nathanson, Neal, et al. *Viral Pathogenesis and Immunity.* 2d ed. Boston: Academic Press/Elsevier, 2007. A compilation of articles on all major viral infections that includes discussions of pathogenesis, host response, virus-host interactions, and the control of viruses.

Stetson D. B., and R. Medzhitov. "Type I Interferons in Host Defense." *Immunity* 25 (2006): 373-381. Summarizes the various roles that interferons play in immune response to pathogens. Discusses the classification of interferons and their role in viral response.

WEB SITES OF INTEREST

Big Picture Book of Viruses
http://www.virology.net/big_virology

Microbiology and Immunology On-line: Immunology
http://pathmicro.med.sc.edu/book/immunol-sta.htm

Virology.net
http://www.virology.net

See also: Antibodies; Autoimmune disorders; Immune response to bacterial infections; Immunity; Immunization; Immunoassay; Immunodeficiency; Opportunistic infections; Pathogenicity; Reinfection; Seroconversion; T lymphocytes; Vaccines: Types; Viral infections; Virology; Virulence; Viruses: Structure and life cycle; Viruses: Types.

Immunity

CATEGORY: Immune response

ALSO KNOWN AS: Acquired (adaptive) immunity, cellular immunity, immune response, inflammatory response, innate immunity

DEFINITION

Immunity is the state, quality, or condition of being resistant to pathogens, parasites, and nonliving harmful substances.

INNATE AND ACQUIRED IMMUNITY

Ubiquitous pathogens are found on surfaces, on food, and in the air. Innate and acquired immunity confer lifelong protective immunity to the body against foreign substances, including harmful toxins, viruses, and bacteria. Three basic components work closely to protect the body: physical barriers such as the various epithelial surfaces, innate immunity, and acquired immune responses. Inherited genes, environment, lifestyle, and acquired characteristics can influence the state of immunity.

Innate, or natural, immunity is the ability inherent from birth to fight infection without adapting to a specific pathogen. Innate immunity is characterized by physical barriers that defend against harmful agents and by more sophisticated defense mechanisms. Sometimes, physical defenses can be triggered through innate immune responses, such as ciliary action or sneezing from histamine production.

Other defenses include bactericidal enzyme action in secreted bodily fluids and more complex complement proteins. The innate immune system is nonspecific, focusing on conserved pathogen-associated molecular patterns so that many organisms are attacked in a similar fashion. Although the quality and efficacy of the initial innate response do not improve after subsequent exposures to the same pathogen, innate immunity includes a number of other defense mechanisms. Epithelial surfaces, including the genitourinary tract, respiratory tract, skin, and gastrointestinal tract, produce antimicrobial peptides such as defensins and cathelicidins that inhibit bacterial and fungal growth. Two nonspecific methods to eliminate microorganisms are phagocytosis and opsonization. In phagocytosis, specialized cells such as neutrophils, monocytes, and macrophages ingest and destroy ingested pathogen particles. In opsonization, phagocytic cells recognize a plasma protein (opsonin) binding to the surface of the pathogen, leading to enhanced phagocytosis.

The hallmark of innate immunity is an inflammatory response (inflammation or edema). Proinflammatory mediators such as cytokines, chemokines, and lipid mediators clear the infection. Inflammation, however, is damaging and painful to tissues, and some chronic diseases possess an inflammatory pathology component. Clinically, drugs can be used to control inflammation. Innate immune response is an early defense mechanism against infection, but it is also essential in boosting subsequent adaptive immune responses.

During adaptive (acquired) immunity, the immune system develops a defense specific to a particular antigen and does so with immunological specificity and long-lasting memory beyond the acute infection. An agent evoking a specific immune response is called an immunogen. Immunogens reacting with antibodies are antigens. Virtually any substance of a certain size, including cell proteins, viral nucleic acids, chemicals, or foreign particles (such as a splinter), can become an antigen. The goal of an acquired immune response is to recognize and destroy substances containing antigens.

To reach this goal, acquired immunity utilizes two sophisticated and flexible mechanisms: cell-mediated immunity and humoral immunity. Cell-mediated response relies on B and T lymphocytes (white blood cells). Following antigen exposure, antigens are taken up and presented to B and T lymphocytes by antigen-presenting cells such as macrophages from the innate system or by dendritic cells from the acquired system. After recognizing their specific matching antigen, B cells differentiate into plasma cells, which then produce and secrete large amounts of antibodies against the specific antigen.

Likewise, T cells differentiate after antigen recognition into helper T cells (Th) or cytotoxic (killer) T cells (Tc); the T cells release lymphotoxins causing cell lysis. Th's secrete lymphokines, which further stimulate Tc and B cells to proliferate and divide, attracting neutrophils and improving phagocytes' ability to engulf and kill pathogens. Although innate immunity is available instantly upon infection, acquired immunity takes approximately seven to ten days to mount an initial response. Parts of the innate system, such as complement or phagocytosis, can also

Components of the Immune System

Major Components	Major Organs	Other Cells
• B lymphocytes (B cells) • T lymphocytes (T cells) • NK (natural killer) cells • Phagocytes (macrophages and neutrophils) • Complement	• Thymus • Liver • Bone Marrow • Tonsils • Lymph nodes • Spleen • Blood	• Stem cells • Immature cells • Effector/cytotoxic cells • T helper cells • Plasma cells • Immunoglobulins (antibodies) • Polymorphonuclear cells • Monocytes • Red blood cells • Platelets • Dendritic cells

be activated by the acquired system through antibody mediation.

Immunoglobulin (Ig) is another term for antibody; it binds specifically to antigenic determinants or epitopes. Immunoglobulins inactivate antigens by complement fixation, neutralization, agglutination, and precipitation. Immunoglobulins are made of two identical heavy chains and identical light chains. They are classified based on their heavy chain as IgM, IgG, IgA, IgE, and IgD.

PASSIVE AND ACTIVE IMMUNITY

Antibody-mediated immunity includes passive and active immunity. Exposure to the pathogen/antigen results in active immunity. For example, during vaccination, the antigen is presented (by injection of a weakened, killed, or recombinant pathogenic antigen), resulting in the vaccinated person's body generating a specific immune response against that antigen.

In passive immunity, "natural" or "artificial," the body does not manufacture its own antibodies; rather, the body gets antibodies from another person. For example, infants undergo natural passive immunity during the transfer of antibodies through the maternal placenta or milk. These infant antibodies disappear between six and twelve months of age with the replacement of breast milk. Passive immunity is short-lived because these antibodies are degraded in the body over time and because no immunological memory exists to produce more antibodies.

Artificial passive immunity involves the transfusion of antiserum or the injection of antibodies that were produced by another person or animal. Immediate protection against an antigen is achieved through these antibodies, although it is a short-lived immunity. Examples of passive immunization include tetanus antitoxin and purified human gammaglobulin.

IMMUNITY DISORDERS AND COMPLICATIONS

Sometimes single components of the immune system are inefficient, absent, or excessive. In these cases, the state of protection is not reached adequately. The impaired immune system is considered immunocompromised, and it could leave the host body vulnerable to various opportunistic infections. Acquired immunodeficiency syndrome (AIDS), for example, is a result of the depletion of helper T cells after a viral infection. The failure of host defense mechanisms can lead to conditions such as autoimmune diseases, immunodeficiencies, allergies, delayed hypersensitivity states, and transplant rejections. Immune responses in the absence of infection include allergy or hypersensitivity reactions, autoimmunity, and graft rejections. An allergic reaction occurs against innocuous substances. Responses to self-antigens are visible in autoimmune diseases. Immunodeficiencies can be inherited (primary) or acquired (secondary).

IMPACT

Vaccination is a preventive measure against morbidity and mortality resulting from infectious diseases such as polio, measles, diphtheria, pertussis, rubella, mumps, tetanus, and *Haemophilus influenzae* type B. It is an artificial method of building immunity by deliberately infecting a person so that the body learns self-protection from a pathogen. Controlling and even eradicating infectious diseases reduces frequent doctor's visits, hospitalizations, and deaths, leading to improved public health, reduced disease burdens, and reduced health care costs. For example, the World Health Organization's immunization campaign from 1967 to 1977 eradicated smallpox.

Another immunization strategy is herd immunity, in which immunization of a high percentage (a herd) of a population provides protection to unvaccinated persons. This type of community immunity tries break the chain of infection by having large sections of a population immune. It slows infectious disease transmission and can even stop outbreaks.

Ana Maria Rodriguez-Rojas, M.S.

FURTHER READING

Baxter, David. "Active and Passive Immunity, Vaccine Types, Excipients, and Licensing." *Occupational Medicine* 57, no. 8 (2007): 552-556. Reviews the concepts of active and passive immunity and discusses the commercially available vaccine types and how they generate an adaptive immune response.

Bonds, M. H., and P. Rohani. "Herd Immunity Acquired Indirectly from Interactions Between the Ecology of Infectious Diseases, Demography, and Economics." *Journal of the Royal Society Interface* 7 (2010): 541-547. Presents a theoretical disease-ecology framework in which fertility, poverty, and disease interact and lead to the acquisition of herd immunity.

DeFranco, Anthony, Richard Locksley, and Miranda Robertson. *Immunity: The Immune Response in Infectious and Inflammatory Disease.* Sunderland, Mass.: Sinauer, 2007. A standard textbook for medical and immunology students that offers a comprehensive overview of the subject. Includes color illustrations.

Keller, M. A., and E. R. Stiehm. "Passive Immunity in Prevention and Treatment of Infectious Diseases." *Clinical Microbiology Reviews* 13, no. 4 (2000): 602-614. Highlights the efficacy of antibodies in the prevention and treatment of infectious diseases.

Murphy, Kenneth, Paul Travers, and Mark Walport. *Janeway's Immunobiology.* 7th ed. New York: Garland Science, 2008. The standard textbook in graduate and medical-school immunology courses because of its clear writing style, organization, and scientific accuracy. Includes color illustrations.

National Library of Medicine. "Immune System and Disorders." Available at http://www.nlm.nih.gov/medlineplus/immunesystemanddisorders.html. Offers updated health information on the immune system and related disorders.

Strugnell, R. A., and O. L. Wijburg. "The Role of Secretory Antibodies in Infection Immunity." *Nature Reviews Microbiology* 8, no. 9 (2010): 656-667. Examines evidence that secretory antibodies offer defense against infection in some animal models. Discusses the evolution of the secretory immune system.

WEB SITES OF INTEREST

Centers for Disease Control and Prevention
http://www.cdc.gov/vaccines

Global Health Council
http://www.globalhealth.org

Microbiology and Immunology On-line: Immunology
http://pathmicro.med.sc.edu/book/immunol-sta.htm

National Network for Immunization Information
http://www.immunizationinfo.org

World Health Organization
http://www.who.int/immunization

See also: Antibodies; Autoimmune disorders; Immune response to bacterial infections; Immune response to fungal infections; Immune response to parasitic diseases; Immune response to prion diseases; Immune response to protozoan diseases; Immune response to viral infections; Immunization; Immunoassay; Immunodeficiency; Opportunistic infections; Reinfection; Seroconversion; T lymphocytes; Vaccines: Types; Virulence.

Immunization

CATEGORY: Prevention
ALSO KNOWN AS: Vaccination

DEFINITION

Immunization, also known as vaccination, is the administration of a substance (a vaccine) through inoculation, ingestion, or nasal inhalation to stimulate a person's immune system in fighting disease. Persons who receive a vaccine are considered immunized against a particular pathogen.

INTRODUCTION

The golden age of immunology occurred from 1870 to 1910, the height of discovery of the biologic basis of immunity and the time when several important vaccines became available. There is renewed interest in vaccine development internationally because of the decreasing effectiveness of antibiotics in treating bacterial infection.

Vaccination remains the most important protection against viral infection, especially because of the lack of effective treatments once a viral infection is established. Also, no useful vaccines exist against malaria, chlamydia, fungi, parasitic protozoa, helminthic parasites, or the human immunodeficiency virus (HIV).

Vaccines for about seventy-five diseases are under development. Early-phase research into numerous vaccines is ongoing for acquired immunodeficiency syndrome (AIDS), malaria, and such common conditions as ear aches. A great deal of research focuses on combining vaccines into a reduced total number of injections in the vaccine schedule (the recommended time line for a given vaccine or vaccines).

Infectious diseases are not the only possible targets of vaccines. Researchers are investigating vaccines' potential for contraception and for treating and preventing diseases such as cocaine addiction, Alzheimer's, and cancer. Researchers also are looking to improve the effectiveness of antigens in stimulating immunity with the use of additives called adjuvants. Only alum, or aluminum hydroxide, has been approved as an adjuvant for human use. In 2011, 349 phase-four vaccine clinical trials were underway.

Before the invention of vaccines, it was known that people who recovered from certain diseases, such as smallpox, were immune to the disease thereafter. Reportedly, Chinese physicians were the first to try to exploit this phenomenon to prevent disease by drying and grinding up smallpox scabs that were then inhaled by children. In England, contaminating a fresh skin cut, called variolation, with scabs from smallpox wounds became common in the eighteenth century. Most often, localized skin reactions occurred; a serious case of smallpox occurred less often. Although only 1 percent of persons became seriously sick after

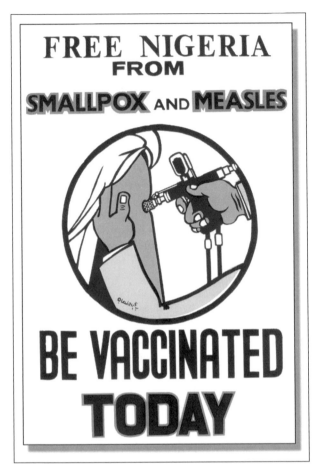

A 1979 poster from health authorities in Nigeria, urging people to get immunized, or vaccinated, against smallpox and measles. (CDC)

variolation, the mortality rate was as high as 50 percent.

Edward Jenner, an English physician, occasionally encountered patients who did not respond with the usual reactions to variolation. One story relates that a milkmaid had told Jenner that she would not get smallpox because she had already had cowpox, a mild disease that causes lesions on the udders of cows. The hands of milkmaids would sometimes become infected. Jenner then began to deliberately inoculate (with cowpox) people with superficial wounds in an attempt to prevent smallpox. The forked, or bifurcated needle, used to scratch the skin and deliver a drop of vaccine is considered the single most successful medical device ever developed because it eliminated the scourge of smallpox. The term "vaccination," from the Latin *vacca*, or "cow," was coined in recognition of Jenner's work.

Because viral diseases cannot be effectively treated once established, vaccination is usually the only practical method of controlling them. Controlling viral disease requires that an entire population be immune to it. A phenomenon called herd immunity is established, however, if most of a population is immune. With herd immunity, disease outbreak is limited to sporadic cases, avoiding epidemic spread of disease. Two centuries after Jenner, smallpox was eliminated worldwide by vaccination.

PRINCIPLES AND RESULTS OF VACCINATION

A vaccine is a suspension of organisms, or pieces of organisms, delivered to the immune system in various ways. Vaccines offer the immune system a biochemical example of the disease microbe that is used by the body to induce immunity. Both antibody-based, or humoral immunity and cell-based immunity depend upon the formation of immunologic memory. Once vaccinated, immunologic memory is responsible for the rapid neutralizing responses that prevent disease after exposure.

It is now known that Jenner's inoculations worked because the cowpox virus, which is not a serious pathogen, is closely related to the smallpox virus. The injection, by skin scratches, provoked a primary immune response against the proteins of the cowpox virus in the recipients, leading to the formation of antibodies and long-term memory cells. Exposure to the smallpox virus and its proteins would lead to the rapid, neutralizing response characteristic of immune people. A vaccinia virus vaccine eventually replaced the cowpox vaccine.

TYPES OF VACCINES AND THEIR CHARACTERISTICS

There are now several basic vaccine types: attenuated microbe vaccines, inactivated whole-agent vaccines, toxoids, subunit vaccines, conjugated vaccines, and nucleic acid vaccines.

Attenuated microbe vaccines. Attenuated microbe vaccines use living but weakened (attenuated) viruses that cannot cause disease in healthy persons. Live attenuated viruses infect and multiply in the cells of the recipient. Attenuated microbes are usually viral strains derived after mutations accumulated during long-term artificial culture or through genetic manipulation. These microbes no longer cause disease, yet they

still are able to cause a low-level infection that generates immunity. Live vaccines more closely mimic an actual infection.

Lifelong immunity is often achieved without booster immunizations, and an effectiveness rate of 95 percent is not unusual. This long-term effectiveness of live viral vaccines probably occurs because the attenuated viruses replicate in the body, increasing the original dose and acting as a series of secondary, or booster, immunizations. Examples of live vaccines include those that protect against smallpox, measles, mumps, and rubella, and the oral polio vaccine, no longer available in the United States. Some newer live-virus vaccines against rotavirus, dengue fever, and other diseases are artificial virus combinations. In development, scientists start with a particular virus's genetic backbone. Genes from a pathogenic virus are added, and those proteins are produced in infected cells of the vaccine recipient.

The best-known example of a live attenuated bacterial vaccine is the Bacille Calmette-Guérin (BCG), a vaccine that has been used for some time, but with limited efficacy, to combat tuberculosis. To make BCG, tuberculosis bacteria from cows were modified in culture to provide immunity without disease. Newer, genetically modified, live-attenuated vaccines against tuberculosis and typhoid fever are in development. The delivery of the microbes' proteins is internal and, therefore, distinct from both oral and injectable vaccines.

Attenuated vaccines are not recommended for people whose immune systems are compromised. Because of advances in chemotherapy treatments for cancer, increases in the number of organ transplant recipients taking immunosuppressive drugs, and an increase in the number of immunocompromised through diseases such as AIDS, the use of attenuated microbe vaccines should be carefully considered. If available, inactivated vaccines are substituted. A separate danger of such vaccines is the theoretical possibility that the live microbes can mutate back to a virulent form.

Inactivated whole-agent vaccines. Inactivated whole-agent vaccines use microbes that have been killed, usually by formalin or phenol chemical treatment. Inactivated virus vaccines used in humans include those for rabies, influenza, and polio, which was adopted for use in the United States after 2003. Inactivated bacterial vaccines include those for pneumococcal pneumonia and cholera. Several long-used inactivated vaccines have been or are being replaced by newer, more effective subunit vaccines; these vaccines are those for pertussis, or whooping cough, and typhoid fever.

Toxoids. Toxoid vaccines are composed of toxins that have been inactivated through chemical or genetic means. As vaccines, they are directed at the toxins produced by a pathogen. The tetanus and diphtheria toxoids have long been part of the standard childhood immunization series. They require a series of injections for full immunity, followed by boosters every ten years. Many older adults have not received boosters, so they are likely to have low levels of protection.

Subunit vaccines. Subunit vaccines use only those molecules or fragments from a microorganism that best stimulates an immune response, referred to as antigenicity. Subunit vaccines that are produced by genetic modification techniques, whereby other microbes are genetically modified to produce the desired antigenic fraction, are called recombinant vaccines. For example, the vaccine against the hepatitis B virus consists of a portion of the viral protein coat that is produced by genetically modified yeast.

Subunit vaccines are inherently safer because they cannot reproduce in the recipient. They also contain little or no extraneous material and, therefore, tend to produce fewer adverse effects. Similarly, it is possible to separate the fractions of a disrupted bacterial cell, retaining the desired antigenic fractions. The newer acellular vaccines for whooping cough contained in the DTaP (diphtheria, tetanus, and pertussis) vaccine use this approach.

Conjugated vaccines. Conjugated vaccines, also referred to as glycoconjugates, have been developed because of the poor immune response of children to vaccines that are based on the capsular polysaccharides surrounding the cell wall of certain bacteria. Polysaccharides are T-independent antigens. This means that a child's immune system responds to the vaccine through his or her B cells (lymphocytes) only. Immunologic memory depends on the contributions of T cells. Therefore, polysaccharides do not stimulate immunity until the age of fifteen to twenty-four months.

In glycoconjugate technology, the polysaccharides are chemically bonded to proteins such as diphtheria or tetanus toxoid. The protein recruits T cells to the vicinity where the polysaccharides and B cells interact.

The B cells receive the chemical signal necessary to form immunologic memory from the T cells. This approach has led to the very successful vaccines for *Haemophilus influenzae* type B, *Streptococcus pneumoniae*, and *Neisseria meningitidis*, which give significant protection, even at two months of age.

Nucleic acid vaccines. Nucleic acid vaccines, or DNA vaccines, are experimental, yet promising, vaccines. Experiments with animals show that small circular DNA (deoxyribonucleic acid) molecules, or plasmids of DNA injected into muscle, results in muscle tissue production of the protein encoded for on the DNA. These proteins stimulate an immune response. While the protein is stable enough to stimulate an immune response, the DNA is degraded rapidly, so the supply of protein is not renewed. RNA (ribonucleic acid), which could be made to replicate in the recipient, might be a more effective vaccine.

VACCINE SAFETY

Variolation, the first attempt to provide immunity to smallpox, sometimes caused the disease it was intended to prevent. At that time, however, the risk was considered worthwhile. The orally delivered live attenuated polio vaccine was effective at reducing polio in the face of an epidemic. On rare occasions, it caused a mild form of the disease. Therefore, the lower-risk inactivated poliovirus vaccine was adopted in the developed world when epidemics were rarer.

In 1999, a vaccine to prevent infant diarrhea caused by rotaviruses was withdrawn from the market because several recipients developed a life-threatening intestinal obstruction called intussusception. Eventually, it was determined that the vaccine was not the cause, and some experts suggested that it be reintroduced where the incidence of rotavirus is high: in developing countries. Eventually, a separate rotavirus vaccine was put into use.

Public reaction to such risks has changed. Most parents have never seen a case of polio or measles and, therefore, tend to view the risk of these diseases as remote. Rumored reports of harmful effects often lead people to avoid certain vaccines. In particular, a contrived connection between the MMR (measles, mumps, rubella) vaccine and autism received widespread publicity. Autism is a poorly understood developmental condition that causes a child, in part, to withdraw from everyday reality, namely other persons. Because autism is usually diagnosed at the age of eighteen to thirty months (the age range in which vaccination is common in the United States and in Europe), some persons claimed a cause-and-effect connection between the vaccines and autism. Medically, however, most experts agree that autism is a condition with a major genetic component, and that is begins before birth. The large increase in autism diagnoses is caused primarily by the greatly expanded definition of "autism spectrum disorder" and not to the adoption of certain vaccines. Testifying to the contrary has been discredited.

Thimerosal is a mercury-containing organic compound. Since the 1930's, it has been widely used as a preservative in vaccines to help prevent bacterial contamination. Concerns about thimerosal have been raised because of an increasing awareness of the theoretical potential for the neurotoxicity of mercury and because of the increased number of thimerosal-containing vaccines added to the immunization schedule. Because of these concerns, the U.S. Food and Drug Administration continues to work with vaccine manufacturers to eliminate thimerosal from vaccines.

CHALLENGES OF VACCINATION

The economics of vaccination. Although interest in vaccine development declined with the introduction of antibiotics, it has intensified in recent years. Fear of litigation contributed to decreased development of new vaccines in the United States and in Europe. However, the passage of the National Childhood Vaccine Injury Act in 1986, which limited the liability of vaccine manufacturers in the United States, helped to reverse this trend. Even so, to the pharmaceutical industry, vaccines are inherently less attractive economically than are drug treatments that last for extended periods of time.

Cultivation of vaccine microbes and antigens. Vaccines can be developed only by growing the pathogen in large quantities. The early successful viral vaccines were developed by animal cultivation. The vaccinia virus for smallpox was grown on the shaved bellies of calves, for example. The introduction of vaccines against polio, measles, mumps, and a number of other viral diseases that would not grow in anything except living human cells awaited the development of cell culture techniques. Cell cultures from human sources enabled the growth of these viruses on a large scale.

A valuable biologic resource for growth of viruses is the chick embryo. Viruses for several vaccines, for ex-

ample, influenza, are grown in the various anatomic compartments of the egg. Interestingly, the first vaccine against hepatitis B virus used viral antigens extracted from the blood of chronically infected humans because no other source was available. Recombinant vaccines and DNA vaccines do not need a cell or animal host to grow the vaccine's microbe. This avoids a major problem with certain viruses that have not been grown in cell culture-hepatitis B, for example.

Distribution and delivery of vaccines. Diarrheal diseases are a major cause of mortality for infants in developing countries, where costs and distribution of vaccines also pose special problems. For example, a vaccine that must be refrigerated would be nearly useless in countries that lack reliable electrical service. As an alternative, edible, plant-derived vaccines of several types are undergoing clinical trials.

IMPACT

Infectious disease places a heavy burden on public health in many parts of the world. The cost in terms of human suffering, social hardship, and economic cost is huge. As a consequence, preventing and combating these diseases are keys to the economic development of many underdeveloped regions.

A number of diseases are vaccine-preventable. The introduction of immunization has been one of the greatest and most cost-effective interventions in human health. The health impact of vaccination programs is tremendous, perhaps surpassed in significance only by measures to prevent poverty and to introduce sanitation systems for clean water.

Kimberly A. Napoli, M.S.

FURTHER READING

Allen, Arthur. *Vaccine: The Controversial Story of Medicine's Greatest Livesaver.* New York: W. W. Norton, 2007. A comprehensive work discussing the vaccine industry. Covers colonial America to the twenty-first century.

Atkinson, W., et al., eds. *Epidemiology and Prevention of Vaccine-Preventable Diseases.* 11th ed. Washington, D.C.: Public Health Foundation, 2009. A comprehensive text on vaccine-preventable diseases. This work is also available at http://www.cdc.gov/vaccines/pubs/pinkbook.

Delves, Peter J., et al. *Roitt's Essential Immunology.* 11th ed. Malden, Mass.: Blackwell, 2006. An excellent textbook on the subject of immunology. Much of the book is detailed and requires some background in biology. Nevertheless, the chapters that deal with infection and immunization are clear and contain much information for general readers.

Hackett, Charles, and Donald Harn. *Vaccine Adjuvants: Immunological and Clinical Principles.* Totowa, N.J.: Humana Press, 2006. Covers additives to vaccines and their effect on immunogenicity.

Plotkin, Stanley A., Walter A. Orenstein, and Paul A. Offit. *Vaccines.* 5th ed. Philadelphia: Saunders/Elsevier, 2008. An excellent description of the role of vaccines in the prevention of disease. Begins with a history of immunization practices. Chapters deal with a specific disease and the role and history of vaccine production in its prevention.

WEB SITES OF INTEREST

ClinicalTrials
http://www.clinicaltrials.gov

College of Physicians of Philadelphia, History of Vaccines
http://www.historyofvaccines.org

Emerging and Reemerging Infectious Diseases Resource Center
http://www.medscape.com/resource/infections

Vaccine Research Center
http://www.niaid.nih.gov/about/organization/vrc

World Health Organization
http://www.who.int/immunization

See also: Antibodies; Centers for Disease Control and Prevention (CDC); Cowpox; Developing countries and infectious disease; Disease eradication campaigns; DTaP vaccine; Emerging and reemerging infectious diseases; Epidemiology; Hepatitis vaccines; Immunity; Malaria vaccine; Microbiology; MMR vaccine; Outbreaks; Polio vaccins; Prevention of bacterial infections; Prevention of viral infections; Public health; Rotavirus vaccine; Smallpox vaccine; T lymphocytes; Tuberculosis (TB) vaccine; U.S. Army Medical Research Institute of Infectious Diseases; Vaccines: Experimental; Vaccines: History; Vaccines: Types; Virology; World Health Organization (WHO).

Immunoassay

CATEGORY: Diagnosis
ALSO KNOWN AS: Bioassay, biochemical assay, immunochemical assay, immunodiagnosis, immunologic test

DEFINITION

An immunoassay is a laboratory technique or method that quantifies the presence or concentration of a substance by immunochemical means.

DIAGNOSIS OF INFECTIOUS AGENTS

Unmanageable infectious disease can be a major burden to global health, even causing societal and civil disruption. Therefore, a key strategy in lessening this burden is rapid, accurate diagnosis of infectious agents, which allows for appropriate intervention by treatment with drugs that slow the spread of infection to others. Today's infectious disease diagnostics still are rooted in classical methods from the twentieth century. Microscopic- and culture-based methodologies are considered the gold standard for the diagnosis of infectious agents, ahead of antigen detection and immunoserology. However, limitations for these classical methodologies include microscopy's poor sensitivity, time-consuming culturing techniques, the biohazard risk of uncultured or fastidious organisms, and skilled worker and manual labor requirements.

Disease-related biomarkers are increasingly used as an alternative diagnostic tool to identify infected persons and populations. A biomarker refers to a specific substance related to the disease in question. The biomarker can be used to examine health status, organ function, and the condition and progression of a disease. Protein and polysaccharide biomarkers are often measured with immunoassays (defined in the following section). Immunoassay detection can accelerate diagnosis or supplement classical microbiology assays by detecting pathogen-associated proteins or host-produced antibodies to the pathogen in an infected person's samples.

While many diagnostic immunoassays are used for infectious disease, some challenges with false-positive and false-negative results remain. These results may come from assay reagents cross-reacting with similar structures in the sample. Also, false results may be caused by nonspecific biomarker expression, or lack thereof. Therefore, these indirect methods tend to be

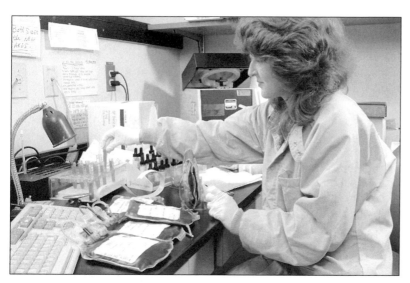

A laboratory technician often applies the immunoassay technique while testing blood samples. (Digital Stock)

undervalued compared with traditional diagnostic tools for infectious agents.

IMMUNOASSAY TECHNOLOGIES AND TECHNICAL CONSIDERATIONS

Diagnostic immunoassays for infectious disease are based on antibody recognition of proteins or peptides specific for the pathogen of interest. The antibodies employed work as a unique analytical reagent equipped with distinct specificity and remarkable binding affinity to detect specific antigens or other antibodies. Immunoassays share four common elements: immobilized capture reagents (usually antibodies), binding of a protein or peptide analyte/antigen of interest, detection with an antibody or antiserum, and an indirect signal readout. Most immunoassays also contain separation steps to remove unbound reagents. The indirect signal readout is directly or inversely proportional to the analyte concentration in the sample. Thus, the signal relates to either the detection of a pathogen-specific antibody or the detection of a pathogenic antigen (or antigens) in the sample. Because of the high specificity and affinity of antibodies used, unpurified blood or other fluid samples can be applied in immunoassays without prior purification. Antibodies can pick out specifically the analyte of interest.

Signal measurement requires a detectable label to quantify the amount of captured antigen or antibody.

The label is a molecule that reacts during the assay producing a quantifiable signal. A variety of labels are available, including enzymes, gold, silver and selenium colloidal particles, radioactive elements, coenzymes, electroactive groups, fluorescent, and phosphorescent and chemiluminescent dyes. Signal interpretation calls for reference to a calibrator that resembles the attributes of the analyte in the sample. Calibrators with known analyte concentrations allow for the correlation of signal strength in the assay with the analyte concentration in the sample.

Independently of their technology, what determines the efficacy of any immunoassay it is the capacity to form antigen-antibody complexes and the ability to detect such immunocomplexes. Highly specific antibody reagents with preferably high affinity are at the heart of successful immunoassays. High specificity allows for minimal cross-reactivity with unrelated proteins while high affinity can translate into high analytical sensitivity.

The first immunoassays were introduced in the 1960's as radioimmunoassays (RIAs) to measure insulin and thyroxine. RIAs typically use radioactive iodine; labels and the amount of radioactivity measured indicate the amount of analyte accounted for. Despite their advantage to detect very low quantities of analytes, the use of RIAs has decreased in clinical laboratories because of issues concerning isotope handling and the disposal of radioactive materials; RIAs were replaced by the enzyme immunoassay (EIA). In EIAs, enzyme labels such as horseradish peroxidase, a-galactosidase, and alkaline phosphatase are utilized instead of radioactive isotopes. During a substrate reaction, the enzyme mediates light emission, color change, or other measurable signals.

Now, enzyme-linked immunosorbent assay (ELISA) is the most common format, in which a solid-phase, bound, capture reagent is combined with an enzyme-labeled detection antibody. The immobilized capture reagent can be an antibody specific for the analyte or a target (such as a receptor), binding the analyte out of the sample. The bound antigen subsequently is recognized by the detection antibody.

In addition to ELISA, the main formats employed in the specific detection of infectious disease agents include lateral flow systems, flow cytometry, and fluorescent polarization. Lateral flow assays, also known as hand-held assays (HHA), are simple immunochromatographic assays, or strip tests. Best known as home pregnancy tests, lateral flow assays are often deployed as point-of-care testing for nose and throat swabs and for urine, fecal, or blood samples because of their simplicity and quick results (within minutes; traditional plate-based assays or immunoanalyzers take much longer).

Many immunoassays are now fully automated on immunoanalyzers. The method of choice (for example, lateral flow, RIA, immunoanalyzer, and flow cytometry) depends on the priorities of the application, such as simplicity versus speed. Molecular diagnostic methods (for example, polymerase chain reaction and microarray technology) have started to complement or even replace immunoassays for the detection of infectious diseases. One example of a molecular diagnostic method is testing for the human immunodeficiency virus (HIV).

VERIFICATION OF ASSAY PERFORMANCE

Assay sensitivity and specificity are essential to accurately determine the presence and concentration of the analyte. Clinical sensitivity and specificity refer to the assay's false-negative and false-positive rates when applied to patient samples. Analytical sensitivity and specificity refer to the assay's ability to recognize the analyte at low concentrations with minimal cross-reactivity.

While clinical assay performance is determined during initial validation, analytical performance is assessed both during validation and during daily quality controls. Quality assessment ensures the collected data are true and accurate. The main issues facing immunoassays include cross-reactivity (that is, nonspecificity) of the reagents used, interferences from sample components, and assay variability within each assay or across repeat measurements. Researchers are working on developing immunoassays with better clinical performance through the development of highly specific reagents, through increased speed with automation, and through novel technologies and greater analytical sensitivity.

IMPACT

The main benefit of any immunoassay is its speed, flexibility, cost efficiency, and relative simplicity, allowing it to be deployed in central laboratories and in the field. Field use is particularly critical to obtaining quick diagnosis of infectious disease and to administering appropriate treatment.

Immunoassay specificity plays a critical role in characterizing and distinguishing methicillin-resistant *Staphylococcus aureus* (MRSA) infections from the methicillin-sensitive (MSSA) strain. MRSA is a multi-drug-resistant aggressive bacterial infection that affects people in hospitals, prisons, and nursing homes. Another advantage of immunoassays is that they are safe to perform and can be adapted to several formats, which range from strip tests to test-tube assays, 96 well microplates, and high throughput analyzers, combined with complex microarray or biosensor systems. Automation has helped streamline workflow and increase productivity in central laboratory settings, while manual versions can be used in universities, colleges, and other low-volume settings.

Although there are several test systems to detect antigens and antibodies, detection methods to diagnose disease differ from those to verify immunity. Therefore, it is critical that the right criteria for the assay selected is clear and appropriate for each application. Thus, detection of antibody can be utilized to verify and measure a person's immunity to bacteria, viruses, and fungi.

Detection of immunity to rubella virus and varicella zoster virus, for example, are common screening tests performed in the health care industry because both viral infections can spread and be fatal in immunocompromised persons, infants, and unvaccinated adults. During prenatal screening, immunity is characterized in addition to past medical history by the TORCH panel, which uses ELISA methodology to test for antibodies against four TORCH organisms: *Toxoplasma gondii* (toxoplasmosis), rubella (German measles), cytomegalovirus (CMV), and herpes simplex virus (HSV). Pretransplant immunity screening for recipients and donors also makes use of immunoassays to determine CMV seroreactivity because transplant recipients are prone to develop CMV infections.

The impact of immunoassay technologies is not restricted to medical diagnosis; it is applied also in pharmaceutical development, veterinary medicine, forensic toxicology, military-based medicine, environmental monitoring, and food sciences. Pregnancy and ovulation home-tests have brought the technology to the general public. Point-of-care diagnostics devices are being improved and expanded in scope, potentially allowing immunoassays to play an even greater role in personalized medicine and infectious disease testing. Tabletop-sized automation and quantitative, sensitive strip tests will improve accurate and early diagnosis and turnaround time, will decrease costs, and will reduce the burdens of infectious diseases and related outbreaks.

Ana Maria Rodriguez-Rojas, M.S.

FURTHER READING

Cavanaugh, Bonita Morrow. *Nurse's Manual of Laboratory and Diagnostic Tests.* 4th ed. Philadelphia: F. A. Davis, 2003. Provides information on hundreds of laboratory and diagnostic tests, with each test presented in two distinct, cross-referenced sections: "Background Information" sections provide a complete description of each test and its purposes; "Clinical Application Data" sections focus on the information nurses most commonly need for patient care.

Pagana, Kathleen Deska, and Timothy J. Pagana. *Mosby's Diagnostic and Laboratory Test Reference.* 9th ed. St. Louis, Mo.: Mosby/Elsevier, 2009. A clinical handbook with alphabetically organized laboratory and diagnostic tests. Each listing includes alternate or abbreviated test names, type of test, normal findings, possible critical values, test explanation and related physiology, and potential complications.

Wild, David, ed. *The Immunoassay Handbook.* 3d ed. Boston: Elsevier, 2005. Includes the following chapters: "Principles," "Product Technology," "Laboratory Management," and "Applications."

WEB SITES OF INTEREST

Lab Tests Online
http://www.labtestsonline.org

Merck Manuals: Laboratory Diagnosis of Infectious Disease
http://www.merckmanuals.com/professional/
sec14/ch168/ch168a.html

Protocolpedia
http://www.protocolpedia.com

See also: Acid-fastness; Bacteriology; Biochemical tests; Diagnosis of bacterial infections; Diagnosis of fungal infections; Diagnosis of viral infections; Gram staining; Microbiology; Microscopy; Pathogenicity; Pathogens; Polymerase chain reaction (PCR) method; Pulsed-field gel electrophoresis; Serology; Virology.

Immunodeficiency

CATEGORY: Immune response

DEFINITION

The immune system defends the body against infections. The impairment or absence of the immune system results in immune deficiencies, or immunodeficiencies, which increase susceptibility to infectious diseases and rare cancers. A normal, healthy immune system confers lifelong protective immunity against harmful toxins, viruses, fungi, bacteria, parasites, and cancer cells. Immune deficiencies predispose a person to persistent and unusual infections, slower healing, and increased incidences of rare cancers. Persons who have immunodeficiency are considered immunocompromised.

For the immunocompromised person, opportunistic infections, especially if left undiagnosed or untreated, increase morbidity and mortality; these infections are typically harmless to a person with a healthy immune system. Because of complex and intertwined regulatory systems in the body, immunodeficiencies that affect either parts of the innate or acquired immune systems can easily lead to serious health complications, even when other parts of the immune system function normally.

Immunocompromised persons often have repeated infections that become serious. Some immunodeficiencies will shorten a person's life, while others, if properly treated, will mainly affect a person's short- or long-term quality of life.

A sore throat or head cold may lead to pneumonia. Severe burns are always associated with complications because the injured skin has lost its mechanical integrity and immune defense properties. Persons with acquired immunodeficiency syndrome (AIDS) are especially susceptible to opportunistic infections and can become critically ill from simple, normally nonthreatening infections.

Medical procedures too are associated with an increased risk of infections. Other complications might present themselves as autoimmune disorders, slowed growth, increased risk of cancer, and damage to lungs, the heart, the nervous system, and the digestive tract.

CONGENITAL AND ACQUIRED IMMUNODEFICIENCIES

Congenital (primary) immunodeficiency (CI) is evident at birth and generally results from genetic defects or disorders. These disorders are relatively rare and are classified based on the immune component that is affected, including B cells, T cells, B and T cells, NK cells, phagocytes, and complement proteins.

Acquired (secondary) immunodeficiency (AI) develops later in life and usually is the result of an infectious process, a complication of another condition or disease, or the use of certain drugs during treatment for another condition. AIs are more common than CIs. Malnutrition, some types of cancer, and infections are the most common causes for AIs. Typical infections that can result in AI are cytomegalovirus, lupus, chronic hepatitis, measles, chickenpox, tuberculosis, German measles (rubella), infectious mononucleosis (Epstein-Barr virus), and certain bacterial and fungal infections.

Certain types of drugs, such as anticonvulsants, immunosuppressants, corticosteroids, some monoclonal antibodies, and chemotherapy drugs, can cause an AI. For example, for tissue or organ transplantation, immunosuppressants are used to prevent organ rejection by intentionally suppressing the immune system. Similarly, immunosuppressants are used to reduce inflammation, as in the case of rheumatoid arthritis. In addition, radiation therapy and some chemotherapy drugs, which are given to treat cancer, destroy the cells of the immune system. Immunosuppressants repress the body's ability to attack infections and, sometimes, to destroy cancer cells. During and sometimes beyond drug treatment, the chance of infection increases.

AI is common among severely sick, hospitalized, and older persons. Almost every lengthy acute disorder or infection can potentially lead to an immunodeficiency. In diabetes, white blood cells malfunction because of high sugar levels in the blood, leading in some cases to AI. The best-known severe AI is AIDS, which is caused by human immunodeficiency virus (HIV) infection.

PREVENTION AND TREATMENT

Treatments exist for preventing and treating infections, for boosting the immune system, and for treating underlying causes. Some immunodeficiencies can be prevented, to a certain extent. These include AIDS, cancer, and diabetes. The risk for HIV infection (and AIDS) can be lessened by avoiding the sharing of drug-injection needles and by practicing safer sex. Decreased use of immunosuppressants by persons with cancer might restore the normal function of the immune system after a successful treatment. In the case of diabetes, balanced blood sugar levels can improve the function of white blood cells and can, consequently, help to prevent infections.

The type of immunodeficiency determines preventive and treatment strategies. Common prevention strategies include eating only cooked food, drinking bottled water, taking one's regular medications, proper vaccination, avoiding exposure to other infectious people, and observing good personal hygiene. Infections can be managed with antibiotics or with the treatment of symptoms.

Immunoglobulin, gamma interferon, and growth factors therapy can help boost the immune system. To properly balance the complex immune regulation systems in the body, immune-related treatments should be applied with careful knowledge of the deficiency. In severe combined immunodeficiency (commonly known as bubble-boy syndrome), stem cell transplantation can offer a permanent cure of this life-threatening condition.

IMPACT

The impact of immunodeficiencies lies in the incidence and prognosis of many infectious diseases, which strongly affect the young, the ill, and the elderly with often devastating outcomes. More research is needed to quantify the impact of infectious disease on immunodeficiencies. Better understanding of the clinical indicators of immune competence may lead to improvements in the prevention, treatment, management, and outcome of infectious diseases and their affect on immunocompromised persons.

Ana Maria Rodriguez-Rojas, M.S.

FURTHER READING

Al-Muhsen, S. Z. "Gastrointestinal and Hepatic Manifestations of Primary Immune Deficiency Diseases." *Saudi Journal of Gastroenterology* 16 (2010): 66-74.

Blaese, R. Michael, and Jerry A. Winkelstein. *Patient and Family Handbook for Primary Immunodeficiency*

Diseases. 4th ed. Towson, Md.: Immune Deficiency Foundation, 2007.

De Bakker, P. I., and A. Telenti. "Infectious Diseases Not Immune to Genome-Wide Association." *Nature Genetics* 42 (2010): 731-732.

Morimoto, Y., and J. M. Routes. "Immunodeficiency Overview." *Primary Care: Clinics in Office Practice* 35 (2008): 159-173.

Sompayrac, Lauren M. *How the Immune System Works*. 3d ed. Hoboken, N.J.: Wiley-Blackwell, 2008.

Strugnell, R. A., and O. L. Wijburg. "The Role of Secretory Antibodies in Infection Immunity." *Nature Reviews Microbiology* 8 (2010): 656-667.

Tolan, Robert W., Jr. "Infections in the Immunocompromised Host." Available at http://emedicine. medscape.com/article/973120-overview.

WEB SITES OF INTEREST

Genetic and Rare Diseases Information Center
http://rarediseases.info.nih.gov/gard

Immune Deficiency Foundation
http://www.primaryimmune.org

International Patient Organisation for Primary Immunodeficiencies
http://www.ipopi.org

See also: Agammaglobulinemia; AIDS; Antibodies; Autoimmune disorders; HIV; Idiopathic thrombocytopenic purpura; Immune response to bacterial infections; Immune response to parasitic diseases; Immune response to viral infections; Immunity; Immunoassay; Infection; Neutropenia; Opportunistic infections; Reinfection; Seroconversion; T lymphocytes; Viral hepatitis.

Impetigo

CATEGORY: Diseases and conditions
ANATOMY OR SYSTEM AFFECTED: Skin

DEFINITION

Impetigo is a highly contagious bacterial skin infection.

CAUSES

Impetigo is caused by one or both of the following types of bacteria: group A *Streptococcus* and *Staphylococcus*. These bacteria are normally found on the skin and in the nose. When small cuts, scratches, or insect bites occur, these bacteria can get under the skin and cause infection. Impetigo is often spread from person to person.

RISK FACTORS

Factors that increase the chance for impetigo include touching a person with impetigo; touching the clothing, towels, sheets, or other items of a person with impetigo; poor hygiene, particularly unwashed hands and dirty fingernails; crowded settings where there is direct person-to-person contact, such as in schools and in the military; a warm, humid environment; and the summer season.

At higher risk are preschool and school-age children; persons in poor health or who have a weakened immune system; and persons who tend to have skin problems, such as eczema, poison ivy, or skin allergy. Other risk factors are getting cuts, scratches, or insect bites, or experiencing other injury or trauma to the skin; having chickenpox; and having a lice infection, such as scabies, head lice, or pubic lice, which cause scratching.

SYMPTOMS

Symptoms of impetigo, which appear four to ten days after exposure, include red spots, sores, or blisters on the skin of the face, arms, legs or other parts of the body that ooze and become covered with a flat, dry, honey-colored crust; itch; and may increase and spread, especially if scratched.

Other symptoms, in more serious cases, include swollen lymph nodes. Normally, impetigo is a fairly mild condition. However, if left untreated, further problems could develop, including pain, swelling, spread of infection, discharge of pus, and fever. In rare cases, people whose impetigo is caused by group A *Streptococcus* may develop glomerulonephritis, scarlet fever, or life-threatening invasive streptococcal disease.

SCREENING AND DIAGNOSIS

A doctor will examine the patient's skin lesions and ask about symptoms and medical history. Initial diagnosis is based on the appearance of the skin lesions. If the patient has impetigo, a culture of his or her skin

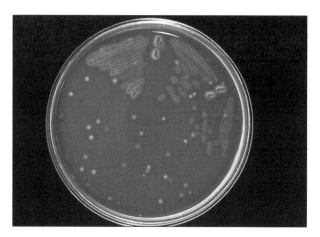

A culture plate containing a species of Streptococcus bacteria, which causes impetigo and other infectious diseases. (CDC)

lesion may be done. The culture will show what specific bacteria are involved.

TREATMENT AND THERAPY

The goals of treatment are to relieve the symptoms and cure the infection. Treatment may include the use of antibiotics. For a mild infection, the patient may get a prescription topical antibiotic, such as mupirocin or retapamulin; an over-the-counter topical antibiotic (significantly less effective), such as neomycin, bacitracin, or polymyxin; or an oral antibiotic, such as cephalosporin or a penicillin. In some cases, staphylococcal infections (such as methicillin-resistant staph infection) may be resistant to these antibiotics. In these cases, other options may be needed.

One should not touch or scratch the lesions. Also, one should wash the skin several times a day with water and an antibiotic soap. The crusts of the lesions are removable by soaking the infected area in warm water for about fifteen minutes. Lesions should be covered loosely with gauze, a bandage, or clothing.

PREVENTION AND OUTCOMES

Prevention of impetigo involves good personal hygiene, including bathing daily with soap and water and washing one's face, hands, and hair regularly; washing hands after caring for someone with impetigo; not sharing towels, clothes, or sheets with a person who has impetigo; keeping fingernails short and clean; changing and washing clothing frequently; not allowing one's children to play or have close contact with someone who may have impetigo; promptly washing wounds, such as cuts, scratches, or insect bites, with soap and water and applying a small amount of antibiotic ointment and a bandage to the affected area.

To help avoid spreading the infection, one should wash hands thoroughly, especially after touching an infected area of the body; should avoid contact with newborns; should stay home until twenty-four hours after the start of treatment; and should not handle food at home until a minimum of twenty-four hours after the start of treatment.

Amy Scholten, M.P.H.;
reviewed by Ross Zeltser, M.D., FAAD

FURTHER READING

Bhumbra, Nasreen A., and Sophia G. McCullough. "Skin and Subcutaneous Infections." In *Update on Infectious Diseases*, edited by Richard I. Haddy and Karen W. Krigger. Philadelphia: W. B. Saunders, 2003.

Crossley, Kent B., Kimberly K. Jefferson, and Gordon L. Archer, eds. *Staphylococci in Human Disease*. Hoboken, N.J.: John Wiley & Sons, 2009.

Koning, S., et al. "Efficacy and Safety of Retapamulin Ointment as Treatment of Impetigo: Randomized Double-Blind Multicentre Placebo-Controlled Trial." *British Journal of Dermatology* 158, no. 5 (2008): 1077-1082.

Swartz, Morton N., and Mark S. Pasternack. "Cellulitis and Subcutaneous Tissue Infection." In *Mandell, Douglas, and Bennett's Principles and Practice of Infectious Diseases*, edited by Gerald L. Mandell, John E. Bennett, and Raphael Dolin. 7th ed. New York: Churchill Livingstone/Elsevier, 2010.

Taylor, Julie Scott. "Interventions for Impetigo." *American Family Physician* 70, no. 9 (November 1, 2004).

WEB SITES OF INTEREST

American Academy of Dermatology
http://www.aad.org

American Osteopathic Association
http://www.osteopathic.org

Dermatologists.ca
http://www.dermatologists.ca

KidsHealth
http://www.kidshealth.org

See also: Acanthamoeba infection; Bacterial infections; Cellulitis; Chickenpox; Children and infectious disease; Contagious diseases; Erythema nodosum; Group A streptococcal infection; Insect-borne illness and disease; Methicillin-resistant staph infection; Pityriasis rosea; Roseola; Rubella; Scarlet fever; Skin infections; Staphylococcal infections; *Staphylococcus*; Streptococcal infections; *Streptococcus*.

Incubation period

CATEGORY: Immune response

DEFINITION

The incubation period is the time between exposure to a virus or bacterium and the development of symptoms.

LENGTH OF INCUBATION PERIODS

Symptom onset is determined by factors such as pathogen growth and invasion, excretion of toxins, and initiation of host-defense mechanisms. The length of incubation time varies greatly and depends on pathogen replication rate, mechanism of disease development, infection route, and other underlying factors. The incubation period of infectious diseases may be as short as a few hours (common in food poisoning) or may last many months (such as with rabies). Incubation periods can also be several years, such as those for leprosy, tuberculosis, and acquired immunodeficiency syndrome, and as long as thirty years, as with variant Creutzfeldt-Jakob disease. Incubation periods for other common diseases are generally shorter and include one to two days for influenza, two to five days for the common cold, two to fourteen days for Rocky Mountain spotted fever, twelve days for smallpox, eight to twelve days for measles, and fourteen to twenty-one days for German measles (rubella).

In infections in which the pathogen travels a short distance before it reaches the target organ, the incubation period is brief (commonly one to three days). Incubation periods of more generalized infections are usually longer because the pathogen needs to move through the body before reaching target organs. Mechanisms involved with long incubation periods, those from months to years, of persistent infections are not well understood. Disease may also result from delayed immune reactions to viral antigen, such as with adenoviruses; from unknown mechanisms during which no immune response can be detected, as in the scrapie-kuru group; or mutations in host genetic material that leads to cell transformation and ultimately, cancer.

CARRIERS

Depending on the disease, a person may or may not be contagious during the incubation period. A person may be a carrier of a disease, such as *Streptococcus* infection, without exhibiting symptoms.

EPIDEMIOLOGY

In the mid-sixteenth century, an Italian physician, Girolamo Fracastoro, provided the first documentation of the incubation period for rabies. The earliest study of the incubation period of pandemic influenza was conducted in 1919. The study, which recorded daily incidence on ships departing from Australian ports, provided estimates of the incubation period of Spanish flu.

IMPACT

The incubation period for infectious disease is directly relevant to prevention and control. Incubation periods provide valuable insight into clinical and public health practices and are important for epidemiologic and ecological studies. In clinical practice, the incubation period can be used to determine causes and sources of infection in individual cases and in developing treatment strategies to extend the incubation period, such as during antiretroviral therapy for human immunodeficiency virus infection, and to project disease prognosis. During an outbreak of emerging diseases, the incubation period can assist in estimating quarantine periods for potentially exposed persons.

C. J. Walsh, Ph.D.

FURTHER READING

Aschengrau, Ann, and George R. Seage. *Essentials of Epidemiology in Public Health.* 2d ed. Sudbury, Mass.: Jones and Bartlett, 2007.

Giesecke, Johan. *Modern Infectious Disease Epidemiology.* 2d ed. London: Hodder Arnold, 2001.

Hawker, Jeremy, et al. *Communicable Disease Control Handbook.* Malden, Mass.: Blackwell, 2005.

Murphy, Kenneth, Paul Travers, and Mark Walport.

Janeway's Immunobiology. 7th ed. New York: Garland Science, 2008.

WEB SITES OF INTEREST

Centers for Disease Control and Prevention
http://www.cdc.gov

U.S. Department of Health and Human Services
http://www.hhs.gov

See also: Antibiotics: Types; Antibodies; Bacterial infections; Contagious diseases; Drug resistance; Epidemiology; Immunity; Infection; Parasitic diseases; Pathogenicity; Pathogens; Public health; Seroconversion; Viral infections.

Infection

CATEGORY: Epidemiology
ALSO KNOWN AS: Contagion, disease

DEFINITION

An infection is a disease state caused by an invasion of the body by pathogenic (disease-causing) microorganisms and by their growth.

INFECTIVE INVADERS

An infection is caused by harmful microorganisms that enter the body through the nose, mouth, ears, eyes, skin pores, and other natural or abnormal openings. Cuts in the skin, for example, are pathways for microorganisms. Once in the body, microorganisms must multiply to cause infection.

The human body mounts a formidable defense against harmful microorganisms. Skin, earwax, and mucous membranes act as barriers against invaders. Tears, mucus, and urine flush away microorganisms. The immune system marshals white blood cells and antibodies to seek and destroy foreign bodies. Nevertheless, microorganisms can still find their way into the body to cause disease, disability, and even death.

Microorganisms begin by attaching themselves to certain cells in the body. The invaders either remain near the invasion site or spread. Some microorganisms produce toxins and other harmful substances, causing such diseases as cholera, botulism, and an-

thrax. Others simply overwhelm the body's defenses with sheer numbers. The most common invaders of the human body are the well-known causes of contagious diseases: bacteria, viruses, fungi, and parasites.

BACTERIAL INFECTIONS

Bacteria are single-celled microorganisms that usually live in colonies of enormous numbers. They thrive in every environment on Earth, including the human body. For bacteria to cause an infection, they must first enter the body. Bacteria access the human body through the following means: inhaled droplets from the coughs or sneezes of an infected person; contact with contaminated body fluids of another person or animal; wounds in the skin; contaminated water or food; contaminated objects, surfaces, and soil; and bites or scratches from insects or other fauna that carry the bacteria.

Once in the body, bacteria seek a friendly environment in which to multiply. If left untreated, bacterial infections tend to worsen. There are a number of diseases caused by bacteria, including strep throat, Lyme disease, *Salmonella* infection, and pneumonia.

VIRAL INFECTIONS

Viruses are microscopically small infectious organisms that enter the body in the same manner as bacteria. Viruses cause such diseases as the common cold, influenza, human immunodeficiency virus infection, chickenpox, and shingles.

A virus infects by invading a living cell, called the host cell. Once inside the host cell, the virus takes control by releasing deoxyribonucleic acid (DNA) or ribonucleic acid (RNA), its genetic material, which forces the host cell to replicate, or reproduce, the virus. The virus usually kills the host cell by preventing it from functioning normally. The newly replicated viruses are released from the dying host cell and then infect other living cells.

Some viruses change the host cell's main functions but do not kill the host cell. One result of this action is that the host cell loses control over normal cell division. Large numbers of abnormal cells amass and spread or form a tumor, which can develop into cancer. Other viruses leave their genetic material in the host cell, where it lies dormant and harmless until the cell is disturbed. The virus might then begin to replicate and cause infection.

Most viruses specialize. That is, they infect only one

particular type of cell. Cold viruses (of which there are hundreds), for example, attack only cells in the human upper respiratory tract. Some viruses infect only humans, and of these, many infect only infants and children.

FUNGAL INFECTIONS

Fungi are single-celled or multicelled organisms that include yeasts and molds. Most grow in damp, warm environments, such as soil, with an abundant food supply. Although many types and species of fungi exist in nature, relatively few infect humans.

Humans pick up fungi from plants, soil, clothing, other people's bodies, animal fur, and many other objects and surfaces. Humans also ingest and inhale fungi. Once on or in the body, fungi seek warm, moist areas such as between the toes, at the corners of the mouth, or in tissue inside the body.

Fungal infections are classified in the following three ways: superficial, systemic, and intermediate. Superficial (cutaneous) infections appear on the surface of the skin, hair, or fingernails and include ringworm and athlete's foot. They are rarely fatal but may be chronic. Systemic infections develop deep within the tissue, often circulating through the blood and often involving vital organs or the nervous system. Some, such as fungal meningitis, can be fatal, particularly in people with weakened immune systems. Intermediate infections occur below the skin (subcutaneous) but do not spread. The most common of this type is vaginal yeast infection.

PARASITIC INFECTIONS

Broadly defined, a parasite is an organism that lives on or inside another organism, called the host. Some parasites, such as amebas, are simple one-celled creatures; others, such as hookworms, have many cells and even internal organs. Infections in humans caused by parasites include malaria, trichinosis, and tapeworm.

Parasites that infect humans are found in the soil, animal waste materials, contaminated food and water, and the bodies of insects. Some parasites produce eggs or larvae that have to develop in their natural environment before they are able to infect humans; others reproduce inside the human body.

Parasites typically enter the body through the skin or mouth. Those that enter through the skin are injected by the bite of an infected insect or bore directly into the skin. Swallowed parasites can remain in the

stomach or burrow through it to invade other internal organs. To survive, parasites gather their nourishment and shelter from their host, usually harming, and sometimes killing, the host. Parasitic infections that harm humans are most common in areas with poor sanitation conditions.

IMPACT

Although no longer the main cause of death in the United States (having been replaced by diseases such as diabetes and stroke), infection continues to take a huge toll on society. Public health experts estimate that the cost of treatment and lost productivity associated with infections is more than $120 billion per year. Other costs to society are inestimable.

Wendell Anderson, B.A.

FURTHER READING

Cohen, Jonathan, William G. Powderly, and Steven E. Opal. *Infectious Diseases*. 3d ed. St. Louis, Mo.: Mosby/Elsevier, 2010. Discusses syndromes by body system, special problems, HIV and AIDS, anti-infective therapy, and clinical microbiology. Includes helpful illustrations, bibliographical references, and an index.

Crawford, Dorothy. *Deadly Companions: How Microbes Shaped Our History*. New York: Oxford University Press, 2009. Nontechnical account of how microorganisms and infections have shaped human civilization.

Farmer, Paul. *Infections and Inequalities: The Modern Plagues*. Berkeley: University of California Press, 2001. An analysis of the link between chronic infectious diseases and poverty, filth, and malnutrition.

Finch, Caleb, and Eileen Crimmins. "Inflammatory Exposure and Historical Changes in Human Life-Spans." *Science* 305 (2004): 1736-1739. Research into the effect of the decline of infectious diseases on human life span.

Ryan, Kenneth J., and C. George Ray, eds. *Sherris Medical Microbiology: An Introduction to Infectious Diseases*. 5th ed. New York: McGraw-Hill, 2010. A textbook presentation of the microbiology of infectious disease.

WEB SITES OF INTEREST

Center for Infectious Disease Research and Policy
http://www.cidrap.umn.edu

Centers for Disease Control and Prevention
http://www.cdc.gov

Infectious Diseases Society of America
http://www.idsociety.org

National Center for Preparedness, Detection, and Control
of Infectious Diseases
http://www.cdc.gov/ncpdcid

National Foundation for Infectious Diseases
http://www.nfid.org

World Health Organization
http://www.who.int/topics/infectious_diseases

See also: Antibiotics: Types; Antibodies; Bacteria: Classification and types; Bacterial infections; Bacteriology; Bloodstream infections; Carriers; Diagnosis of fungal infections; Drug resistance; Epidemiology; Fungal infections; Fungi: Classification and types; Hospitals and infectious disease; Hosts; Iatrogenic infections; Microbiology; Opportunistic infections; Parasitic diseases; Pathogenicity; Pathogens; Primary infection; Public health; Secondary infection; Superbacteria; Viral infections; Virology; Wound infections.

Infectious colitis

CATEGORY: Diseases and conditions
ANATOMY OR SYSTEM AFFECTED: Colon, digestive system, gastrointestinal system, intestines
ALSO KNOWN AS: *Clostridium difficile* infection

DEFINITION

Infectious colitis is inflammation of the colon caused by a bacterial or viral infection.

CAUSES

Infectious colitis is caused by viruses and bacteria that are introduced into the body or develop from antibiotic use that allows an overgrowth of normal bacteria in the colon. Food-borne illnesses, commonly called food poisoning, deliver bacteria that may include *Escherichia coli*, *Salmonella*, *Shigella*, and *Campylobacter*. Pseudomembranous colitis, now referred to as *Clostridium difficile* infection, occurs when antibiotics

alter the normal bacteria in the colon, allowing for an overgrowth of *C. difficile*.

RISK FACTORS

Eating spoiled or unclean food and drinking unclean water may lead to food poisoning and could increase the risk for infectious colitis in any age group. The use of antibiotics may cause the normal bacteria of the colon to be affected, leading to an overgrowth of bacteria. International travel may expose persons to unclean conditions and bacteria. Women and older adults are at greater risk of *C. difficile* infection. Drugs that are used for indigestion, such as proton pump inhibitors, or drugs that limit the ability of the colon to move waste, such as some pain medicines, may also increase the risk for infection.

SYMPTOMS

Symptoms depend on the cause of the infectious origin of the colitis. Colitis related to food poisoning usually includes bloody diarrhea and may lead to dehydration. Infection with *C. difficile* includes a fever and the production of a toxin that causes nonbloody diarrhea. In both cases, persons may have abdominal pain, may always feel the need to have a bowel movement, and may have other signs of infection, such as sore joints and a general, overall poor feeling. Blood work usually shows an elevated white-blood-cell count, which often indicates infection in the body.

SCREENING AND DIAGNOSIS

No screening test exists for colitis of infectious origin. Diagnosis is made based on presenting symptoms. Because both bloody and nonbloody diarrhea are symptoms of a variety of diseases, the doctor will ask specific questions designed to narrow possible causes. The doctor will feel the affected person's abdomen, do a rectal examination, order a blood stool test, and order blood work, which will include a complete blood count that measures white blood cells and electrolyte levels. More severe cases may need a colonoscopy or radiology tests, such as a computed tomography (CT) scan.

TREATMENT AND THERAPY

The goal of therapy is to rest the bowel. A clear liquid diet and rest are often all that is needed for most cases of infectious colitis. The body will rid itself of the causative bacteria or virus. If the causative agent is found to be *C. difficile*, however, the causative antibiotic is usually stopped and an antibiotic specific to *C. difficile* is prescribed. Hospitalization and intravenous fluids may be given to combat severe dehydration, and antidiarrheal medicines and pain medicines may be prescribed.

PREVENTION AND OUTCOMES

Preventive measures include ingesting safe food, drinking clean water, and using antibiotics appropriately. One should ensure that food is carefully prepared and stored at appropriate temperatures, ensure that one's drinking water is from safe sources (or has been boiled), and ensure that one's hands are washed frequently. Also, one should report any diarrhea while on antibiotics or other medicines.

C. difficile infection, which is caused by an overgrowth of bacteria from antibiotic overuse or misuse, is more difficult to prevent because persons may need to take antibiotics to treat other infections in the body.

Patricia Stanfill Edens, R.N., Ph.D., FACHE

FURTHER READING

EBSCO Publishing. *DynaMed: "Clostridium difficile" colitis.* Available through http://www.ebscohost.com/dynamed.

Feldman, Mark, Lawrence S. Friedman, and Lawrence J. Brandt, eds. *Sleisenger and Fordtran's Gastrointestinal and Liver Disease: Pathophysiology, Diagnosis, Management.* New ed. 2 vols. Philadelphia: Saunders/Elsevier, 2010.

Johnson, Leonard R., ed. *Gastrointestinal Physiology.* 7th ed. Philadelphia: Mosby/Elsevier, 2007.

Walsh, Christopher. *Antibiotics: Actions, Origins, Resistance.* Washington, D.C.: ASM Press, 2003.

Weese, J. S. "*Clostridium difficile* in Food: Innocent Bystander or Serious Threat?" *European Society of Clinical Microbiology and Infectious Diseases* 16 (2009): 3-10.

WEB SITES OF INTEREST

American College of Gastroenterology
http://www.acg.gi.org

Canadian Association of Gastroenterology
http://www.cag-acg.org

National Digestive Diseases Information Clearinghouse
http://digestive.niddk.nih.gov

See also: Alliance for the Prudent Use of Antibiotics; Amebic dysentery; Antibiotic-associated colitis; Antibiotics: Types; Bacteria: Classification and types; Bacterial infections; *Clostridium; Clostridium difficile* infection; Diverticulitis; Enteritis; Food-borne illness and disease; Hookworms; Inflammation; Intestinal and stomach infections; Norovirus infection; Viral gastroenteritis; Viral infections.

Infectious disease specialists

CATEGORY: Epidemiology

DEFINITION

An infectious disease specialist (IDS) is generally a medical doctor who has trained in internal medicine (or possibly pediatrics) and who specializes in diagnosing, treating, and managing infectious diseases. Infectious diseases are those diseases that are passed from person to person and not those caused by genetic or environmental influences. Infectious diseases can be caused by bacteria, fungi, parasites, prions, or viruses.

FUNCTIONS

An IDS usually has eight to ten years of specialized training beyond high school. This training focuses first on internal medicine and then on bacteriology, epidemiology, immunology, parasitology, and virology. After training, an IDS can then seek certification in internal medicine and infectious diseases by passing the examinations given by the American Board of Internal Medicine. The IDS performs diagnosis and medical treatment; he or she does not perform surgery.

An IDS studies how infectious diseases enter the body; how they spread through the body; how the body's defenses fight different types of infection (immunology); what effect these infections have on the body and its systems; how antibiotics and other agents fight, control, or minimize the effects of the infection; and how infections spread throughout the general population or a specific population (epidemiology). An IDS has specific insight into the use or overuse of antibiotics and knows the potential adverse effects of such drugs and may help track and control difficult diseases such as methicillin-resistant *Staphylococcus aureus* and other antibiotic-resistant infections. An IDS has specialized knowledge that may also include helping persons with compromised immune systems, such as those with multiple sclerosis or human immunodeficiency virus (HIV) infection or those participating in chemotherapy.

The patients of an IDS may have diseases as widespread as influenza, malaria, measles, meningitis, mumps, and tuberculosis. Certain infections, such as measles or yellow fever, affect the entire body. However, other infections may affect only one organ or one system in the body. For example, the common cold usually affects only the upper respiratory tract. Other infectious diseases may affect only the digestive system, the urinary tract, or the ears. An IDS works to counteract the effects of these infections.

An IDS often works in a hospital setting, which allows for timely consultation with other doctors. An IDS is often called in to cases in which an infection is suspected (usually from the presence of a fever), but in which the cause or source of that infection is unclear (even after testing and treatment). In this sense, an IDS becomes a sort of disease detective, who may also be consulted when the disease is unusual, as when a doctor without detailed knowledge of infectious diseases faces, for example, a tropical disease in a nontropical area.

A pediatric IDS may work in a children's hospital in conjunction with other types of pediatricians. Generally, a pediatric IDS treats children from birth through the teenage years and has further training in the unique signs, symptoms, and treatments involving children with infections (which can be quite different from the treatments for adults). An IDS may also assist public health organizations such as the Centers for Disease Control and Prevention in tracking and reporting infectious diseases and their spread.

IMPACT

Most often, infectious diseases are diagnosed and treated by primary care doctors. However, in cases in which the diagnosis is particularly difficult or in which commonly prescribed treatments have failed, an IDS can be contacted for consultation.

An IDS also helps travelers, for example, prepare for their visits to countries known for certain infectious diseases, especially those that are not common to the United States. Travelers will be informed about safe sanitation practices peculiar to a certain country and about certain recommended immunizations before travel. Finally, an IDS interacts with public health agencies to track and control outbreaks of infections at both the local and global levels.

Marianne M. Madsen, M.S.

FURTHER READING

Editors of *Scientific American. Infectious Disease: A "Scientific American" Reader.* Chicago: University of Chicago Press, 2008.

Kasper, Dennis, Fauci, Anthony. *Harrison's Infectious Diseases.* New York: McGraw-Hill Professional, 2010.

Nagami, Pamela. *The Woman with a Worm in Her Head and Other True Stories of Infectious Disease.* New York: St. Martin's Griffin, 2002.

Pendergrast, Mark. *Inside the Outbreaks: The Elite Medical Detectives of the Epidemic Intelligence Service.* Boston: Houghton Mifflin Harcourt, 2010.

WEB SITES OF INTEREST

Association for Professionals in Infection Control and Epidemiology
http://www.knowledgeisinfectious.org

Center for Infectious Disease Research and Policy
http://www.cidrap.umn.edu

Infectious Diseases Society of America
http://www.idsociety.org

National Foundation for Infectious Diseases
http://www.nfid.org

World Health Organization
http://www.who.int/topics/infectious_diseases

See also: Biosurveillance; Centers for Disease Control and Prevention (CDC); Disease eradication campaigns; Emerging and reemerging infectious diseases; Emerging Infections Network; Epidemic Intelligence Service; Epidemics and pandemics: Causes and management; Epidemiology; National Institute of Allergy and Infectious Diseases; National Institutes of Health; Outbreaks; Public health; Social effects of infectious disease; U.S. Army Medical Research Institute of Infectious Diseases; World Health Organization (WHO).

Infectious Diseases Society of America

CATEGORY: Epidemiology

DEFINITION

The Infectious Diseases Society of America (IDSA) is a scientific association focusing on identifying, treating, and preventing infectious diseases.

FOUNDING AND MISSION

In the early 1960's, medical researchers, recognizing the need to establish an organization specifically for infectious diseases professionals, formed the IDSA. It was founded in October, 1963. Pneumonia expert Maxwell Finland served as the group's first president and was joined by 125 charter members. By 2010, approximately nine thousand persons, primarily scientists, doctors, and medical personnel, were members of the IDSA. Throughout IDSA's history, leading infectious diseases researchers, including several Nobel Prize winners, served as IDSA officers. Many served on committees that helped shape national and industry policies on infectious diseases and the use of antibiotics.

Members participate in annual meetings and in workshops that focus on specific infectious disease concerns, including bioterrorism. They contribute articles and commentary discussing infectious diseases research in the society's periodicals, including *Clinical Infectious Diseases*. The IDSA issues and updates clinical practice guidelines for numerous infectious diseases, such as community acquired pneumonia. The IDSA established its Emerging Infections Network for medical professionals to notify colleagues regarding unique infections or pathogens they have treated. Stressing public health, the IDSA helped establish the National Network for Immunization Information to educate people concerning vaccinations that are essential in preventing the contracting and spread of infectious diseases.

The IDSA recognizes members' achievements, presenting awards for diverse roles in the infectious diseases field. Through the IDSA Education and Research Foundation, the society encourages young physicians to specialize in infectious diseases by offering postdoctoral fellowships to train with experts. IDSA members often serve as mentors.

Aware that many infectious disease strains become resistant to antibiotics, the IDSA encourages research into the development of new antibiotic formulas to counter these resistant strains. In 2004, the IDSA released the report "Bad Bugs, No Drugs: As Antibiotic Discovery Stagnates, a Public Health Crisis Brews," which identifies microbes posing the most significant health risks. These microbes are methicillin-resistant *Staphylococcus aureus*, vancomycin-resistant enterococci, floroquinclone-resistant *Pseudomonas aeruginosa*, *Acinetobacter baumannii*, *Aspergillus* species, and *Escherichia coli* and *Klebsiella* species. The IDSA supported federal legislation, including the Strategies to Address Antimicrobial Resistance Act, which would improve federal support for research and development of more powerful antibiotics.

In early 2010, the IDSA announced its 10 x '20 Initiative, urging pharmaceutical industries to create ten antibiotics to combat emerging resistant pathogens within one decade (2020). A July, 2010, IDSA statement warned that antibiotics associated with livestock and plants raised for food were linked to humans becoming resistant to antibiotics. Critical of the U.S. Food and Drug Administration's procedures to approve new antibiotics, the IDSA created its Antimicrobial Availability Task Force.

DISEASES

The IDSA has addressed influenza pandemic threats and the need for adequate vaccine supplies to protect populations. Leaders stressed the responsibility of governments to control influenza. In the fall of 2005, Walter E. Stamm, IDSA president, wrote Michael Leavitt, secretary of the U.S. Department of Health and Human Services, stating that the federal government should procure more antiviral drugs to combat the H5N1 avian influenza. In summer, 2009, IDSA leaders suggested procedures for medical professionals to fight H1N1 flu.

In 2000, IDSA formed the HIV Medicine Association (HIVMA) within its administrative structure to provide support to medical professionals focusing on treating adults and children infected with the human immunodeficiency virus (HIV) or living with acquired immunodeficiency syndrome (AIDS). The approximately 3,600 HIVMA members are also members of IDSA. Through HIVMA, IDSA sponsors the AIDS Training Program, in which members teach (at Uganda's Makerere University) physicians from developing countries about HIV and AIDS prevention and treatment. The program is part of the Academic Alliance for AIDS Care and Prevention in Africa.

The guidelines of the Lyme Disease Review Panel of the IDSA provoked controversy because it states that Lyme disease is not a chronic condition and does not require intensive antibiotic treatment. The panel warned that prolonged antibiotics exposure might cause medical complications or result in resistance to antibiotic drugs. Connecticut attorney general Richard Blumenthal questioned the panel's scientific credibility. Panel chair Gary Wormser defended the IDSA's position. In 2010, an autonomous review panel declared that the IDSA panel's conclusions were sound.

Impact

The IDSA has been at the forefront of efforts to strengthen public health standards, to implement improved prevention programs, to improve the treatment of people suffering from infectious diseases, and to encourage innovative research that analyzes pathogens and develops the means to destroy them. The society's resources have aided infectious disease professionals to perform their work effectively and to enhance that specialty. By 2010, the IDSA helped train more than 360 African doctors participating in the AIDS Training Program to help mitigate the impact of HIV/AIDS on that continent.

Frequently interacting with all levels of government, the IDSA asserts the importance of access to scientifically based health care and effective antibiotics. For example, the IDSA intervened when state drug programs' limitations deprived patients of sufficient medications for infectious diseases. Furthermore, IDSA educational material increases the public's awareness of infectious diseases and demonstrates the need for governments and medical professionals to prepare for potential health threats by new pathogens.

Elizabeth D. Schafer, Ph.D.

Further Reading

Boucher, Helen, et al. "Bad Bugs, No Drugs, No ES-KAPE! An Update from the Infectious Diseases Society of America." *Clinical Infectious Diseases* 48, no. 1 (January 1, 2009): 1-12. Emphasizes the need for diverse groups' collaboration with IDSA to achieve potent antibiotics to control the most dangerous infectious diseases pathogens.

Kass, Edward H., and Katherine Murphey Hayes. *A*

History of the Infectious Diseases Society of America. Chicago: University of Chicago Press, 1988. A comprehensive history of the IDSA and its activities through 1987. Photographs, figures, appendices, endnotes.

Spellberg, Brad, et al. "The Epidemic of Antibiotic-Resistant Infections: A Call to Action for the Medical Community from the Infectious Diseases Society of America." *Clinical Infectious Diseases* 46, no. 2 (January 15, 2008): 155-164. Looks at what impedes the prevention and control of infectious diseases. Suggests ways to resolve this public health crisis.

Talbot, George H., et al. "Bad Bugs Need Drugs: An Update on the Development Pipeline from the Antimicrobial Availability Task Force of the Infectious Diseases Society of America." *Clinical Infectious Diseases* 42, no. 5 (March 1, 2006): 657-668. Provides details about antimicrobial resistant diseases posing the greatest public health risks.

Web Sites of Interest

Association for Professionals in Infection Control and Epidemiology
http://www.knowledgeisinfectious.org

Infectious Diseases Society of America
http://www.idsociety.org

HIV Medicine Association
http://www.hivma.org

National Foundation for Infectious Diseases
http://www.nfid.org

National Network for Immunization Information
http://www.immunizationinfo.org

See also: Centers for Disease Control and Prevention (CDC); Disease eradication campaigns; Emerging and reemerging infectious diseases; Emerging Infections Network; Epidemiology; Infectious disease specialists; National Institute of Allergy and Infectious Diseases; National Institutes of Health; Outbreaks; Public health; Social effects of infectious disease; U.S. Army Medical Research Institute of Infectious Diseases; World Health Organization (WHO).

Infectiousness. *See* Virulence.

Inflammation

CATEGORY: Diseases and conditions
ANATOMY OR SYSTEM AFFECTED: All

DEFINITION

Inflammation generally refers to the short-term swelling and redness associated with the body's healing process in response to some type of injury caused by an external source. Typical examples of external inflammation include a sprained ankle, rash, sore throat, or hives. However, internal inflammation that is not visible can be chronic and can eventually lead to a range of diseases and other health problems, including autoimmune disease, human immunodeficiency virus (HIV) infection, pneumonia, hepatitis A and B, pancreatitis, cancer, asthma, gastrointestinal disorders, mumps, allergies, and arthritis. Other conditions, including cardiovascular problems, diabetes, Parkinson's disease, and Alzheimer's disease are also believed to be caused by inflammation.

During the inflammation process, plasma proteins and white blood cells called phagocytes are brought to the injured area through the blood to attack the foreign substance and begin the process of tissue repair. The process of inflammation involves seven general steps, beginning with the entry of the foreign stimulant or other damage, followed by a widening of the blood vessels to allow more blood to flow, which then allows for an increase in vascular permeability to facilitate the fluid flow. Increased fluid flow occurs, followed by the entrance of white blood cells into the affected tissue. These white blood cells then destroy any microbes that may have invaded the body; finally, repair of the tissue takes place.

CAUSES

Inflammation is caused by a foreign substance's entrance into the body. This action triggers the immune system, which is the defensive system of the body. Because inflammation refers to a general biological response by an organism to some type of injury or harm, there can be many causes. These causes range from physical injury to the tissues, including cuts, burns, frostbite, or splinters, to chemical injury from an ingested toxin or irritant, resulting in an autoimmune response. Inflammation can also be caused by some type of foreign invader, such as a virus, a fungus, a bacterium, or other para-

site, and can even be caused by prolonged exposure to radiation.

RISK FACTORS

Long-term risk factors for developing inflammation include a diet high in refined sugars, starches, simple carbohydrates, trans fats, saturated fats, omega-6 fats found in corn oil and margarine, and gluten, which is a protein found in wheat, barley, and rye. Additional lifestyle risks include stress, a lack of exercise, exposure to cigarette smoke or environmental pollutants, and excessive ultraviolet rays from the sun.

Additional risk factors include accidents, trauma, surgery, insect bites or stings, and infection from foreign invaders, such as bacteria, parasites, and viruses. Steroid medications, estrogen, and acetaminophen are sometimes linked to incidents of inflammation.

SYMPTOMS

One of the key external symptoms of inflammation is redness of the skin, which is often accompanied by pain, loss of function, swelling and stiffness in the joints, and heat in the area of the redness. Occasionally, inflammation can affect internal organs, so that the appearance of redness and swelling may not be visible. In these cases of hidden inflammation, additional internal symptoms include headaches, fever, backaches, coughs, chills, and fatigue.

SCREENING AND DIAGNOSIS

The most common diagnostic methods include a physical exam to locate any painful joints, a medical history, X rays, and a blood test called the C-reactive protein level test. If this blood test indicates a level of 0.7 or above, then inflammation in the blood system is diagnosed. If untreated, this type of inflammation can lead to cardiovascular problems. Ultrasound and computed tomography (CT) scans can detect small cysts and calcium deposits created by prolonged inflammation.

TREATMENT AND THERAPY

Nonsteroidal anti-inflammatory drugs, such as aspirin, ibuprofen, and naproxen, are often effective against inflammation. Additional treatments include corticosteroids, such as prednisone, and medications such as leflunomide or sulfasalazine, which are often used to treat conditions such as cancer and to treat

In the News: Low-Grade Inflammation as a Trigger for Heart Attacks and Strokes

Researchers have suspected for some time that the body's inflammatory response may play a critical role in heart attacks and strokes. It is well known that risk factors for heart attack and stroke include obesity, high cholesterol levels, high blood pressure, and smoking. Blood tests in a 1988 study in Finland, however, showed the presence of the bacterium *Chlamydia pneumoniae* inside the cells of people with coronary artery disease. It seemed apparent, however, that *C. pneumoniae* alone was not a risk factor or cause of heart disease.

Researchers in the Helsinki Heart Study also looked for the presence of human heat-shock protein 60 (hHsp60), indicating an immune response that could possibly lead to atherosclerosis, and of C-reactive protein (CRP), which sends white blood cells to the site of injury or infection but can cause harm if prolonged or excessive. An eight-year follow-up of this study showed that the risk for heart disease increased when levels of *C. pneumoniae* or hHsp60 antibodies were high. However, the risk was greatest when all three factors were elevated, indicating a possible synergistic effect. The study concluded that chronic infection, autoimmunity, and inflammation in combination contributed to coronary events in the study population.

Scientific research continues to establish definitive links between heart disease and chronic infections, inflammation, and autoimmune conditions. These links could lead to attacking the basic processes of atherosclerosis, to treatment with anti-inflammatory drugs, and to the prevention of heart attacks and stroke.

Martha Loustaunau, Ph.D.

tuna, herring, sardines, and mackerel, all of which contain the omega-3 fatty acids. These omega-3 fatty acids reduce the action of prostaglandins, which are hormones that increase inflammation. High-fiber foods, unprocessed foods, oils such as those found in avocados and nuts, and olive oil, green tea, and vitamins D and E, also have anti-inflammatory properties.

One should avoid simple carbohydrates because these sugars cause a rapid rise in blood-sugar levels, which is the cause of glycosylation, also called the Browning reaction. During this reaction, sugar attaches to the collagen in any cell, leading to an increase in inflammation. Regular exercise is also recommended to prevent inflammation. Sunscreen is recommended to prevent the sun's ultraviolet rays from causing damage to the cell walls that can lead to inflammation. Small, daily dosages of aspirin and ibuprofen can reduce the inflammatory stimulus, especially the one that can lead to atherosclerosis and other cardiovascular disorders. Benzyl isothiocyanide can prevent the accumulation of the superoxide anion.

Jeanne L. Kuhler, Ph.D.

FURTHER READING

Black, Jessica. *The Anti-inflammation Diet and Recipe Book: Protect Yourself and Your Family from Heart Disease, Arthritis, Diabetes, Allergies, and More.* New York: Hunter House, 2006. This book is written by a naturopathic doctor who emphasizes a particular diet to prevent inflammation and other conditions and disorders.

Challem, Jack. *The Inflammation Syndrome: Your Nutrition Plan for Great Health, Weight Loss, and Pain-Free Living.* New York: Wiley, 2010. Explores the cumulative effect of low-grade inflammation that grows into chronic, debilitating diseases, including heart disease, diabetes, syndrome X, obesity, arthritis, allergies, and asthma. Covers anti-inflammatory drugs and the impact of nutrition.

Górski, Andrzej, Hubert Krotkiewski, and Michał Zimecki, eds. *Inflammation.* Boston: Kluwer Academic, 2001. A series of papers review current understandings of inflammatory processes and re-

persons who have received organ transplants. Antihistamine drugs can block the production of histamine, which increases the inflammation response. Disease-modifying antirheumatic drugs, such as methotrexate, minocycline, and cyclosporine, are effective treatments. External hot and cold therapy can also be effective. Hot therapy can decrease muscle cramps and cold therapy can narrow blood vessels, resulting in decreased inflammation.

PREVENTION AND OUTCOMES

To help limit one's chance of getting inflammation, one should eat antioxidants, which prevent free-radicals, such as superoxide, from forming and damaging cell walls. Foods and herbs that are rich in antioxidants are broccoli, berries, tomatoes, cherries, ginger, garlic, rosemary, onion, ground flax seeds, and fish oil from cold water fish such as salmon, anchovy, sponses, from allergies to life-threatening sepsis, and evaluate therapeutic strategies aimed at combating inflammatory diseases.

Murphy, Kenneth, Paul Travers, and Mark Walport. *Janeway's Immunobiology.* 7th ed. New York: Garland Science, 2008. An excellent text that provides a lucid and comprehensive examination of the immune system, covering such topics as immunobiology and innate immunity, the adaptive immune response, and the evolution of the immune system.

Meggs, William Joel, and Carol Svec. *The Inflammation Cure.* New York: McGraw-Hill, 2003. Examines research linkages between inflammation and heart disease and diseases associated with aging, including arthritis, Alzheimer's, osteoporosis, and some cancers. Covers causes, treatments, and lifestyle changes to promote wellness.

Parkham, Peter. *The Immune System.* 2d ed. New York: Garland Science, 2005. A basic immunology text that details how cells and molecules work together in defending the body against invading microorganisms, describes situations in which the immune system cannot control disease, and examines what happens when the immune system overreacts.

Pillai, Sreekumar, Christopher Oresajo, and James Hayward. "Ultraviolet Radiation and Skin Aging: Roles of Reactive Oxygen Species, Inflammation, and Protease Activation, and Strategies for Prevention of Inflammation-Induced Matrix Degradation." *International Journal of Cosmetic Science* 27 (2004): 17-34. A review article that discusses the impact of ultraviolet radiation on inflammation.

Miyoshi, Noriyuki, et al. "Benzyl Isothiocyanate Inhibits Excessive Superoxide Generation in Inflammatory Leukocytes: Implication for Prevention Against Inflammation-Related Carcinogenesis." *Carcinogenesis* 25 (2004): 567-575. This research article details the effects of inflammation on cancer.

WEB SITE OF INTEREST

Centers for Disease Control and Prevention
http://www.cdc.gov

See also: Bacterial infections; Infection; Pathogenicity; Pathogens; Viral infections.

Influenza

CATEGORY: Diseases and conditions
ANATOMY OR SYSTEM AFFECTED: Lungs, muscles, nose, respiratory system, throat
ALSO KNOWN AS: The flu, grip, grippe, seasonal flu

DEFINITION

Influenza (commonly known as the flu) is a disease that affects the respiratory system. It is caused by a variety of viruses in the Orthomyxovirus family. Influenza infections are not unique to people; they also occur in other animals, most notably birds and pigs. Infection with an influenza virus leads to illness that can be mild or life-threatening, depending on the person's age, general health, and immunity to the particular infecting virus. Every year, the influenza viruses that infect people can differ from those that infected people the previous year.

CAUSES

There are two significant types of influenza viruses: A and B (influenza virus type C causes minor infections). Each influenza A or B virus carries on its outer surface two types of protein: hemagglutinin (H) and neuraminidase (N). Influenza A viruses are classified into subtypes based on the type of HA and NA proteins they carry. There are sixteen types of HA and nine types of NA. When scientists talk about H1N1 influenza, for example, they mean an influenza type A virus that carries HA type 1 and NA type 1 on its surface.

Influenza B viruses, and influenza A subtypes, are further classified into strains. There are hundreds of influenza virus strains, but not all can infect people.

The genes that code for the H and N proteins tend to mutate (change) somewhat each year. This mutation is called antigenic drift, and it is the reason a new flu vaccine has to be made each year. Antigenic drift changes the virus enough so that it reduces a person's natural immunity to it.

Every few decades or so, an influenza A virus will undergo antigenic shift. This is a major change in the virus, which basically leads to the appearance of a completely new flu virus, against which people have no immunity. The emergence of H1N1 influenza in 2009 is thought to be the result of such a shift. Viruses that appear because of antigenic shifts may cause pandemics (worldwide epidemics), as did the 2009 H1N1 influenza virus. (The word "pandemic" does not mean

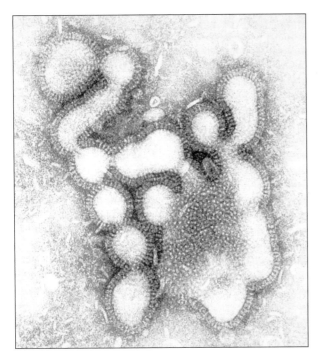

The influenza virus. (Digital Stock)

"severe illness." It means the infecting microbe can easily cause illness that spreads across the globe.)

Viruses are normally specific to a species. This means, for example, that a bird flu (avian influenza) virus normally cannot cause infection in a human. There have been several cases, however, in which bird flu viruses have infected humans. The best-known avian influenza virus is H5N1, which has caused more than five hundred confirmed cases in humans. Of these cases, 297 were fatal, making H5N1 the deadliest bird flu virus in humans.

The virus can be transmitted to humans only by handling sick or uncooked dead birds. Health authorities around the world remain concerned that if the virus develops the ability to jump among people (instead of, only, from birds to people), it will cause a major pandemic with many deaths.

RISK FACTORS

For the seasonal flu, people younger than age five or older than age sixty-five years are most at risk for contracting the flu, as are health care workers. Crowding increases the risk of virus transmission between people.

In addition, several groups of people are at high risk for complications from the flu. According to the Centers for Disease Control and Prevention (CDC), high risk groups include pregnant women, people with certain chronic medical conditions (for example, heart disease or diabetes), people whose immune system is weakened or suppressed, young children, and people older than age fifty years.

H5N1 avian influenza remains a problem in certain parts of the world. People living or traveling in areas where the virus is active are at risk if they handle sick birds or if they eat uncooked birds that are infected.

SYMPTOMS

It can take up to four days (in adults) from the time of infection until symptoms appear. The classic symptoms of the flu are fever and chills, sore throat, cough, runny nose, muscle aches, and headache. The headache can be severe enough to cause sensitivity to light. Muscle aches are most common in the legs, though they can appear anywhere in the body. Extreme fatigue is another common symptom.

Nausea, vomiting, and diarrhea can occur in people with the flu and are especially common in children and people who are infected with the 2009 H1N1 flu strain. Most flu symptoms disappear in five to six days, though full recovery takes longer; the fatigue may last several weeks.

Pneumonia is a common complication of influenza. It can be primary (caused by the flu virus) or secondary (caused by another virus or by bacteria). Because influenza weakens the body and its immune system, infections by other microbes can occur in a person who is fighting the flu. Symptoms of pneumonia include cough that gets worse instead of better, difficulty breathing, and, sometimes, bloody phlegm. A person who is recovering from the flu and redevelops fever and cough most likely has bacterial pneumonia.

People with chronic medical conditions should watch for signs that their condition is worsening because of the flu. This is not uncommon, especially in people with heart disease or respiratory conditions such as asthma or emphysema.

SCREENING AND DIAGNOSIS

Most of the time, the flu is inferred from the symptoms, and no special testing is required. There are some situations in which knowing the exact subtype of flu virus can influence treatment decisions. There are also situations when doctors need to determine if an outbreak of respiratory illness in the population has been caused by influenza. For that purpose, rapid testing is available.

There áre eleven approved rapid tests in the United States. These tests give results in fifteen minutes, but their sensitivity and accuracy vary. Rapid testing is usually done using a swab from nose or throat secretions. (The location of the swab may also affect the test's accuracy in some tests.) Rapid testing can be done only within the first four days of symptom appearance.

The most accurate way of testing for the specific type of flu virus is through a technique called reverse transcription polymerase chain reaction (RT-PCR). Testing with RT-PCR can take up to four hours and is not always available for diagnostic tests.

A viral culture can be done on swabs taken from affected persons. In a viral culture, the virus obtained from the persons is allowed to multiply in the laboratory, where large quantities allow for typing. Viral cultures are not used to determine treatment because they take three to ten days to grow and provide results. However, they can be used to determine the type of flu virus that is circulating in a given population.

A test for the presence of H5 flu virus is available to state and public health authorities. The test, known as influenza A/H5 (Asian lineage) virus real-time RT-PCR primer and probe set, is available when suspected human cases of avian influenza appear in the United States. It takes four hours to get the results. If H5 virus is detected, further testing needs to be done to check if the virus is indeed the H5N1 avian flu virus.

TREATMENT AND THERAPY

For most people who are otherwise healthy, the treatment of influenza consists of treating the symptoms. Treatment includes pain relievers for body aches and headaches and medicine to reduce fever. Many over-the-counter (OTC), multisymptom flu treatments are available. They treat the worst cold symptoms and can bring relief, though they will not cure the flu. OTC products contain a mixture of medications. To avoid overdosing, one should know what medicines the OTCs contain. For example, many OTC products contain acetaminophen, the active ingredient in Tylenol. People who take acetaminophen in addition to multisymptom OTC treatments risk building up a dangerous level of acetaminophen in their body.

Children younger than eighteen years of age should not be given aspirin. Aspirin in children can cause Reye's syndrome, a potentially fatal disorder that often follows a viral infection. Medications against the flu virus are called antiviral medications. Two classes of antivirals are available against the flu virus: Neuraminidase inhibitors are effective against influenza A and B. They interfere with the release of the virus from infected cells. Two drugs are available in this class: oseltamivir (Tamiflu) and zanamivir (Relenza). Amantadines are effective against (some) influenza A viruses only, and viral resistance to this class of antivirals is high. Two drugs are available in this class: amantadine (Symmetrel) and rimantadine (Flumadine).

Taking these medications within the first forty-eight hours after symptoms appear will reduce the length and severity of the symptoms. Treatment with antiviral drugs is especially important in people at high risk for complications, as this type of treatment has been shown to reduce or prevent the occurrence of such complications. Antiviral drugs can also be used to prevent the flu if a person knows he or she has been exposed. However, these medications should never be used in place of vaccination.

Of the neuraminidase inhibitors, zanamivir is given through an inhaler. Because inhaling the medicine can cause strong airway spasms, using zanamivir is not recommended for people with certain airway diseases, such as asthma. Use of the inhaler can be difficult for elderly people or people with certain physical or mental limitations.

Oseltamivir is approved for persons age one year and older. Zanamivir is approved as a treatment for persons age seven years and older and for prevention in persons age five years and older. Amantadine and rimantadine are approved for prevention of flu in people one year of age and older. Amantadine is also approved for flu treatment in persons one year and older. Rimantadine is approved for treating persons age thirteen years and older.

While drug resistance to amantadines has been a growing problem, resistance to oseltamivir is a newer phenomenon. Because oseltamivir is the most used antiviral flu treatment, resistance is a worrisome development. It is therefore more important than ever to limit the use of antiviral flu drugs to high-risk groups.

PREVENTION AND OUTCOMES

Vaccination is the best protection against the flu. In early 2010, the CDC's Advisory Committee on Immunization Practices recommended a universal influenza vaccine every year for everyone age six months and older. (The previous recommendation called for yearly vaccinations for children six months to eighteen years of age and for certain high-risk groups.)

Because the flu viruses that circulate in the population change every year, it is important to get the flu vaccine each year. The vaccines change each year according to early testing results that show what virus subtypes are starting to appear. Vaccination is especially important in people who are at high risk for serious complications from influenza. It is also important that people who care for or live with a person in any of the risk groups be vaccinated to prevent giving the disease to the high-risk person. Health care workers are also strongly encouraged to receive the vaccine every year to protect themselves and their patients.

There are two types of influenza vaccines: a killed virus vaccine given by injection and a live, weakened virus given as a nasal spray. The live virus vaccine can be given to healthy (nonpregnant) persons between the age of two and forty-nine years. The vaccine is marketed as FluMist or LAIV (live attenuated influenza vaccine). Side effects from the injected vaccine are usually mild and include redness and soreness in the area of the injection. Allergic reactions to the vaccine may also occur, though they are uncommon. (People allergic to eggs should not receive the injected flu vaccine.) On rare occasions, some people who received the injected flu vaccine developed a paralysis disorder known as Guillain-Barré syndrome.

Regardless of the type of vaccine received, a person is not protected against the flu until approximately two weeks after vaccination. People at high risk for flu complications (who receive the injected, killed vaccine) may be given antiviral drugs during the two-week period. The live vaccine can cause mild flulike symptoms for several days.

Good hygiene is an important part of protection against the flu. Washing hands frequently or using alcohol-based hand sanitizers will reduce the risk of getting the flu. It is especially important to wash hands before eating and before touching areas on the face, especially the nose and mouth. People should be sure to wash their hands after blowing their nose or coughing into their hands. Covering the nose and mouth while coughing or sneezing reduces the risk of spreading influenza virus particles through the air.

Adi R. Ferrara, B.S., ELS

FURTHER READING

Barry, John M. *The Great Influenza: The Story of the Deadliest Pandemic in History*. New York: Viking Penguin, 2005. Woven into this fascinating story of the world's deadliest flu pandemic is a look at the virus and the science of the flu. This book also provides an interesting look at the politics behind the response to major epidemics.

Beigel, John, and Mike Bray. "Current and Future Antiviral Therapy of Severe Seasonal and Avian Influenza." *Antiviral Research* 78 (2008): 91-102. Article that discusses the use of antiviral medications against influenza viruses.

EBSCO Publishing. *Health Library: Flu*. Available through http://www.ebscohost.com. A concise look at influenza.

"Influenza." In *The Merck Manual Home Health Handbook*, edited by Robert S. Porter et al. 3d ed. Whitehouse Station, N.J.: Merck Research Laboratories, 2009. A concise, easily understood look at all aspects of influenza.

Strauss, James, and Ellen Strauss. *Viruses and Human Disease*. 2d ed. Boston: Academic Press/Elsevier, 2008. Detailed discussion of animal viruses with emphasis on those associated with human disease. Includes accounts of the history of human viruses.

WEB SITES OF INTEREST

Centers for Disease Control and Prevention
http://www.cdc.gov/flu

Clean Hands Coalition
http://www.cleanhandscoalition.org

Flu.gov
http://flu.gov

World Health Organization
http://www.who.int/topics/influenza

See also: Antiviral drugs: Types; Avian influenza; Common cold; Diagnosis of viral infections; Fever; H1N1 influenza; Home remedies; Infection; Influenza vaccine; Over-the-counter (OTC) drugs; Pharyngitis and tonsillopharyngitis; Prevention of viral infections; Respiratory route of transmission; Seasonal influenza; Strep throat; Treatment of viral infections; Viral infections; Viral pharyngitis; Viral upper respiratory infections.

Influenza vaccine

CATEGORY: Prevention
ALSO KNOWN AS: Flu vaccine

DEFINITION

The influenza vaccine helps to protect against infection with the influenza virus. Influenza is an acute viral respiratory illness with abrupt onset and is spread primarily by respiratory droplets from person to person (mainly through inhalation of virus-containing droplets). Influenza is caused by a group of viruses of the Orthomyxoviridae family, which are separated into three strain types (A, B, and C) according to their nuclear material.

Vaccination is the most effective protection against influenza. It is recommended for unhealthy persons and for persons who are likely to transmit influenza to unhealthy persons in a given community. Moreover, the vaccine may be administered to anyone wishing to reduce the risk of influenza.

Influenza vaccines are designed to trigger an immune response to hemagglutinin and neuraminidase, the two proteins found on the surface of the influenza virus. These proteins are always changing (mutating), so every year, seasonal influenza vaccines have to be reformulated with the three strains that are likely to be more effective in fighting new influenza strains.

The World Health Organization's Global Influenza Programme monitors the influenza viruses circulating among humans worldwide and quickly identifies new strains so that new, appropriate vaccines can be made for a particular year.

TYPES OF INFLUENZA VACCINES

The trivalent inactivated influenza vaccine (TIV) has been available since the mid-twentieth century. TIV is administered by intramuscular or intradermal routes and contains three inactivated viruses: type A

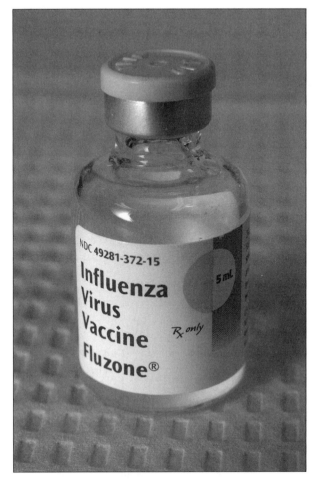

A vial containing Fluzone, an influenza virus vaccine. (CDC)

(H1N1), type A (H3N2), and type B. The influenza vaccine viruses are grown in chicken egg, thus the final product contains residual egg protein. The vaccines are also available in both pediatric- and adult-dose formulations and can be preservative-free in a single vial or in a multidose vial with thimerosal as a preservative.

The live attenuated influenza vaccine (LAIV), which contains the same three influenza viruses as TIV, is administered by intranasal route. LAIV viruses are also grown in chicken egg. LAIV is preservative-free and is provided in a single-dose sprayer unit with one-half the dosage sprayed into each nostril.

Improved technology and innovation has enabled improved methods of administering influenza vaccines, including a reduced-dose injectable made possible by the addition of adjuvants, and the use of a cell culture vaccine. Scientists are also exploring new routes of administration, such as intradermal (with or without needle) and transcutaneous, in which a patch delivers the vaccine through micro-needles that may barely penetrate the skin before dissolving and releasing the vaccine.

Most vaccinated persons develop postvaccination hemagglutination inhibition antibody titers. These antibodies are protective against illness caused by strains similar to those in the vaccine or by related variants that may emerge during outbreaks.

Oladayo Oyelola, Ph.D., SC(ASCP)

FURTHER READING

Betts, R. F. "Influenza Virus." In *Mandell, Douglas, and Bennett's Principles and Practice of Infectious Diseases,* edited by Gerald L. Mandell, John E. Bennett, and Raphael Dolin. 7th ed. New York: Churchill Livingstone/Elsevier, 2010.

Delves, Peter J., et al. *Roitt's Essential Immunology.* 11th ed. Malden, Mass.: Blackwell, 2006.

Hak, E., et al. "Influence of High-Risk Medical Conditions on the Effectiveness of Influenza Vaccination Among Elderly Members of Three Large Managed-Care Organizations." *Clinical Infectious Diseases* 35 (2002): 370-377.

Plotkin, Stanley A., Walter A. Orenstein, and Paul A. Offit. *Vaccines.* 5th ed. Philadelphia: Saunders/Elsevier, 2008.

WEB SITES OF INTEREST

Centers for Disease Control and Prevention
http://www.cdc.gov/vaccines

College of Physicians of Philadelphia, History of Vaccines
http://www.historyofvaccines.org

Global Health Council
http://www.globalhealth.org

Vaccine Research Center
http://www.niaid.nih.gov/about/organization/vrc

See also: Antiviral drugs: Types; Avian influenza; Common cold; H1N1 influenza; Home remedies; Immunity; Immunization; Infection; Influenza; Prevention of viral infections; Respiratory route of transmission; Seasonal influenza; Vaccines: Types; Viral infections; Viral pharyngitis; Viral upper respiratory infections.

Insect-borne illness and disease

CATEGORY: Transmission
ALSO KNOWN AS: Arthropod-borne illness and disease, vector-borne illness and disease

DEFINITION

An insect-borne illness or disease is a disease transmitted by an insect that carries bacteria or viruses from one host to another. Many types of insects can extract bacteria and viruses from infected birds, animals, and humans while feeding on blood. Pathogens are transmitted when these insects bite the animal or human, causing illness, disease, and sometimes death. Several of these diseases are found worldwide and others are regional.

MOSQUITO-BORNE DISEASES

The majority of insect-borne diseases and illnesses is transmitted by mosquitoes. As a group, these diseases lead to millions of deaths each year, with infants, children, and pregnant women showing particular vulnerability to illness and mortality. Controlling mosquito populations and avoiding mosquito bites are the two most important ways to avoid these diseases. The main preventive mechanisms include getting rid of standing water, using larvicidal chemicals or bacteria in standing water that cannot be drained (such as rice paddies), wearing protective clothing, avoiding being outdoors during times when mosquitoes are prevalent, and having secure screens on all windows and doors. Additional protective measures include spraying pesticides in the home (if necessary), soaking bed nets in pyrethroid pesticide, and using a repellant containing NN-diethyl metatoluamide (DEET). A major issue in fighting insect-borne diseases, however, is insect resistance to pesticides.

For many of the mosquito-borne diseases, there is a cycle between birds and mammals that involves the mosquito picking up the virus from a bird or mammal and transmitting it to a human. For some of these illnesses, vaccines or prophylactic drugs are available, but for many others, the search for preventive medication remains.

One particularly severe and widespread mosquito-borne disease is malaria, which is caused by four species of *Plasmodium: falciparum, vivax, malariae,* and *ovale,* the former of which is responsible for the most deaths, particularly in Africa. It is estimated that three billion people live in areas where they are at risk for malaria. In 2006, about one-half billion people suffered from malaria and more than one million died from it. *Plasmodia* are transmitted by the *Anopheles* mosquito, and the incubation period lasts from seven to thirty days, depending on the *Plasmodium* species transmitted. Symptoms of malaria include shivering, fever, headache, vomiting, and sweating. Severe malaria can involve such symptoms as impaired con-

sciousness, seizures, coma, anemia, pulmonary edema, and cardiovascular collapse. Drug treatments for malaria include chloroquine, mefloquine, quinine, and doxycycline, but some of these are ineffective. Certain pathogens have developed resistance to antibiotics, and more will develop resistance in the future.

Preventing malaria infection is a top priority for many health and research organizations, which are trying to establish vaccines and better treatments for those suffering from the disease. In areas such as sub-Saharan Africa, where malaria is hyperendemic, anti-malaria therapy is recommended for pregnant women and children because of their increased susceptibility; however, this therapy decreases the chance of becoming infected only and does not ensure immunity. In 2006, the World Health Organization reassessed the risks versus the benefits of dichloro-diphenyl-trichloroethane (DDT) use and deemed indoor residual spraying of homes to be one of the major mechanisms of controlling malaria. Bed nets soaked in pesticide are also recommended to reduce exposure to mosquito bites, as is the use of a DEET-containing repellant.

Another mosquito-borne illness is dengue fever, a viral infection that occurs in approximately one hundred million people each year, leading to thousands of deaths. Dengue fever is endemic to Southeast Asia and Latin America (including Puerto Rico) and is rarely found in the United States. It is most commonly transmitted by the mosquito *Aedes aegypti.* There are four viruses from the Flaviviridae family (DENV 1, 2, 3 and 4) that cause dengue, which has a three-to-eight-day incubation period. Symptoms of dengue include high fever, rash, nosebleeds, and pain in the muscles, joints, and bones. Most persons recover from these symptoms after seven to ten days. The more severe form, dengue hemorrhagic fever (DHF), has additional symptoms of vomiting, abdominal pain, and the failure of the circulatory system when the capillaries become too permeable. No vaccine exists for dengue fever. Reducing exposure to mosquito bites is the recommended prevention.

West Nile virus (of the Flaviviridae family) has been reported in recent years in Europe, North America, Africa, and the Middle East. Most people (80 percent) who are infected with West Nile virus do not experience any symptoms. About 20 percent of those infected have symptoms such as fever, aches, swollen lymph nodes, a rash, and vomiting, and the incubation period is three to fourteen days after being bitten. Less than 1 percent of people infected suffer from the most severe symptoms, which include vision loss, disorientation, convulsions, and coma; these symptoms are caused by encephalitis (brain swelling) and can lead to death.

Yellow fever virus (of the Flaviviridae family) is chiefly transmitted by the mosquitoes *A. aegypti* and *A. africanus*. Yellow fever is present in many countries of South America and sub-Saharan Africa, regions with an estimated six hundred million people. The incubation period is three to six days. Mild cases involve fever, aches, and muscle weakness, which typically dissipate within forty-eight hours. Severe cases result in hemorrhagic symptoms such as black vomit, nosebleeds, and bleeding gums. The disease gets its name from the skin-yellowing jaundice caused by liver failure in severe cases, as cellular necrosis occurs in the liver. There is a vaccine available for yellow fever; however, it continues to carry a significant disease burden, especially in poor areas. During epidemics, the fatality rate for those infected is 15 to 50 percent.

Japanese encephalitis virus is also a member of the Flaviviridae family and is typically carried by the mosquito *Culex tritaeniorhynchus*. This illness is found primarily in Asia and affects about fifty thousand people each year; approximately one-third of these cases are fatal. Outbreaks generally occur in rural areas. The incubation period is generally five to fifteen days. The disease involves acute-onset encephalitis and other manifestations, including seizures, paralysis, coma, and death. The fatality rate ranges widely, between 0.3 and 60 percent. Vaccines are available but are quite costly and come with adverse side effects.

St. Louis encephalitis is a member of the Flaviviridae family and is transmitted mainly by the *Culex* species of mosquitoes. The incubation period for the virus is between five and fifteen days. Symptoms include fever, headache, stiff neck, disorientation, coma, and convulsions, depending on the severity of the infection. The fatality rate is between 3 and 30 percent. There is no vaccine or therapy, other than supportive care, for St. Louis encephalitis.

Chikungunya is a member of the genus *Alphavirus* in the family Togaviridae and is present mainly in Asia and Africa. The mosquito *A. aegypti* as the primary vector, but *A. albopictus* is also known to transmit the virus. The incubation period ranges from two to twelve days but usually averages two to four days. Symptoms include fever, headache, nausea, vomiting, rash, and joint pain. Recovery usually takes about seven to ten days, and the disease is not usually fatal. Supportive care such as rest, fluids, and nonsteroidal anti-inflammatory drugs is recommended. Arthritic symptoms, particularly in the wrists, hands, and ankles but sometimes in the larger joints, continue in about one-third of cases. Chikungunya is one of the few mosquito-borne diseases that has a milder course in children than in adults. No vaccine or antiviral treatment is available for Chikungunya virus.

TICKBORNE DISEASES

Tickborne diseases are caused by tick bites and are most commonly contracted in heavily wooded areas. Measures to prevent tickborne diseases involve the evasion of ticks, primarily, and the avoidance of tick bites. Measures include wearing light-colored protective clothing, checking for ticks after being outdoors, and using an insect repellant containing 20 to 30 percent DEET. Another measure is to maintain yards and gardens in a way that keeps ticks away. This includes applying acaricide pesticides in May or June, using wood chips between wooded areas and grassy areas to minimize tick migration into the yard, and ensuring that patio and playground equipment is away from trees and bushes. Controlling the deer population by erecting fences and by not feeding deer help to reduce the incidence of deer ticks. Tick removal should be done with fine-tipped tweezers, grasped as close to the tick head as possible. This method reduces the chance that an infected tick will release more bacteria-containing saliva into the bloodstream when removed from the skin.

Lyme disease is caused by the bacterium *Borrelia burgdorferi* and is transmitted by *Ixodes scapularis* (black-legged tick/deer tick) and *I. pacificus* (Western black-legged tick) and is carried by deer, squirrels, and mice. Most cases in the United States occur on the East Coast and in the Midwest. Symptoms of Lyme disease include fever, headache, fatigue, and a skin rash that often looks like a bulls eye (erythema migrans); a rash occurs in about 80 percent of cases. The incubation period lasts between three and thirty-two days. Lyme-infected tick season typically runs from May through July. Early detection is critical to avoid infection of the joints and the cardiac and nervous systems. A course of antibiotics administered for a few weeks is typically effective against Lyme disease. If left untreated, severe arthritis, meningitis, heart palpitations, and Bell's palsy (loss of muscle tone on one or both sides of the face) can occur. Most persons recover after a course of antibiotics; however, some people experience long-term effects of fatigue, arthritis, and cognitive deficits. A Lyme disease vaccine was available until 2002, when the company making it discontinued production, citing a lack of demand.

Rocky Mountain spotted fever is caused by the bacterium *Rickettsia rickettsii* and is typically transmitted by *Dermacentor variabilis* (American dog tick) or *D. andersoni* (Rocky Mountain wood tick). The incubation period is typically five to fifteen days after the tick bite. Early symptoms of the disease include fever, muscle pain, loss of appetite, and severe headache. Later symptoms of Rocky Mountain spotted fever are rash, joint pain, and diarrhea. The majority of cases in the United States have been reported in the southeast. Other regions affected include North, Central, and South America. Treatment with tetracycline antibiotics for five to ten days is usually successful.

FLEABORNE DISEASE

One fleaborne disease is plague, which is caused by the bacterium *Yersinia pestis*. The bacterium is usually transmitted by infected rodent fleas, with an incubation period of two to six days. Plague, also called the Black Death, killed millions of people across Europe in the fourteenth century. Fleas also carry infection between squirrels, chipmunks, rabbits, and prairie dogs, resulting in transmission to humans. Each year there are one thousand to two thousand cases. In Asia, South America, and Africa, the most common carrier is the flea species *Xenopsylla cheopis*. Plague is found in the western United States and in parts of South America, Asia, and Africa. One of the telltale symptoms is a painful, hot, and swollen lymph node. Additional symptoms are fever, headache, and exhaustion. Antibiotics can be used to treat plague if treatment starts early enough. Without antibiotics, the disease continues to progress to infection of the bloodstream and lungs (plague pneumonia) and has a high fatality rate. Plague vaccine is not commercially available in the United States.

IMPACT

Insect-borne diseases affect hundreds of millions of people each year and kill millions, especially children in tropical countries. Determining mechanisms for fighting the diseases and the insects that carry them is a top research priority worldwide.

Dawn M. Bielawski, Ph.D.

FURTHER READING

Enayati, A., and J. Hemingway "Malaria Management: Past, Present, and Future." *Annual Review of Entomology* 55 (2010): 569-591. This article describes the history of malaria control, vaccines, vector control, and modern innovations for control.

Gratz, Norman G. *Vector- and Rodent-Borne Diseases in Europe and North America: Distribution, Public Health Burden, and Control.* New York: Cambridge University Press, 2006. This book examines insect- and rodent-borne diseases, mechanisms to control them, and their epidemiology in Europe, the United States, and Canada. The author is a former director of Vector Biology and Control for the World Health Organization.

Ligon, B. Lee. "Infectious Diseases that Pose Specific Challenges After Natural Disasters." *Seminars in Pediatric Infectious Diseases* 17 (2006): 36-45. This article focuses on the many diseases that tend to be more prevalent after earthquakes, floods, hurricanes, and other natural disasters. Includes a section on insect-borne diseases.

Shah, Sonia. *The Fever: How Malaria Has Ruled Humankind for 500,000 Years.* New York: Farrar, Straus and Giroux, 2010. This investigative study looks at how malaria has helped shape the history of humankind and how human limitations have prevented its eradication.

Sherman, Irwin W. *The Elusive Malaria Vaccine: Miracle or Mirage?* Washington, D.C.: ASM Press, 2009. Looks at attempts to develop a vaccine for malaria and explains why a useful vaccine still does not exist. Scientific literature and interviews with scientists working on vaccines provide the book's foundation.

Tolle, Michael A. "Mosquito-Borne Diseases." *Current Problems in Pediatric and Adolescent Health Care* 39 (2009): 97-140. A thorough review of the life cycles of insects as disease agents. Includes discussion of the diagnoses, treatments, and vaccines for several mosquito-borne diseases. Special focus on the impact of the diseases on pregnant women and on children.

WEB SITES OF INTEREST

Centers for Disease Control and Prevention, Division of Vector Borne Infectious Diseases
http://www.cdc.gov/ncidod/dvbid

Malaria Foundation International
http://www.malaria.org

National Institute of Allergy and Infectious Diseases
http://www.niaid.nih.gov/topics/vector

See also: Arthropod-borne illness and disease; Blood-borne illness and disease; Fleas and infectious disease; Flies and infectious disease; Hosts; Mosquitoes and infectious disease; Ticks and infectious disease; Transmission routes; Vectors and vector control.

Insecticides and topical repellants

CATEGORY: Prevention

DEFINITION

Insecticides and topical repellants are chemical or biological substances (pesticides) used to kill adult or larval-stage insects and to prevent troublesome (and disease-causing) insect behavior, such as biting. Through genetic engineering, biotechnology has developed insecticides that are produced within plant species.

Insects that feed on crops and stored foods are targeted by insecticides. Also targeted are insect vectors, including mosquitoes and ticks, that transmit human diseases such as malaria, yellow fever, West Nile virus, Lyme disease, and dengue fever.

CHEMICAL INSECTICIDES

Carbamate insecticides affect the nervous system of insects. These insecticides block the regulation of the neurotransmitter acetylcholine by inhibiting the vital enzyme cholinesterase.

Organochlorine insecticides, such as dichloro-diphenyl-trichloroethane (DDT), were used in the past. They were withdrawn from the market because of their harmful health effects and their persistence in the environment.

Like carbamate insecticides, organophosphate pesticides affect the nervous system of insects by blocking the regulation of the neurotransmitter acetylcholine. However, organophosphates are not persistent in the environment. Some are poisonous nerve agents.

Organosulfer pesticides have very low toxicity in insects and are used only to control mites. The chemical structure of organosulfer pesticides is similar to DDT, with sulfur used in place of carbon as the central atom.

BIOLOGICAL INSECTICIDES

Pyrethroid pesticides are synthetic versions of the natural chrysanthemum pesticide pyrethrin. The ground, dried flowers were used in the early nineteenth century to control body lice among soldiers in the Napoleonic wars. The synthetic versions have been modified to increase their stability in sunlight. Pyrethroids are generally effective against most agricultural insect pests when used at very low concentrations of 0.01 to 0.1 pound per acre. Some synthetic pyrethroids are toxic to the insect's nervous system.

The formamidine insecticides are used in the control of organophosphate-resistant and carbamate-resistant pests. Nicotinoid pesticides are chemically similar to nicotine. They are used to treat soil, stored seeds, and the foliage of cotton, rice cereals, peanuts, potatoes, vegetables, fruits, and nuts.

Limonene is extracted from citrus peel. It is effective against the pests of domestic animals (or pets); these pests include fleas, lice, mites, and ticks. Eugenol extracted from cloves and cinnamaldehyde extracted from cinnamon are used on ornamental plants and on many crops to control various insects.

Neem seed oil extracts are chemically similar to limonene. The oil has insecticidal, fungicidal, and bactericidal properties when insects consume or come in contact with it. The oil disrupts molting by inhibiting the juvenile molting hormone.

Spinosad, a product of the soil bacterium *Saccharopolyspora spinosa*, is effective against various caterpillar pests, which come in contact with or consume crops that have been treated. Crops treated include cotton, vegetables, tree fruits, and ornamentals.

Rotenoids (rotenone) are produced in the roots of beans. Used to treat the foliage of crops, rotenoids are both a stomach and contact insecticide used to control leaf-eating caterpillars.

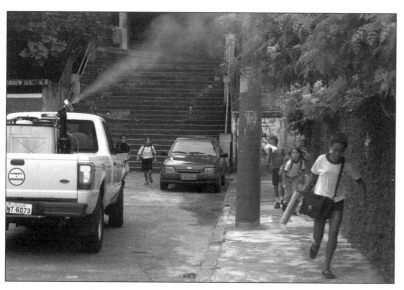

City workers spray mosquito insecticide in a Rio de Janeiro, Brazil, neighborhood, as children are near. (AP/Wide World Photos)

LARVICIDES

Larval control can be used when insect breeding sites are within flying range of communities. Frequently, they are used to supplement the effects of other control methods. The control of mosquitoes is the most common use of larvicides. Spores from several serotypes of the bacterium *Bacillus thuringiensis* are specific to various species of mosquito larvae. The gene for the toxic *B. thuringiensis* protein has been added to the deoxyribonucleic acid (DNA) of leafy plants through genetic engineering. The plant manufactures the substance that destroys the mosquito larvae.

Larva-eating fish, too, can be used for the control of mosquito larvae. When confined in water containers, larva-eating fish have been used for malaria control by reducing the numbers of malaria-carrying mosquitoes.

PHYSICAL BARRIERS

Floating layers of expanded polystyrene beads prevent mosquito breeding when used in isolated sites such as cesspools and water tanks. The barriers are used in areas where malaria is common.

CHEMICAL INSECT REPELLANTS

The mechanisms of action of insect repellents are not well understood. The active ingredients DEET (NN-diethyl metatoluamide), Merck IR3535, and Pi-

caridin are the most commonly available synthetic repellants. Each has efficacy against a broad range of insects.

DEET is used to repel biting pests such as mosquitoes and ticks that carry Lyme disease. Products containing DEET include a variety of liquids, lotions, sprays, and impregnated materials such as wristbands.

BIOLOGICAL INSECT REPELLENTS

Produced by wild tomato plants as a natural pesticide is 2-Undecanone. Oil of lemon eucalyptus also has pesticide qualities. The chemically synthesized version, methyl nonyl ketone, is applied to skin or clothing to repel mosquitoes, biting flies, and gnats. Synthetic insect repellent is available as a lotion and as a spray. Oil of citronella comes from dried, cultivated grasses and has a distinctive floral scent that masks the carbon dioxide humans exhale and the lactic acid of human bodies, to which mosquitoes and other biting insects are attracted.

INSECT ATTRACTANTS

Insect attractants are signal-carrying chemicals known as pheromones. Sex pheromones encourage sexual behavior. Thus, a male insect may be attracted to and attempt to copulate with an object covered with sex pheromones; this interrupts the insect's reproductive cycle. Insect pheromone has been used in high concentrations in insect-breeding grounds. As a result, insect populations diminish, making it difficult for insects to locate mates; mating behavior is further affected and reproduction is further interrupted.

Another type of attractant, the insect bait, is used to control cockroaches and ants and must be eaten by the insects to be effective. The baits are formulated with food or other insect attractant, which is eaten by the ants or cockroaches and then transported back to their respective colonies. Baits, because they confine the insecticide to a small, secure area, help lower the risk of human or pet exposure to the chemicals within.

IMPACT

Insecticides are essential to the success of agriculture, and without topical insect repellents, humans would be highly susceptible to infectious diseases transmitted by a huge vector population.

Kimberly A. Napoli, M.S.

FURTHER READING

Centers for Disease Control and Prevention. *Fourth National Report on Human Exposure to Environmental Chemicals* (2009). Available at http://www.cdc.gov/exposurereport. A U.S. government report on the effects of insecticides and other chemicals on human health.

Ware, George W., and David M. Whitacre. *The Pesticide Book.* 6th ed. Willoughby, Ohio: MeisterPro Information Resources, 2004. Comprehensive coverage of chemical and biological insecticides and repellents.

World Health Organization. *Pesticides and Their Application for the Control of Vectors and Pests of Public Health Importance.* 6th ed. Geneva: Author, 2006. A report of the WHO Pesticide Evaluation Scheme of the Department of Control of Neglected Tropical Diseases.

WEB SITES OF INTEREST

Centers for Disease Control and Prevention, Agency for Toxic Substances and Disease Registry
http://www.atsdr.cdc.gov

National Pesticide Information Center
http://npic.orst.edu

World Health Organization: Pesticide Evaluation Scheme
http://www.who.int/whopes

See also: Biochemical tests; Chemical germicides; DDT; Developing countries and infectious disease; Insect-borne illness and disease; Sleeping nets; Vectors and vector control; Water treatment.

Integrase inhibitors

CATEGORY: Treatment

DEFINITION

Integrase inhibitors are a new class of antiretroviral drugs developed to treat human immunodeficiency virus (HIV) infection and could theoretically be applied to other retroviruses. Integrase inhibitors block the action of an enzyme that catalyzes an important step in retroviral infection.

RETROVIRAL LIFE CYCLE

Retroviruses store their genetic material in the form of ribonucleic acid (RNA). Upon entering the target host cell, the reverse transcriptase enzyme uses the RNA genome as a template to synthesize a deoxyribonucleic acid (DNA) strand. In the cytoplasm, integrase binds to the viral DNA and begins processing the 3 end by removing nucleotides. Then, the integrase-DNA complex translocates to the cell nucleus, where the enzyme makes a staggered cut in the host DNA. Integrase joins the 3 end of the viral DNA to the 5 end of the host DNA by base pairing. The enzyme fills in the gaps of missing nucleotides and ligates the joined ends by forming covalent bonds.

Upon integration, the viral genome is copied and transcribed as part of the human chromosome. The enzyme protease cleaves peptides expressed from the viral genome into mature proteins that can be assembled into new virions, which are released from the host cell to complete the retroviral life cycle.

ANTIRETROVIRAL DRUGS

Older therapies block the activity of reverse transcriptase (with nucleoside and nucleotide reverse transcriptase inhibitors or with non-nucleoside reverse transcriptase inhibitors) or block maturation of viral proteins with protease inhibitors. Retroviruses can easily develop resistance to these drugs, because the reverse transcriptase and protease genes can undergo many base substitutions and still produce functional enzymes. These mutational changes alter protein conformation, making the enzymes harder to inhibit with a single drug.

When the integrase is inhibited, host enzymes circularize the provirus, which is then degraded, preventing stable integration into the host genome. There is no known human equivalent of the integrase enzyme, suggesting that this class of drugs is not likely to be toxic to the human cell.

CLINICAL USE

Raltegravir was the first integrase inhibitor to be approved by the U.S. Food and Drug Administration (2007). It has been shown to reduce the amount of virus in the body (viral load) and to increase the number of CD4-positive T cells, which is one type of immune cell invaded by HIV.

Raltegravir is a derivative of diketobutanoic acid. HIV resistance to raltegravir is caused by mutations in locations near the active site; therefore, other diketobutanoic acids are being modified to tightly bind mutated integrases from resistant strains. Quinolone derivatives also appear to have anti-integrase effects.

IMPACT

Resistance to antiretroviral agents has complicated efforts to treat HIV; therefore, the emergence of a new class of drugs that uses a different mechanism of action and carries a lower risk of resistance is welcome news for persons with multidrug-resistant strains.

Kathleen LaPoint, M.S.

FURTHER READING

Berger, Daniel S. "The Dawn of a New Treatment: A Look at Experimental HIV Integrase Inhibitors." *Positively Aware: The Monthly Journal of the Test Positive Aware Network* 17 (2006): 44-45.

Fangman, John J. W., and Martin S. Hirsch. "Integrase Inhibitors and Other New Drugs in Development." In *AIDS Therapy*, edited by Raphael Dolin, Henry Masur, and Michael S. Saag. 3d ed. New York: Churchill Livingstone/Elsevier, 2008.

Rockstroh, Jürgen K. "Integrase Inhibitors: Why Do We Need a New Drug Class for HIV Therapy?" *European Journal of Medical Research* 14, suppl. 3 (2009): 1-3.

WEB SITES OF INTEREST

AIDSinfo
http://aidsinfo.nih.gov

AIDS.org
http://www.aids.org

See also: AIDS; Antibodies; Antiviral drugs: Mechanisms of action; Antiviral drugs: Types; Autoimmune disorders; Blood-borne illness and disease; HIV; Immunity; Maturation inhibitors; Protease inhibitors; Quinolone antibiotics; Retroviral infections; Retroviridae; Reverse transcriptase inhibitors; T lymphocytes; Treatment of viral infections; Viral infections.

Intestinal and stomach infections

CATEGORY: Diseases and conditions
ANATOMY OR SYSTEM AFFECTED: Abdomen, digestive system, gastrointestinal system, intestines, stomach
ALSO KNOWN AS: Food poisoning, food-borne illness, gastroenteritis, gastrointestinal infections, GI infections, stomach bug, stomach flu

DEFINITION

Gastrointestinal (GI) infections are caused by the overgrowth of resident or foreign bacteria, viruses, fungi, or parasites that can lead to vomiting, diarrhea, bloating, fever, and abdominal pain. GI infections occur with a wide range of symptoms, including none, minor or mild, and those requiring hospitalization for treatment; infections can also be fatal. The elderly, the very young, and the immunocompromised are more likely to develop serious complications from a GI infection.

CAUSES

Certain bacteria, viruses, fungi, and parasites can cause GI infections. In the United States, the most common cause of GI infection is the consumption of food infected with bacteria or food containing toxins released by those organisms (often referred to as food poisoning). Bacteria associated with food poisoning include *Campylobacter jejuni*, *Salmonella*, and *Shigella* species, and enterohemorrhagic *Escherichia coli* O157:H7.

Botulism is a potentially fatal GI infection caused by consuming food contaminated with a toxin produced by *Clostridium botulinum*; this infection is often associated with consuming improperly canned or prepared foods. Inflammatory diarrhea (also referred to as bloody diarrhea) can be caused by *Shigella* or *Salmonella* spp., *C. jejuni*, or *E. coli*. Inflammation of the colon can be life-threatening if it is accompanied by obstruction or rupture of the bowel. *Clostridium difficile* and *Enterococcus fecalis* can cause hospital-acquired GI infections.

Causing no symptoms is *Helicobacter pylori*, a spiral-shaped bacterium. Persons become carriers of the bacteria without knowing they are carriers. In some cases, long-term infection with *H. pylori* can cause the development of an ulcer.

Cholera is an acute diarrheal illness caused by infection of the intestine with the bacterium *Vibrio cholerae*.

Facts: Diarrheal Diseases and Children, Worldwide

- Second leading cause of death in children younger than age five years.

- Kills 1.5 million children every year.

- About 2 billion cases of diarrheal disease are reported each year.

- Mainly affects children younger than age two years.

- A leading cause of malnutrition in children younger than age five years.

Source: World Health Organization

Although rare and easily treated in the United States, cholera can decimate a population in underdeveloped countries. An outbreak began in Haiti in the fall of 2010 among persons living in poor conditions following a deadly earthquake earlier in the year.

Viral gastroenteritis (referred to as a stomach bug or stomach flu) is a GI infection caused by a virus. These infections are common in the United States and can be acquired by consuming improperly prepared food (raw or undercooked) that also contains a virus and by contact with contaminated saliva or feces. Many viruses cause gastroenteritis, including rotaviruses, noroviruses, adenoviruses, enteroviruses, and hepatitis A, with rotaviruses being the most common cause of severe gastroenteritis in infants and young children worldwide.

Generally, GI infections are mild, and most healthy people recover from infection without complications. Noninflammatory diarrhea, which is usually caused by a rotavirus or an adenovirus, is typically self-limiting. Viral gastroenteritis, however, can be life-threatening for those who are unable to drink enough fluids to replace those fluids lost through vomiting and diarrhea. Infants, young children, and immunocompromised, disabled, and elderly persons are at risk for dehydration from the loss of fluids.

Some viruses are seasonal or are found only in certain environments. In the United States, rotavirus and astrovirus infections occur most commonly between October and April, while adenovirus infections can occur anytime during the year. Outbreaks of noro-

virus infections can occur in schools, child-care facilities, and nursing homes, and they have been associated with outbreaks in banquet halls, on cruise ships, in dormitories, and at campgrounds.

In underdeveloped countries with poor sanitation, parasites are the most common cause of GI infections; however, these infections may also be found in urban areas, depending on the social habits of residents. Parasites that infect humans and cause GI infections include protozoa and helminths.

In the United States, the most common protozoa that infect humans are *Giardia intestinalis* (also known as *G. lamblia*) and *Cryptosporidium* species. These protozoa may be consumed by hikers who drink untreated water from a lake, river, or stream. Protozoa can multiply inside the human body, leading to serious infection. Tapeworms (cestodes) are among the most common helminths that infect people in the United States. *Dipylidium* is a tapeworm found in cats and dogs. People become infected after accidentally swallowing a flea infected with a tapeworm larvae. Most reported cases involve children. Tapeworms are also found in raw or undercooked pork, beef, and fish. In many cases, the serious health problems that tapeworms cause occur when these parasites pass through the intestines and infect other organs, such as the skin, muscles, eyes, and brain.

RISK FACTORS

Risk factors for an intestinal or stomach infection include consuming improperly prepared food, such as raw or undercooked beef, pork, chicken, eggs, shellfish, or fish. Another risk factor is drinking water from untreated or contaminated sources or consuming raw food prepared or cleaned with untreated or contaminated water. *C. difficile* and *E. fecalis* are associated with recent antibiotic use and long-term hospitalization. GI infections can be very contagious, and pathogens are easily transferred from an infected person to another by touching a contaminated surface such as a door knob, faucet handle, or other common surface. Frequent and proper handwashing reduces the risk of transfer of the bacteria.

Consuming eggs laid by hens infected with *Salmonella* can cause a GI infection. Hens get infected with *Salmonella* by consuming contaminated feed. The feed usually acquires *Salmonella* by contact with flies and rodent feces. *Salmonella* bacteria may be present on the surface of infected eggs and can also penetrate the

The Organs and Structures of the Abdomen

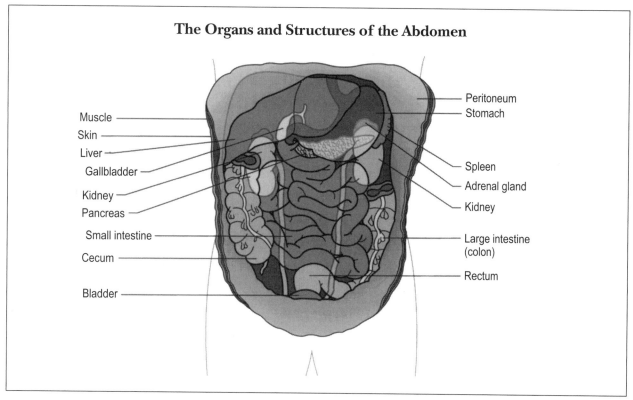

Abdominal organs and structures are located between the rib cage and the pelvic bone.

shell and infect the egg contents. Therefore, washing the surface of the egg and hands after touching eggs will remove most bacteria. In addition, a hen infected with *Salmonella* can carry the bacteria in its ovaries. Eggs then become infected with *Salmonella* as the eggs are forming; bacteria are contained within the shells. The most common site of bacterial contamination is the egg white. Thoroughly cooking the egg until the yolk and egg white are solid will kill the bacteria.

Consuming raw or undercooked contaminated beef can cause bacterial infections with *Salmonella* and *E. coli* O157:H7. Risk factors include improper and unsanitary handling of animals at the time of slaughter, of meat products at the time of processing, and of food being prepared at home.

Produce-related outbreaks have become more common in the United States. Cases of *E. coli*-contaminated spinach and lettuce have led to hospitalizations, death, and the recall of thousands of pounds of produce. It remains unclear exactly how fields of leafy green vegetables, such as spinach and lettuce, become reservoirs for these pathogens, although it is believed that the sources of the pathogens are animal waste and by-products. Also, commercially processed foods that contain contaminated meat or produce, such as frozen pot pies, vegetable snacks, frozen pepperoni pizzas, and canned hot dog chili sauce, have been sources of bacterial GI infections.

Consuming improperly prepared pork or wild game infected with the roundworm *Trichinella spiralis* can cause GI infections in humans. The incidence of *Trichinella* infection has declined markedly in the United States since the availability of home freezers and the use of proper food preparation and cooking. *Taenia solium* is a pork tapeworm that can cause a GI infection if tapeworm eggs are consumed in food or water, are obtained from surfaces contaminated with feces, or are obtained through autoinfection (self-re-infection). After being consumed, the eggs hatch and penetrate the intestine. Once in the bloodstream, the eggs may develop into cysticerci in the muscles, brain, or eyes; they can then cause an infection in these organs known as cysticercosis.

Consuming infected raw or undercooked shellfish

or fish may cause an infection with hepatitis A, other hepatitis viruses, several types of bacteria, and cholera. Some soft cheeses and some ready-to-eat foods (such as hot dogs and cold cuts from delicatessen counters) may contain the bacterium *Listeria* and cause listeriosis in severely immunocompromised persons. To prevent listeriosis, shellfish and fish should be heated until the point of steaming before consumption.

Children in particular may acquire waterborne infections from lakes or pools after swallowing water during recreational activities. Public swimming pools and lakes may be contaminated with pathogens from infected swimmers; exposure to infected feces or soiled diapers can be avoided with proper hygiene, handwashing, and disposal of waste. It is generally recommended, however, that infected persons avoid using public swimming pools and other such recreational sites until the infection has resolved.

SYMPTOMS

Symptoms of GI infections depend on the pathogen and the amount consumed. In general, symptoms can develop quickly (within thirty minutes) or more slowly (within hours) and can worsen over days to weeks. Usually the infection is self-limiting and runs its course within forty-eight hours. GI infections can cause nausea, diarrhea, vomiting, fever, abdominal cramping, bloating, loss of appetite (anorexia), and dysentery (blood or mucus in the stool). If these symptoms continue for many days or if good hydration is not maintained, weight loss and dehydration may occur. Other flulike symptoms include chills, headache, muscle aches, and malaise.

Viral GI infections tend to be self-limited. These symptoms typically begin one to two days after exposure and can last for up to ten days, depending on the type of virus. Self-limited infections are typically noninflammatory; however, inflammatory diarrhea (also referred to as bloody diarrhea) can be life-threatening if obstruction or rupture of the bowel occurs. In some people, *E. coli* O157:H7 infection can cause a complication called hemolytic uremic syndrome, a life-threatening condition. Prolonged diarrhea can occur when persons are infected with parasites, *E. fecalis*, or *C. difficile*.

Each year, rotaviruses cause about one-half million deaths among young children worldwide, with the majority of deaths in developing countries (where access to treatment is limited). Infection with hepatitis

A causes a sudden onset of fever, loss of appetite, and malaise, followed by jaundice (yellowing of the eyes and skin). Symptoms of giardiasis (infection with *Giardia*) normally begin one to two weeks (with an average seven days) after infection and may last two to six weeks in otherwise healthy persons.

Some GI infections may have little or no GI symptoms. Other than passing of eggs and adult tapeworms (which can be quite dramatic), symptoms associated with infection by the pork tapeworm *T. solium* usually involve the muscles, brain, or eyes (infected with cysticerci or cysts). *H. pylori* infection often does not cause any symptoms until the person has developed a stomach ulcer.

SCREENING AND DIAGNOSIS

Generally, in the United States, GI infections are diagnosed by a physician after a physical examination and on the basis of symptoms. Stool specimens are collected for the diagnosis of some GI infections. Various laboratory tests can be conducted on stool specimens, including bacterial culture, microscopic analysis, pathogen isolation, serology (to check for antibodies), or antigen detection, which aids in identifying the causative pathogen. Some viruses, such as adenoviruses, may be excreted in the stool for prolonged periods even after resolution of the infection; therefore, presence of the virus does not necessarily indicate active infection. In the case of bacterial infections, antibiotic susceptibility testing may be used to determine microbial resistance to antibiotic therapy.

TREATMENT AND THERAPY

Most infections are mild and require only symptomatic treatment and adequate hydration. Dehydration can lead to kidney and other organ failure. Severe dehydration may require hospitalization and treatment with intravenous fluids. To prevent dehydration, one should drink 8 ounces of fluids every two hours until diarrhea and vomiting stop. Oral rehydration fluids are formulated to replace lost electrolytes and nutrients. Drinks containing caffeine or alcohol should be avoided.

Antidiarrheal medications that contain loperamide are generally not recommended for treatment of GI infections because these drugs prevent the body from eliminating the pathogen through the stool, which may make the infection worse. Drugs that reduce symptoms of nausea and vomiting (anti-emetics) but do not reduce bowel movement are helpful and may minimize fluid loss.

Antiparasitic drugs, such as praziquantal or niclosimide, are used to treat tapeworm infections. Antibiotics should not be used to treat most food-borne infections, including those caused by bacteria, because these infections are typically self-limiting. Serious bacterial GI infections, however, which do not respond to hydration and require hospitalization for treatment should receive antibiotic therapy. Bacteria such as *E. coli* and *C. difficile* have developed resistance to certain antibiotics, which makes these infections more difficult to treat. No effective antiviral medication is available to treat serious viral illnesses; therefore, only symptomatic treatment is provided for these infections.

Prevention and Outcomes

Most GI infections can be avoided by maintaining frequent and good handwashing technique, by drinking clean water, and by following safe food-storage and food-preparation practices. Two live, oral rotavirus vaccines are available for use in infants in the United States that can prevent rotavirus gastroenteritis.

Good handwashing technique involves wetting hands with clean, warm, running water; applying soap; then rubbing hands together to make a lather and scrubbing for a minimum of twenty seconds. Finally, hands should be rinsed well under running water and dried using a paper towel or air dryer. One should also use a paper towel to turn off the faucet.

Many GI infections can be prevented by drinking only clean, treated water and by using uncontaminated water to wash all food that is to be eaten raw. All raw fruits and vegetables should be washed or peeled (or both) before eating. Persons should avoid consuming uncooked foods when traveling in countries with minimal water treatment and sanitation systems. Persons also should avoid direct contact of the skin with soil or sand (by wearing shoes and protective clothing and using towels on beaches) in areas where fecal contamination of soil is likely, and should wash hands and exposed skin with soap and clean water as soon as possible to avoid oral contact. When camping or backpacking, persons should bring a supply of clean water or should treat water from lakes or streams by boiling (a rolling boil for a minimum of one minute) or by combining disinfection and filtration if the water is to be used for drinking or food preparation. Persons should avoid swimming in water that is likely to be contaminated with human or animal waste and should avoid swallowing water when swimming.

Safe storage and preparation of food means keeping cold food cold and hot food hot. Cold food should be stored in a refrigerator (at 40° Fahrenheit or below) or a freezer (0° F or below). One should cook food to a safe minimum internal temperature. All cuts of pork, ground beef, veal, and lamb should be cooked to a minimum internal temperature of 160° F, while all poultry should be cooked to 165° F. One should maintain hot cooked food at 140° F or above and should reheat cooked food to 165° F. Eggs should be cooked until both the white and the yolk are firm and should be consumed promptly after cooking. One should refrigerate unused or leftover foods promptly, should discard food that is past its expiration date, and should discard cracked or dirty eggs. Raw meat or eggs should not be consumed. After contact with raw meat or eggs, one should wash hands, cooking utensils, and food preparation surfaces with soap and water. The U.S. Centers for Disease Control and Prevention (CDC) has developed the food safety motto, "remember to clean, separate, cook, and chill."

The two rotavirus vaccines available in the United States differ in composition and schedule of administration. No preference, however, is given to either vaccine by the CDC's Advisory Committee on Immunization Practices. Additional studies are needed to evaluate the safety and efficacy of rotavirus vaccine administered to infants who are born preterm, who have immune deficiencies, who live in households with immunocompromised persons, who have chronic GI disease, or who start the vaccine series later than recommended.

Beatriz Manzor Mitrzyk, Pharm.D.

Further Reading

Centers for Disease Control and Prevention. "Clean Hands Save Lives." Available at http://www.cdc.gov/cleanhands. Information from the CDC on good hygiene and handwashing technique.

_____. "A Guide to Drinking Water Treatment and Sanitation for Backcountry and Travel Use." Available at http://www.cdc.gov/healthywater/drinking. Recommendations from the CDC on safe drinking-water practices for outdoor enthusiasts and travelers.

_____. "Prevention of Rotavirus Gastroenteritis Among Infants and Children: Recommendations of the Advisory Committee on Immunization Practices." *Morbidity and Mortality Weekly Report* 58 (February 6, 2009): 1-25. Also available at http://www.cdc.gov/mmwr/preview/mmwrhtml/rr5802a1.htm. Recommendations from the CDC on the safety and efficacy of the rotavirus vaccine.

Feldman, Mark, Lawrence S. Friedman, and Lawrence J. Brandt, eds. *Sleisenger and Fordtran's Gastrointestinal and Liver Disease: Pathophysiology, Diagnosis, Management.* New ed. 2 vols. Philadelphia: Saunders/Elsevier, 2010. An excellent textbook on gastroenterology, intestinal pathology, and treatment protocols.

Johnson, Leonard R., ed. *Gastrointestinal Physiology.* 7th ed. Philadelphia: Mosby/Elsevier, 2007. This book contains a variety of specialized topics dealt with by experts on gastrointestinal physiology.

National Center for Immunization and Respiratory Diseases. "Viral Gastroenteritis." Available at http://www.cdc.gov/ncidod/dvrd/revb/gastro/faq.htm. Information from a center of the CDC on viral gastroenteritis symptoms and management.

U.S. Department of Agriculture. "Foodborne Illness: What Consumers Need to Know." Available at http://www.fsis.usda.gov/fact_sheets. A fact sheet for consumers about symptoms, pathogens, and prevention of food-borne illnesses.

WEB SITES OF INTEREST

American Gastroenterological Association
http://www.gastro.org

Centers for Disease Control and Prevention
http://www.cdc.gov

U.S. Department of Agriculture: Food Safety and Inspection Service
http://www.fsis.usda.gov

See also: Amebic dysentery; Antibiotic-associated colitis; Ascariasis; Balantidiasis; Campylobacteriosis; Cholera; Cryptosporidiosis; Developing countries and infectious disease; *Escherichia coli* infection; Fecal-oral route of transmission; Food-borne illness and disease; Gastritis; Giardiasis; *Helicobacter pylori* infection; Protozoan diseases; Rotavirus infection; Salmonellosis; Shigellosis; Travelers' diarrhea; *Vibrio*; Waterborne illness and disease; Worm infections; Zoonotic diseases.

Intestinal trichomoniasis

CATEGORY: Diseases and conditions
ANATOMY OR SYSTEM AFFECTED: Gastrointestinal system, intestines

DEFINITION

Intestinal trichomoniasis is a protozoan infection of the large intestine of mammals. Although scarcely reported in the medical literature, it has been found in humans (extremely rare), monkeys, rats, dogs, cats, ducks, tree shrews, birds, and guinea pigs. Trichomoniasis also exists in the female and male reproductive systems of humans (as one of the most common sexually transmitted diseases) and mouth (common in persons with deficient oral hygiene practices), albeit caused by parasites different from the parasite that causes intestinal trichomoniasis.

CAUSES

Human intestinal trichomoniasis is associated with an overabundance of the parasite *Pentatrichomonas hominis*. Intestinal trichomoniasis in animals is caused by a variety of species-dependent trichomonads (a kind of protozoa). Usually nonpathogenic, these parasites are responsible for the diarrheal havoc of intestinal trichomoniasis.

RISK FACTORS

P. hominis is a worldwide, naturally occurring, normally harmless parasite residing in mammalian intestinal tracts. However, because the parasites are excreted through fecal matter, intestinal trichomoniasis is more prevalent in mammals in underdeveloped parts of the world, particularly in equatorial and subtropical regions. An overabundance of this parasite may occur when the host comes in contact with fresh fecal matter and subsequently ingests it through contaminated water or food or ingests it through hand-to-mouth transmission.

Similarly, children age five years and younger are also at a higher risk for developing an infection. Persons with a compromised immune system also may be at a greater risk of parasitic proliferation.

Symptoms

Intestinal trichomoniasis disrupts normal abdominal functioning. Symptoms include diarrhea, abdominal discomfort, nausea, vomiting, and subsequent loss of appetite.

Screening and Diagnosis

Freshly passed diarrheic samples are taken from the host and analyzed through stool cultures, light microscopy, and smear examinations.

Treatment and Therapy

Given that the cause of intestinal trichomoniasis is a nonpathogenic parasite, no effective treatment exists for the infection. Metronidazole, a medication used to treat genital trichomoniasis, does not cure intestinal trichomoniasis.

The infection may last from one month up to one year or more. To avoid dehydration during the infection, one should drink a sufficient amount of uncontaminated water.

Prevention and Outcomes

Stringent handwashing technique, eating uncontaminated food, and drinking uncontaminated water are the best ways to keep the normally harmless parasite from proliferating.

Alicia Williams, M.A.

Further Reading

Chomicz, Lidia, et al. "Anti-*Pentatrichomonas hominis* Activity of Newly Synthesized Bensimidazole Derivatives: In Vitro Studies." *Acta Parasitologica* 54 (2009): 165-171.

Crucitti, T., et al. "Detection of *Pentatrichomonas hominis* DNA in Biological Specimens by PCR." *Letters in Applied Microbiology* 38 (2004): 510-516.

Feldman, Mark, Lawrence S. Friedman, and Lawrence J. Brandt, eds. *Sleisenger and Fordtran's Gastrointestinal and Liver Disease: Pathophysiology, Diagnosis, Management.* New ed. 2 vols. Philadelphia: Saunders/Elsevier, 2010.

Ortega, Ynes. "Food- and Waterborne Protozoan Parasites." In *Foodborne Pathogens: Microbiology and Molecular Biology*, edited by Pina M. Fratamico, Arun K. Bhunia, and James L. Smith. Norwich, England: Caister Academic Press, 2005.

Web Sites of Interest

American Gastroenterological Association
http://www.gastro.org

Global Health Council
http://www.globalhealth.org/infectious_diseases

U.S. Department of Agriculture: Food Safety and Inspection Service
http://www.fsis.usda.gov

See also: Cholera; Developing countries and infectious disease; Fecal-oral route of transmission; Foodborne illness and disease; Hookworms; Intestinal and stomach infections; Isosporiasis; Oral transmission; Parasitic diseases; Protozoan diseases; Travelers' diarrhea; Tropical medicine; Typhoid fever; Viral gastroenteritis; Waterborne illness and disease.

Isosporiasis

Category: Diseases and conditions
Anatomy or system affected: Abdomen, gastrointestinal system, intestines

Definition

Isosporiasis is an uncommon human parasitic infection of the intestines characterized by profuse watery diarrhea and cramping abdominal pain.

Causes

Isosporiasis is caused by the coccidian protozoan parasite *Isospora belli* (taxonomically related to *Cryptosporidium, Cyclospora*, and *Toxoplasma* species), which infects the epithelial cells of the small intestine. Humans are the only known host for this parasite. Infection is typically acquired by the ingestion of oocysts in food or water contaminated with the feces of infected humans (fecal-oral mode of transmission).

Risk Factors

Isosporiasis has a worldwide distribution but is more common in tropical and subtropical regions, particularly in areas with poor sanitation. Endemic areas include Africa, Australia, the Caribbean Islands, Latin America, and Southeast Asia. Males and females are equally susceptible to isosporiasis. The disease can affect both adults and children and can cause severe diarrhea in infants. The exact prevalence of isosporiasis is unknown.

Isosporiasis is more common in persons with acquired immunodeficiency syndrome (AIDS). Reports suggest infection rates of up to 3 percent in persons with AIDS in the United States and of 8 to 20 percent in persons with AIDS in Haiti and Africa; these rates, however, may be underestimated. Isosporiasis has also been reported in persons with lymphoma and leukemia and in recipients of renal and liver transplants.

SYMPTOMS

The incubation period ranges from three to fourteen days. Clinical manifestations may include a variety of symptoms, including profuse diarrhea with watery, nonbloody, foamy, mucus-containing, offensive-smelling diarrhea (suggestive of a malabsorption process); cramping abdominal pain; vomiting; malaise; anorexia; weight loss; and low-grade fever. In protracted cases, steatorrhea (an excess of fat in the feces) may occur. Clinical presentation may mimic inflammatory bowel disease and irritable bowel syndrome. Complications are rare and include dehydration, hemorrhagic colitis, and disseminated extraintestinal disease.

In immunocompetent persons, the disease is usually self-limiting within two to three weeks. Occasionally, chronic illness occurs in infants or in otherwise healthy adults. In persons with immune dysfunction, especially AIDS, isosporiasis can persist for months and years, or it can persist indefinitely and can be a life-threatening diarrheal illness.

SCREENING AND DIAGNOSIS

Diagnosis is made by appropriate staining techniques and by microscopic examination of the stool specimen for ova. Routine laboratory tests are not diagnostic. However, peripheral eosinophilia may be a clue to infection because mild peripheral eosinophilia is found in one-half of infected persons.

TREATMENT AND THERAPY

Oral cotrimoxazole (sulfamethoxazole at 800 milligrams [mg] and trimethoprim at 160 mg) is the drug of choice (four times daily for one to four weeks). This treatment ameliorates the diarrhea and eliminates the parasite in majority of cases. In persons who cannot take sulfonamides, pyrimethamine with folinic acid or ciprofloxacin may be used. Persons with AIDS who develop isosporiasis may need lifelong suppressive treatment with cotrimoxazole. Only those persons with chronic isosporiasis that is associated with severe dehydration should require continued inpatient care.

PREVENTION AND OUTCOMES

Because isosporiasis is typically spread by ingesting contaminated food or water, preventive measures include improved personal hygiene and sanitation to eliminate possible fecal-oral transmission from food, water, and environmental surfaces. Appropriate isolation measures may help in preventing transmission because the shedding of oocysts may last for weeks.

Katia Marazova, M.D., Ph.D.

FURTHER READING

Farthing, Michael J. G. "Treatment Options for the Eradication of Intestinal Protozoa." *Nature Clinical Practice Gastroenterology and Hepatology* 3 (2006): 436-445.

Goodgame, Richard W. "Understanding Intestinal Spore-Forming Protozoa: Cryptosporidia, Microsporidia, Isospora, and Cyclospora." *Annals of Internal Medicine* 124 (1996): 429-441.

Marshall, M. M., et al. "Waterborne Protozoan Pathogens." *Clinical Microbiology Reviews* 10 (1997): 67-85.

Minnaganti, Venkat R. "Isosporiasis." Available at http://emedicine.medscape.com/article/219776-overview.

Ortega, Ynes. "Food- and Waterborne Protozoan Parasites." In *Foodborne Pathogens: Microbiology and Molecular Biology*, edited by Pina M. Fratamico, Arun K. Bhunia, and James L. Smith. Norwich, England: Caister Academic Press, 2005.

WEB SITES OF INTEREST

American Gastroenterological Association
http://www.gastro.org

Global Health Council
http://www.globalhealth.org/infectious_diseases

U.S. Department of Agriculture: Food Safety and Inspection Service
http://www.fsis.usda.gov

See also: Amebic dysentery; Antiparasitic drugs: Types; Cryptosporidiosis; Diagnosis of protozoan diseases; Enteritis; Fecal-oral route of transmission; Food-borne illness and disease; *Giardia*; Giardiasis; Intestinal and stomach infections; Norovirus infection; Parasitic diseases; Peritonitis; Prevention of protozoan diseases; Protozoa: Classification and types; Protozoan diseases; Sexually transmitted diseases (STDs); Soilborne illness and disease; Treatment of protozoan diseases; Waterborne illness and disease.

J

Japanese encephalitis

CATEGORY: Diseases and conditions
ANATOMY OR SYSTEM AFFECTED: Brain, central nervous system

DEFINITION

Japanese encephalitis is a mosquito-borne virus that leads to swelling of the brain. It can affect the central nervous system and cause severe complications, even death.

CAUSES

Japanese encephalitis is caused by the bite of a mosquito infected with the virus.

RISK FACTORS

The factors that increase the chance of being exposed to Japanese encephalitis include living or traveling in certain rural parts of Asia. According to the Centers for Disease Control and Prevention, outbreaks of Japanese encephalitis have occurred in China, Korea, Japan, Taiwan, and Thailand. These countries have controlled the disease through vaccinations. Other countries that still have periodic epidemics include Vietnam, Cambodia, Myanmar, India, Nepal, and Malaysia. Also, laboratory workers who might be exposed to the virus are at high risk for developing Japanese encephalitis.

SYMPTOMS

Symptoms of Japanese encephalitis, which usually appear five to fifteen days after the bite of an infected mosquito, include agitation, brain damage, chills, coma, confusion, convulsions (especially in infants), fever, headache, nausea, neck stiffness, paralysis, tiredness, tremors, and vomiting.

SCREENING AND DIAGNOSIS

A doctor will ask about symptoms and medical history and will perform a physical exam. Tests may include blood tests to look for antibodies, a magnetic resonance imaging (MRI) scan (a scan that uses radio waves and a powerful magnet to produce detailed computer images), a computed tomography (CT) scan (a detailed X-ray picture that identifies abnormalities of fine tissue structure), and cerebrospinal fluid tests.

TREATMENT AND THERAPY

Because there is no specific treatment for Japanese encephalitis, care is concentrated on treating specific symptoms and complications.

PREVENTION AND OUTCOMES

A Japanese encephalitis vaccine is recommended for people who live or travel in certain rural parts of Asia and for laboratory workers who are at risk of exposure to the virus. Also, to protect against mosquito bites and to prevent the disease, one should remain in well-screened areas, wear clothes that cover most of the body, and use on skin and clothing those insect repellents that contain up to 30 percent NN-diethyl metatoluamide (DEET).

Krisha McCoy, M.S.;
reviewed by David L. Horn, M.D., FACP

FURTHER READING

Booss, John, Margaret Esiri, and Margaret M. Esin, eds. *Viral Encephalitis in Humans*. Washington, D.C.: ASM Press, 2003.

Centers for Disease Control and Prevention. "Japanese Encephalitis." Available at http://www.cdc.gov.

EBSCO Publishing. *DynaMed: Japanese Encephalitis*. Available through http://www.ebscohost.com/dynamed.

Goddard, Jerome. *Physician's Guide to Arthropods of Medical Importance*. 4th ed. Boca Raton, Fla.: CRC Press, 2003.

Marquardt, William C., ed. *Biology of Disease Vectors*. 2d ed. New York: Academic Press/Elsevier, 2005.

National Institute of Neurological Disorders and Stroke. "Meningitis and Encephalitis Fact Sheet." Available at http://www.ninds.nih.gov.

Peters, C. J. "Infections Caused by Arthropod- and

Rodent-Borne Viruses." In *Harrison's Principles of Internal Medicine*, edited by Anthony Fauci et al. 17th ed. New York: McGraw-Hill, 2008.

United Nations International Children's Emergency Fund. "Vaccine Is Key to Preventing Outbreaks of Japanese Encephalitis." Available at http://www.unicef.org/infobycountry/india_28555.html.

WEB SITES OF INTEREST

Encephalitis Society
http://www.encephalitis.info

National Center for Emerging and Zoonotic Infectious Diseases
http://www.cdc.gov/ncezid

Public Health Agency of Canada
http://www.phac-aspc.gc.ca

U.S. Department of State, International Travel
http://travel.state.gov/travel

See also: Arthropod-borne illness and disease; Bacterial meningitis; Eastern equine encephalitis; Encephalitis; Encephalitis vaccine; Insect-borne illness and disease; Mosquito-borne viral encephalitis; Mosquitoes and infectious disease; Sleeping nets; Sleeping sickness; Subacute sclerosing panencephalitis; Vectors and vector control; Viral infections; West Nile virus.

Jock itch

CATEGORY: Diseases and conditions
ANATOMY OR SYSTEM AFFECTED: Skin
ALSO KNOWN AS: Tinea cruris

DEFINITION

Jock itch is a fungal infection of the skin on the groin, upper inner thighs, or buttocks. It most commonly occurs in hot, humid conditions. Doctors often refer to jock itch as tinea cruris.

CAUSES

Jock itch is caused by common fungal organisms that grow best in warm, moist areas. Jock itch can affect women but most commonly affects men, especially men who perspire heavily. The fungus that causes jock

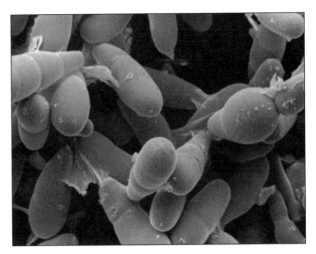

The fungus Epidermophyton floccosum, *which causes tinea cruris, or jock itch.*

itch most often results from wearing wet, damp, or unlaundered clothing (such as underwear or an athletic supporter); sharing towels that are infected with jock itch fungus; and infrequent showering, especially after exercising or perspiring heavily from work.

RISK FACTORS

Risk factors for jock itch include hot, humid conditions; heavy perspiration; obesity; tight clothing; wearing clothes, especially underwear or athletic supporters, that have not been cleaned; changing underwear infrequently; infrequent showering; sharing towels or clothing with other people; using public showers or locker rooms; and having an immune system disorder.

SYMPTOMS

Jock itch causes a chafed, itchy, sometimes painful rash in the groin, upper inner thigh, or buttock. The rash is usually red, tan, or brown; usually defined clearly at the edges; and often slightly scaly.

SCREENING AND DIAGNOSIS

Jock itch often can be diagnosed based on the appearance and location of the rash. However, other skin problems may look like jock itch. If uncertain of the diagnosis, one should contact a doctor, who will ask about symptoms and medical history and perform a physical exam. In some cases, the doctor will order a lab test of the infected skin area. Testing usually consists of a skin scraping that can be viewed under a microscope or cultured.

TREATMENT AND THERAPY

Over-the-counter antifungal creams can usually treat jock itch. Creams or lotions work better on jock itch than do sprays. In severe or persistent cases, a doctor may prescribe stronger creams or oral medication. One should use the prescription for the entire time that the doctor recommends. This will help prevent recurrence of the rash. If the rash does not resolve within a month of treatment, one should contact the doctor.

Antifungal creams for jock itch include miconazole, clotrimazole, econazole, oxiconazole (Oxistat), keto-conazole, terbinafine (Lamisil), tolnaftate, ciclopirox (Penlac), haloprogin (Halotex), naftifine (Naftin), and undecylenic acid. While all these medications can effectively treat jock itch, terbinafine may lead to a more rapid cure than some of the others. It is also more expensive than most of the foregoing medications. Tolnaftate and undecylenic acid may be less effective than some of the other medications, but as generics, they are generally among the least expensive treatments available. Creams are usually applied twice daily for two to four weeks. One should follow the instructions given on the package or by the pharmacist or physician.

One should not use antifungal creams that are recommended specifically for athlete's foot. These creams may be too harsh for the groin. In some cases, over-the-counter antifungal creams may not work or effectively treat the rash. In these cases, the doctor can prescribe a stronger antifungal cream.

If the jock itch rash begins to ooze, one should contact the doctor. This symptom may indicate that the rash could be secondarily infected with bacteria. If the doctor confirms that it is infected, he or she may prescribe an antibiotic.

PREVENTION AND OUTCOMES

To help prevent jock itch and its recurrence, one should shower regularly and shower soon after exercising or perspiring heavily. After showering, one should dry the groin area thoroughly and apply absorbent powder to help keep the groin area dry; wear loose-fitting, breathable clothing; wear cotton underwear; avoid wearing clothing that chafes the groin; always launder clothing, such as underwear and athletic supporters; avoid sharing towels or clothing with others; avoid wearing wet swimsuits for long periods of time; and avoid storing damp clothing in a locker or in a gym bag.

Rick Alan; reviewed by John C. Keel, M.D.

FURTHER READING

American Academy of Family Physicians. "Tinea Infections: Athlete's Foot, Jock Itch, and Ringworm." Available at http://www.aafp.org/afp/980700ap/980700b.html.
Berger, T. G. "Dermatologic Disorders." In *Current Medical Diagnosis and Treatment 2011*, edited by Stephen J. McPhee and Maxine A. Papadakis. 50th ed. New York: McGraw-Hill Medical, 2011.
Fleischer, Alan B., Jr. *The Clinical Management of Itching.* New York: Parthenon, 2000.
Nadalo, D., et al. "What Is the Best Way to Treat Tinea Cruris?" *Journal of Family Practice* 55, no. 3 (2006): 256-258.
Porter, Robert S., et al., eds. *The Merck Manual Home Health Handbook.* 3d ed. Whitehouse Station, N.J.: Merck Research Laboratories, 2009.
Richardson, Malcolm D., and Elizabeth M. Johnson. *The Pocket Guide to Fungal Infection.* 2d ed. Malden, Mass.: Blackwell, 2006.

WEB SITES OF INTEREST

American Academy of Dermatology
http://www.aad.org

American Academy of Family Physicians
http://familydoctor.org

Canadian Dermatology Association
http://www.dermatology.ca

DoctorFungus.org
http://www.doctorfungus.org

See also: Antifungal drugs: Mechanisms of action; Antifungal drugs: Types; Athlete's foot; Chromoblastomycosis; Diagnosis of fungal infections; Fungal infections; Fungi: Classification and types; Men and infectious disease; Onychomycosis; Prevention of fungal infections; Ringworm; Skin infections; Tinea capitis; Tinea corporis; Tinea versicolor; Treatment of fungal infections; *Trichophyton.*

Joint infections. *See* Prosthetic joint infections.

K

Kaposi's sarcoma

CATEGORY: Diseases and conditions
ANATOMY OR SYSTEM AFFECTED: Blood, lymphatic system, mouth, nose, skin, throat

DEFINITION

Kaposi's sarcoma (KS), first described by the Hungarian dermatologist Moritz Kaposi in 1872, is a cancer of the endothelium of lymphatic and blood vessels. It commonly manifests as a series of lesions under the skin and in the lining of the mouth, nose, and throat. The lesions appear as purple, red, or brown blotches. KS can also result in lesions of the gastrointestinal tract, lungs, and liver.

There are several types of KS, which are defined by the population affected: classic KS, which is seen primarily in older men of Mediterranean, Eastern European, or Middle Eastern origin; epidemic KS, which is seen in persons with acquired immunodeficiency syndrome (AIDS); African KS, which is endemic to equatorial Africa and affects mostly men under age forty years; Iatrogenic or transplant-associated KS, which is seen in immune-suppressed persons who have had transplants; and non-epidemic-related KS, a rarer type of KS that is seen in men who test negative for human immunodeficiency virus (HIV) and who have sex with men.

CAUSES

Kaposi's sarcoma is caused by the human herpesvirus-8 (HHV-8), which is also known as Kaposi's sarcoma-associated herpesvirus (KSHV). Approximately 1 to 5 percent of the U.S. population carries the virus.

RISK FACTORS

The greatest risk factor in developing KS is being HHV-8 positive (and, thus, immunosuppressed). Most cases do not progress to KS unless the carrier is also immunosuppressed because of HIV infection (persons who are HIV-positive have about a 50 percent chance of developing KS), organ transplantation (iatrogenic KS),

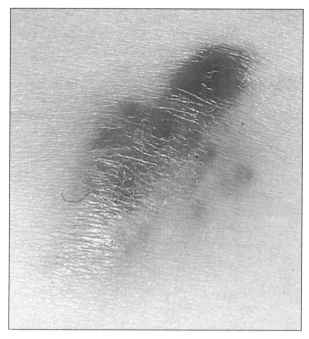

A Kaposi's sarcoma lesion on a person with acquired immunodeficiency syndrome, or AIDS. (SIU School of Medicine)

or aging (classic KS). The HHV-8 virus is sexually transmitted, but virus titers are highest in saliva and may be transmitted through deep kissing.

SYMPTOMS

The appearance of colored skin blotches is the typical KS symptom. The skin form may cause edema, especially of the legs, because of lymphatic blockage. Shortness of breath is found in cases involving the lungs. Cases involving the gastrointestinal (GI) system will show weight loss, nausea, vomiting, and rectal bleeding.

SCREENING AND DIAGNOSIS

A skin examination for typical KS lesions and a sexual history is the most common method of diagnosis. Cytological examination of a skin biopsy can confirm diagnosis. For lung involvement, a doctor will order X rays and a bronchoscopy with biopsy. Suspected GI cases are checked through occult blood testing and a rectal examination, followed by an endoscopy and a biopsy to confirm the GI diagnosis.

TREATMENT AND THERAPY

Treatment for KS focuses on the underlying immune deficiency. In persons with HIV/AIDS, treatment will include highly active antiretroviral therapy (HAART), in which three or more anti-HIV drugs are used simultaneously. KS skin lesions are reduced and may disappear. In persons who have received a transplant, an effective treatment is to reduce the level of immune suppressive drugs already being taken by the transplant recipient. Surgery is possible when only a few small lesions are present, and often, the doctor will order cryosurgery.

Local treatment with alitretinoin has good results for some persons. Intralesion injection of chemotherapy agents, such as vinblastine, has also been used. When widespread lesions are present, systemic chemotherapy can be employed with liposomal anthracyclines (doxorubicin or daunorubicin). Other agents (bleomycin, etoposide, vincristine, vinblastine, paclitaxel, and vinorelbine) may also be used. Electron-beam radiation therapy has been effective on facial lesions. Experimental treatments include angiogenesis inhibitors and interferon alpha.

PREVENTION AND OUTCOMES

Avoiding HIV infection is the most effective way to prevent the development of KS. Preventive methods include maintaining a strong and healthy immune system, practicing safer sex (such as using condoms during sexual intercourse) or abstaining from sex, and avoiding intravenous drug use, especially if it involves using shared needles.

Ralph R. Meyer, Ph.D.

FURTHER READING

Brown, Elizabeth E., et al. "Virologic, Hematologic, and Immunologic Risk Factors for Classic Kaposi Sarcoma." *Cancer* 107, no. 9 (2006): 2282-2290.

Di Lorenzo, Giuseppe, et al. "Management of AIDS-Related Kaposi's Sarcoma." *Lancet Oncology* 8 (2007): 167-176.

Galanda, Claudia D., ed. *AIDS-Related Opportunistic Infections.* New York: Nova Biomedical Books, 2009.

Ganem, Don. "KSHV Infection and the Pathogenesis of Kaposi's Sarcoma." *Annual Review of Pathology* 1 (2006): 273-296.

Murphy, Kenneth, Paul Travers, and Mark Walport. *Janeway's Immunobiology.* 7th ed. New York: Garland Science, 2008.

Parker, James N., and Philip M. Parker, eds. *The Official Patient's Sourcebook on Kaposi's Sarcoma.* San Diego, Calif.: Icon Health, 2003.

WEB SITES OF INTEREST

AIDSinfo
http://aidsinfo.nih.gov

American Cancer Society
http://www.cancer.org

American Social Health Association
http://www.ashastd.org

National Cancer Institute
http://www.cancer.gov/cancertopics/types/aids

See also: AIDS; Antiviral drugs: Types; Autoimmune disorders; Blood-borne illness and disease; Contagious diseases; Herpesviridae; Herpesvirus infections; HIV; HIV vaccine; Iatrogenic infections; Men and infectious disease; Opportunistic infections; Saliva and infectious disease; Sexually transmitted diseases (STDs); Skin infections; Viral infections.

Kawasaki disease

CATEGORY: Diseases and conditions
ANATOMY OR SYSTEM AFFECTED: Arteries, blood vessels, immune system, lymph nodes, skin
ALSO KNOWN AS: Kawasaki syndrome, mucocutaneous lymph node syndrome

DEFINITION

Kawasaki disease (KD) is a rare childhood disease that causes inflammation of the blood vessels. First described by Japan's Tomisaku Kawasaki in 1967, the disease occurs worldwide. All arteries are affected, including coronary arteries, which send blood to the heart muscle. KD is an autoimmune disease, and it usually involves the skin, lymph nodes, and the membranes inside the throat, mouth, and nose.

CAUSES

Scientists do not know what causes KD, but they speculate that it may be caused by a virus, a bacterial infection, or even toxins. It occurs mostly during early spring and late winter. It affects boys, mostly, and girls age two to five years. KD affects the heart and the walls of blood vessels and causes inflammation.

RISK FACTORS

The risk factors vary, but, in addition to higher rates for boys, KD is more likely in persons of Asian descent and persons of all ethnic backgrounds living in Asian countries.

SYMPTOMS

Symptoms of KD range from fever and rash to inflammation of the mouth, lips, and throat. Other symptoms include swollen lymph glands, redness and irritation of the whites of the eyes, and peeling skin. A high fever can last five days to two weeks.

SCREENING AND DIAGNOSIS

The disease can be difficult to diagnose. There are no tests that screen for the disease, so diagnosis comes after other diseases are ruled out. A doctor will order blood and urine tests and may order an echocardiography, which is the most useful tool to monitor potential coronary artery abnormalities.

TREATMENT AND THERAPY

There are some types of medicines helpful in treating symptoms of KD. For example, aspirin may be helpful in treating an associated high fever, especially in children, who must begin an aspirin regimen as soon as they exhibit a high fever. The goal is to lower the fever and inflammation as quickly as possible to prevent heart damage. High doses of aspirin can be used also to prevent clots in the arteries.

An immune protein called gammaglobulin, which is given intravenously (through a vein), helps lower the risk of coronary problems. About 25 percent of children develop heart disease if treatment is delayed or not prescribed.

PREVENTION AND OUTCOMES

There is no known way to prevent this disorder. Doctors and scientists continue to study the long-term implications of this disease.

Marvin L. Morris, M.P.A.

FURTHER READING

Anderson, M. S., et al. "Erythrocyte Sedimentation Rate and C-reactive Protein Discrepancy and High Prevalence of Coronary Artery Abnormalities in Kawasaki Disease." *Pediatric Infectious Disease Journal* 20 (2001): 698-702.

Hoffman, Gary S., and Cornelia M. Weyland, eds. *Inflammatory Diseases of Blood Vessels.* New York: Marcel Decker, 2002.

"Kawasaki Disease." In *Nelson Essentials of Pediatrics,* edited by Karen J. Marcdante et al. 6th ed. Philadelphia: Saunders/Elsevier, 2011.

Parker, James N., and Philip M. Parker. *Kawasaki Disease: A Bibliography, Medical Dictionary, and Annotated Research Guide to Internet References.* San Diego, Calif.: Icon Health, 2004.

Wooditch, A. C., and S. C. Aronoff. "Effect of Initial Corticosteroid Therapy on Cononary Artery Aneurysm Formation in Kawasaki Disease: A Meta-analysis of 862 Children." *Pediatrics* 116 (2005): 989-995.

WEB SITES OF INTEREST

American Academy of Pediatrics
http://www.healthychildren.org

Genetic and Rare Diseases Information Center
http://rarediseases.info.nih.gov/gard

National Heart, Lung, and Blood Institute
http://www.nhlbi.nih.gov

See also: Autoimmune disorders; Children and infectious disease; Inflammation.

Keratitis

CATEGORY: Diseases and conditions
ANATOMY OR SYSTEM AFFECTED: Eyes, vision

DEFINITION

Keratitis is the inflammation of the cornea. There are many forms of keratitis, including acanthamoeba, dendritic, diffuse lamellar, disciform, exposure, filamentary, fungal, herpetic, microbial, neurotrophic, punctate, rosacea, sclerosing, and superficial punctate. Keratitis sicca is also known as dry eye syndrome.

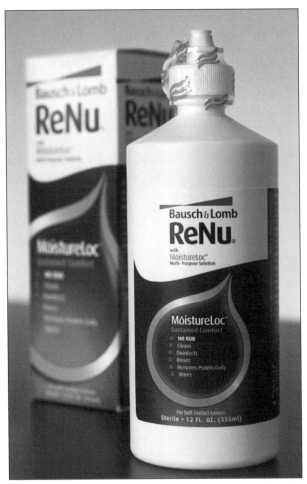

The contact lens solution ReNu was recalled in 2006 after an outbreak of eye infections with the fungus Fusarium *keratitis.* (AP/Wide World Photos)

CAUSES

Causative organisms involved in keratitis include bacteria, fungi, viruses, and acanthamoeba. Bacterial species that have frequently been associated with this disease include *Staphylococcus aureus, S. epidermidis, Streptococcus pneumoniae, S. viridans, Propionibacterium* sp., *Mycobacterium* sp., *Pseudomonas aeruginosa, Serratia marcescens, Proteus mirabilis, Moraxella* sp., and *Haemophilus influenzae.*

RISK FACTORS

The following are some of the more important factors that can increase the likelihood of developing keratitis: contact lens wear, previous ocular surgery, ocular trauma, ocular surface disease, corneal epithe-lial abnormalities, and systemic conditions such as diabetes and malnourishment.

SYMPTOMS

The typical symptoms of keratitis include blurred vision, photophobia, ocular pain, foreign body sensation, redness, tearing, and discharge.

SCREENING AND DIAGNOSIS

A detailed medical history is critical to achieve an accurate diagnosis. This history should include ocular symptoms, previous contact lens wear, systemic diseases, and current medications. The physical examination involves an assessment of visual acuity, a thorough external examination, and slit-lamp biomicroscopy. Smears and cultures can be useful in cases that involve a corneal infiltrate, that are chronic in nature or unresponsive to traditional broad spectrum antibiotic therapy, or that have clinical features that indicate amebic, fungal, or mycobacterial keratitis.

TREATMENT AND THERAPY

Some of the common agents used to treat bacterial keratitis include cefazolin, tobramycin, gentamicin, fluoroquinolones (such as besifloxacin, ciprofloxacin, gatifloxacin, levofloxacin, and moxifloxacin), ceftazidime, ceftriaxone, amikacin, carithromycin, azithromycin, sulfacetamide, and trimethoprim/sulfamethoxazole. Alternative delivery forms such as ointments and collagen shields can be used to enhance drug delivery of the chosen antibiotic. Severe cases of keratitis can benefit from a loading dose (every five to fifteen minutes for the first one to three hours) followed by frequent administration (every thirty to sixty minutes). Patients suffering from keratitis sicca are frequently treated with one or more of the following agents: artificial tears, cyclosporine, corticosteroids, or systemic omega-3 fatty acids.

PREVENTION AND OUTCOMES

Minimizing a person's exposure to certain risk factors may reduce the likelihood of this eye infection. One should be educated in proper contact lens care and about the risks associated with overnight wear of contact lenses. The risk of ocular trauma can be reduced through the use of protective eye wear. Ocular surface disease should be treated with agents such as artificial tears or cyclosporine.

Julie Y. Crider, Ph.D.

FURTHER READING

Awwad, Shady T., et al. "Updates in Acanthamoeba Keratitis." *Eye and Contact Lens* 33 (2007): 1-8.

Johnson, Gordon J., et al., eds. *The Epidemiology of Eye Disease.* 2d ed. New York: Oxford University Press, 2003.

Mueller, J. B., et al. "Ocular Infection and Inflammation." *Emergency Medicine Clinics of North America* 26 (2008): 57.

Parker, James N., and Philip M. Parker, eds. *The Official Patient's Sourcebook on Keratitis.* San Diego, Calif.: Icon Health, 2002.

Riordan-Eva, Paul, and John P. Whitcher. *Vaughan and Asbury's General Ophthalmology.* 17th ed. New York: Lange Medical Books/McGraw-Hill, 2007.

Schlech, Barry A. "New Anti-infectives for Ophthalmology." In *Ocular Therapeutics: Eye on New Discoveries*, edited by Thomas Yorio, Abbot F. Clark, and Martin B. Wax. New York: Academic Press, 2008.

Sutton, Amy L., ed. *Eye Care Sourcebook: Basic Consumer Health Information About Eye Care and Eye Disorders.* 3d ed. Detroit: Omnigraphics, 2008.

WEB SITES OF INTEREST

American Academy of Ophthalmology
http://www.aao.org

American Optometric Association
http://www.aoanet.org

Canadian Ophthalmological Society
http://www.eyesite.ca

National Foundation for Eye Research
http://www.nfer.org

See also: Acanthamoeba infection; Bacterial infections; Conjunctivitis; Eye infections; Hordeola; Inflammation; Ophthalmia neonatorum; Trachoma.

Ketolide antibiotics

CATEGORY: Treatment

DEFINITION

Ketolide antibiotics are semisynthetic derivates of erythromycin A and members of the macrolide class of antibiotics. Broadly, ketolides are inhibitors of bacterial protein synthesis.

MECHANISM OF ACTION

The inhibition of bacterial protein synthesis by ketolides is produced though reversible binding close to the peptidyl transferase site of the 50S ribosomal subunit, specifically the II and V domains of the 23S rRNA (ribosomal ribonucleic acid). The binding affinity is reported to be ten to one hundred times greater than that seen with erythromycin. One of the most notable chemical structural changes between macrolides and ketolides is the absence of an L-cladinose from the 3 position of the erythonolide ring, which functionally is important in increasing the compound's acid stability. Additionally, in its place, a keto-functional group is formed. Like macrolides, ketolides exhibit bacteriostatic activity, although bactericidal activity has been achieved at higher levels. Ketolides that are being investigated, including cethromycin (ABT-773), utilize various other chemical modifications.

SUSCEPTIBLE AND NONSUSCEPTIBLE ORGANISMS

Ketolides were introduced as an alternative to macrolides in the treatment of respiratory tract infections. The increasing use of macrolides (including azithromycin, erythromycin, and clarithromycin) and the subsequent resistance to macrolide antibiotics, coupled with increasing resistance to other antibiotics such as beta-lactams, has highlighted the need for new antibiotics to treat these resistant strains.

Common bacteria responsible for respiratory infections against which ketolides are active include nonresistant and resistant gram-positive aerobic bacteria (*Streptococcus pneumoniae*, *S. pyogenes*, Viridans group streptococci, *Staphylococcus aureus*, and coagulase-negative staphylococci). Gram-negative bacteria against which ketolides are active include *Haemophilus influenzae*, *Moraxella catarrhalis*, *Chlamydophila pneumoniae*, *Legionella pneumoniae*, *Mycoplasma pneumoniae*, *Neisseria* species, *Bordetella pertussis*, and *Ureaplasma urealyticum*. Organisms against which ketolides are not active include *Pseudomonas aeruginosa*, Enterobacteriacae, and *Clostridium difficile*.

CLINICAL SIGNIFICANCE

The only ketolide approved by the U.S. Food and Drug Administration is telithromycin (Ketek). Telithromycin is approved for the treatment of mild-to-moderate community acquired pneumonia caused by susceptible strains of *S. pneumoniae* (including resistant strains), *H. influenzae*, *C. pneumoniae*, *M. catarrhalis*, and *M. pneumoniae*. Telithromycin carries a black-box warning that it should not be used in persons with myasthenia gravis because of reports of fatal and life-threatening respiratory failure. To slow the growth of resistant microorganisms, ketolides should be reserved for persons in whom susceptible strains are known or presumed.

IMPACT

In an era of increasing antibiotic use and increasing patterns of resistance, antibiotics with the ability to target microorganisms that are resistant to older antibiotics are critical. Respiratory tract infections are a time and health burden on both patients and the medical system. Antibiotics such as ketolides provide an additional tool for practitioners to combat resistant bacteria.

Allison C. Bennett, Pharm.D.

FURTHER READING

Sanford, Jay P., et al. *The Sanford Guide to Antimicrobial Therapy.* 18th ed. Sperryville, Va.: Antimicrobial Therapy, 2010.

Walsh, Christopher. *Antibiotics: Actions, Origins, Resistance.* Washington, D.C.: ASM Press, 2003.

Zhanel, George. "The Ketolides: A Critical Review." *Drugs* 62 (2002): 1771-1804.

Zhanel, George, and Daryl Hoban.. "Ketolides in the Treatment of Respiratory Infections." *Expert Opinion on Pharmacotherapy* 3 (2002): 277-297.

Zuckerman, Jerry, Fozia Qamar, and Batholomew Bono. "Macrolides, Ketolides, and Glycylcyclines: Azithromycin, Clarithromycin, Telithromycin, Tigecycline." *Infectious Disease Clinics of North America* 23 (2009): 997-1026.

WEB SITES OF INTEREST

eMedicineHealth: Antibiotics
http://www.emedicinehealth.com/antibiotics

Todar's Online Textbook of Bacteriology
http://www.textbookofbacteriology.net

See also: Alliance for the Prudent Use of Antibiotics; Aminoglycoside antibiotics; Antibiotic-associated colitis;

Antibiotics: Types; Bacteria: Classification and types; Bacterial infections; Bacteriology; Cephalosporin antibiotics; Drug resistance; Glycopeptide antibiotics; Lipopeptide antibiotics; Macrolide antibiotics; Methicillin-resistant staph infection; Microbiology; Oxazolidinone antibiotics; Penicillin antibiotics; Quinolone antibiotics; Tetracycline antibiotics; Treatment of bacterial infections.

Kidney infection

CATEGORY: Diseases and conditions
ANATOMY OR SYSTEM AFFECTED: Genitourinary tract, kidneys
ALSO KNOWN AS: Pyelonephritis

DEFINITION

Kidney infection occurs when there is a bacterial infection in one or both kidneys. The kidneys remove waste (in the form of urine) from the body. They also balance the water and electrolyte content in the blood by filtering salt and water.

CAUSES

Kidney infection may be caused by, most commonly, a bladder infection that was not treated or inadequately treated; conditions that slow the flow of urine from the bladder, such as an enlarged prostate or kidney stones; having a cystoscopy done to examine the bladder; surgery of the urinary tract; use of a catheter to drain urine from the bladder; and, rarely, bacteria from another part of the body that has entered the kidneys.

RISK FACTORS

The factors that increase the chance of developing kidney infection include sexual activity; pregnancy; diabetes; birth disorder of the urinary tract, including vesicoureteral reflux; blockage of the urinary tract, including tumors, an enlarged prostate gland, kidney stones, or a catheter or stent placed in the urinary tract; polycystic kidneys; sickle cell anemia; previous kidney transplant; and a weakened immune system. Also, girls and women are at greater risk for kidney infection.

SYMPTOMS

Symptoms include pain in the abdomen, lower back, side, or groin; frequent urination; urgent urination

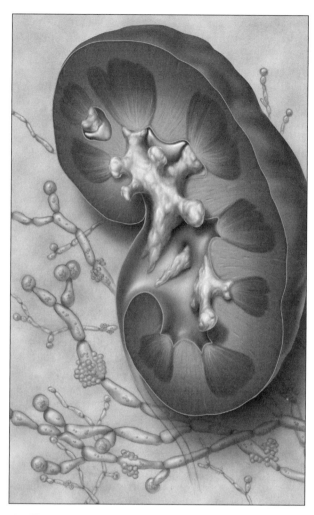

An illustration of a kidney infected with Candida fungi.

that produces only a small amount of urine; sensation of a full bladder, even after urination; burning pain with urination; fever and chills; nausea and vomiting; pus and blood in the urine; and loss of appetite.

SCREENING AND DIAGNOSIS

A doctor will ask about symptoms and medical history and will perform a physical exam. Kidney infection is diagnosed with urine tests. The urine is examined for bacteria, white blood cells, blood, and other abnormal elements.

If the infection does not go away after treatment or if the person has had several kidney infections, other tests might be ordered to see if there are problems with the kidney, ureters, and bladder. These tests in-

clude a kidney ultrasound (a test that uses sound waves to examine the kidney); an abdominal computed tomography (CT) scan (a detailed X-ray picture that identifies abnormalities of fine tissue structure); and a voiding cystourethrography (an X ray of the urinary bladder and urethra made after injection with a contrast medium).

TREATMENT AND THERAPY

Kidney infections are treated with antibiotics. If the infection is not treated correctly or is left untreated, the condition can lead to septicemia (a blood infection that has spread throughout the body), chronic infection, scarring of the kidney, or permanent kidney damage. In some cases, the infected person may need to be hospitalized and may need to receive antibiotics intravenously.

PREVENTION AND OUTCOMES

Because kidney infection is often a complication of a bladder infection, the chance of getting a bladder infection can be lessened by drinking increased amounts of fluids (about eight to ten 8-ounce glasses per day); this includes drinking cranberry juice, which may help prevent bladder infection too. Other preventive measures are to practice good hygiene, to urinate when the need arises, and to take showers rather than baths. Women should wipe from the front to the back after using the toilet, should urinate before and after having sex, and should avoid douches and genital deodorant sprays.

Diane Savitsky; reviewed by Adrienne Carmack, M.D.

FURTHER READING

Brenner, Barry M., ed. *Brenner and Rector's The Kidney.* 8th ed. Philadelphia: Saunders/Elsevier, 2008.

Greenberg, Arthur, et al., eds. *Primer on Kidney Diseases.* 4th ed. Philadelphia: Saunders/Elsevier, 2005.

Kiel, Raphael, et al. "Does Cranberry Juice Prevent or Treat Urinary Tract Infection?" *Journal of Family Practice* 52, no. 2 (February, 2003): 154-155.

O'Callaghan, C. A., and Barry M. Brenner. *The Kidney at a Glance.* Malden, Mass.: Blackwell Science, 2000.

Parker, James N., and Philip M. Parker, eds. *The 2002 Official Patient's Sourcebook on Pyelonephritis.* San Diego, Calif.: Icon Health, 2002.

Walsh, Patrick C., et al., eds. *Campbell-Walsh Urology.* 4 vols. 9th ed. Philadelphia: Saunders/Elsevier, 2007.

See also: Acute cystitis; Acute interstitial nephritis; Bacterial infections; Pelvic inflammatory disease; Urethritis; Urinary tract infections.

Koch's postulates

CATEGORY: Epidemiology

DEFINITION

Koch's postulates are a set of experimental guidelines used to determine if a particular microorganism is the causative agent of a particular disease.

HISTORICAL OVERVIEW

In the nineteenth century, Robert Koch, a German physician and bacteriologist, played a significant role in determining the etiology (cause) of an infectious disease. Through his work with *Bacillus anthracis* (the causative agent of anthrax), he linked a specific microorganism to a specific infectious disease. Koch conducted experiments showing that *B. anthracis* was always present in diseased animals, that healthy animals inoculated with the bacterium would develop the disease, and that cultivation of the bacterium in artificial media followed by inoculation resulted in the disease.

Koch also discovered the causative organisms for several other diseases, including tuberculosis and cholera. In describing the etiology of tuberculosis, Koch proposed a set of guidelines for establishing a cause and effect relationship between a given microorganism and a specific disease. These scientific criteria are known as Koch's postulates.

THE POSTULATES

Koch's postulates are a set of four experimental criteria used to establish the etiology of a disease. The first criterion states that the pathogen must be present in all infected persons and absent in all healthy persons. The second criterion states that the pathogen must be isolated from the diseased person and cultivated in the laboratory. The third criterion states that the cultivated pathogen must cause the disease in a healthy person after inoculation. The fourth criterion states that the pathogen must be isolated again from the infected person and identified as identical to the original isolate.

EXCEPTIONS

There are some exceptions to Koch's postulates. Certain pathogens and fastidious microorganisms have complex and unusual growth requirements and can survive only within living host cells. Such microorganisms cannot be cultured on artificial media. Numerous pathogens infect a specific species only while others become transformed in vitro. Some infectious diseases have unclear origins while others cause multiple disease conditions. Many infections develop from the combined effects of several different microorganisms. Various diseases do not originate from a microorganism and may be the result of poor nutrition, chromosomal abnormality, organ failure, or environmental influences. These exceptions have stimulated the need for modifications to Koch's postulates.

IMPACT

Koch's contributions were invaluable in the advancement of medical microbiology and in the understanding of the nature of a disease. Koch's postulates still provide the essential principles for determining the causative agents of emerging infectious diseases and the basic foundation within which to address disease and public health.

Rose Ciulla-Bohling, Ph.D.

FURTHER READING
Daniel, Wayne W. *Biostatistics: A Foundation for Analysis in the Health Sciences.* 9th ed. Hoboken, N.J.: John Wiley & Sons, 2009.
Engelkirk, Paul G., and Gwendolyn R. W. Burton. *Burton's Microbiology for the Health Sciences.* 8th ed. Baltimore: Lippincott Williams & Wilkins, 2007.

Hardy, Simon P. *Human Microbiology*. New York: Taylor and Francis, 2003.

Murray, Patrick R., Ken S. Rosenthal, and Michael A. Pfaller. *Medical Microbiology*. 6th ed. Philadelphia: Mosby/Elsevier, 2009.

Straus, Eugene, and Alex Straus. *Medical Marvels: The One Hundred Greatest Advances in Medicine*. Amherst, N.Y.: Prometheus Books, 2006.

Tortora, Gerard J., Berdell R. Funke, and Christine L. Case. "Koch's Postulates." In *Microbiology: An Introduction*. 10th ed. San Francisco: Benjamin Cummings, 2010.

WEB SITES OF INTEREST

Association for Professionals in Infection Control and Epidemiology
http://www.knowledgeisinfectious.org

Centers for Disease Control and Prevention
http://www.cdc.gov

Collection of Biostatistics Research Archive
http://biostats.bepress.com/repository

National Institutes of Health
http://www.nih.gov

See also: Bacteriology; Diagnosis of bacterial infections; Diagnosis of viral infections; Epidemiology; Microbiology; Pathogens; Public health; Virology.

Kuru

CATEGORY: Diseases and conditions
ANATOMY OR SYSTEM AFFECTED: Brain, central nervous system
ALSO KNOWN AS: Acquired prion disease, laughing death, transmissible human spongiform encephalopathy

DEFINITION

Kuru is a rare, progressively degenerative, ultimately fatal, chronic, neurological ailment caused by an infectious protein (now called a prion). Scientists initially discovered kuru through studies of cannibalistic rituals of the Fore peoples of Papua New Guinea,

who consumed the brains of dead tribal members. In the Fore language, the word *kuru* meant shaking, but it became associated with the disease because trembling was a characteristic symptom.

Although this brain infection is nonexistent or extremely rare in most countries, it reached epidemic proportions among the Fore in the 1950's and 1960's when more than one thousand deaths occurred (in a population of about eight thousand persons). Deaths increased in the 1970's and 1980's before dramatically declining in the 1990's and the first decade of the twenty-first century.

CAUSES

The cause of kuru was a riddle until researchers, including American physician Daniel Carleton Gajdusek, found that the disease was connected with the cannibalistic burial customs of the Fore and was transmissible to chimpanzees. These discoveries had important implications for such human maladies as Creutzfeldt-Jakob disease and for animal illnesses such as bovine spongiform encephalopathy (so called because of the large holes in infected brains). In 1976, Gajdusek received the Nobel Prize in Physiology or Medicine for his breakthrough discoveries.

In 1997, Stanley B. Prusiner won the Nobel Prize in Physiology or Medicine for his research on infectious proteins, which he called prions (derived from the terms "protein" and "infectious"). This research further deepened understanding of the cause of kuru and other diseases by showing that they were caused by prions. Lacking nucleic acids, prions are unable to reproduce, but they can be transmitted through the ingestion of prion-infected tissue, such as human brain tissue. Another route of transmission is genetic inheritance, thereby distinguishing prions from such infectious agents as viruses.

RISK FACTORS

The riskiest behavior is consuming prion-infected tissue. At the disease's peak, kuru was about eight times more prevalent among women and children than among men, most likely because women were the major consumers of dead brain tissue.

SYMPTOMS

Because of kuru's long incubation period, symptoms can take several months to several years to appear (some researchers extend the period to thirty or fifty years). According to Gajdusek, kuru's symptoms emerge in three main stages. The first or ambulant stage is characterized by excessive fatigue and unsteadiness of stance, speech, and limbs, which are prone to shivering; the second or sedentary stage is distinguished by more extreme tremors, lack of coordination, and deep depression, followed by fits of laughter (kuru is also known as laughing death); the third or terminal stage is marked by the person's inability to sit or stand, by incontinence, and by difficulty swallowing (leading to malnutrition, which often factors into the ultimate cause of death).

SCREENING AND DIAGNOSIS

A doctor (generally a neurologist) will question an infected person and those who know him or her about the onset of symptoms, especially changes in the ability to walk and the slurring of speech. Other indications, such as tremors of the head, trunk, and limbs, will also form part of the diagnosis.

TREATMENT AND THERAPY

Because no treatment for kuru exists and the prognosis is always fatal, the best treatment is supportive care and ameliorative medicines. However, scientist Prusiner believes that a comprehensive understanding of the three-dimensional structure of infectious proteins will lead to anti-gene therapies for persons with prion diseases.

PREVENTION AND OUTCOMES

Kuru can be prevented by not ingesting prion-infested brains.

Robert J. Paradowski, Ph.D.

FURTHER READING

Anderson, Warwick. *The Collectors of Lost Souls: Turning Kuru Scientists into Whitemen.* Baltimore: Johns Hopkins University Press, 2008.

Klitzman, Robert. *The Trembling Mountain: A Personal Account of Kuru, Cannibals, and Disease.* New York: Plenum Press, 2001.

Prusiner, Stanley B., ed. *Prion Biology and Diseases.* 2d ed. Cold Spring Harbor, N.Y.: Cold Spring Harbor Laboratory Press, 2004.

Zigas, Vincent. *Laughing Death: The Untold Story of Kuru.* Clifton, N.J.: Humana Press, 1990.

WEB SITES OF INTEREST

Genetic and Rare Diseases Information Center
http://rarediseases.info.nih.gov/gard

National Organization for Rare Disorders
http://www.rarediseases.org

See also: Creutzfeldt-Jakob disease; Encephalitis; Fatal familial insomnia; Food-borne illness and disease; Gerstmann-Sträussler-Scheinker syndrome; Guillain-Barré syndrome; Iatrogenic infections; Prion diseases; Prions; Progressive multifocal leukoencephalopathy; Subacute sclerosing panencephalitis; Variant Creutzfeldt-Jakob disease.

L

Labyrinthitis

CATEGORY: Diseases and conditions
ANATOMY OR SYSTEM AFFECTED: Auditory system, ears

DEFINITION

Labyrinthitis is an inflammation of the labyrinth in the inner ear. The labyrinth is a system of cavities and canals in the inner ear that affects hearing, balance, and eye movement.

CAUSES

The most common causes of labyrinthitis include viral or bacterial infection. Other causes are head injury, tumor in the brain or head, disease of blood vessels, stroke, nerve problems, and side effects of drugs, including aminoglycoside antibiotics, aspirin, and quinine.

RISK FACTORS

Risk factors for labyrinthitis include current or recent viral infection (especially a respiratory infection), allergies, smoking, drinking too much alcohol, and stress.

SYMPTOMS

The symptoms can range from mild to severe and can last days or weeks. Symptoms are usually temporary but rarely can become permanent. The most common symptoms are vertigo (spinning sensation) and dizziness, and other symptoms include fatigue, nausea and vomiting, hearing loss, involuntary eye movement, and ringing in the ear (tinnitus).

SCREENING AND DIAGNOSIS

A doctor will ask about symptoms and medical history and will perform a physical exam. Initial diagnosis is based on the symptoms and the results of the exam. Tests include an examination of the middle ear for signs of a viral or bacterial infection; hearing tests; an electronystagmogram (a test of eye movement); a magnetic resonance imaging (MRI) scan (a scan that uses radio waves and a powerful magnet to produce detailed computer images); and a computed tomography (CT) scan (a detailed X-ray picture that identifies abnormalities of fine tissue structure).

TREATMENT AND THERAPY

Treatment may include antibiotics (only for bacterial infection); medication to control the symptoms, including antiemetics (to control nausea and vomiting); vestibular suppressants, such as meclizine, to help control loss of balance and dizziness; steroids, in limited situations, to help control inflammation; antiviral medication (such as Acyclovir), which may be prescribed by a physician. Without antibiotic treatment, bacterial labyrinthitis can lead to permanent hearing loss or permanent problems with balance.

Self-care measures include rest and lying still with eyes closed in a darkened room during acute attacks. The patient also should avoid movement, especially sudden movement, as much as possible, and should avoid reading. One can resume normal activities gradually after the symptoms have cleared.

In some cases, nausea and vomiting cannot be controlled. This can result in severe dehydration, which may require hospitalization to receive intravenous fluids. Rarely, labyrinthitis may be caused by a break in the membranes between the middle and inner ear. Surgery to repair the break may be required. If a tumor is causing the condition, surgery may also be needed.

PREVENTION AND OUTCOMES

To reduce the risk of getting labyrinthitis, one should seek prompt treatment for any ear problems or infection, get medical advice on treating respiratory infections, avoid head injury by wearing seat belts and safety helmets, and avoid alcohol. One should take steps to prevent blood vessel disease or stroke by eating a low fat and low cholesterol diet, by not smoking, by treating high blood pressure, by controlling diabetes, and by exercising regularly.

Rick Alan; reviewed by Elie Edmond Rebeiz, M.D., FACS

FURTHER READING

Barkdull, G. C., et al. "Cochlear Microperfusion: Experimental Evaluation of a Potential New Therapy for Severe Hearing Loss Caused by Inflammation." *Otology and Neurotology* 26 (2005): 19-26.

Brandt, Thomas. *Vertigo: Its Multisensory Syndromes.* 2d ed. New York: Springer, 2003.

Ferrari, Mario. *PDxMD Ear, Nose, and Throat Disorders.* Philadelphia: PDxMD, 2003.

Gelfand, Stanley A. *Essentials of Audiology.* 3d ed. New York: Thieme, 2009.

Polensek, S. H. "Labyrinthitis." In *Ferri's Clinical Advisor 2011: Instant Diagnosis and Treatment*, edited by Fred F. Ferri. Philadelphia: Mosby/Elsevier, 2011.

WEB SITES OF INTEREST

Health Canada
http://www.hc-sc.gc.ca

National Library of Medicine
http://www.nlm.nih.gov

Vestibular Disorders Association
http://www.vestibular.org

See also:: Inflammation; Middle-ear infection; Pharyngitis and tonsillopharyngitis; Viral pharyngitis.

Laryngitis

CATEGORY: Diseases and conditions
ANATOMY OR SYSTEM AFFECTED: Larynx, throat, upper respiratory tract

DEFINITION

Laryngitis is swelling of the mucous membrane of the larynx (voice box). This swelling usually involves the vocal cords and leads to hoarseness or even complete loss of voice.

CAUSES

Common causes of laryngitis, hoarseness, or voice loss are upper respiratory tract infection (most often caused by a virus, such as the common cold), irritation caused by voice overuse (overuse by yelling, singing, and speaking loudly for extended periods of time), airborne irritants (includes cigarette smoke, pollen, dust, and mold allergens), and vocal nodules (benign lesions, like calluses, that are caused by thickening of the epithelial tissue of the vocal cords). Other causes of laryngitis are vocal polyps (soft, fluid-filled lesions on the vocal cords, which can be caused by one episode of voice overuse), which can become cancerous, particularly in smokers; infections including tuberculous laryngitis and fungal laryngitis; and gastroesophageal reflux disease, or GERD, in which stomach acid rises up in the esophagus and, in the case of laryngitis, irritates the vocal folds.

Other less common causes of hoarseness or voice loss include functional dysphonia (abnormal use of the vocal mechanisms despite normal anatomy), laryngeal papilloma (growths on the larynx caused by human papilloma viral infection), muscle tension dysphonia (a voice disorder caused by excessive or unequal tension while speaking), Reinke's edema (an accumulation of fluid in the vocal cords, usually associated with smoking), spasmodic dysphonia (a condition resulting in irregular voice breaks), vocal cord paralysis (weakness or immobility of the vocal cords), and side effects from inhaled medications used for asthma.

RISK FACTORS

Risk factors for laryngitis include smoking and exposure to secondhand smoke; excessive use of the voice, as in singing, public speaking, or yelling or screaming; allergies to dust, mold, and pollen; excessive alcohol consumption; respiratory infection; uncontrolled GERD; dehydration; and stress.

SYMPTOMS

Symptoms of laryngitis include hoarseness (raspiness, breathiness, and strain) or loss of voice, changes in volume (loudness) or in pitch (how high or low the voice is), sore throat, and a sensation of a lump in the throat.

SCREENING AND DIAGNOSIS

One should consult a doctor if experiencing hoarseness that has no obvious cause or has lasted more than two to three weeks, has hoarseness with difficulty swallowing or breathing, is coughing up blood, has a lump in the neck, or has throat pain out of proportion to that usually experienced with the common cold. For some of these symptoms, persons should seek emergency medical care, especially if experiencing a complete loss of voice or a severe change in voice lasting more than a few days.

A doctor will ask about symptoms and medical history, will perform a physical exam, and may refer the patient to an otorhinolaryngologist, also called an ear, nose, and throat (ENT) doctor, if the laryngitis does not have an easily identified cause or cure. An ENT doctor will examine the patient's larynx using a flexible, lighted scope that is passed through the nose and down the back of the throat. In some cases, the doctor will place a mirror in the back of the mouth to see the larynx. Under some circumstances, other tests may be indicated to evaluate swallowing mechanisms or other processes related to normal voice functioning.

TREATMENT AND THERAPY

Laryngitis caused by seasonal allergies, cold or flu, or other viral respiratory infections usually resolves within two weeks. To relieve symptoms during this time, one should rest the voice, drink increased amounts of fluids, avoid smoking, take nonprescription pain relievers (such as acetaminophen and ibuprofen) as needed, and try steam inhalation.

Managing underlying illnesses, such as GERD or viral infections, often relieves laryngitis. Surgery may be performed to treat growths on the vocal cords, treat vocal cord paralysis, or treat some other laryngeal disorders. Laryngitis from voice overuse usually resolves within a few days. Voice therapy is often used to treat voice problems, especially those related to vocal overuse. Voice therapy consists of voice education, healthy use of the voice, instruction in proper voice technique and use of the breathing muscles, and the Alexander technique (a method to treat voice impairment by practicing proper breathing and posture).

PREVENTION AND OUTCOMES

Some of the illnesses and disorders that can cause laryngitis are not preventable. However, to prevent and treat mild hoarseness related to laryngitis, the American Academy of Otolaryngology–Head and Neck Surgery recommends that one should quit smoking; avoid secondhand smoke; avoid agents that can dehydrate the body, such as alcohol and caffeine; drink increased amounts of fluids; humidify one's home; avoid acidic or spicy foods if prone to GERD;

avoid using one's voice for too long or too loudly; seek professional voice training; and avoid speaking or singing when one's voice is hoarse.

Laurie LaRusso, M.S., ELS;
reviewed by Rosalyn Carson-DeWitt, M.D.

FURTHER READING

American Academy of Otolaryngology–Head and Neck Surgery. "Fact Sheet: Common Problems That Can Affect Your Voice." Available at http://www.entnet.org/healthinformation/throat.cfm.

Colton, Raymond H., Janina K. Casper, and Rebecca Leonard. *Understanding Voice Problems: A Physiological Perspective for Diagnosis and Treatment.* 3d ed. Philadelphia: Lippincott Williams & Wilkins, 2006.

Icon Health. *Laryngitis: A Medical Dictionary, Bibliography, and Annotated Research Guide to Internet References.* San Diego, Calif.: Author, 2004.

Lustig, L. R., et al. "Common Laryngeal Disorders." In *Current Medical Diagnosis and Treatment 2011*, edited by Stephen J. McPhee and Maxine A. Papadakis. 50th ed. New York: McGraw-Hill Medical, 2011.

Ossoff, Robert H., et al., eds. *The Larynx.* Philadelphia: Lippincott Williams & Wilkins, 2003.

Sataloff, Robert T., ed. *Reflux Laryngitis and Related Disorders.* 3d ed. San Diego, Calif.: Plural, 2006.

WEB SITES OF INTEREST

American Academy of Family Physicians
http://familydoctor.org

American Academy of Otolaryngology–Head and Neck Surgery
http://www.entnet.org

Public Health Agency of Canada
http://www.phac-aspc.gc.ca

See also:: Bronchiolitis; Bronchitis; Common cold; Croup; Epiglottitis; Inflammation; Influenza; Mononucleosis; Nasopharyngeal infections; Pharyngitis and tonsillopharyngitis; Pneumonia; Strep throat; Tuberculosis (TB); Viral infections; Viral pharyngitis; Viral upper respiratory infections.

Lassa fever

CATEGORY: Diseases and conditions
ANATOMY OR SYSTEM AFFECTED: All

DEFINITION

First described in 1969, Lassa fever is a viral hemorrhagic fever endemic to West Africa, principally Nigeria, Sierra Leone, Guinea, and Liberia.

CAUSES

Lassa fever is caused by a strain of Lassa virus, a single-stranded ribonucleic acid (RNA) arenavirus and a member of the family Arenaviridae. The viral reservoir and disease vector is *Mastomys natalensis*, a species of ubiquitous African rodent.

RISK FACTORS

Contact with *Mastomys* rodents in the human settlements they frequent is the primary infection source. Mud-walled huts built directly on the ground offer the rodents easy entry. Once a dwelling is infested with rats, the inhabitants come into contact with the virus-laden excretions of those rats.

Human-to-human contact is also a major risk factor, documented by hospital-based Lassa fever outbreaks. Largely responsible to these outbreaks is poor attention to infection-control measures, such as not reusing syringes. Hospitalized persons represent the severe end of the clinical spectrum, and outbreaks of this kind generally confer high mortality. Household contact with a symptomatic person is also a significant risk factor.

SYMPTOMS

The clinical course of Lassa fever varies from mild illness to severe hemorrhagic disorder, with blood loss too profuse to sustain life. Initially, however, symptoms mirror those of other febrile illnesses, such as influenza.

The striking clinical features of Lassa fever are poorly understood neurologic complications. Sensorineural deafness frequently occurs, most often during convalescence. Hearing may become distorted or characterized by tinnitus, chronic ringing in the ears. Other neurologic symptoms can include involuntary eye movements (nystagmus) and loss of consciousness. Lassa fever also causes neuropsychiatric complications: among them psychosis, hallucinations, and dementia.

SCREENING AND DIAGNOSIS

Given the lack of definitive initial symptoms, Lassa fever requires a laboratory-based diagnosis. Several techniques are available. The indirect fluorescent-antibody (IFA) test, long a mainstay, identifies antibodies in a person's blood serum specific to Lassa virus infection. Diagnosis through IFA is not dependably rapid, however. Enzyme-linked immunosorbent assays have been developed that quantify Lassa virus antigens in the serum of infected persons. This method is rapid and reliable, early in the disease course.

A molecular technique, polymerase chain reaction (PCR), directly identifies Lassa virus RNA in infected cells and in urine. Viral RNA is first transcribed to deoxyribonucleic acid (DNA) by a process called reverse transcription PCR.

TREATMENT AND THERAPY

Ribavirin is a broad-spectrum antiviral drug that significantly reduces the case-fatality rate when given early in the disease course. It is less effective, however, in limiting late-onset neurologic complications. Researchers are looking at potential treatments using alternative antiviral strategies.

PREVENTION AND OUTCOMES

Political instability and sparse economic resources are among the factors that have stood in the way of vaccine development. Meanwhile, instituting standard infection-control measures would help prevent hospital outbreaks. To the extent possible, quarantine would impede the spread of Lassa fever in local areas.

To meet the public health threat that Lassa fever raises in West Africa, the Mano River Union has been established in Sierra Leone, Liberia, and Guinea to provide national and regional surveillance, control, and prevention.

Judith Weinblatt, M.S., M.A.

FURTHER READING

Crawford, Dorothy. *The Invisible Enemy: A Natural History of Viruses*. New York: Oxford University Press, 2000.

Donaldson, Ross I. *The Lassa Ward: One Man's Fight Against One of the World's Deadliest Diseases*. New York: St. Martin's Press, 2009.

Howard, Colin R., ed. *Viral Haemorrhagic Fevers*. Boston: Elsevier, 2005.

Oldstone, Michael B. A. *Viruses, Plagues, and History:*

Past, Present, and Future. New York: Oxford University Press, 2010.

WEB SITES OF INTEREST

American Society of Tropical Medicine and Hygiene
http://www.astmh.org

International Committee on Taxonomy of Viruses
http://www.ictvonline.org

World Health Organization
http://www.who.int

See also:: Bubonic plague; Developing countries and infectious disease; Hantavirus infection; Hemorrhagic fever viral infections; Iatrogenic infections; Plague; Rabies; Rat-bite fever; Rodents and infectious disease; Tropical medicine; Viral infections.

Legionella

CATEGORY: Pathogen
TRANSMISSION ROUTE: Ingestion, inhalation

DEFINITION

Legionella pneumophila, the bacterium that causes Legionnaires' disease, leads to severe pneumonia and is the most commonly known form of *Legionella* disease worldwide.

Taxonomic Classification for *Legionella*

Kingdom: Bacteria
Phylum: Proteobacteria
Order: Gammoproteobacteria
Family: Legionellales
Genus: *Legionella*
Species:
L. pneumophila
L. longbeachae

NATURAL HABITAT AND FEATURES

Legionella are gram-negative rod-shaped bacteria that proliferate in water, mud, streams, and within some aquatic devices, such as decorative water fountains. Whirlpool spas have also been found to harbor *Legionella*, as have air conditioning systems and water heaters. Some forms of *Legionella* are known to infect such amebas as *Acanthamoeba castellanii* or *Hartmanella* species. Several cases of *L. longbeachae* have been identified in potting compost in Scotland. The transmission was believed to occur through the inhalation of droplets from the compost.

When not infecting humans or animals, *Legionella* reside within fresh-water protozoa and amebas, and within biofilm, which is an aggregate of different types of bacteria that link together, as on a water surface. Legionellae have been proven to reproduce with fourteen different types of amebas, two species of protozoa, and one species of slime mold. Legionellae alternate between two states, the reproductive state and the transmissive state.

L. pneumophila thrives best at temperatures ranging from 60° to 107.6° Fahrenheit (20° to 42° Celsius). The incubation period for *Legionella* ranges from two to nineteen days. Most outbreaks occur in warm weather.

PATHOGENICITY AND CLINICAL SIGNIFICANCE

Legionella invades the host lungs, and the microbes are immediately attacked by the host macrophages. However, *Legionella* converts these macrophages into compartments in which the bacteria then multiply. This is similar to the means *Legionella* employ when they grow within protozoa, which are usually their hosts. Each year up to eighteen thousand people are hospitalized for Legionnaires' disease in the United States. Up to 30 percent of these cases are fatal.

The presence of this pathogen in humans can be detected with sputum cultures or with urinary antigen assays. A second test may be needed several days later if the first test is negative and patients still present with symptoms that are indicative of *Legionella* infection, such as vomiting, high fever, chills, cough, diarrhea, and confusion. *Legionella* infection is more likely to occur in persons who have already been hospitalized for another illness and who then contract *Legionella*; it is also common in those persons with compromised immune systems, such as persons with cancer or with human immunodeficiency virus (HIV) infection. In addition, persons who take immunosuppressive drugs, such as those who have had organ transplants, have an elevated risk of *Legionella* infection.

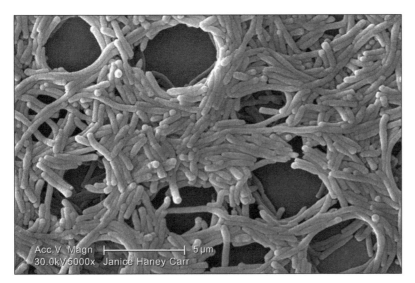

Legionella pneumophila *bacteria*. (CDC)

Legionella infection may present in hospitals in which patients live in close quarters. All patients diagnosed with pneumonia while in the hospital should be tested for *Legionella*.

Guinea pigs were the first species in which *Legionella* was isolated in 1943, but the genus was not established until 1979, three years after the 1976 outbreak, when more than two hundred persons attending an American Legion conference at a hotel in Philadelphia became severely ill; twenty-nine attendees died. The pathogen was traced to the air conditioning system of the hotel. A milder form of this infection is referred to as Pontiac fever, named after the city in Michigan where an outbreak of *Legionella* infection occurred in 1968, infecting more than sixty county health workers. This discovery was made retrospectively after the 1976 identification of *Legionella*. The source of the infection in the Pontiac case was found to be the air conditioning system. In contrast to Legionnaires' disease, Pontiac fever may develop in healthy persons.

Legionella can be isolated in the blood, lung tissue, sputum, and stool. It has also been cultured from bone marrow.

DRUG SUSCEPTIBILITY

Erythromycin is a common drug of choice for eradicating infection with *Legionella*, although other macrolide antibiotics, such as azithromycin or levofloxacin, have been approved by the U.S. Food and Drug Administration for the treatment of this infection. *Legionella* infection may initially be misdiagnosed as *Streptococcus pneumoniae* infection, the most common cause of pneumonia, if laboratory testing is not performed.

Christine Adamec, M.B.A.

FURTHER READING

Bitar, Dina M., et al. "Legionnaires' Disease and Its Agent *Legionella pneumophila*." In *Community-Acquired Pneumonia*, edited by Norbert Suttorp, Tobias Welte, and Reinhard Marre. Boston: Birkhäuser, 2007. Covers Legionnaires' disease while the rest of the book covers other forms of pneumonia that can develop in persons living in communities other than nursing homes or hospitals.

Dirven, Kristien, et al. "Comparison of Three Legionella Urinary Antigen Assays During an Outbreak of Legionellosis in Belgium." *Journal of Medical Microbiology* 54 (2005): 1213-1216. Compares and contrasts the use of urinary antigen tests to identify the presence of *Legionella*.

Fields, Barry S., Robert F. Benson, and Richard E. Besser. "*Legionella* and Legionnaires' Disease: Twenty-five Years of Investigation." *Clinical Microbiology Reviews* 15 (2002): 506-526. This article discusses the clinical presentation, life cycle, diagnosis, and epidemiologic trends of *Legionella*.

Pravinkumar, S. J., et al. "A Cluster of Legionnaires' Disease Caused by *Legionella longbeachae* Linked to Potting Compost in Scotland, 2008-2009." *European Surveillance* 15 (2010). Available at http://www.eurosurveillance.org/viewarticle.aspx?articleid=19496. Discusses the finding of a form of *Legionella* that was identified in potting soil rather than in the aquatic environment with which it was usually associated.

WEB SITES OF INTEREST

American Lung Association
http://www.lungusa.org

Centers for Disease Control and Prevention
http://www.cdc.gov

National Institute of Environmental Health Sciences
http://www.niehs.nih.gov

See also:: Airborne illness and disease; Antibiotics: Types; Atypical pneumonia; Bacterial infections; Bronchiolitis; Bronchitis; Infection; Influenza; Legionnaires' disease; Leptospirosis; Melioidosis; Pleurisy; Pneumocystis pneumonia; Pneumonia; Pontiac fever; Respiratory route of transmission; Soilborne illness and disease; Tuberculosis (TB); Waterborne illness and disease; Whooping cough.

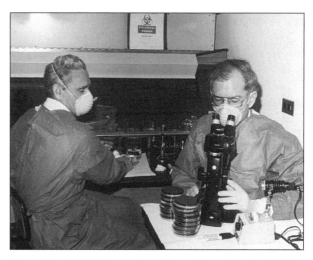

Researchers in 1978 examine culture plates isolating the bacteria that causes what came to be known as Legionnaires' disease. (CDC)

Legionnaires' disease

CATEGORY: Diseases and conditions
ANATOMY OR SYSTEM AFFECTED: Lungs, respiratory system
ALSO KNOWN AS: Legionnaires' pneumonia, legionella disease, legionellosis

DEFINITION

Legionnaires' disease is a lung infection and a form of pneumonia. The disease is named for an outbreak of a particular type of pneumonia at the American Legionnaires Convention in Philadelphia in 1976.

CAUSES

This disease is caused by the bacterium *Legionella pneumophilia*. The bacterium is most often found in sources of standing water, such as that in cooling towers and air conditioners, and in heating, ventilating, and air conditioning (HVAC) systems. The bacterium can also be found in soil.

Legionnaires' disease can be contracted by breathing into the lungs the water vapor from a standing water source that contains *Legionella* bacteria and by breathing into the lungs the dust from soil containing *Legionella* bacteria. The infection does not move from one person to another.

RISK FACTORS

Factors that increase the chance for Legionnaires' disease include advanced age, smoking, excessive alcohol intake, chronic lung disease, weakened immune system (as with acquired immunodeficiency syndrome), kidney failure, diabetes, taking cortisone or other immunosuppressive drugs, organ transplant, and working with soil, especially newly tilled soil or potting soil. Also, men are at higher risk for the disease.

SYMPTOMS

Symptoms include fatigue, fever (often high), chills and muscle aches, dry cough, chest pain with coughing or breathing, loss of appetite, and headache. Symptoms that develop if the infection becomes serious include shortness of breath; abdominal pain; nausea, vomiting, or diarrhea; mental problems; confusion and memory loss.

SCREENING AND DIAGNOSIS

A doctor will ask about symptoms and medical history and will perform a physical exam. Tests may include blood tests to look for high or rising antibodies to *Legionella* bacteria, sputum tests (which examines mucus from deep inside the lungs to identify the cause of the infection), kidney function tests (poor kidney function is often seen with *Legionella* infection), urine tests to check for *Legionella* proteins in the urine, and a chest X ray to diagnose pneumonia or lung infection.

TREATMENT AND THERAPY

This disease is usually treated with antibiotics such as quinolones, macrolides (azithromycin, clarithromycin, or erythromycin), and tetracycline. In severe cases, a drug called rifampin may be given. Initial therapy may be given by vein.

PREVENTION AND OUTCOMES

Proper design, maintenance, and cleaning of high-risk areas can reduce the risk of spreading the disease. This includes any area with standing water. One can reduce the risk of getting Legionnaires' disease by not smoking, by limiting the amount of alcohol intake, by wearing gloves and a mask if working with freshly tilled soil or potting soil, by not inhaling dust from the soil, and by moistening the soil to lower the amount of dust.

Rick Alan; reviewed by David L. Horn, M.D., FACP

FURTHER READING

Arcavi, L., and N. L. Benowitz. "Cigarette Smoking and Infection." *Archives of Internal Medicine* 164 (2004): 2206-2216.

Centers for Disease Control and Prevention. "Patient Facts: Learn More About Legionnaires' Disease." Available at http://www.cdc.gov/legionella/patient_facts.htm.

Corrin, Bryan, and Andrew G. Nicholson. *Pathology of the Lungs.* 2d ed. New York: Churchill Livingstone/Elsevier, 2006.

Cunha, B. A. "The Atypical Pneumonias: Clinical Diagnosis and Importance." *Clinical Microbiology and Infection* 12, suppl. 3 (2006): 12-24.

_____. "Atypical Pneumonias: Current Clinical Concepts Focusing on Legionnaires' Disease." *Current Opinion in Pulmonary Medicine* 14 (2008): 183-194.

Hoebe, Christian J. P. A., and Jacob L. Kool. "Control of *Legionella* in Drinking-Water Systems." *The Lancet* 355 (June 17, 2000): 2093-2094.

Levitzky, Michael G. *Pulmonary Physiology.* 7th ed. New York: McGraw-Hill Medical, 2007.

Mason, Robert J., et al., eds. *Murray and Nadel's Textbook of Respiratory Medicine.* 5th ed. Philadelphia: Saunders/Elsevier, 2010.

Neil, K., et al. "Increasing Incidence of Legionellosis in the United States, 1990-2005: Changing Epidemiologic Trends." *Clinical Infectious Diseases* 47 (2008): 591.

Ryan, Kenneth J., and C. George Ray, eds. *Sherris Medical Microbiology: An Introduction to Infectious Diseases.* 5th ed. New York: McGraw-Hill, 2010.

Springston, John. "*Legionella* Bacteria in Building Environments." *Occupational Hazards* 61, no. 8 (August, 1999): 51-56.

WEB SITES OF INTEREST

American Lung Association
http://www.lungusa.org

Canadian Centre for Occupational Health and Safety
http://www.ccohs.ca

Centers for Disease Control and Prevention
http://www.cdc.gov

National Institute of Environmental Health Sciences
http://www.niehs.nih.gov

See also:: Airborne illness and disease; Antibiotics: Types; Atypical pneumonia; Bacterial infections; Bronchiolitis; Bronchitis; Infection; Influenza; *Legionella*; Leptospirosis; Melioidosis; Pleurisy; Pneumonia; Pontiac fever; Respiratory route of transmission; Soilborne illness and disease; Tuberculosis (TB); Waterborne illness and disease; Whooping cough.

Leishmaniasis

CATEGORY: Diseases and conditions
ANATOMY OR SYSTEM AFFECTED: All
ALSO KNOWN AS: Black fever, espundia, kala-azar, post kala-azar dermal leishmaniasis

DEFINITION

Leishmaniasis is the umbrella term for a heterogeneous group of protozoan parasitic diseases designated as cutaneous, mucocutaneous, or visceral.

CAUSES

As part of the life cycle of the protozoan genus *Leishmania*, the organisms are injected into the bloodstream of human hosts through the bite of vector sandflies. They proliferate within phagocytes (immune system cells) to continue their existence as obligate parasites. More than twenty disease-causing species of *Leishmania*, borne by some thirty species of blood-feeding sandflies, account for the striking epidemiologic and clinical diversity of leishmaniasis.

RISK FACTORS

Perhaps the most significant risk factor for leishmaniasis is extreme poverty, which translates as malnutrition, lessened resistance to infection, and poor housing. Cattle and other livestock may increase sandfly density, and sanitation is generally inadequate in endemic areas. Large-scale migrations, whether economic or war-driven, expose vulnerable populations to new *Leishmania* strains. On a global scale, urbanization, deforestation, and climate change introduce human migrants to new routes of infection.

SYMPTOMS

The form of infection depends on the locale and on the *Leishmania* species encountered. The clinical spectrum varies from self-limiting skin lesions (cutaneous leishmaniasis) to lethal systemic infection (visceral leishmaniasis).

The skin surface nodules or ulcers of cutaneous leishmaniasis often heal without treatment. Once healed, however, the infection can invade facial mucous membranes up to years later, causing the mucocutaneous form of the disease. Mucosal structures of the face and throat may be destroyed, mutilating facial features.

Visceral leishmaniasis, or kala-azar, is the most severe form of the disease. Progressive fever, body wasting, anemia, and enlarged liver and spleen are characteristic. Untreated, the case-fatality rate is more than 90 percent; the rate is about 10 percent with treatment.

Visceral leishmaniasis can also reappear after recovery as post-kala-azar dermal leishmaniasis (PKDL). Between 5 and 60 percent of cured persons develop the chronic, unsightly PKDL. Large numbers of parasites in exposed skin of those with PKDL offer ready access to sandflies, contributing to the transmission of visceral leishmaniasis between epidemics.

SCREENING AND DIAGNOSIS

The World Health Organization, among other agencies, is active in leishmaniasis screening and identification. Often an entire village or district in an endemic area is surveyed, ideally with house-to-house screening.

The diagnostic gold standard is detection of the DNA (deoxyribonucleic acid) of the responsible *Leishmania* species. The molecular techniques are limited to well-equipped laboratories rarely available in endemic countries.

Diagnosis of cutaneous leishmaniasis is confirmed by microscopic examination of skin scrapings, if fea-sible. Samples that can be analyzed later are collected directly from skin lesions. The characteristic appearance of mucocutaneous leishmaniasis often suffices for diagnosis.

Symptoms of visceral leishmaniasis resemble those of malaria, and coinfection with acquired immunodeficiency syndrome also complicates diagnosis. Accurate and early diagnosis of visceral leishmaniasis has been advanced by the development of serologic tests that can be used in real-world field settings. In general, these tests detect levels of antibodies in the blood of those thought to be infected. Another immunologic test can detect antigens in the urine of infected persons.

An important development in serologic testing is the use of a recombinant antigen that corresponds to the partial sequence of a *Leishmania* protein. A fingerstick blood sample means the test result can be determined in twenty minutes.

TREATMENT AND THERAPY

An effective, inexpensive, and widely available therapy does not exist. Parenteral administration of antimony compounds has been successfully used for decades, and it is still the most common treatment for cutaneous and mucocutaneous leishmaniasis. It is, however, toxic and expensive. Oral antifungal agents have met with some recent success. Among the available treatments for cutaneous leishmaniasis that do not require drugs are cauterization, cryotherapy, and topical creams.

Drug options for visceral leishmaniasis are generally toxic, expensive, and difficult to administer. Lengthy treatment and the need for frequent laboratory monitoring add limitations. Spreading parasitic resistance to antimonial drugs is a major problem, to the degree that antimonial treatment may fail in some locales. Where they are still useful, antimony compounds require thirty days of painful intramuscular injections.

Amphotericin B is also effective, but it is administered intravenously and requires a month's hospitalization. A liposomal formulation is a major advance in that it is well-tolerated and shortens treatment, but the drug is beyond the financial reach of most endemic countries. Miltefosine, an anticancer drug, is the first oral drug for visceral leishmaniasis; it cannot be given to pregnant women, however. Two treatment approaches for visceral leishmaniasis are advocated to counter drug resistance: Combination therapy with available drugs would reduce the dose of each and shorten the treatment course. Immunotherapy (developing ways to strengthen the host immune response) is being pursued as a research strategy.

PREVENTION AND OUTCOMES

Prevention must consider variables that include the *Leishmania* species, regional geography, and vector biology. A combination of approaches is required: sandfly control, spraying of dwellings and animal shelters, treating sleeping nets with an insecticide, and applying insect repellents to skin and fabrics. Active, early case detection and rapid treatment can inhibit infection spread.

Leishmaniasis is one of the few parasitic diseases that vaccination could theoretically control. However, protection achieved with animal models has not carried over into successful field studies. Development of vaccines using recombinant methods continues.

Judith Weinblatt, M.S., M.A.

FURTHER READING

Clark, David P. *Germs, Genes, and Civilization: How Epidemics Shaped Who We Are Today.* Upper Saddle River, N.J.: FT Press, 2010. Argues that infectious diseases have influenced human culture in ways not usually recognized.

Cliff, Andrew, Peter Haggett, and Matthew Smallman-Raynor. *World Atlas of Epidemic Diseases.* New York: Oxford University Press, 2004. Beautifully illustrated, this book brings together basic information on fifty of the great epidemic diseases spanning five thousand years.

Marquardt, William, ed. *Biology of Disease Vectors.* 2d ed. Burlington, Mass.: Academic Press/Elsevier, 2005. An excellent reference for understanding the roles of flies and other insects in the transmission of infectious disease. Discusses prevention and control strategies and future implications.

Parker, James M., and Philip M. Parker, eds. *The Official Patient's Sourcebook on Leishmaniasis: A Revised and Updated Directory for the Internet Age.* San Diego, Calif.: Icon Health, 2002. This book is part research primer, part medical resource. Chapters include research summaries and glossaries.

WEB SITES OF INTEREST

Centers for Disease Control and Prevention
http://www.cdc.gov/parasites

International Leishmania Network
http://leishnet.net

World Health Organization
http://www.who.int

See also:*:* Arthropod-borne illness and disease; Developing countries and infectious disease; Diagnosis of protozoan diseases; Fleas and infectious disease; Flies and infectious disease; Insect-borne illness and disease; Malaria; Parasitic diseases; Pathogens; Prevention of protozoan diseases; Protozoa: Classification and types; Protozoan diseases; Skin infections; Treatment of protozoan diseases; Vectors and vector control.

Leprosy

CATEGORY: Diseases and conditions
ANATOMY OR SYSTEM AFFECTED: Peripheral nervous system, skin, upper respiratory tract
ALSO KNOWN AS: Hansen's disease

DEFINITION

Leprosy is a chronic disease of the peripheral nerves and mucosa of the upper respiratory tract that shows skin lesions primarily. Leprosy is caused by the bacilli (bacteria) *Mycobacterium leprae.* The rod-shaped *M. leprae* is about 2.7 micrometers (μm) long and 0.3 to 0.4 μm wide. Although the exact mode of transmission of *M. leprae* remains debatable, the bacteria are observed in the inflammatory cells of the skin lesions and the peripheral nerves. Children, adolescents, and adults can contract the disease.

In certain ways, leprosy resembles tuberculosis and granuloma. In all three, the immune response of the body plays a vital role in disease development. If the immune system, in persons with leprosy, destroys *M. leprae* (in a process called high host resistance), the infected person will have tuberculoid leprosy (also called paucibacillary leprosy, meaning "few *M. leprae*"). If the infected person's body is unable to defend against *M. leprae* (low host resistance), the result is lepromatous leprosy (or multibacillary leprosy, meaning "many *M. leprae*"). Another type is borderline leprosy, which can develop into lepromatous leprosy.

The bacterium that causes leprosy was first discovered in 1873 by Norwegian doctor Gerhard Armauer Hansen (the disease is also known as Hansen's disease), but the disease existed long before this discovery and infected persons in many parts of the world, including China, Japan, India, Nepal, Egypt, Europe, and Brazil. Persons with leprosy often suffer deep social stigma, including physical isolation, because the disease is believed to be highly contagious.

CAUSES

Infection with *M. leprae* causes leprosy. Children are more susceptible to the disease, which can be contracted through frequent contact with the skin lesions of a person with active or untreated leprosy or through inhalation. A person can inhale the bacteria that are emitted through the cough or sneeze of a person with active, untreated leprosy (*M. leprae* can remain in the atmosphere for months). A genetic cause of leprosy has been offered, but this possible cause remains debatable.

RISK FACTORS

Risk factors for developing leprosy include contacting the skin of a person with untreated, active leprosy and inhaling *M. leprae* through an infected person's cough or sneeze. Persons living in the tropics and subtropics are most at risk for developing the disease.

SYMPTOMS

Symptoms appear several months after the person is infected with the bacterium that causes leprosy. Clinical and pathological symptoms can further differentiate into either tuberculoid leprosy or lepromatous leprosy.

In the tuberculoid form, one or a few well-hypopigmented (paler color) or reddish skin lesions with defined borders appear on the arms, legs, and back; this form also includes a loss of sensation. In the lepromatous form, multiple yellowish or brown nodular skin lesions (papules) with poorly defined borders appear on the body; this form also includes sensory loss. Advanced symptoms of the lepromatous form include facial nerve damage, thickened peripheral nerves, distinguishable thickened and disfigured face (leonine facies), swollen ear lobes, loss of eye lashes, disappearance of eye brows, muscle paralysis, expanded nostrils, clawed hands, foot drops, dry skin, and ulceration. In the borderline form of leprosy, which is an intermediate form, the poorly defined single or multiple skin lesions appear with early involvement of nerve damage.

SCREENING AND DIAGNOSIS

There are no blood tests to detect the disease; however, the following laboratory tests are used to confirm

Registered Prevalence of Leprosy and Number of New Cases Detected, by World Health Organization (WHO) Region (2008-2009)

WHO region	Registered prevalence (rate per 10,000 persons), early 2009	New cases detected (rate per 100,000 persons), 2008
Africa	30,557 (0.45)	29,814 (4.37)
Americas	47,069 (0.54)	41,891 (4.85)
South-East Asia	120,689 (0.69)	167,505 (9.60)
Eastern Mediterranean	4,967 (0.10)	3,938 (0.80)
Western Pacific	9,754 (0.05)	5,859 (0.33)
Total	**213,036**	**249,007**

Source: Weekly Epidemiological Record, 2009, World Health Organization

or disconfirm leprosy: lepromin test, which distinguishes tuberculoid leprosy from lepromatous leprosy; serological tests, which can detect antibodies in the blood; stained skin scrapings, which can help identify acid-fast *M. leprae*; and a skin lesion biopsy, in which a tissue sample of a skin lesion is surgically removed, sectioned, stained, and analyzed under a microscope.

TREATMENT AND THERAPY

The World Health Organization (WHO) has approved multidrug therapy using the antibiotics dapsone, rifampicine, and clofazimine, all of which are effective in killing *M. leprae*. Using one of these drugs alone, however, is not recommended because of the risk of developing immunity to that drug. Side effects of the treatment include inflammation, which is caused by the host's response to dead *M. leprae* in the body. The inflammation, more specifically known as erythema nodosum leprosum, causes fever and can be controlled by anti-inflammatory drugs such as corticosteroids and aspirin.

PREVENTION AND OUTCOMES

Most people have a natural immunity to leprosy. Because *M. leprae* cannot be cultured in the laboratory, an antileprosy vaccine cannot be made to help those who do not have a natural immunity. The Bacille Calmette-Guérin vaccine, which is used primarily against tuberculosis, may be useful against the development of leprosy.

Another preventive measure is to avoid contact with the skin lesions of a person with leprosy, but it is not necessary to isolate a person with leprosy. Persons not infected who live with an infected person should get regular check ups by a physician.

Active, widespread awareness about the disease and its prevention has led to a significant drop in the number of cases of leprosy worldwide. In 1966, for example, there were eleven million reported cases; in the early twenty-first century, that number was one-half million.

Arun S. Dabholkar, Ph.D.

FURTHER READING

Dastur, D. K., Y. Ramamohan, and A. S. Dabholkar. "Some Neuropathologic and Cellular Aspects of Leprosy." *Progress Research* 18 (1974): 53-75.

Gould, Tony. *A Disease Apart: Leprosy in the Modern World.* New York: St. Martin's Press, 2005.

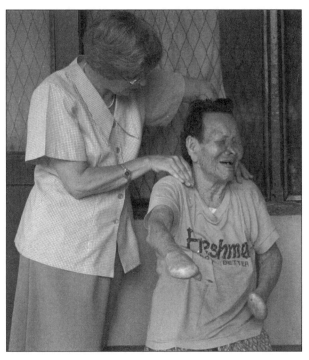

A man with leprosy receives massage therapy at a rehabilitation center in Thailand. (AP/Wide World Photos)

Hastings, Robert C., ed. *Leprosy.* 2d ed. New York: Churchill Livingstone, 1994.

International Federation of Anti-Leprosy Associations. "How to Diagnose and Treat Leprosy." Available at http://www.ilep.org.uk/library-resources/ilep-publications/english.

WEB SITES OF INTEREST

American Leprosy Missions
http://www.leprosy.org

International Federation of Anti-Leprosy Associations
http://www.ilep.org.uk

New Zealand Dermatological Society
http://dermnetnz.org

Stigma Research and Action
http://stigmaj.org

World Health Organization
http://www.who.int/lep

See also:: Acid-fastness; Bacterial infections; Cellulitis; Erythema nodosum; Mycobacterial infections; *Mycobacterium*; Quarantine; Skin infections; Social effects of infectious disease.

Leptospira

CATEGORY: Pathogen
TRANSMISSION ROUTE: Direct contact, ingestion

DEFINITION

Leptospira are gram-negative, motile, obligate, and aerobic spirochete that use only long-chain fatty acids as an energy source. Both free-living and parasitic forms of *Leptospira* exist.

**Taxonomic Classification
for *Leptospira***

Kingdom: Bacteria
Phylum: Spirochaetes
Class: Spirochaetes
Order: Spirochaetales
Family: Leptospiraceae
Genus: *Leptospira*
Species:
L. biflexa
L. borgpetersenii
L. inadai
L. interrogans
L. meyeri
L. noguchii
L. wolbachii

NATURAL HABITAT AND FEATURES

The name *Leptospira* was derived from the Greek words *leptos* and *spira*, meaning "thin coil." Leptospires are 10 to 20 micrometers (μm) long and 0.1 μm thick and are tightly coiled in a right-handed manner around a central cylinder; they are highly motile. Motility is derived from two periplasmic flagella that, as in other spirochetes, are attached to opposite ends of the protoplasmic cylinder, unattached at the other end, and extend about two-thirds of the way along the cylinder. The membrane-cell wall of the cylinder is rigid, while the complex outer sheath is flex-ible. When the flagella rotate in the space between the sheath and the cylinder, the entire organism rotates in the opposite direction, allowing for motility.

Because *Leptospira* are so thin, they are difficult to visualize under a normal light microscope; most can be seen using dark field or phase contrast microscopy. All strains grow best at a pH (acid) level of 7.2 to 7.6. Pathogenic strains do best at a temperature between 82.4° and 86° Fahrenheit (28 and 30° Celsius), but some can grow at temperatures as low as 55.4° F (13° C).

Visible growth on agar often takes four to seven days. Nonpathogenic strains, which are saprobic, do best at slightly lower temperatures, and many have minimal growth temperatures in the 41° to 50° F (5° to 10° C) range. Visible growth on agar is usually apparent after two to three days. All species require long-chain fatty acids, which they break down through beta-oxidation, as their energy source. These fatty acids are usually supplied in vitro by the Ellinghausen-McCullough-Johnson-Harris medium.

No leptospires are able to use sugars as energy sources, but they can build needed sugars through Krebs cycle intermediates. Most pathogenic strains also require vitamins B_1 and B_{12}, and all strains require iron. The genome size is usually about four million base pairs forming more than four thousand genes. The genome of *L. interrogans* consists of a larger 4.3 megabase chromosome and a smaller 359 kilobase chromosome. The *Leptospira* genome is larger than those found in most other pathogenic spirochetes.

Taxonomic separation for many years has been by serotypes, and more than 240 serovars of *Leptospira* have been discovered. Genotypic DNA analysis has shown that strains that share the same serotype may be genetically distant, while closely related strains may show different serotypes. Modern *Leptospira* taxonomy uses genotyping and has placed most pathogenic serovars in *L. interrogans* and most saprobic serovars in *L. biflexa*. However, fifteen to twenty other less common, genetically distinct, species have been postulated by genotyping.

Nonpathogenic strains can be found in many aquatic and damp habitats throughout the world, excluding polar regions. Pathogenic strains are parasitic or commensal in many animal species, including humans, but rodents, especially mice and rats, seem to serve as primary reservoirs for many pathogenic strains. In commensal or parasitized animals, the bacteria usually reside in the kidneys and bacteria are usually introduced into the environment through urine. The leptospires can remain alive for several weeks outside their host as long as they remain damp and warm. Infections occur year round in the tropics, but mainly in the summer, when the weather is warmer. In more temperate regions, infections occur mainly in winter, when rodents are more likely to enter homes for shelter. It has been postulated that human infections in temperate regions may increase with global warming.

PATHOGENICITY AND CLINICAL SIGNIFICANCE

Leptospirosis, caused by infection with *Leptospira*, is considered a zoonotic disease that affects a variety of animals, including mammals, birds, reptiles, and insects. Humans are only occasionally infected, mostly in the tropics and mostly by contact with dogs or small rodents. The most severe form of human leptospirosis is also known as Weil's disease, named for Adolph Weil, who first described it in the late nineteenth century. The bacteria usually enter a host when contaminated water comes in contact with abraded skin or with mucous membranes.

Early symptoms of leptospirosis in humans include fever, chills, and headache, which are often mistaken for flu. During this time, bacteria can be isolated from the blood. After a brief asymptomatic phase, bacteria become ensconced in the endothelium of internal organs, such as the liver, nervous system, lungs, heart, and, especially, the kidneys. This can lead to liver damage, which leads to jaundice, meningitis, pulmonary hemorrhage, kidney failure, and, occasionally, cardiovascular problems and delirium. Mortality is common, especially in untreated persons, and is usually caused by pulmonary problems or kidney failure.

DRUG SUSCEPTIBILITY

Early in the infection, oral doxycycline is the drug of choice. In acute infections, hospitalization and intravenous penicillin G are the preferred treatments. For persons allergic to penicillins, erythromycin is an effective alternative. Third generation cephalosporins, such as cefotaxime and ceftriaxone, have also been shown to be effective treatments, but dosage must be monitored carefully if the infected person is in renal failure, because these drugs can build up to toxic levels if not cleared properly by the kidneys.

Immunizations for humans are not routine in the United States because the immunizations are serotype specific, and there are many different serotypes. Out-side the United States, however, some at-risk workers are immunized against locally endemic serotypes. Immunization of pets, especially dogs, against the more common serotypes can reduce the chance that dogs will become infected and then pass the bacteria to humans.

Richard W. Cheney, Jr., Ph.D.

FURTHER READING

Krieg, Noel R., et al., eds. *Bergey's Manual of Systematic Bacteriology*. Vol. 4. 2d ed. New York: Springer, 2010. This volume describes the Spirochaetes in detail.

Madigan, Michael T., and John M. Martinko. *Brock Biology of Microorganisms*. 12th ed. Upper Saddle River, N.J.: Pearson/Prentice Hall, 2010. This text outlines many common bacteria, describing natural history, pathogenicity, and other topics.

World Health Organization. *Human Leptospirosis: Guidance for Diagnosis, Surveillance, and Control*. Malta: World Health Organization, 2003. Information on culturing, serotyping, and genotyping *Leptospira*, and information on leptospirosis.

WEB SITES OF INTEREST

Leptospirosis Information Center
http://www.leptospirosis.org

Todar's Online Textbook of Bacteriology
http://www.textbookofbacteriology.net

See also:: Bacterial infections; Dogs and infectious disease; Leptospirosis; Rodents and infectious disease; Soilborne illness and disease; Tropical medicine; Waterborne illness and disease.

Leptospirosis

CATEGORY: Diseases and conditions
ANATOMY OR SYSTEM AFFECTED: All
ALSO KNOWN AS: Cane-cutter fever, canicola fever, hemorrhagic jaundice, icterohemorrhagic fever, mud fever, rice-field fever, Stuttgart disease, swamp fever, swineherd's disease, Weil's disease

DEFINITION

Leptospirosis is a rare and contagious bacterial infection caused by the bacterium *Leptospira*. Leptospirosis is most common in warm, tropical conditions and can affect any part of the body. With prompt and proper treatment, prognosis is usually good. If untreated, complications may develop that can potentially be fatal.

CAUSES

Leptospirosis is caused by contact with fresh water, wet or dampened soil, or vegetation that has been soiled by urine from an infected animal. When contact is made with the contaminated material, bacteria enter the body through open sores or wounds in the skin, or through mucous membranes. Humans can also contract leptospirosis by drinking water that has been contaminated by the urine of an infected animal. Once the bacteria have entered the body, they flow into the bloodstream and throughout the body, causing infection.

RISK FACTORS

Anyone can contract leptospirosis, but people who are at an increased risk are canoeists, rafters, swimmers (in lakes, rivers, and streams); workers in flood plains; workers in wet agricultural settings; people who have pets (particularly dogs or livestock); people who work with the land (including farmers, ranchers, loggers, and rice-field workers); and people, including veterinarians and veterinary staff, who work with animals.

SYMPTOMS

Symptoms typically appear about ten days after infection and include one or more of the following: sudden fever, rigors, pain, and headache; dry cough; nausea, vomiting, and diarrhea; conjunctivitis (pinkeye); aching joints; sore throat; painful bones; abdominal pain; enlarged spleen, liver, or lymph glands; rigid muscles; and a rash on the skin.

SCREENING AND DIAGNOSIS

A doctor will ask about symptoms and medical history and will perform a physical exam. Tests may include a blood test to determine the presence of antibodies to the *Leptospira* bacterium, and cultures or other laboratory tests.

TREATMENT AND THERAPY

Treatment options include medications such as antibiotics, including penicillin, tetracycline, chloramphenicol, and erythromycin.

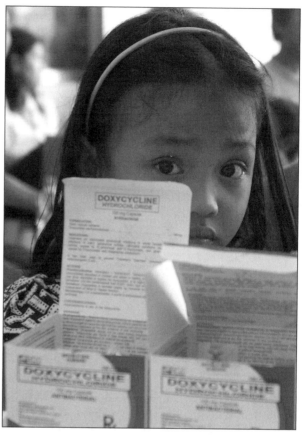

An outbreak of leptospirosis in the Philippines in 2009 was met with the wide distribution of antibiotics to treat the disease. (AP/Wide World Photos)

PREVENTION AND OUTCOMES

To help reduce the chance of getting leptospirosis, one should reduce contact with soil, vegetation, and water that could possibly be contaminated with infected animal urine, including urine from rodents. If working with materials that could be contaminated, one should wear protective clothing, including waterproof boots or waders, that covers the skin. Persons working in an especially high-risk area should consult a doctor about beginning antibiotic treatment before potential exposure.

Diana Kohnle; reviewed by David L. Horn, M.D., FACP

FURTHER READING

Centers for Disease Control and Prevention. Division of Bacterial and Mycotic Diseases. "Leptospirosis." Available at http://www.cdc.gov.

Forbes, Betty A., Daniel F. Sahm, and Alice S. Weiss-
    feld. *Bailey and Scott's Diagnostic Microbiology.* 12th
    ed. St. Louis, Mo.: Mosby/Elsevier, 2007.
New York State Department of Health. "Leptospi-
    rosis (Weil's Disease)." Available at http://www.
    nyhealth.gov/diseases.
Ryan, Kenneth J., and C. George Ray, eds. *Sherris Med-
    ical Microbiology: An Introduction to Infectious Diseases.*
    5th ed. New York: McGraw-Hill, 2010.

WEB SITES OF INTEREST

American Society of Tropical Medicine and Hygiene
http://www.astmh.org

Canadian Health Network
http://www.canadian-health-network.ca

Leptospirosis Information Center
http://www.leptospirosis.org

National Library of Medicine
http://www.nlm.nih.gov

See also:: Bacterial infections; Botulism; Cholera;
Hantavirus infection; *Leptospira*; Malaria; Melioidosis;
Q fever; Rodents and infectious disease; Soilborne illness and disease; Tetanus; Tropical medicine; Waterborne illness and disease; Zoonotic diseases.

Lipopeptide antibiotics

CATEGORY: Treatment

DEFINITION

Lipopeptide antibiotics are molecules that are synthesized primarily by soil bacteria through nonribo-
somal metabolic pathways. These molecules typically
consist of a fatty acid connected to a short linear or
cyclic amino acid chain, and they are generally acidic,
making them highly soluble in water. In addition to
naturally occurring lipopeptide antibiotics, synthetic
and semisynthetic analogues have been developed.
This class of antibiotics includes polymyxins, daptomycin, and echinocandins. Many require calcium for
maximum antimicrobial activity, and most are active
against gram-positive, but not gram-negative bacteria.

MECHANISM OF ACTION

Lipopeptide antibiotics bind to the cell membranes of specific microbial species and increase their
permeability. As the cell membrane becomes less
stable, the cell contents leak out and the bacterium or
fungus dies.

SPECIFIC COMPOUNDS

The best studied lipopeptide antibiotics are polymyxin B and polymyxin E (colistin), which were discovered in the 1940's. Isolated from the soil bacterium *Bacillus polymyxa*, polymyxins are used to treat a
variety of gram-negative organisms, including *Pseudomonas aeruginosa, Escherichia coli, Klebsiella pneumoniae,
Enterobacter aerogenes*, and *Haemophilus influenzae*. These
compounds bind specifically to the lipopolysaccharide component of the outer membrane and disrupt
the phospholipid bilayer. This detergent effect is effective against difficult-to-treat bacterial biofilms.

Commonly used commercial antibiotic ointments
for wound healing combine polymyxin B with other
antibiotics. An aerosolized form of polymyxin E is
used to treat chronic *P. aeruginosa* infections in persons with cystic fibrosis. Polymyxin M (mattacin) is a
later discovered polymyxin isolated from *Paenibacillus
kobensis*. It is effective against both gram-positive and
gram-negative bacteria.

Daptomycin, produced by *Streptomyces roseosporus*, is
a relatively new lipopeptide antibiotic used for hard-
to-treat infections of skin and skin structures, bacterial infections of the blood (bacteremia), and right-
sided endocarditis. It is thought to bind to the cell
membrane in a calcium-dependent manner, forming
transmembrane channels that promote the leakage
of ions. The resulting depolarization of the cell inhibits the synthesis of protein, deoxyribonucleic acid
(DNA), and ribonucleic acid (RNA), leading to rapid
cell death. Daptomycin appears to be effective against
virtually all gram-positive organisms, but it is too large
to cross the outer membrane of gram-negative bacteria. Resistance to daptomycin is rare because of its
nonspecific mechanism of action.

Echinocandins are large natural and semisynthetic compounds that are effective against *Candida*
and *Aspergillus* species. They include caspofungin, micafungin, and anidulafungin, which are administered
as intravenous injections. These antifungal compounds prevent the synthesis of (1,3)beta-D-glucan,
an essential component of the fungal cell wall. The

semisynthetic antifungal compound anidulafungin, derived from a fermentation product of *A. nidulans*, also targets (1,3)beta-D-glucan synthesis.

IMPACT

Lipopeptide antibiotics are fast-acting bactericidal and antifungal compounds that do not tend to cause resistance. The problem of antimicrobial resistance and the lack of new antibiotics has renewed interest in lipopeptide antibiotics, and they are often used for serious infections when other therapies fail. Daptomycin in particular is effective against methicillin-resistant and vancomycin-resistant *Staphylococcus aureus*. The main limitations of these compounds are their poor solubility, their accumulation in tissues, and their risk of toxicity.

Kathleen LaPoint, M.S.

FURTHER READING

Cottagnoud, Philippe. "Daptomycin: A New Treatment for Insidious Infections Due to Gram-Positive Pathogens." *Swiss Medical Weekly* 138 (2008): 93-99.

Fischbach, Michael, et al. "Antibiotics for Emerging Pathogens." *Science* 325 (2009): 1089-1093.

Pirri, Giovanna, et al. "Lipopeptides as Anti-infectives: A Practical Perspective." *Central European Journal of Biology* 4 (2009): 258-273.

WEB SITES OF INTEREST

eMedicineHealth: Antibiotics
http://www.emedicinehealth.com/antibiotics

National Institute of Allergy and Infectious Diseases
http://www.niaid.nih.gov/topics/antimicrobialresistance

Todar's Online Textbook of Bacteriology
http://www.textbookofbacteriology.net

See also: Alliance for the Prudent Use of Antibiotics; Aminoglycoside antibiotics; Antibiotic resistance; Antibiotics: Types; Bacteria: Classification and types; Bacterial infections; Cephalosporin antibiotics; Drug resistance; Glycopeptide antibiotics; Ketolide antibiotics; Macrolide antibiotics; Microbiology; Oxazolidinone antibiotics; Penicillin antibiotics; Quinolone antibiotics; Superbacteria; Tetracycline antibiotics; Treatment of bacterial infections.

Listeria

CATEGORY: Pathogen
TRANSMISSION ROUTE: Ingestion

DEFINITION

The bacterium *Listeria monocytogenes* commonly contaminates foods. It is difficult to detect and, in rare cases, causes listeriosis, a serious and often fatal disease in humans.

Taxonomic Classification for *Listeria*

Kingdom: Monera
Domain: Bacteria
Phylum: Firmicutes
Class: Bacilli
Order: Bacillales
Family: Listeriaceae
Genus: *Listeria*
Species:
L. monocytogenes
L. innocua
L. seeligeri
L. ivanovii
L. welshimeri
L. grayi
L. murrayi

NATURAL HABITAT AND FEATURES

Listeria species are found in soil, decaying vegetation, water, sewage, and field crops such as alfalfa. The only pathogenic species, *L. monocytogenes*, occurs in humans, other mammals, birds, fish, crustaceans, and insects. *L. monocytogenes* also occurs in foods such as vegetables, poultry, fresh and processed meats (such as bologna and hot dogs), soft cheeses (such as feta, farmer's cheese, and *queso blanco*), and salad dressings. It occurs in raw foods and in processed products. The first three confirmed outbreaks of listeriosis, in the 1980's, were reported from ingesting coleslaw, milk, and Mexican-style cheese (*queso fresco*), respectively.

Listeria spp. are characterized as gram-positive, non-spore-forming rods, which may occur in short chains or in coccoid forms. They are facultative anaerobes, are catalase-positive, always ferment, and ferment sugars to produce acid. Their cell walls contain teichoic acids but not mycolic acids. An unusual property of *L. monocytogenes* is that it can be intracellular in animal cells.

L. monocytogenes grows slowly under refrigerated conditions and is resistant to cold, acid, and salt. These properties increase the risk of infection from ingesting processed and stored foods that may be contaminated.

L. innocua has a significantly larger genome than *L. monocytogenes* (3.01 megabases compared with 2.94 megabases), though *L. innocua* lacks some virulence genes and is nonpathogenic. Both genomes code for about 3,000 proteins, with perhaps 100 to 120 more in *L. innocua*. Thus, *L. innocua* grows in a wide variety of environments and is easier than *L. monocytogenes* to detect. Because of many genetic and metabolic similarities, and because they are often found together in a variety of situations, *L. innocua* could be used as an indicator of *L. monocytogenes* in quality control and regulatory analyses of foods. The two species grow slowly and indistinguishably on many laboratory media but can be distinguished by PCR (polymerase chain reaction) and colony morphology on special blood agars. Pulse-field gel electrophoresis of genomic deoxyribonucleic acid (DNA) and ribotyping are also used to distinguish *Listeria* spp.

Of the thirteen serovars of *L. monocytogenes*, listeriosis is most often caused by strains of just three: serovars 4b, 1/2a, and 1/2b. In the lab, serovars are distinguished by serotyping and phagetyping.

PATHOGENICITY AND CLINICAL SIGNIFICANCE

Even as a food-borne disease, listeriosis is not mainly a gastrointestinal illness. Instead, severe symptoms include meningitis, sepsis, and abortion in women in late-term pregnancy. Many people who ingest *L. monocytogenes* do not show any symptoms but may carry bacteria and act as a source of food contamination. The disease is especially risky for infants, the elderly and bedridden, and persons with acquired immunodeficiency syndrome (AIDS) or other immune disorders. Incidence of listeriosis is about five cases per million people per year, probably worldwide. Case fatality is quite severe at 20 to 30 percent. Thus, the United States reports about five hundred deaths per year from listeriosis. Most cases are sporadic, and epidemics are rare.

The virulence of *L. monocytogenes* is an inherent property of the bacterium because of virulence genes carried in its genome. After entering the gastrointestinal tract, bacteria are attacked by phagocytes but resist destruction. Instead, they persist intracellularly, proliferate inside phagocytes, and release progeny when phagocytes lyse, or break apart. The bacterial pore-forming protein listeriolysin O facilitates cell lysis of phagocytic cells. The bacterial surface protein internalin (InlA) aids in the crossing of the intestinal barrier to enter the nervous system. Other bacterial virulence proteins are InlB, ActA, PlcA, and PlcB. These proteins (with InlA and listeriolysin O) are encoded by virulence genes, some linked in a 10-kilobase region of the *L. monocytogenes* genome, absent from *L. innocua*.

DRUG SUSCEPTIBILITY

Listeria spp. are susceptible to many different antibiotics, though resistant strains are emerging. *L. monocytogenes* infection in humans can usually be treated with ampicillin, especially if treatment starts early. No vaccine is available.

R. L. Bernstein, Ph.D.

FURTHER READING

Bell, Chris, and Alec Kyriakides. *Listeria: A Practical Approach to the Organism and Its Control in Foods.* 2d ed. Ames: Iowa State University Press, 2005. One of a series on pathogenic food-borne microorganisms, this book gives biological and pathogenic details on *Listeria* and includes discussion of listeriosis outbreaks.

Bibek, Ray, and Arun Bhunia. *Fundamental Food Microbiology.* 4th ed. Boca Raton, Fla.: CRC Press, 2007. Description of food-borne microbial diseases, including pathogenic processes and emerging pathogens.

Doumith, Michel, et al. "New Aspects Regarding Evolution and Virulence of *Listeria monocytogenes* Revealed by Comparative Genomics and DNA Arrays." *Infection and Immunity* 72 (2004): 1072-1083. DNA data imply that *L. innocua* evolved from a strain of *L. monocytogenes* serovar 4 by several processes, including loss of virulence genes.

Glaser, Philippe, et al. "Comparative Genomics of *Listeria* Species." *Science* 294 (2001): 849-852. A research report on complete genomic DNA sequences of *L. monocytogenes* and *L. innocua*, identifying numerous genes in common and some unique to each organism.

Montville, Thomas J., and Karl R. Matthews. *Food*

Microbiology: An Introduction. 2d ed. Washington, D.C.: ASM Press, 2008. Introductory textbook with a major section on pathogenic organisms, including *Listeria*, in foods.

WEB SITES OF INTEREST

Centers for Disease Control and Prevention, Division of Foodborne, Bacterial, and Mycotic Diseases
http://www.cdc.gov/nczved/divisions/dfbmd

PathoSystems Resource Integration Center
http://www.patricbrc.org

U.S. Department of Agriculture, Food Safety and Inspection Service
http://www.fsis.usda.gov

See also:: Bacteria: Classification and types; *Campylobacter*; *Clostridium*; *Escherichia*; Food-borne illness and disease; *Giardia*; Intestinal and stomach infections; Listeriosis; Pregnancy and infectious disease; *Salmonella*; Sepsis; *Shigella*; Soilborne illness and disease; *Staphylococcus*; Waterborne illness and disease; *Yersinia*.

Listeriosis

CATEGORY: Diseases and conditions
ANATOMY OR SYSTEM AFFECTED: Blood, brain, central nervous system

DEFINITION

Listeriosis is a food-borne illness that can lead to death in newborns and in persons with compromised immune systems. Infants born to women infected with listeriosis may have meningitis (brain infection) or bacteremia (bacterial blood infection). Infected infants who survive may suffer neurological damage and developmental delays. Listeriosis can cause the death of a fetus of an infected pregnant woman.

Up to 65 percent of deaths from food-borne illnesses in the United States are caused by listeriosis. About twenty-five hundred people become ill with listeriosis per year in the United States, and, of these, five hundred die. The numbers of the infected may be greater, but such cases have not been identified, likely because symptoms were mild.

CAUSES

Listeriosis is caused by the bacterium *Listeria monocytogenes*, a pathogen that lives in water and soil. It is resistant to refrigeration and is found in ill-prepared or subsequently contaminated meats and vegetables, particularly in luncheon meats, hot dogs, soft cheeses, cole slaw, and unpasteurized milk.

RISK FACTORS

Pregnant women have twenty times the risk of developing listeriosis as others, according to the Centers for Disease Control and Prevention, and an estimated one-third of listeriosis cases occur during pregnancy. Other persons at risk are those with compromised immune systems, such as persons with the acquired immune deficiency syndrome (AIDS), who have a three hundred times greater risk for listeriosis compared with healthy persons. In addition, others who are at risk include persons with cancer, kidney disease, or diabetes; persons who have had an organ transplant and who take immunosuppressant drugs; persons taking glucocorticosteroids; and persons age sixty years and older.

SYMPTOMS

Infected persons may present with nausea, vomiting, diarrhea, and fever. Newborn infants may have jaundice, pneumonia, skin rash, lethargy, and vomiting. Symptoms may occur anytime from two to seventy days from when the contaminated food was consumed. Healthy people may have mild symptoms or no symptoms. Pregnant women may have mild symptoms, but her fetus remains at risk for infection.

SCREENING AND DIAGNOSIS

If listeriosis is suspected, the blood, urine, or feces is screened for *L. monocytogenes*. Also, a spinal fluid test may be used for screening, and the amniotic fluid of a pregnant woman may be tested.

TREATMENT AND THERAPY

Treatment is with antibiotics such as ampicillin. Infected newborns are also treated with antibiotics.

PREVENTION AND OUTCOMES

Active measures can help to avoid infection. One should thoroughly cook all meats, wash all vegetables, and avoid unpasteurized milk products. Uncooked

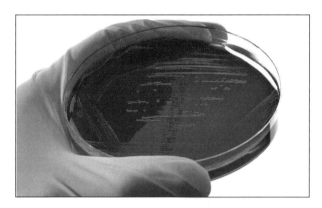

A culture plate contains Listeria, *the bacterium that causes listeriosis.*

meats should be separated from vegetables and other foods during food preparation.

As soon as possible after food preparation, the preparer should wash his or her hands and any cutting boards and knives used to prepare uncooked foods.

Persons at high risk for listeriosis should avoid soft cheese unless the label on the product indicates the cheese was made with pasteurized milk. Deli meat, cold salad, soft cheese, and pâté should be avoided by pregnant women.

Christine Adamec, M.B.A.

FURTHER READING

Bortolussi, Robert. "Listeriosis: A Primer." *CMAJ: Canadian Medical Association Journal* 179 (2008): 795-797.

Cheung, Vincent Y., and Wilma L. Sirkin. "Listeriosis Complicating Pregnancy." *CMAJ: Canadian Medical Association Journal* 181 (2009): 821-822.

Khare, Manjiri. "Infectious Disease in Pregnancy." *Current Obstetrics and Gynaecology* 15 (2005): 149-156.

U.S. Department of Health and Human Services. National Toxicology Program. "Listeria and Food Poisoning." Available at http://cerhr.niehs.nih.gov/common/listeria.html.

U.S. National Institutes of Health. "Listeriosis." Available at http://www.nlm.nih.gov/medlineplus/ency/article/001380.htm.

WEB SITES OF INTEREST

Centers for Disease Control and Prevention, Food Safety Program
http://www.cdc.gov/foodsafety

U.S. Department of Agriculture, Food Safety and Inspection Service
http://www.fsis.usda.gov

See also:*:* Bacteria: Classification and types; Bacterial infections; Children and infectious disease; Foodborne illness and disease; *Listeria*; Pathogens; Pregnancy and infectious disease; Soilborne illness and disease; Waterborne illness and disease.

Liver cancer

CATEGORY: Diseases and conditions
ANATOMY OR SYSTEM AFFECTED: Liver, tissue
ALSO KNOWN AS: Hepatocarcinoma, hepatocellular cancer, malignant hepatoma, primary liver cancer

DEFINITION

Hepatocellular (*hepato* means "liver" and "cellular" means "pertaining to the cell") cancer is defined as a primary liver cancer that originates in the liver. Mutations (changes in deoxyribonucleic acid, or DNA) can occur in hepatocytes (principal cells of the liver), which can become cancer cells (malignant). Primary liver cancer can spread (metastasize) to other organs of the body. Similarly, cancers from other organs can metastasize to the liver. This spreading cancer in the liver is called secondary liver cancer. Related conditions include hepatoblastoma, a liver cancer in children; cholangiocarcinoma, a cancer of bile ducts in the liver; and angiosarcoma or hemangiosarcoma, a cancer of blood vessels in the liver.

CAUSES

Liver cancer is caused by existing liver disease, such as hepatitis or cirrhosis; hereditary metabolic disorders, such as hemochromatosis; aflatoxins, which are toxins produced by certain molds; and diabetes.

RISK FACTORS

Viral hepatitis, an inflammation of the liver caused by a virus, is a risk factor for developing liver cancer. Hepatitis, which can become progressive and chronic, is also caused by toxins and by heavy drinking of alcohol. If chronic hepatitis remains untreated, it can cause liver failure.

Chronic cirrhosis is a progressive degenerative condition in which there is diffuse destruction of hepatocytes and an increase in fats and connective tissue. Chronic cirrhosis can develop into liver cancer as hepatocytes are transformed into cancer cells. Nonalcoholic cirrhosis is a greater risk than is alcoholic cirrhosis.

Hereditary factors are responsible for certain storage diseases, such as hemochromatosis. Genetic hemochromatosis is a condition of impaired iron metabolism causing iron deposits in the tissues of the liver, pancreas, heart muscle, and other organs. The iron from the food is absorbed by the intestine in excess and is then circulated to the organs by arteries. In the liver, accumulated iron in hepatocytes can cause cirrhosis. Cirrhosis then develops into liver cancer.

Environmental factors that increase the risk for liver cancer include the toxins produced by the fungi *Aspergillus favus* and *A. parasiticus*. These toxins, called aflatoxins, often grow on wet grains. They can induce mutations that cause hepatocellular cancer. Exposure to chemicals such as nitrites, arsenic, organochlorine, polyvinyl chloride, and pesticides also can cause liver cancer. Diabetes may be related to the condition called nonalcoholic fatty liver, which may lead to cirrhosis and then to primary liver cancer.

SYMPTOMS

The symptoms of liver cancer include fatigue, weakness, abdominal pain, enlarged liver, loss of appetite, nausea, and vomiting. By the time symptoms appear, the condition is advanced.

SCREENING AND DIAGNOSIS

Diagnosis of liver cancer is made using the following screening methods:

Ultrasound. A noninvasive technique in which ultrasound waves are used to identify liver tumors. Because this is not an X-radiation technique, no radiation is involved; also, no injections are required.

Computed tomography (CT) scan. With this technique, computer-generated cross-sectional images of the liver are obtained with X rays to identify liver tumors; therefore, radiation is involved. Contrast material is injected into a vein; the tumor has different contrast than that of adjacent normal tissue. Triphasic CT scans are better for diagnosis of liver cancer. During a triphasic scan, images are obtained at three different times during the blood flow.

Magnetic resonance imaging (MRI). An imaging tech-

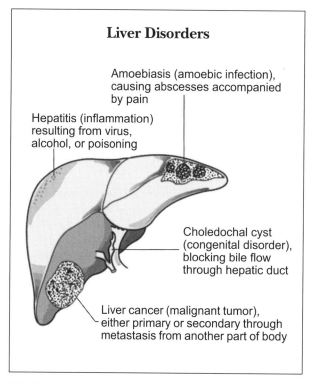

Liver Disorders

Amoebiasis (amoebic infection), causing abscesses accompanied by pain

Hepatitis (inflammation) resulting from virus, alcohol, or poisoning

Choledochal cyst (congenital disorder), blocking bile flow through hepatic duct

Liver cancer (malignant tumor), either primary or secondary through metastasis from another part of body

The liver's unique structure and functions leave it vulnerable to many diseases, including liver cancer.

nique that uses a magnetic field to detect liver tumors. Contrast material is injected through a vein to differentiate tumors from normal tissue.

All of these imaging techniques can detect large enough tumors, but nanotechnology, still in development, would be able to detect even a single cancer cell.

Biopsy. In liver biopsy, a piece of liver is sectioned, stained, and examined under a microscope. Liver biopsy can confirm the diagnosis.

Staging system. Progressive stages of the disease are classified 1 through 4 and are based on the number and size of tumors, blood vessels, lymph nodes, organs around the liver, and pathology.

TREATMENT AND THERAPY

Treatment of liver cancer includes chemotherapy, surgery, biological and targeted therapy, and tumor ablation.

Chemotherapy. Certain liver cancer cells can be destroyed only with chemotherapy. In chemotherapy, drugs are usually administered intravenously. Common drugs used are sorafenib (Nexavar) and doxorubicin (Adriamycin and Rubex).

Surgery. If a liver is only partly cancerous, only the tumor is surgically removed, in a procedure called partial hepatectomy or liver resection. If the entire liver is cancerous, the whole liver is surgically removed and replaced with a nondiseased liver from a donor. This procedure is call liver implantation.

Biologic and targeted therapy. Drugs such as sorafenib are used to target the dividing cells of the tumor and the tumor's blood supply.

Tumor ablation. A procedure for destroying the tumor without the use of drugs. In hepatic artery embolization, the tumor will be deprived of nutrition; this leads to the death of the tumor cells. In radio frequency ablation, a "hot" metal probe is used to kill tumor cells. In cryotherapy, a "frozen" metal probe is used to kill tumor cells.

PREVENTION AND OUTCOMES

Persons with hepatitis and cirrhosis are predisposed to primary liver cancer, so preventive measures should especially be followed by those with these diseases. A vaccine is available for preventing hepatitis B, but not for hepatitis C.

Long exposure to cancer-causing chemicals should be avoided. Hereditary factors, however, cannot be avoided. In persons with diabetes or for those who have alcoholism, the liver needs to be screened to check for fatty deposits.

Arun S. Dabholkar, Ph.D.

FURTHER READING

Abou-Alfa, Ghassan K., and Ronald P. DeMatteo. *One Hundred Questions and Answers About Liver Cancer.* 2d ed. Sudbury, Mass.: Jones and Bartlett, 2009.

Boyer, Thomas D., Teresa L. Wright, and Michael P. Manns, eds. *Zakim and Boyer's Hepatology: A Textbook of Liver Disease.* 5th ed. Philadelphia: Saunders/Elsevier, 2006.

Feldman, Mark, Lawrence S. Friedman, and Lawrence J. Brandt, eds. *Sleisenger and Fordtran's Gastrointestinal and Liver Disease: Pathophysiology, Diagnosis, Management.* New ed. 2 vols. Philadelphia: Saunders/Elsevier, 2010.

Stevens, Alan, James S. Lowe, and Barbara Young. *Wheater's Basic Histopathology: A Colour Atlas and Text.* 4th ed. London: Elsevier Health Sciences, 2002.

WEB SITES OF INTEREST

American Cancer Society
http://www.cancer.org

American Liver Foundation
http://www.liverfoundation.org

Liver Cancer Network
http://www.livercancer.com

National Cancer Institute
http://www.cancer.gov

See also:: Cancer and infectious disease; Hepatitis A; Hepatitis C; Hepatitis D; Hepatitis E; Hepatitis vaccines; Vaccines: Experimental; Viral hepatitis; Viral infections.

Lockjaw. *See* Tetanus.

Lyme disease

CATEGORY: Diseases and conditions
ANATOMY OR SYSTEM AFFECTED: All

DEFINITION

Lyme disease is the most common tickborne disease in the United States and is caused by a corkscrew-shaped bacterium called *Borrelia burgdorferi.*

CAUSES

Lyme disease is a bacterial infection resulting from the bite of an infected deer tick. An infected tick transmits the bacterium to humans by biting the skin. If untreated, the bacterium can travel through the bloodstream, settle in various body tissue, and cause a number of acute and persistent symptoms, ranging from mild to severe.

RISK FACTORS

Persons who live in areas where there are ticks have a risk of being bitten by a disease-infected tick. An increased risk is usually directly related to the amount of time a person spends outdoors in areas where there are many ticks.

Geographic location. Lyme disease is found most often in three geographic locations in the United States: northeastern and mid-Atlantic region: Maine to Maryland; upper north-central region: Minnesota and Wisconsin; and northwest region: northwestern California and Oregon.

Time of year. Ticks are most active during the warmer months of the year. Peak at-risk times vary from region to region, based on the temperature. For the northeast and north-central United States, increased risk is between April and November, with the peak occurring in July. For the southern United States, ticks are active year-round. Other areas can be variable, based on the temperature.

Activity. People who work outdoors in jobs such as surveying, landscaping, forestry, gardening, and utility service have a higher risk of Lyme disease. Participating in outdoor recreational activities such as hiking, camping, and hunting also can increase a person's risk.

Landscape condition. The ticks that carry Lyme disease are more likely to live in wet, green, brushy, or wooded areas. They are less likely to be near pruned, well-cared-for plants, but more likely to be near shrubby or brushy plants that are not maintained. Living near or visiting wooded or brushy areas can increase a person's risk.

Age. Lyme disease occurs more often in children under the age of fifteen years and in adults between the ages of twenty-five and forty-four years. Persons in these age ranges participate at a higher rate in outdoor activities that expose them to ticks.

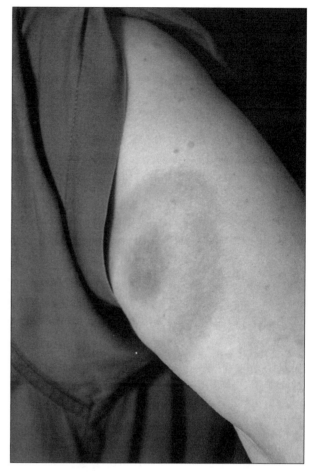

The characteristic bull's-eye rash on the arm of a woman with Lyme disease. (CDC)

SYMPTOMS

The symptoms of Lyme disease can be confusing, and they differ among infected persons both in their nature and in their severity. Some people may not have any symptoms, but Lyme disease may still be diagnosed through a blood test.

Lyme disease progresses through different stages with varying and sometimes overlapping symptoms. Symptoms, which typically occur within three to thirty-two days of a tick bite (early infection), include the following:

Rash. A red rash, known as erythema migrans (EM), starts as a small red spot at the site of the tick bite and expands over a period of days or weeks, forming a circular- or oval-shaped rash. The rash often resembles a bull's eye: a red ring surrounding a clear or bluish area with a red center. The size of the rash can range from dime-sized to the entire width of a person's back. More than one ring may develop. Typically, the rash disappears within four weeks.

Although Lyme disease is often associated with this rash, many people do not have the rash right away or at all, or they may have a red rash but one without the bull's eye pattern. If having symptoms that resemble those of Lyme disease, the person should see a doctor; avoid waiting for a rash to appear.

Flulike symptoms. Muscle and joint aches, headache, fever (100° to 103° Fahrenheit), stiff neck, swollen glands, and fatigue may occur with or without the rash. These symptoms usually last about five to twenty-one days.

For early widespread infection, the symptoms include the following:

Multiple EM lesions. The rash may appear in several places on the body.

Arthritis and general joint pain. Joint pain symptoms are sometimes the first noticeable symptoms. They include stiffness and swelling of the joints, particularly in the large joints, such as the knee, elbow, and shoulder.

Nervous system problems. The bacteria can affect the brain, spinal cord, and other nerves of the body. Symptoms of this include weakness and drooping of the face and eyelid on one side (Bell's palsy). It may also occur on both sides of the face. Other symptoms are low back pain; widespread numbness, tingling, and burning; impaired motor coordination; persistent headache; stiff neck; mood changes; difficulty concentrating or sleeping; generalized weakness; conjunctivitis (eye redness and inflammation); and problems with the heart, liver, lymph nodes, and testes.

All symptoms of early manifestation usually occur with the first rash or within about six weeks of it. They may disappear on their own within a few weeks or months.

Symptoms of late infection include joint pain (such as painful inflammation of the joints and intermittent or chronic arthritis), chronic nervous system problems (such as memory problems, dementia, depression, sleep disorder, nerve pain), and chronic skin problems (such as thinning, thickening, or discoloration of the skin, usually of the hands and feet).

SCREENING AND DIAGNOSIS

The purpose of screening is early diagnosis and treatment. Screening tests are usually administered to people without current symptoms, but who may be at high risk for certain diseases or conditions. Routine screening for Lyme disease is not recommended if one has no symptoms.

Persons who have removed an attached tick from their body should consult a doctor. For thirty days after being bitten, the person should watch closely for fever and for the characteristic bulls-eye rash at the site of the bite. If these symptoms develop, one should consult a doctor immediately.

One is much less likely to develop Lyme disease if the tick had been attached for less than twenty-four hours. Treatment with appropriate antibiotics after a tick bite, while not endorsed by all experts, may also reduce risk.

There are no tests that are completely accurate in diagnosing Lyme disease. However, a doctor may order one or more of the following tests to support the diagnosis of Lyme disease:

Antibody test. Antibodies are the body's defense against an infection. If one has been infected with the Lyme disease bacteria, the body will release specific antibodies to fight it. It takes about four weeks or more for these antibodies to become detectable. Antibody tests include antibody titer (enzyme-linked immunoabsorbent assay), which measures the level of Lyme disease antibodies in the blood. If this test is equivocal or positive, the person will need to have a Western blot to confirm the results

Western blot. This test detects the presence of the antibody to specific Lyme disease proteins in the blood.

Both of these tests, however, can have false-negative results or false-positive results. False negatives may occur if the test is performed too soon after infection, if too few antibodies are made by the body, or if the test is performed incorrectly. False positives may occur if the test is performed incorrectly. Also, the immune system produces unrelated antibodies that appear in the test as if they were produced in response to Lyme disease, resulting in a false positive.

Direct detection test. These tests look directly for the bacterium, or pieces of it, in the blood and other fluids of the body, such as urine and spinal fluid. One main type of direct detection test is the antigen detection test. This test looks for a unique protein from the Lyme disease bacteria that may be in body fluids and is useful for detecting Lyme disease if the person is already taking antibiotics or for needs to be tested for a later flare-up of symptoms

Another direct detection test is polymerase chain reaction, which identifies specific deoxyribonucleic acid (DNA) from the Lyme bacteria and is able to detect small amounts of bacterial DNA.

Culture. A laboratory culture is done by growing the Lyme bacteria from fluid taken from an open sore or other source of body fluids. If the bacteria grow, the test is considered positive. Cultures often take many weeks to grow the bacteria and are rarely used today.

Analysis of spinal fluid. This test is done when a person's symptoms indicate that Lyme disease is affecting the nervous system. Spinal fluid is removed by spinal tap (inserting a needle into the spinal column) and is tested for bacteria using one of the foregoing tests.

Single photon emission computed tomography. This test

is rarely used but may be done in certain cases with symptoms that involve the nervous system. It is a kind of brain scan that looks for brainwave patterns that may indicate Lyme disease infection.

TREATMENT AND THERAPY

The specific treatment for Lyme disease depends on how long one has had the disease, when it is diagnosed, and whether there are any complications. In all stages, medications are used to kill the Lyme bacteria in the body in an effort to eliminate the disease or reduce the symptoms and complications.

Lyme disease responds well to antibiotics. Antibiotics, including doxycycline (Vibramycin, Adoxa, and others) and amoxicillin (Amoxil, Dispermox, and Trimox), are usually effective. The infected person will need to take antibiotics for ten days to four weeks. Some symptoms may continue after treatment.

For persistent or severe cases that do not respond to oral antibiotics, the doctor may prescribe intravenous antibiotic treatments (usually ceftriaxone). Chronic arthritis may require anti-inflammatory medication or joint injection with steroids. There are no surgical options for treating the disease.

PREVENTION AND OUTCOMES

To help prevent Lyme disease, one should avoid areas that are likely to be infested with deer ticks (moist, shaded, wooded, or grassy areas, especially in northeastern, mid-Atlantic, and upper north-central regions of the United States and northwestern California). When going to wooded grassy areas, especially in spring and summer, one should wear light-colored clothing with a tight weave to spot ticks easily; wear enclosed shoes and a long sleeve shirt; tuck the shirt into the pants; tuck pants into socks or boot tops; and wear a hat. One should apply insect repellent containing NN-diethyl metatoluamide (DEET) to clothes and exposed skin. Insect repellents containing permethrin can be applied to pants, socks, and shoes, but not to skin. Both products can cause eye irritation and DEET can cause skin reactions, so one should follow label directions for application; should avoid applying near eyes, nose, or mouth (children should avoid applying to their hands); and wash skin after returning indoors. Persons also should stay on cleared, well-traveled paths and walk in the center of trails to avoid overgrown grass and brush; avoid sitting on the ground or stone walls; and remove leaf litter, brush,

---

Speaking with a Healthcare Provider About Lyme Disease

SPECIFIC QUESTIONS TO ASK ABOUT LYME DISEASE
What is Lyme disease?
How do you get Lyme disease?
What does a tick that carries Lyme disease look like?
What should I do if I get a tick on me?
How do I safely remove a tick if I find one?
Can you test the tick to see if it carries Lyme disease?

SPECIFIC QUESTIONS ABOUT THE RISK OF DEVELOPING LYME DISEASE
Based on my medical history and lifestyle, am I at risk for Lyme disease?
How do I best prevent Lyme disease?
How do I know if I might have Lyme disease?
Is there a test for Lyme disease?

SPECIFIC QUESTIONS ABOUT TREATMENT OPTIONS
How do I best treat Lyme disease?
What medications are available to help me?
What are the benefits and side effects of these medications?
Will these medications interact with other medications, over-the-counter products, or dietary and herbal supplements?
Will the medications cure me of the disease?
Are there any alternative or complementary therapies that will help me?

SPECIFIC QUESTIONS ABOUT LIFESTYLE CHANGES
Can I continue my regular activities?
What can I do to prevent being bitten by a tick?

SPECIFIC QUESTIONS ABOUT OUTLOOK
How do I know that my prevention or treatment program is effective?
Once I am treated, can Lyme disease come back?
Is Lyme disease contagious?
Can I get the disease again if another tick bites me?

---

and woodpiles from around the home and the edges of the yard.

To manage ticks, one should put clothes that have been worn outdoors in a clothes dryer for twenty minutes to kill unseen ticks. Deer ticks are unlikely to infect unless they remain in contact with the skin for at least twenty-four hours. This leaves ample time to do a full-body check for ticks at the end of a day spent outdoors. Pets should be checked for ticks too.

Not all ticks carry Lyme disease. Deer ticks are small, approximately the size of a poppy seed. If a tick is found, one should remove it by using a pair of tweezers and grasping the tick by the head or mouthparts as close to the skin as possible, and by pulling directly outward, gently but firmly, with steady, even force. One should not twist the tick out, crush the tick's body, or handle it with bare fingers because this can spread infection. One should not put a hot match to the tick or cover it with petroleum jelly, nail polish, or any other substance. After the tick is removed, one should swab the site thoroughly with an antiseptic to prevent infection.

Antibiotics, including a single dose of doxycycline, have been shown to reduce the risk of contracting Lyme disease after a known tick bite. The risk of catching Lyme disease after a single tick bite is low, and many experts do not necessarily recommend preventive antibiotic treatment, even in parts of the United States with a relatively high risk of Lyme disease.

Mary Calvagna, M.S.;
reviewed by David L. Horn, M.D., FACP

FURTHER READING

Atkinson, P. W., ed. *Vector Biology, Ecology, and Control.* New York: Springer Science, 2010. This book is a good source for the reader who needs a detailed study of vectors, including ticks, and the latest methods for effective vector control.

Edlow, Jonathan A. *Bull's Eye: Unraveling the Medical Mystery of Lyme Disease.* 2d ed. New Haven, Conn.: Yale University Press, 2004. A look at Lyme disease from the perspective of scientific mystery and understanding.

Edlow, Jonathan A., and Robert Moellering, Jr., eds. "Tick-Borne Diseases, Part 1: Lyme Disease." *Infectious Disease Clinics of North America* 22, no. 2 (2008). Special issue on Lyme disease, from a respected journal.

Service, M. W., ed. *Encyclopedia of Arthropod-Transmitted Infections.* New York: CABI, 2001. Offers basic information related to the transmission, symptoms, treatment, and control of infections transmitted by biting midges, ticks, lice, and related organisms.

Vanderhoof-Forschner, Karen. *Everything You Need to Know About Lyme Disease and Other Tick-Borne Disorders.* 2d ed. Hoboken, N.J.: John Wiley & Sons, 2003. A consumer guide that aims to provide basic

knowledge and useful insights into the prevention and management of Lyme disease.

Weiner, H. R. "Lyme Disease: Questions and Discussion." *Comprehensive Therapy* 32 (2006): 17-19. Brief but informative article on Lyme disease and therapeutics.

WEB SITES OF INTEREST

American Lyme Disease Foundation
http://www.aldf.com

Lyme Disease Association
http://www.lymediseaseassociation.org

See also:: Acariasis; Anaplasmosis; Arthropod-borne illness and disease; Babesiosis; Bell's palsy; *Borrelia*; Cat scratch fever; Colorado tick fever; Ehrlichiosis; Immunoassay; Mediterranean spotted fever; Mites and chiggers and infectious disease; Rocky Mountain spotted fever; Skin infections; Ticks and infectious disease; Vectors and vector control.

Lymphadenitis

CATEGORY: Diseases and conditions
ANATOMY OR SYSTEM AFFECTED: Immune system, lymph nodes, lymphatic system

DEFINITION

Lymphadenitis is inflammation of a lymph node. The condition is common in children.

CAUSES

Lymphadenitis usually results from a bacterial infection, but can also occur in response to a virus, fungus, or cancer. Lymph nodes filter infection and cancer cells, which are then drained by way of the lymphatic system, an interconnecting network of channels that move lymph fluid through the body to the blood. The nodes become inflamed in response to a buildup of bacteria or other inflammatory triggers. Lymphadenitis is commonly caused by members of the *Mycobacterium* species of bacteria, either tuberculosis-causing (tuberculous) or nontuberculous *Mycobacterium*. In children, infection with nontuberculous *Mycobacterium* is usually responsible for lymph node swelling; the bacteria are common to water and soil and to dairy products.

RISK FACTORS

Risk factors for lymphadenitis include any recent viral, fungal, or bacterial infection or cancer. Recent infections caused by *Staphylococcus* or *Streptococcus* bacteria can result in lymphadenitis, even if the initial infection is successfully treated. Underlying chronic illness can predispose a person to lymphadenitis, but healthy people can also be affected.

SYMPTOMS

Swelling of one or more lymph nodes is the primary symptom. The nodes may be painless or tender, and feel rubbery or hard. The overlying skin may appear normal or may be bruised or inflamed. In children, infection with nontuberculous *Mycobacterium* results in inflammation of nodes in the face, neck (cervical), collarbone (clavicular), or under the jaw (submandibular), which may drain infectious fluid (pus) through the skin.

SCREENING AND DIAGNOSIS

Lymphadenitis can be diagnosed based upon symptoms in persons who have had a recent infection in the area of the swollen node. If there is no known history of infection, a more thorough work up may be warranted. Common diagnostic procedures include biopsy (microscopic analysis) of lymph tissue following surgical removal (excision) of the lymph node and fine needle aspiration, a procedure in which a small needle is inserted into the node to remove lymph cells. A chest X ray, a computed tomography (CT) scan, or a magnetic resonance imaging (MRI) test may be performed to evaluate the area of the body containing the enlarged node.

TREATMENT AND THERAPY

Treatment may involve surgical excision of all involved nodes, an extended course of antibiotics, and simple observation for lymphadenitis to resolve on its own. Treatment decisions are made based upon the cause of lymphadenitis, whether the lymph node or nodes can be removed with minimal scarring or damage to underlying nerves or blood vessels, and the potential benefit or risks of months-long antibiotic therapy. One should have any collection of pus (abscess) surgically drained.

PREVENTION AND OUTCOMES

Based on the multitude of potential causes, lymphadenitis cannot be prevented. The primary concern should be early medical attention and treatment.

Carita Caple, M.S.H.S., R.N.

FURTHER READING

Amir, J. "Non-tuberculous Mycobacterial Lymphadenitis in Children: Diagnosis and Management." *Israel Medical Association Journal* 12 (2010): 49-52.

Harris, Robert L., et al. "Cervicofacial Nontuberculous *Mycobacterium* Lymphadenitis in Children: Is Surgery Always Necessary?" *International Journal of Pediatric Otorhinolaryngology* 73 (2009): 1297-1301.

"Lymphatic Disorders." In *The Merck Manual Home Health Handbook,* edited by Robert S. Porter et al. 3d ed. Whitehouse Station, N.J.: Merck Research Laboratories, 2009.

McDowell, Julie, and Michael Windelsprecht. *The Lymphatic System.* Santa Barbara, Calif.: Greenwood Press, 2004.

Schmitt, D. B. "Swollen Lymph Nodes: Brief Version." In *Pediatric Advisor,* edited by J. Burley et al. Broomfield, Colo.: Clinical Reference Systems, 2008.

WEB SITES OF INTEREST

About Kids Health
http://www.aboutkidshealth.ca

American Academy of Family Physicians
http://familydoctor.org

Centers for Disease Control and Prevention
http://www.cdc.gov

National Library of Medicine
http://www.nlm.nih.gov

See also:: Bacterial infections; Children and infectious disease; Inflammation; Mycobacterial infections; *Mycobacterium*; Skin infections; *Staphylococcus*; *Streptococcus*.

Lymphocytes. *See* T lymphocytes.

M

Macrolide antibiotics

CATEGORY: Treatment

DEFINITION

Macrolide antibiotics are well-established, broad-spectrum, antibacterial agents derived from *Streptomyces* bacteria. Macrolides are a large, structurally diverse group of antibiotics composed of different-sized macrocyclic lactones attached to sugar moieties. The best-known macrolide antibiotic is erythromycin. Newer semisynthetic derivatives of erythromycin include azithromycin, clarithromycin, and dirithromycin. Macrolide antibiotics are especially useful as a treatment option for persons who are allergic to penicillin.

MODE OF ACTION

Macrolide antibiotics are generally bacteriostatic agents that disrupt bacterial growth without causing cell death. These agents inhibit bacterial growth by suppressing protein synthesis. This mechanism occurs with the antibiotic reversibly binding to the 50S bacterial ribosomal subunit and inhibiting translocation by dissociating peptidyl-transfer ribonucleic acid (RNA) from the ribosome. This process prevents peptide chain elongation, cell growth, and reproduction. At high concentrations, macrolides have been known to exhibit bactericidal properties and cause cell death by interfering with deoxyribonucleic acid (DNA) replication.

PHARMACOLOGY

The pharmacological properties of an antibiotic dictate its effectiveness in inhibiting bacterial infections. Macrolides are typically administered orally but are generally poorly absorbed. Newer erythromycin derivatives exhibit broader activity and effectiveness against intracellular pathogens. Their most important attributes include improved lung and tissue absorption, higher intracellular concentrations and bioavailability, fewer dosing regimens, and less frequent drug-drug interactions.

INDICATIONS

Macrolides primarily display antibacterial activity toward most aerobic and anaerobic gram-positive bacteria with the exception of enterococci. Macrolides also inhibit some *Mycoplasma* species and anaerobic gram-negative pathogens. These antibiotics are effective in treating respiratory tract infections such as Legionnaires' disease, community acquired pneumonia, pertussis (whooping cough), and diphtheria. Other indications include skin and soft tissue infections and sexually transmitted diseases, including chlamydia, syphilis, and gonorrhea. Macrolides also are potent against *Helicobacter pylori* infections of the stomach, penicillin-resistant staphylococcal infections, and group A streptococcal and pneumococcal infections in persons allergic to penicillin. Macrolides are not recommended for the treatment of meningitis.

SIDE EFFECTS

Macrolides are considered one of the safest and best tolerated classes of antibiotics, even in children. The most common side effects include gastrointestinal upsets such as abdominal pain, dyspepsia (indigestion), diarrhea, nausea, and vomiting. More serious side effects can occur depending on the prescribed antibiotic and include allergic and dermatologic reactions, hepatic (liver) dysfunction, drug-drug interactions, cardiac and ventricular arrhythmias, and dose-related complications such as tinnitus and hearing loss.

IMPACT

Macrolide antibiotics have been essential in the treatment of infectious diseases for many years. Their discovery has provided a safe alternate therapy option for persons with an allergy to penicillin, one of the most frequent causes of severe allergic drug reactions.

Rose Ciulla-Bohling, Ph.D.

FURTHER READING

Kirst, Herbert A. "Antibiotics: Macrolides." In *Van Nostrand's Encyclopedia of Chemistry*, edited by Glenn D.

Considine. 5th ed. Hoboken, N.J.: Wiley-Interscience, 2010.

Sanford, Jay P., et al. *The Sanford Guide to Antimicrobial Therapy.* 18th ed. Sperryville, Va.: Antimicrobial Therapy, 2010.

Schönfeld, W., and H. A. Kirst, eds. *Macrolide Antibiotics.* Boston: Birkhäuser, 2002.

WEB SITES OF INTEREST

Alliance for the Prudent Use of Antibiotics
http://www.tufts.edu/med/apua

Centers for Disease Control and Prevention
http://www.cdc.gov

U.S. Food and Drug Administration
http://www.fda.gov

See also: Alliance for the Prudent Use of Antibiotics; Aminoglycoside antibiotics; Antibiotics: Types; Bacteria: Classification and types; Cephalosporin antibiotics; Glycopeptide antibiotics; Ketolide antibiotics; Lipopeptide antibiotics; Oxazolidinone antibiotics; Penicillin antibiotics; Prevention of bacterial infections; Quinolone antibiotics; Reinfection; Secondary infection; Superbacteria; Tetracycline antibiotics; Treatment of bacterial infections.

Mad-cow disease. *See* Variant Creutzfeldt-Jakob disease.

Malaria

CATEGORY: Diseases and conditions
ANATOMY OR SYSTEM AFFECTED: All

DEFINITION

Malaria is a disease passed through the blood. It is caused by a parasite that is typically passed to humans through the bite of an infected mosquito.

CAUSES

Malaria is caused by one of the following four types of parasites: *Plasmodium falciparum, P. vivax, P. ovale,* and *P. malariae.*

An *Anopheles* mosquito becomes infected when it

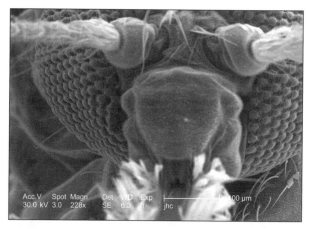

Magnified image of the Anopheles *mosquito, a carrier of the protozoan parasite that causes malaria.* (CDC)

bites someone with malaria. In turn, the mosquito passes the malaria to a new person through a new bite. Malaria can also be passed from a pregnant girl or woman to her fetus. It can also be passed through a blood transfusion from an infected donor.

P. falciparum is by far the most dangerous of the forms of malaria. In most areas it is also the most common form.

RISK FACTORS

Risk factors that increase the chance of getting malaria include living in or traveling to hot, humid climates where *Anopheles* mosquitoes are prevalent; failing to use insect repellants containing NN-diethyl metatoluamide (DEET) when outdoors; failing to use sleeping nets (especially nets treated with permethrin); failing to use medications to prevent malaria infection; and visiting or living in Africa, Asia, or Latin America. Malaria occurs regularly in tourists who fail to follow recommended precautions. The majority of fatal cases of malaria seem to be acquired by tourists visiting game parks and other rural areas in East Africa.

SYMPTOMS

Once inside the bloodstream, parasites travel to the liver and then multiply there (the hepatic phase). During this phase, the infected person has no symptoms. After several days, the parasites' offspring are released into the bloodstream, where they infect red blood cells. Within forty-eight hours, the infected red blood cells burst, and the parasites infect more red blood cells. This process leads to recurrent fevers (as high as 106° Fahrenheit), chills, diffuse muscles aches, headaches, nausea and vomiting (or both), diarrhea, anemia, and jaundice (yellow coloring of the skin or eyes).

Without treatment, the cycle of red blood cell destruction and fever will continue. This can lead to death. Symptoms usually begin within ten days to four weeks of being bitten by an infected mosquito. *P. malariae* may not produce symptoms for a year or more. *P. falciparum* infections, which tend to cause more severe symptoms, are associated with higher death rates.

SCREENING AND DIAGNOSIS

A doctor will ask about symptoms, medical history, and travel history, and will perform a physical exam. A blood test will analyze the affected person's blood for parasites.

TREATMENT AND THERAPY

Prescription drugs are used to treat malaria by killing the parasites. Choice of antimalarial agent depends on the type of parasite and the severity and stage of the infection. The following medications are used alone or in combination: chloroquine (in many parts of the world, *P. falciparum* is resistant to this drug), mefloquine (Lariam), doxycycline, clindamycin, malarone, quinidine, quinine, combination of pyrimethamine and sulfadoxine (Fansidar), primaquine (for hepatic, or first, phase of *P. vivax* and *P. ovale*), and artemisinin. All these medications, except chloroquine and primaquine, are commonly used to treat resistant strains of *P. falciparum*.

PREVENTION AND OUTCOMES

To reduce the chance of getting malaria when in an area where malaria is prevalent, one should take antimalarial medication before, during, and after travel. One should use DEET insect repellent (a minimum of 30 to 35 percent DEET) when outside and should use proper mosquito netting (sleeping nets) at night. Electronic mosquito repellents, which are supposed to repel mosquitoes by emitting a sound, do not prevent mosquito bites. One should use flying-insect spray in non-air-conditioned rooms while sleeping, should wear clothing that covers as much skin as possible, and should avoid being outdoors from dusk to dawn, when mosquitoes are most prevalent.

Michelle Badash, M.S.;
reviewed by David L. Horn, M.D., FACP

FURTHER READING

Crompton, Peter D., Susan K. Pierce, and Louis H. Miller. "Advances and Challenges in Malaria Vaccine Development." *Journal of Clinical Investigation* 120 (2010): 4168-4178.

Enayati, A., J. Hemingway, and P. Garner. "Electronic Mosquito Repellents for Preventing Mosquito Bites and Malaria Infection." *Cochrane Database of Systematic Reviews* (2009): CD005434. Available through *EBSCO DynaMed Systematic Literature Surveillance* at http://www.ebscohost.com/dynamed.

Jong, Elaine C., and Russell McMullen, eds. *Travel and Tropical Medicine Manual.* 4th ed. Philadelphia: Saunders/Elsevier, 2008.

Mandell, Gerald L., John E. Bennett, and Raphael Dolin, eds. *Mandell, Douglas, and Bennett's Principles and Practice of Infectious Diseases.* 7th ed. New York: Churchill Livingstone/Elsevier, 2010.

O'Hanlon, Leslie Harris. "Tinkering with Genes to Fight Insect-Borne Disease: Researchers Create Genetically Modified Bugs to Fight Malaria, Chagas', and Other Diseases." *The Lancet* 363 (April 17, 2004): 1288.

WEB SITES OF INTEREST

American Society of Tropical Medicine and Hygiene
http://www.astmh.org

Centers for Disease Control and Prevention
http://www.cdc.gov/parasites

Malaria Vaccine Initiative
http://www.malariavaccine.org

Multilateral Initiative on Malaria
http:///www.mimilaria.org

World Health Organization
http://www.who.int

See also: Arthropod-borne illness and disease; Blood-borne illness and disease; Chikungunya; Dengue fever; Developing countries and infectious disease; Malaria vaccine; Mosquitoes and infectious disease; Parasites: Classification and types; Parasitic diseases; Quinolone antibiotics; Rift Valley fever; Sleeping nets; Tropical medicine; Yellow fever.

Malaria vaccine

CATEGORY: Prevention

DEFINITION

Malaria vaccine is a preparation designed to provide immunity against infection by the parasite *Plasmodium,* which leads to malaria.

BACKGROUND

Malaria is caused by four species of *Plasmodium*: *P. falciparum, P. vivax, P. malariae,* and *P. ovale. P. falciparum* causes about 90 percent of malaria cases and is responsible for the most deaths, particularly in Africa. It is estimated that 3 billion people are at risk for malaria exposure. About 500 million people suffer from malaria worldwide, and 1 million children in Africa die each year from the disease.

Plasmodia are transmitted by the *Anopheles* mosquito; the incubation period lasts between seven and thirty days, depending on the *Plasmodium* species transmitted. Symptoms of malaria include shivering, fever, headache, vomiting, and sweating. Severe malaria can involve such symptoms as impaired consciousness, seizures, coma, anemia, pulmonary edema, and cardiovascular collapse.

VACCINE STATUS

Preventing malaria infection is a top priority for many health and research organizations around the world, as they are trying to establish vaccines to protect against the disease. No commercially available vaccine for malaria exists, despite decades of research on the topic. Many researchers are focusing on developing vaccines against *P. falciparum,* while a few groups are working on a vaccine for *P. vivax.* The life cycle of *P. falciparum* is quite complex, as it provides several stages on which to focus vaccine development.

The most advanced vaccine is RTS,S, which has been studied in phase-three trials in several countries in sub-Saharan Africa since 2009; the phase-two trial for this drug showed 30 to 50 percent efficacy in reducing malaria in infants and children. Based on these results, it appears that the vaccine will only partially protect those immunized.

Another promising vaccine is FMP2.1/AS02A, which has shown efficacy in children in Mali. Numerous clinical trials have attempted to select safe, effective vaccines. Because of the complexity of the parasite's life cycle, it is likely that multiple types of vaccines will be necessary to interrupt that life cycle.

IMPACT

A viable, disease-preventing malaria vaccine has the potential to save millions of lives by providing protection against *Plasmodium* infection.

Dawn M. Bielawski, Ph.D.

FURTHER READING

Crompton, Peter D., Susan K. Pierce, and Louis H. Miller. "Advances and Challenges in Malaria Vaccine Development." *Journal of Clinical Investigation* 120 (2010): 4168-4178.

Enayati, A., and J. Hemingway. "Malaria Management: Past, Present, and Future." *Annual Review of Entomology* 55 (2010): 569-591.

Mahamadou, A. Thera, et al. "Safety and Immunogenicity of an AMA1 Malaria Vaccine in Malian Children." *PLoS* 5 (2010): e9041.

Sherman, Irwin W. *The Elusive Malaria Vaccine: Miracle or Mirage?* New York: ASM Press, 2009.

WEB SITES OF INTEREST

Centers for Disease Control and Prevention
http://www.cdc.gov/malaria

Emerging and Reemerging Infectious Diseases Resource Center
http://www.medscape.com/resource/infections

Laboratory of Malaria Immunology and Vaccinology
http://www.niaid.nih.gov/topics/malaria/research/pages/mvdb.aspx

Malaria Vaccine Initiative
http://www.malariavaccine.org

Vaccine Resource Library
http://www.path.org/vaccineresources/malaria

World Health Organization
http://www.who.int/immunization/topics/malaria

See also: Arthropod-borne illness and disease; Blood-borne illness and disease; Chikungunya; Dengue fever; Developing countries and infectious disease; Emerging and reemerging infectious diseases; Malaria; Mosquitoes and infectious disease; Parasites: Classification and types; Parasitic diseases; Rift Valley fever; Sleeping nets; Tropical medicine; Vaccines: Types; Yellow fever.

Malassezia

CATEGORY: Pathogen
TRANSMISSION ROUTE: Direct contact

DEFINITION

Malassezia are lipophilic, dimorphic fungi that are found as normal flora on the skin of humans and other mammals. These fungi can cause a variety of skin conditions and systemic infections in special circumstances.

**Taxonomic Classification
for *Malassezia***

Kingdom: Fungi
Phylum: Basidiomycota
Subphylum: Ustilaginomycotina
Class: Exobasidiomycetes
Order: Malasseziales
Genus: *Malassezia*
Species:
  M. dermatis
  M. furfur
  M. globosa
  M. japonica
  M. obtusa
  M. restricta
  M. slooffiae
  M. sympodialis
  M. yamatoensis

NATURAL HABITAT AND FEATURES

Malassezia are lipophilic yeasts. Most species depend upon saturated fatty acids for growth. They are found as part of the normal flora of the skin of humans and other mammals in areas where sebaceous glands secreting sebum are located. Sebum is composed of triglycerides and esters. *Malassezia* lipases degrade triglycerides into both unsaturated and saturated fatty acids. The *Malassezia* consume the specific saturated fatty acids and leave the unsaturated fatty acids on the skin.

Since discovery of the fungi in 1874, thirteen *Malassezia* sp. have been described. Four species, *caprae*, *equina*, *nana*, and *pachydermatis*, are associated with animals, and the other species are found as human commensals and as opportunistic pathogens. Human colonization begins shortly after birth and is maintained throughout adulthood. Certain diseases, such as diabetes mellitus or human immunodeficiency virus infection, may encourage the yeasts to grow, as may treatment with drugs, such as corticosteroids or cancer chemotherapy, that impair the immune system. Systemic infection may occur in association with vascular catheters, particularly when intravenous lipids are administered.

While *Malassezia* are classified as yeasts, they are dimorphic fungi occurring as both saprophytic yeasts and parasitic mycelia. The yeast forms vary from spherical to ovoid and reach diameters of 8 micrometers (μm). The yeasts multiply by monopolar budding. The presence of a prominent collarette at the budding site helps to distinguish them from *Candida glabrata*, which is otherwise similar in appearance. The hyphae are short and septate with occasional branching and are 2.5 to 4 μm in diameter. Parker's ink, Gomori's methenamine silver, or periodic acid-Schiff (PAS) stains can all be used to aid in microscopic visualization of the organisms from specimens such as skin scrapings or punch biopsies.

The fungi are difficult to culture; a source of lipid must be added to meet their growth requirements. Sabouraud's dextrose agar can be overlaid with sterile olive oil or other media, including Leeming-Norman, Dixon agar; Littman oxgall may be employed. Colonies comprising budding yeasts grow slowly, maturing in five days at 86° to 98.6° Fahrenheit (30° to 37° Celsius). They initially appear as small, smooth, creamy colonies and later become dull and wrinkled with a tan or brownish coloration. Colonial and microscopic morphology, growth requirements, biochemical tests, and molecular tests have all been used for the identification of various species.

PATHOGENICITY AND CLINICAL SIGNIFICANCE

Sebaceous glands cover the human body, with the exception of the palms of the hands and the soles of the feet. The secretion of sebum is under glandular control. Activity begins at birth under control of maternal androgens and then declines until puberty. Secretion remains steady until middle age, when androgens decrease and sebum production declines. In women, the decline is linked to menopause, but in men the decline occurs somewhat later.

Dandruff and seborrheic dermatitis are superficial infections with *Malassezia* species that are associated with the hyperproliferation of the cells of the epidermis, which results in flaking of the skin. When *Malassezia* shift the composition of sebum to a preponderance of unsaturated fatty acids, these fatty acids alter the skin barrier and create inflammation and ultimately hyperproliferation and flaking of the skin. These two conditions affect up to 50 percent of the population at some time in their lives, and they are most common during those years of highest sebaceous gland activity. While dandruff affects only the scalp, seborrheic dermatitis can involve the scalp, eyebrows, nose, external ears, and even the trunk and groin areas. *M. globosa* and *M. restricta* are the most common species identified. The diagnosis may be confirmed by microscopic examination of skin scrapings that reveal the round yeasts.

Pityriasis versicolor is a superficial infection of the skin covering the trunk and proximal extremities in young adults. The infection is associated with transformation of the yeast to the mycelial phase, but the factor or factors inciting the change is unknown. A fatty acid metabolite of *Malassezia*, azeleic acid, is responsible for the depigmentation of the skin lesions. *M. globosa* is the species found in the majority of infected persons. In most cases the diagnosis is made clinically, but confirmation can be obtained by observing round yeast forms accompanied by short hyphae elements on microscopic examination of skin scrapings.

Neonatal cephalic pustulosis, or neonatal acne, occurs in about 3 percent of hospitalized neonates. The condition is a pustular eruption involving the face, neck, and scalp. Maternal hormones stimulate neonatal sebum production, facilitating *Malassezia* growth after being introduced to the fetus during pregnancy or passed on by health care workers. The diagnosis is made on the basis of the clinical appearance of the skin lesions, smears showing yeasts on microscopic examination, and response to topical antifungal therapy. *M. sympodialis* has been the species associated with more severe cases, while *M. furfur* is found in mild cases or in asymptomatic infants.

Severely ill neonates or adults receiving infusions of intravenous lipids to provide parenteral nutrition are at risk for systemic infection through the bloodstream by *Malassezia*. While the lipid emulsions are not intrinsically contaminated, they do support the growth of *Malassezia* by providing them with fatty acids. The impaired immune systems of severely ill persons may allow systemic spread of the infection.

Most conventional blood culture systems have poor cultural yields for these organisms. Lysis-centrifugation with subsequent culture onto lipid supplemented media, or the addition of lipids to the broth used for blood culture, may provide a higher yield. Blood cultures obtained through the central venous catheter used for hyperalimentation are more likely to be positive than are peripheral vein samples. Additionally, buffy coat smears have revealed yeast forms in the blood of some infants. *M. furfur* is the species usually found.

Domestic pets, especially dogs, are colonized and sometimes infected with *Malassezia*. Canine ear and skin infections are commonly observed and treated by veterinarians. *M. pachydermatis* is the usual species, and because this species is uncommon in human infections, canine transmission is thought to be of minimal importance.

DRUG SUSCEPTIBILITY

Malassezia are uniformly susceptible to the azole class of antifungal agents. Ketoconazole is the most commonly used azole in the treatment of the various types of infection caused by these organisms. Ketoconazole shampoo and cream are employed for superficial infections such as dandruff, seborrheic dermatitis, and neonatal cephalic pustulosis. Ketoconazole cream may also be successfully used for the treatment of pityriasis versicolor, but more extensive or persistent cases should be treated with oral itraconazole or fluconazole. In cases of systemic infection associated with lipid infusions, the contaminated central venous catheter should be removed and intravenous antifungal therapy with an agent such as fluconazole commenced.

H. Bradford Hawley, M.D.

FURTHER READING

Hibbett, David S., et al. "A Higher-Level Phylogenetic Classification of the Fungi." *Mycological Research* 111 (2007): 509-547. A complete classification of fungi.
Inamadar, A. C., and A. Palit. "The Genus *Malassezia* and Human Disease." *Indian Journal of Dermatology, Venereology, and Leprology* 69 (2003): 265-270. A

short general review of diseases caused by *Malas-sezia.*

Larone, Davise H. *Medically Important Fungi: A Guide to Identification.* 4th ed. Washington, D.C.: ASM Press, 2002. A standard guide with illustrations.

Naldi, Luigi, and Alfredo Rebora. "Seborrheic Dermatitis." *New England Journal of Medicine* 360 (2009): 387-396. Comprehensive review of effective treatments for dandruff and seborrheic dermatitis.

Ro, Byung In, and Thomas L. Dawson. "The Role of Sebaceous Gland Activity and Scalp Microfloral Metabolism in the Etiology of Seborrheic Dermatitis and Dandruff." *Journal of Investigative Dermatology Symposium Proceedings* 10 (2005): 194-197. An excellent scientific explanation of the metabolic relationship of *Malassezia* to the skin.

WEB SITES OF INTEREST

Microbiology and Immunology On-line: Mycology
http://pathmicro.med.sc.edu/book/mycol-sta.htm

Systematic Mycology and Microbiology Laboratory
http://www.ars.usda.gov

See also: Dandruff; Dermatophytosis; Fungi: Classification and types; Mycosis; *Piedraia*; Pityriasis rosea; Skin infections.

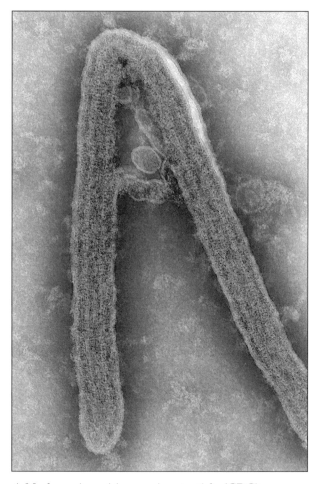

A Marburg virus virion, or virus particle. (CDC)

Marburg hemorrhagic fever

CATEGORY: Diseases and conditions
ANATOMY OR SYSTEM AFFECTED: All

DEFINITION

Marburg hemorrhagic fever is a highly infectious, deadly viral disease endemic to sub-Saharan Africa. The disease is characterized by massive hemorrhaging from all body orifices and by high mortality.

CAUSES

Marburg fever was first identified in 1967 in Marburg, Germany, from which it gets its name. It arose among personnel in a laboratory using African green monkeys to prepare polio vaccine. The agent for the fever is Marburg virus, characterized by a single linear negative-sense ribonucleic acid (RNA) genome and a filamentous appearance of the virion particles in the electron microscope. Marburg fever arises sporadically every couple of years. The normal viral reservoir is the Egyptian fruit bat (*Rousettus aegyptiacus*) and possibly some other bat species. How the virus is passed from bats to humans is not understood.

RISK FACTORS

The Marburg virus is highly infective and is spread by direct contact with the bodily fluids of an infected person. Anyone in contact with such persons is at risk. The African episodes often occur near caves or mines that harbor bats. In 2008, two cases in the Western world were reported, including one in the state of Colorado. The case involved tourists who had recently visited Python Cave in Uganda.

Medical personnel who treat persons with Marburg

hemorrhagic fever must exercise extreme caution. Research staff who work with primates or primate tissues from African species are at risk. Because of the high infectivity of Marburg virus, related research must be done in a level-P4 containment laboratory.

SYMPTOMS

The incubation period is five to ten days, with a sudden onset of flulike symptoms (fever, chills, headache, sore throat, and myalgia). The symptoms get progressively worse, and by the fifth day, persons infected will experience symptoms such as anorexia; the development of a rash, especially on the trunk; nausea; vomiting; diarrhea; and chest pain. These symptoms progress to moderate weight loss, anuria, delirium, hypovolemic shock, coma, multiorgan failure, and severe hemorrhaging from all body orifices. Those persons who recover from the infection often continue to have one or more conditions, including orchitis, recurrent hepatitis, uveitis, myelitis, and inflammation of the parotid gland.

SCREENING AND DIAGNOSIS

In Africa, the symptoms may be confused with other endemic diseases such as malaria or typhoid fever. Medical personnel must be particularly cautious of mine workers and those persons living near caves. The virus can be identified through various testing methods, including enzyme-linked immunoabsorbent assay (ELISA), polymerase chain reaction, and virus isolation. Upon autopsy, diagnosis is confirmed by immunohistochemistry.

TREATMENT AND THERAPY

Treatment includes supportive hospital therapy with barrier nursing in isolation. The disease will run its course, as there is no cure or effective treatment. In some cases, transfusion of fresh-frozen plasma to replace blood-clotting proteins has had some limited success in reducing hemorrhaging. An experimental vaccine has been developed. Mortality has ranged from 23 percent (in a 1967 incident in Europe) to 88 percent (in a 2005 outbreak in urban Angola).

PREVENTION AND OUTCOMES

One should avoid caves and mining areas in Africa and avoid contact with the bodily fluids of persons with Marburg hemorrhagic fever.

Ralph R. Meyer, Ph.D.

FURTHER READING

Hartman, Amy L., Jonathan S. Towner, and Stuart T. Nichol. "Ebola and Marburg Hemorrhagic Fever." *Clinical Laboratory Medicine* 30 (2010): 161-177.

Mahanty, Siddhartha, and Mike Bray. "Pathogenesis of Filoviral Haemorrhagic Fevers." *The Lancet: Infectious Diseases* 4 (2004): 487-498.

Slenczka, Werner, and Hans Dieter Klenk. "Forty Years of Marburg Virus." *Journal of Infectious Diseases* 196 (2007): S131-135.

Wagner, Edward K., and Martinez J. Hewlett. *Basic Virology*. 3d ed. Malden, Mass.: Blackwell Science, 2008.

WEB SITES OF INTEREST

Centers for Disease Control and Prevention
http://www.cdc.gov

International Committee on Taxonomy of Viruses
http://www.ictvonline.org

Universal Virus Database
http://www.ictvdb.org

See also: Bats and infectious disease; Dengue fever; Developing countries and infectious disease; Ebola hemorrhagic fever; Fever; Filoviridae; Hemorrhagic fever viral infections; Plague; Primates and infectious disease; Vaccines: Experimental; Viral infections; West Nile virus; Zoonotic diseases.

Mastitis

CATEGORY: Diseases and conditions
ANATOMY OR SYSTEM AFFECTED: Breasts, skin, tissue
ALSO KNOWN AS: Breast infection

DEFINITION

Mastitis is painful swelling and redness in the breast. It is especially common among women who are breast-feeding. While it is most common in just one breast, it can occur in both.

CAUSES

Mastitis is often caused by trapped breast milk in a milk duct. The trapped breast milk can irritate the tissue around it and cause swelling and pain. Mastitis also can be caused by a bacterial infection in the breast tissue. Milk ducts or cracked skin around the nipple can allow bacteria to enter the breast and cause an infection.

Mastitis often occurs during breast-feeding, but it is possible to get mastitis at other times. This article focuses on symptoms and treatment of lactation-associated mastitis.

RISK FACTORS

Risk factors for mastitis include previous mastitis; abrasion or cracking of the breast nipple; wearing a bra or clothing that is too tight; missed breast-feeding (causing overdistention of the breast); irregular breast-feeding; pressure on the breasts caused by sleeping on the stomach, holding the breast too tightly during feeding, or baby sleeping on the breast; and exercising (especially running) without a support bra.

Other factors include too much milk remaining in the breast. This can be caused by a baby's teething, the use of an artificial nipple or pacifier, incorrect positioning of the baby during feedings, and abrupt weaning.

Still other risk factors include yeast infection of the breast, low resistance to infection or an immune deficiency disorder, psoriasis or other skin conditions that affect the nipple, diabetes mellitus, rheumatoid arthritis, the use of cortisone drugs, prior breast surgery or implants, and smoking.

SYMPTOMS

Symptoms may include fever; fatigue; nausea or vomiting; aches, chills, or other flulike symptoms; redness, tenderness, or swelling of the breast; a burning feeling in the breast; a hard feeling or tender lump in the breast; pus draining from the nipple; and swollen lymph glands in the armpit or above the collar bones.

SCREENING AND DIAGNOSIS

A doctor will ask about symptoms and medical history and will perform a physical exam of the affected breast. If the diagnosis is uncertain, or if mastitis recurs, the doctor may order a culture of breast milk or nipple discharge, a biopsy of the affected area, a breast ultrasound, a mammography, or an X ray of the breast.

TREATMENT AND THERAPY

Treatment includes clearing blocked breast ducts. Relieving the blockage in the milk duct is an effective

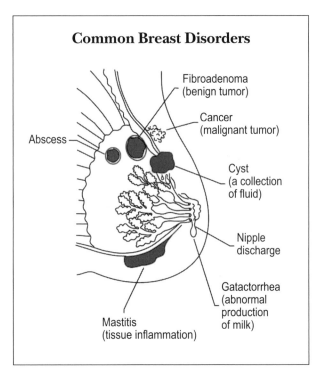

In addition to mastitis, a number of diseases and disorders can affect the breast.

way to decrease the pain and swelling. To clear blocked breast ducts, one should breast-feed frequently (breast-feeding with mastitis is not harmful to the baby). One should consult a doctor if also taking medicines to ensure the medicines are not harmful to the baby; offer the baby the infected breast first (to promote complete emptying of the infected breast); use a breast pump to express milk; and apply warm compresses to breasts before feeding (to stimulate milk ejection reflex).

To reduce pain and swelling in the breast, one should apply ice compresses to the affected area after breast-feeding. If the mastitis is not caused by breast-feeding, one should consider using over-the-counter pain relievers as recommended by the doctor and should ask the doctor what pain relievers are safe for the mother and the baby. Taking aspirin is not advised during pregnancy or breast-feeding. Also, one should drink large amounts of fluids and get extra rest.

Antibiotics may be used to treat the infection. They may help cure the infection or reduce the risk of more serious but rare complications, such as blood infection. If breast-feeding, one should consult the doctor about which antibiotics are best to take while breast-feeding.

The bacterium known as *Staphylococcus aureus* is responsible for many cases of bacterial mastitis. Some forms of staph have become resistant to many of the commonly used antibiotics. The resistant bacterium has been rare in cases of mastitis. If mastitis does not respond to antibiotics, a localized collection of pus (an abscess) might be present. This is usually treated with other antibiotics and a drainage procedure or surgery.

PREVENTION AND OUTCOMES

Strategies to help prevent mastitis include preventing engorgement of the breast with milk by frequent breast-feeding and by using a breast pump. Other measures include washing hands and nipples before breast-feeding, avoiding bras or clothing that are too tight, not sleeping on breasts, and not allowing a baby to sleep on breasts. If the nipples crack, one should apply lotion or cream as recommended by a doctor.

Rick Alan;
reviewed by Ganson Purcell, Jr., M.D., FACOG, FACPE

FURTHER READING

Amir, L. "Breastfeeding and *Staphylococcus aureus*: Three Case Reports." *Breastfeeding Review* 10 (2002): 15-18.

Barbosa-Cesnik, C., K. Schwartz, and B. Foxman. "Lactation Mastitis." *Journal of the American Medical Association* 289 (2003): 1609-1612.

Bland, Kirby I., and Edward M. Copeland III. *The Breast: Comprehensive Management of Benign and Malignant Diseases*. 4th ed. Philadelphia: Saunders/Elsevier, 2009.

Chinyama, Catherine N. *Benign Breast Disease: Radiology, Pathology, Risk Assessment*. New York: Springer, 2004.

Crossley, Kent B., Kimberly K. Jefferson, and Gordon L. Archer, eds. *Staphylococci in Human Disease*. Hoboken, N.J.: John Wiley & Sons, 2009.

Dixon, J. Michael, ed. *ABC of Breast Diseases*. 3d ed. Hoboken, N.J.: BMJ Books-Wiley, 2006.

Laibl, V. R., et al. "Clinical Presentation of Community-Acquired Methicillin-Resistant *Staphylococcus aureus* in Pregnancy." *Obstetrics and Gynecology* 106 (2005): 461-465.

Love, Susan, and Karen Lindsey. *Dr. Susan Love's Breast Book*. Rev. 4th ed. Cambridge, Mass.: Da Capo Press, 2005.

National Library of Medicine. "Breast Infection." Available at http://www.nlm.nih.gov/medlineplus/ency/article/001490.htm.

Reddy, Pavani. "Postpartum Mastitis and Community-Acquired Methicillin-Resistant *Staphylococcus aureus*." *Emerging Infectious Diseases* 13, no. 2 (February 1, 2007): 298.

Riordan, Jan, ed. *Breastfeeding and Human Lactation*. 4th ed. Sudbury, Mass.: Jones and Bartlett, 2010.

WEB SITES OF INTEREST

American Academy of Dermatology
http://www.aad.org

La Leche League International
http://www.llli.org

Our Bodies Ourselves
http://www.obos.org

Women's Health Matters
http://www.womenshealthmatters.ca

Women's Health.gov
http://www.womenshealth.gov

See also: Bacterial infections; Breast milk and infectious disease; Brucellosis; Endometritis; Inflammation; Methicillin-resistant staph infection; Skin infections; Staphylococcal infections; *Staphylococcus*; Thrush; Women and infectious disease.

Mathematical modeling

CATEGORY: Epidemiology
ALSO KNOWN AS: Epidemic modeling, mathematical epidemiology

DEFINITION

Mathematical modeling is the use of a complex mathematical formula or algorithm to predict the outcome of a disease, to hypothesize its likely spread, and to determine what public health actions could limit its transmission.

Epidemiologists, health care workers, public health

officials, and the general public all have a vested interest in whether and how a particular infectious disease will spread, in what portions of the population it will affect, and in whether it will turn into an epidemic. Scientists have created sophisticated statistical, mathematical, and computer programming methods to develop hypotheses as to how a disease might spread through a population and whether any factors are likely to inhibit its growth. Scientists also run mathematical calculations to determine if and how vaccination against a disease will affect its spread.

HISTORY

In 1911, British doctor Sir Ronald Ross was one of the first to determine that mathematics could be used to study disease transmission. He believed that epidemiology, which is the study of the variation of disease from time to time and place to place, to be considered scientifically, it must be considered mathematically. Doing so, he argued, is the only way to apply careful reasoning to epidemiology's methods. Accordingly, Ross attempted to apply the law of mass action, a mathematical model used in chemistry, to explain how an epidemic was transmitted. Another mathematical model of epidemics was constructed in the 1920's by Lowell Reed and Wade Hampton Frost of Johns Hopkins University. Since this time, scientists have applied many mathematical models from different disciplines and have created a few new models to explain disease transmission.

BASIC IDEAS

An infinite number of assumptions can be made and many variables can be factored into a model to predict the transmission of an infectious disease. However, the following four fundamental ideas are most often used in mathematical modeling:

Reproduction. The average number of people a person with a given disease would infect if no one had immunity to that disease

Susceptibility. The proportion of people in the population who do not have immunity and do not have the disease

Age. The average age at which a person in the general population is likely to get the disease

Life expectancy. The average life expectancy of the population in the transmission path of the disease

Modelers add many other factors to their calculations, such as the proportion of children to adults in the population, how close people live to one another in the area, and whether or not school is in session. They may also add real-world examples of how another, possibly related, epidemic occurred to ensure their model is as close to reality as possible. A person's contact pattern may also need to be considered. For example, an infectious disease would have a very different pattern of spreading if two different people contracted the disease: one who lived alone and went immediately to the hospital to be isolated, and another who died at home, undiagnosed, after exposing his or her multigenerational family (as happened in Canada with the introduction in 2003 of the virus that causes SARS).

LIMITATIONS

In any type of modeling, the model created is only as good as the assumptions with which the creator populated the model. If a model is correctly constructed mathematically, yet the results are still out of line with the disease's observed patterns, the assumptions may need to be revisited. Real-world issues also come into play; a mathematical model is, at its best, a highly likely scenario. Genetic mutations of a disease or a shift in human behavior can alter how the scenario actually evolves. These factors, for example, can lead to the development of a vaccine for influenza that seemed, at the beginning of flu season, to cover all likely influenza viruses but, in fact, did not cover all the actual viruses that were active that year, or can lead to the development of a vaccine that did not account for the particular virulence of a given strain.

IMPACT

By using well-reasoned and highly accurate mathematical models to predict the spread of infectious diseases, scientists using mathematical modeling inform public health policymakers and public health workers of the factors that affect the spread of disease. Mathematical models can determine what diseases are likely in a particular population and thus can help determine what types of vaccines are necessary to prevent the occurrence or recurrence of a given disease.

Marianne M. Madsen, M.S.

FURTHER READING

Castillo-Chavez, Carlos, ed. *Mathematical Approaches for Emerging and Reemerging Infectious Diseases: Models, Methods, and Theory.* New York: Springer, 2002. Contains essays about mathematical modeling by some of the leaders in the field.

Daley, D. J., and J. Gani. *Epidemic Modeling: An Introduction.* Reprint. New York: Cambridge University Press, 2005. Provides a general introduction to mathematical techniques used in modeling for infectious diseases.

Diekmann, O., and J. A. P. Heesterbeek. *Mathematical Epidemiology of Infectious Diseases: Model Building, Analysis, and Interpretation.* New York: John Wiley & Sons, 2000. Introduces basic questions, key ideas, and fundamental mathematical concepts. Presents theory and includes examples.

Keeling, M. J., and L. Danon. "Mathematical Modelling of Infectious Diseases." *British Medical Bulletin* 92 (2009): 33-42. Discusses the application of mathematical models to determine the current state of an epidemic, to predict the future progress of the disease, and to quantify uncertainty about predictions.

Keeling, Matt J., and Peiman Rohani. *Modeling Infectious Diseases in Humans and Animals.* Princeton, N.J.: Princeton University Press, 2007. Discusses mathematical modeling as it relates to public health planning.

Ma, Stefan, and Yingcun Xia, eds. *Mathematical Understanding of Infectious Disease Dynamics.* Hackensack, N.J.: World Scientific, 2008. Covers the basic mathematics for epidemic modeling with real examples related to public health policy applications.

Ma, Zhien, and Jia Li, eds. *Dynamical Modeling and Analysis of Epidemics.* Hackensack, N.J.: World Scientific, 2009. Discusses the quantitative analysis of models. Uses examples such as SARS and tuberculosis to show transmission.

Sokolowski, John A., and Catherine M. Banks, eds. *Principles of Modeling and Simulation: A Multidisciplinary Approach.* Hoboken, N.J.: John Wiley & Sons, 2009. Explores a wide range of modeling simulations and techniques.

WEB SITES OF INTEREST

Association for Professionals in Infection Control and Epidemiology
http://www.knowledgeisinfectious.org

Imperial College of London, Mathematical Models of the Epidemiology and Control of Infectious Diseases
http://www.infectiousdiseasemodels.org

See also: Biostatistics; Biosurveillance; Centers for Disease Control and Prevention (CDC); Disease eradication campaigns; Emerging and reemerging infectious diseases; Emerging Infections Network; Epidemic Intelligence Service; Epidemiology; Infectious disease specialists; Koch's postulates; Outbreaks; Public health.

Maturation inhibitors

CATEGORY: Treatment

DEFINITION

Maturation inhibitors make up a newer, investigational, antiviral drug class that attacks the human immunodeficiency virus (HIV), a retrovirus, in the last stage of development. This attacks prevents the continued retroviral infection of the body's T cells.

PATIENT POPULATION AND PLANNED USE

The first-in-class maturation inhibitor, bevirimat (also known as PA-457), reached phase-two clinical studies in 2010, but the population being considered for treatment expanded as quickly as research on bevirimat progressed. Maturation inhibitors were initially considered for people infected with HIV who were treatment naïve, that is, had not previously taken this or any other medication for HIV. However, the surprising and high levels of resistance to bevirimat in early studies led researchers to begin developing additional maturation inhibitors that could withstand initial resistance instead. Resistance to bevirimat appeared linked to resistance that developed in people who had used protease inhibitors, which work on a similar area of HIV as maturation inhibitors. Most studied maturation inhibitors, including the lead compound bevirimat and vivecon (also known as MPC-9055), a maturation inhibitor in earlier clinical studies, are given once daily.

MECHANISM OF ACTION

Maturation inhibitors block viral replication of HIV, a retrovirus, at viral maturation, the final stage of virus production before budding, when the infectious cell spreads through the body. During maturation, proteins gather and are released from cells to spread to other T cells in the body. Unlike protease inhibitors, which target protease enzymes at this viral stage, the target of maturation inhibitors is in the Gag (group-specific antigen) region of the HIV cell. To keep the virus noninfectious, maturation inhibitors work at the polyprotein precursor, the primary protein that assembles the virions into mature particles that can be sent to infect other cells

ADVANTAGES

Maturation inhibitors have many theoretical and actual advantages compared with existing treatment options for persons with HIV, whether these persons are treatment naïve or treatment experienced. The pharmacokinetics of maturation inhibitors, such as bevirimat, allow for once-daily dosing. This feature alone greatly increases adherence, especially in treatment-experienced persons who typically have undergone difficult and complicated dosing regimens. Maturation inhibitors as a class are generally easy to tolerate, with few side effects and drug interactions noted. The goal of treatment with maturation inhibitors is to add a new drug class to existing options for highly active antiretroviral therapy (HAART) of HIV, so as to provide new and successful treatment options for people with resistant disease.

IMPACT

The addition of a new antiretroviral class can reinvigorate treatment of resistance disease and can contribute to successful adherence with easier dosing schedules and a good side effect profile, which improve the adherence potential of drugs in this class. The development of bevirimat provided a new opportunity for treatment-resistant persons to lower their viral loads. Phase-two studies of bevirimat, however, identified a greatly reduced effect in persons who were resistant to protease inhibitors, possibly because protease inhibitor activity altered the Gag area of HIV to render bevirimat inactive. Drug manufacturers continued to experiment with other investigational compounds in the maturation inhibitor class, such MPC-9055, but in 2010, these studies were placed on hold.

Nicole M. Van Hoey, Pharm.D.

FURTHER READING

Hicks, Charles B. "Resistance to Maturation Inhibitors: Will Bevirimat Find a Role?" *AIDS Clinical Care*, February, 2010. Available at http://www.medscape.com/viewarticle/715614.

Martin, David E., Karl Salzwedel, and Graham P. All-
away. "Bevirimat: A Novel Maturation Inhibitor for the Treatment of HIV-1 Infection." *Antiviral Chemistry and Chemotherapy* 19, no. 3 (2008): 107-113.

Salzwedel, Karl, David E. Martin, and Michael Sakalian. "Maturation Inhibitors: A New Therapeutic Class Targets the Virus Structure." *AIDS Review* 9, no. 3 (2007): 162-172.

Wit, Ferdinand W. N. M., Joep M. A. Lange, and Paul A. Volberding. "New Drug Development: The Need for New Antiretroviral Agents." In *Global HIV/AIDS Medicine*, edited by Paul A. Volberding et al. Philadelphia: Saunders/Elsevier, 2008.

WEB SITES OF INTEREST

AIDSinfo
http://aidsinfo.nih.gov

Canadian AIDS Treatment Information Exchange
http://www.catie.ca

Centers for Disease Control and Prevention
http://www.cdc.gov/hiv

See also: AIDS; Antibodies; Antiviral drugs: Mechanisms of action; Antiviral drugs: Types; Autoimmune disorders; Blood-borne illness and disease; HIV; Immunity; Integrase inhibitors; Protease inhibitors; Quinolone antibiotics; Retroviral infections; Retroviridae; Reverse transcriptase inhibitors; T lymphocytes; Treatment of viral infections; Viral infections.

Measles

CATEGORY: Diseases and conditions
ANATOMY OR SYSTEM AFFECTED: All
ALSO KNOWN AS: Rubella, rubeola

DEFINITION

Measles is a viral infection that is highly contagious. It causes fever, cough, and a rash. It was once a common childhood illness. Measles is now seen less often in the United States because of the use of the measles vaccine.

CAUSES

The measles virus is spread by direct contact with nasal or throat secretions of infected people and by

Facts: Measles

- Measles is one of the leading causes of death among young children even though a safe and cost-effective vaccine is available.

- In 2008, there were 164,000 measles deaths globally: nearly 450 deaths per day, or 18 deaths per hour.

- More than 95 percent of measles deaths occur in developing countries with inadequate health-care infrastructures.

- Measles vaccination led to a 78 percent drop in measles deaths between 2000 and 2008 worldwide.

- In 2008, about 83 percent of the world's children received one dose of measles vaccine by their first birthday through routine health services, up from 72 percent in 2000.

Source: World Health Organization

airborne transmission (less frequently). Measles is communicable from one to two days before onset of symptoms, three to five days before the rash, and four days after the appearance of the rash.

RISK FACTORS

The factors that increase the chance of developing measles include being unvaccinated or inadequately vaccinated, living in crowded or unsanitary conditions, and traveling to developing countries where measles is common. Also, measles is most common in winter and spring.

Other risk factors include compromised immunity (for example, untreated human immunodeficiency virus infection), even if vaccinated; being born after 1956 and having received no diagnosis of measles; and receiving a vaccine before 1968, without additional vaccination.

SYMPTOMS

Symptoms, which usually occur eight to twelve days following exposure, include a fever (often high), runny nose, red eyes, hacking cough, sore throat, exhaustion, and small spots inside the mouth (two to four days after initial symptoms). Three to five days after initial symptoms appear, a raised, itchy rash will start around the ears, face, and side of the neck and then generally spread to the arms, trunk, and legs over the next two days (and then last about four to six days). Full recovery, without scarring, generally takes seven to ten days from the onset of the rash.

SCREENING AND DIAGNOSIS

Diagnosis is made from the symptoms and the appearance of the rash. Laboratory tests are usually not needed to diagnose measles.

TREATMENT AND THERAPY

Measles is caused by a virus, so it cannot be treated with antibiotics. The focus of treatment is on relieving symptoms. Gargling with warm salt water will often relieve the sore throat. Using a humidifier can provide some relief.

A high fever can be treated with nonaspirin medication, which includes acetaminophen. Aspirin is not recommended for children or teens with a current or recent viral infection because of the risk of Reye's syndrome. One should consult the doctor about medicines that are safe for children.

Other treatment includes getting extra rest, drinking increased amounts of liquids, and eating a soft, bland diet. Cold sponge baths may also help with symptoms.

In most cases, complications are rare, but persons with severe cases may need to be hospitalized. Complications may include encephalitis (inflammation of the brain) and bacterial pneumonia (a lung infection).

PREVENTION AND OUTCOMES

Getting vaccinated is the best way to prevent measles, as the vaccine contains live viruses that can no longer cause disease. The vaccine is usually given in combination form and includes vaccines against measles, mumps, and rubella (MMR). The MMR vaccine is given twice: at age twelve to fifteen months and at age four to six years (or at age eleven to twelve years).

In some cases, the vaccine is given within three days after exposure. This can prevent or reduce symptoms. Immunoglobulin is given to certain unvaccinated people within six days of exposure. This is usually for infants and pregnant women.

In general, one should avoid the vaccine if he or she has had severe allergic reactions to vaccines or vaccine components, is pregnant (a woman should avoid pregnancy for one to three months after receiving the vaccine), has a weakened immune system, or has a high

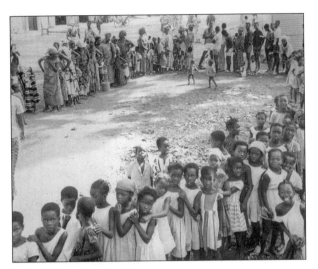

Children in Niger wait in line for the measles vaccination in 1988. (CDC)

fever or severe upper respiratory tract infection. If not vaccinated, one should avoid contact with anyone who has measles.

Rick Alan; reviewed by David L. Horn, M.D., FACP

Further Reading

Bernstein, David, and Gilbert Schiff. "Viral Exanthems and Localized Skin Infections." In *Infectious Diseases*, edited by Sherwood L. Gorbach, John G. Bartlett, and Neil R. Blacklow. Philadelphia: W. B. Saunders, 2004.

Centers for Disease Control and Prevention. "Vaccine Safety: Measles, Mumps, and Rubella (MMR) Vaccine." Available at http://www.cdc.gov/vaccinesafety.

EBSCO Publishing. *Health Library: Measles Vaccine.* Available through http://www.ebscohost.com.

"Measles." In *Epidemiology and Prevention of Vaccine-Preventable Diseases*, edited by W. Atkinson et al. 11th ed. Washington, D.C.: Public Health Foundation, 2009.

Peter, G., and P. Gardner. "Standards for Immunization Practice for Vaccines in Children and Adults." *Infectious Disease Clinics of North America* 15 (2001): 9-19.

Pickering, Larry K., et al., eds. *Red Book: 2009 Report of the Committee on Infectious Diseases.* 28th ed. Elk Grove Village, Ill.: American Academy of Pediatrics, 2009.

Weedon, David. *Skin Pathology.* 3d ed. New York: Churchill Livingstone/Elsevier, 2010.

Web Sites of Interest

Caring for Kids
http://www.caringforkids.cps.ca

Centers for Disease Control and Prevention
http://www.cdc.gov

National Foundation for Infectious Diseases
http://www.nfid.org

Public Health Agency of Canada
http://www.phac-aspc.gc.ca

See also: Airborne illness and disease; Chickenpox; Children and infectious disease; Contagious diseases; Croup; Encephalitis; Epiglottitis; Impetigo; MMR vaccine; Mononucleosis; Mumps; Paramyxoviridae; Pityriasis rosea; Rubella; Shingles; Skin infections; Subacute sclerosing panencephalitis; Vaccines: Types; Viral infections; Viral meningitis.

Measles, mumps, and rubella vaccine. *See* MMR vaccine.

Mediterranean spotted fever

CATEGORY: Diseases and conditions
ANATOMY OR SYSTEM AFFECTED: All
ALSO KNOWN AS: Boutonneuse fever, Marseilles fever

Definition

Mediterranean spotted fever (MSF) is a condition caused by the bacterium *Rickettsia conorii*, which is transmitted through the bite of a tick. In the spring and summer, MSF is endemic to countries that border the Mediterranean and Black seas and to parts of central Africa, South Africa, and India. In a few cases, MSF is particularly serious and can lead to death.

Causes

MSF is usually transmitted by the bite of the brown dog tick, *Rhipicephalus sanguineus*, although it can be transmitted through the skin or eyes when an infected tick is crushed. *Rickettsia conorii* is considered a parasite because it can survive only within the cells of a host insect, animal, or human. The parasite is usually found in the cells lining the blood vessels.

RISK FACTORS

The risk factors are contact with a brown dog tick and living in areas where MSF is endemic. Farmers and persons who participate in outdoor activities, such as hiking and camping, are at increased risk for contact with ticks. Another risk factor is crushing a tick between one's fingers.

SYMPTOMS

MSF has a five-to-seven-day incubation period. The usual symptoms of the condition are the characteristic black spot at the site of the tick bite and fever, headache, chills, muscle and joint pain, malaise, anorexia, nausea and vomiting, diarrhea, rash on the palms of the hands and the soles of the feet, conjunctivitis, and visual problems. If treatment is delayed, MSF can cause vasculitis, difficulty breathing, nerve and brain damage, kidney failure, enlarged liver, Guillain-Barré syndrome, and death. The severe form of MSF is more common in the elderly, in alcoholics, in persons with glucose-6-phosphatase dehydrogenase deficiency, and in persons with a suppressed immune system.

SCREENING AND DIAGNOSIS

There is no routine screening for MSF. A diagnosis of MSF is suspected based on the presence of the symptoms. It is usually confirmed by immunofluorescence assay, which identifies the antibodies to *R. conorii*. Cultures of *R. conorii* may be taken from the bloodstream.

TREATMENT AND THERAPY

MSF is treated with doxycycline (200 milligrams daily) orally or intravenously for ten to fourteen days. If there is central nervous system involvement, the antibiotic josamysin may be used because doxycycline may not penetrate the central nervous system. Other antibiotics that can be used are chloramphenicol, levoquin, cipro, and clarithromycin.

PREVENTION AND OUTCOMES

MSF can be prevented by avoiding contact with the brown dog tick. This means avoiding wild dogs that may be carrying ticks. When working in fields or when hiking or camping, one should wear long pants and high socks. Also, one should apply DEET (NN-diethyl metatoluamide) spray.

Christine M. Carroll, R.N.

FURTHER READING

Bratton, R. L., and G. R. Corey. "Tick-Borne Disease." *American Family Physician* 71 (2005): 2323.

Colomba, Claudia, et al. "Mediterranean Spotted Fever: Clinical and Laboratory Characteristics of 415 Sicilian Children." *BMC Infectious Diseases* 6 (2006). Available at http://www.biomedcentral.com/1471-2334/6/60.

Hechemy, Karim E., et al., eds. *Rickettsiology and Rickettsial Diseases.* New York: Blackwell, 2009.

Raoult, Didier, and Philippe Parola, eds. *Rickettsial Diseases.* New York: Informa Healthcare, 2007.

WEB SITES OF INTEREST

Centers for Disease Control and Prevention, Division of Vector Borne Infectious Diseases
http://www.cdc.gov//ncidod/dvbid

Microbiology and Immunology On-line: Parasitology
http://pathmicro.med.sc.edu/book/parasit-sta.htm

University of Florida, Department of Entomology and Nematology
http://entomology.ifas.ufl.edu/creatures/urban/medical/brown_dog_tick.htm

See also: Acariasis; Arthropod-borne illness and disease; Babesiosis; Bacterial infections; Blood-borne illness and disease; Colorado tick fever; Fleas and infectious disease; Insect-borne illness and disease; Lyme disease; Mites and chiggers and infectious disease; Parasitic diseases; *Rickettsia*; Rocky Mountain spotted fever; Ticks and infectious disease; Vectors and vector control.

Melioidosis

CATEGORY: Diseases and conditions
ANATOMY OR SYSTEM AFFECTED: Lungs, respiratory system, skin
ALSO KNOWN AS: Nightcliff gardener disease, paddy-field disease, pseudoglanders, Whitmore disease

DEFINITION

Melioidosis is an infectious disease of humans and animals. It is caused by the bacterium *Burkholderia pseudomallei*, a natural inhabitant of soil and water commonly found in Southeast Asia, Australia, India, China, and regions of Africa. Although melioidosis may be asymptomatic, it commonly manifests as an infection of the skin and lungs. *B. pseudomallei* has been listed as a potential biological warfare agent.

CAUSES

B. pseudomallei is ubiquitous in the soil, stagnant waters, and rice paddies of endemic areas of the world. Humans become infected by exposure of abraded skin to contaminated soil or water, by inhaling contaminated dust particles, or by ingestion of contaminated food or water. The incidence of melioidosis is higher during the rainy season. In nonendemic regions, such as the United States, rare cases of melioidosis are associated with travel to affected regions.

RISK FACTORS

Although healthy persons may develop melioidosis, the most important risk factor associated with this disease is diabetes mellitus. Other risk factors include immune deficiencies, kidney disease, chronic lung disease, the blood disorder thalassemia, occupational hazards such as rice paddy cultivation, and travel in endemic areas.

SYMPTOMS

The clinical presentation of melioidosis varies. It can be either acute (short term) or chronic (a minimum two months' duration). The incubation period usually ranges from two to five days but may last years. Symptoms of acute localized infection usually include skin abscesses, muscle aches, and fever. Cough and chest pain, suggestive of pulmonary infection, may also be present. Severe symptoms include blood infection (sepsis) with high fever, abdominal pain, severe headaches, and respiratory distress. This form of the disease has a high mortality rate. Chronic melioidosis involves multiple-organ infection and usually manifests as joint and muscle pain.

SCREENING AND DIAGNOSIS

A definitive diagnosis is made when the culture from any clinical specimen (blood, urine, sputum samples, aspirated pus, or throat swabs) has *B. pseudomallei* organisms. Chest radiography and a computed tomography scan may be used to diagnose pulmonary

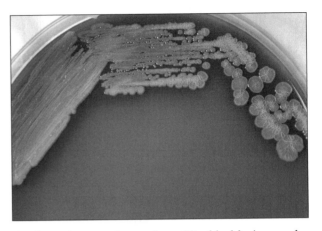

A culture plate contains a colony of Burkholderia pseudomallei *bacteria, the pathogen that causes melioidosis.* (CDC)

melioidosis and abscess formation in body organs, respectively.

TREATMENT AND THERAPY

Treatment consists of antibiotic therapy. Mildly ill persons usually receive one or more oral antibiotics for a course of a minimum of thirty days. Moderately or severely ill persons receive antibiotics intravenously for about fourteen days, after which a maintenance treatment with oral antibiotics is recommended for a period of up to one year.

PREVENTION AND OUTCOMES

To reduce exposure to *B. pseudomallei* organisms, people living in endemic areas and travelers to these regions should avoid contact with soil, mud, and water; avoid drinking untreated water; practice adequate food hygiene and personal hygiene; and disinfect skin after contact with any suspected contaminated source.

Anna Binda, Ph.D.

FURTHER READING

Falade, Oluwaseun O., et al. "Clinical Problem-Solving: Beware of First Impressions." *New England Journal of Medicine* 359 (2008): 628-634.

Gibney, Katherine B., et al. "Cutaneous Melioidosis in the Tropical Top End of Australia." *Clinical Infectious Diseases* 47, no. 5 (2008): 603-609.

Levitzky, Michael G. *Pulmonary Physiology.* 7th ed. New York: McGraw-Hill Medical, 2007.

Shih, H-I, et al. "Sporadic and Outbreak Cases of Melioidosis in Southern Taiwan: Clinical Features and

Antimicrobial Susceptibility." *Infection* 37, no. 1 (2009): 9-15.

WEB SITES OF INTEREST

Center for Biosecurity
http://www.upmc-biosecurity.org

Centers for Disease Control and Prevention, Division of Foodborne, Bacterial, and Mycotic Diseases
http://www.cdc.gov/nczved/divisions/dfbmd

See also: Biological weapons; *Burkholderia*; Glanders; Skin infections; Soilborne illness and disease; Waterborne illness and disease.

Men and infectious disease

CATEGORY: Epidemiology

DEFINITION

Infectious diseases that are unique to men primarily involve the reproductive and urinary tracts and the immune system. Bacterial infections can result in prostatitis and epididymitis. Viral infections are responsible for orchitis and for human immunodeficiency virus (HIV) infection and acquired immunodeficiency syndrome (AIDS).

BACTERIAL INFECTIONS

The bacterial infections that are unique to men include prostatitis and epididymitis.

Prostatitis. Prostatitis is an infection of the prostate gland. It is the most common urologic diagnosis in males younger than age fifty years and the third most common diagnosis in men older than age fifty years. The disease is classified as acute bacterial prostatitis or chronic bacterial prostatitis.

The most common causal organisms of bacterial prostatitis include gram-negative members of the Enterobacteriaceae family, which include *Escherichia coli, Proteus mirabilis, Klebsiella* species, *Enterobacter* species, *Pseudomonas aeruginosa, Staphylococcus, Serratia* species, and *Trichomonas* species. About 80 percent of chronic bacterial prostatitis is caused by *E. coli.*

Symptoms of prostatitis may include pain or burning sensation when urinating (dysuria), difficulty urinating, frequent urination (particularly at night), pain in the penis or testicles, and painful ejaculation. In acute bacterial prostatitis, symptoms associated with the sudden onset of infection include high fever, chills, and nausea. In chronic bacterial prostatitis, symptoms include a clear-to-milky urethral discharge, ejaculatory pain, hematospermia (blood in the semen), and sexual dysfunction.

Initial therapy is directed at gram-negative enteric bacteria. The best antibiotic choices for treatment include antibiotics such as ciprofloxacin, ofloxacin, ampicillin with gentamicin, gatifloxacin, and moxifloxacin. Other useful agents include fluoroquinolones and trimethoprim-sulfamethoxazole.

Epididymitis. Epididymitis is an inflammation of the coiled tube (epididymis) at the back of the testicle that stores and carries sperm. Males of any age can get epididymitis, but it is most common in men between the ages of twenty and thirty-nine years.

Epididymitis has a number of causes. *Chlamydia trachomatis* and *Neisseria gonorrhoeae* are the most common causes of epididymitis in males younger than age thirty-five years. Members of the Enterobacteriaceae family and *Enterococcus* are frequent pathogens in older men. Sexually transmitted diseases (STDs), particularly gonorrhea and chlamydia, are the most common cause of epididymitis in young, sexually active men.

Epididymitis symptoms can include a tender, swollen, or red scrotum; testicle pain and tenderness; painful urination or an urgent or frequent need to urinate; painful intercourse or ejaculation; chills and fever; a lump on the testicle; enlarged lymph nodes in the groin; discharge from the penis; and blood in the semen. Epididymitis is treated with antibiotic medications such as ceftriaxone, ciprofloxacin, doxycycline, and azithromycin.

VIRAL INFECTIONS

The viral infections that are unique to or that often affect men include orchitis and HIV infection and AIDS.

Orchitis. Orchitis is an inflammation of one or both testicles, most commonly associated with the virus that causes mumps. At least one-third of males who contract mumps after puberty develop orchitis. Other causes of orchitis usually are bacterial, including STDs such as gonorrhea or chlamydia.

Orchitis can be either bacterial or viral. Most often, bacterial orchitis is the result of epididymitis. Primary orchitis is one of the few genitourinary infections resulting from viral pathogens. Mumps, coxsackie B, Epstein-Barr, and varicella reach the testis through the bloodstream. Most cases of viral orchitis are the result of mumps in males who were not immunized against the disease. High-risk sexual behaviors that can lead to STDs also put one at risk of sexually transmitted orchitis.

Orchitis symptoms usually develop suddenly. They may include testicular swelling on one or both sides, pain ranging from mild to severe, tenderness in one or both testicles that may last for weeks, fever, discharge from the penis, and blood in the ejaculate.

Treatment for viral orchitis, the type associated with mumps, is aimed at relieving symptoms. A physician may prescribe nonsteroidal anti-inflammatory drugs and may recommend bed rest, elevation of the scrotum, and application of cold packs.

HIV and AIDS. AIDS is a chronic, potentially life-threatening disease. It is estimated that more than one million people are living with HIV infection, which causes AIDS, in the United States, and that more than one-half million people have died after developing AIDS. More than one-half (53 percent) of new infections occur in gay and bisexual men.

HIV destroys CD4 cells, white blood cells that are essential in helping the body fight disease. By damaging the immune system, HIV interferes with the body's ability to fight disease-causing organisms. A man may become infected if he has unprotected anal or oral sex with an infected partner whose blood or semen enters his body. The virus can enter the body through mouth sores or small tears that sometimes develop in the rectum during sexual activity.

Unprotected anal sex (that is, anal sex without the use of a condom) greatly increases the chance of infection. The risk increases if a person has multiple sexual partners. Open sores on the genitals act as doorways for HIV to enter the body. HIV also can be transmitted through shared needles and syringes (as in intravenous drug use) contaminated with infected blood.

Initial infection with HIV may produce no symptoms, although the infected person is contagious. An infected person may remain symptom-free for years, but the virus continues to multiply and destroy immune cells. Without treatment, the infection typically progresses to AIDS in about ten years, by which time the immune system has been severely damaged,

making the person susceptible to opportunistic infections. The signs and symptoms of these infections may include night sweats, chills or high fever, cough and shortness of breath, chronic diarrhea, oral lesions, persistent fatigue, and weight loss.

Opportunistic infections include pneumonia caused by *Pneumocystis* or brain infection with toxoplasmosis, which can cause cognitive and psychological sequelae. A weakened immune system can increase susceptibility to lymphoma, a form of brain cancer, and a cancer of soft tissues called Kaposi's sarcoma.

There is no vaccine to prevent HIV infection and no cure for AIDS, but a variety of drugs can be used in combination to control the HIV virus. These drugs include non-nucleoside reverse transcriptase inhibitors, nucleoside reverse transcriptase inhibitors, protease inhibitors, entry or fusion inhibitors, and integrase inhibitors.

Protection from infection is possible by avoiding any behavior that allows HIV-infected fluids, such as blood or semen, to enter the body. A new condom should be used for each act of anal or oral sex. Injection-drug users should avoid sharing needles or syringes.

IMPACT

Infectious diseases of the male reproductive system, of which there are as many as twenty, remain a major cause of illness. Initial symptoms of disease may be relatively mild, causing many men to underestimate the potential affect on their health. If the particular disease continues to develop untreated, it can have serious consequences and may cause irreversible damage.

In addition to causing local organ dysfunction, reproductive system infections can trigger a series of systemic symptoms such as headache, fatigue, nausea, or insomnia, which may lead to erectile dysfunction or infertility. Most of these diseases are curable with antibiotics, and they normally produce no lasting problems.

By contrast, AIDS is a chronic, life-threatening disease for which there is no cure. More than one million people are living with HIV infection in the United States, and more than one-half million people have died after developing AIDS.

Gerald W. Keister, M.A.

Further Reading

Kumar, Vinay, et al. "Immunodeficiency Syndromes." In *Robbins and Cotran Pathologic Basis of Disease*, edited by Vinay Kumar, Abul K. Abbas, and Nelson Fausto. 8th ed. Philadelphia: Saunders/Elsevier, 2010. This chapter in a standard medical textbook clearly presents information on immunodeficiency disorders and diseases, including HIV infection and AIDS.

Nickel, J. C. "Inflammatory Conditions of the Male Genitourinary Tract: Prostatitis and Related Conditions, Orchitis, and Epididymitis." In *Campbell-Walsh Urology*, edited by Patrick C. Walsh et al. 4 vols. 9th ed. Philadelphia: Saunders/Elsevier, 2007. Discusses the features, diagnoses, and treatment of diseases of the male reproductive and genitourinary systems.

Taguchi, Yosh, and Merrily Weisbord, eds. *Private Parts: An Owner's Guide to the Male Anatomy*. 3d ed. Toronto: McClelland & Stewart, 2003. A guide to male genital and sexual health, covering topics such as prostate disease, erectile dysfunction, cancer, and sexually transmitted diseases.

Tracy, C. R., et al. "Diagnosis and Management of Epididymitis." *Urologic Clinics of North America* 35 (2008): 101. A study describing the epidemiology, causes, symptoms, diagnosis and management of epididymitis.

Web Sites of Interest

Centers for Disease Control and Prevention, Men's Health
http://www.cdc.gov/men

Prostatitis Foundation
http://www.prostatitis.org

UrologyHealth.org
http://www.urologyhealth.org

See also: AIDS; Antibiotics: Types; Bacterial infections; Bloodstream infections; *Chlamydia*; Cholecystitis; Epididymitis; Gonorrhea; HIV; Kidney infection; Opportunistic infections; Prostatitis; Urethritis; Urinary tract infections; Viral infections.

Meningococcal meningitis

CATEGORY: Diseases and conditions
ANATOMY OR SYSTEM AFFECTED: Brain, central nervous system, spinal cord
ALSO KNOWN AS: Meningococcal disease

Definition

Meningococcal meningitis (MM) is an invasive bacterial form of meningitis, an infection that causes swelling and inflammation of the thin lining (membrane) that surrounds the brain and spinal cord. MM, which can cause severe brain damage and is fatal if untreated, was first described clinically in 1805 in Switzerland following an outbreak in Geneva.

Causes

MM is caused by several different bacteria, including *Neisseria meningitidis*, a gram-negative diplococcus bacterium found exclusively in humans. A minimum of thirteen different serogroups of *N. meningitidis* have been identified, based on the capsular polysaccharide. Serogroups A, B, and C have been recognized as significant causes of meningococcal disease.

Risk Factors

Risk factors for the invasive disease may be a combination of host, environment, and organism strain. Recent respiratory tract infection, low socioeconomic status, and a susceptible population increase vulnerability. Climatic factors also influence seasonal outbreaks. In Africa, epidemics begin during the dry season; in temperate countries, sporadic illness and epidemics appear during the late winter and early spring.

MM is spread through direct contact with respiratory droplets of infected people. Therefore, it can be spread through close and prolonged contact with others, through sneezing or coughing, and by living close to an infected person.

Symptoms

The clinical manifestations of meningococcal disease can be quite varied, ranging from transient fever and the presence of bacteria in the blood (bacteremia) to fulminate disease and death occurring within hours of clinical onset. Symptoms include intense headache, fever, nausea, vomiting, photophobia, stiff neck, lethargy, myalgia, and a characteristic petechial rash.

SCREENING AND DIAGNOSIS

MM is difficult to diagnose outside epidemics because symptoms mimic many other illnesses. Initial diagnosis can be made by clinical examination followed by a lumbar puncture showing a purulent spinal fluid. The bacteria can sometimes be seen in microscopic examinations of the spinal fluid.

TREATMENT AND THERAPY

Antimicrobial chemoprophylaxis is the primary means of preventing transmission of invasive meningococcal disease from patients to close contacts. The identification of the *N. meningitidis* serogroups and their susceptibility test to antibiotics are important for treatment and for control measures. A range of antibiotics, including penicillin, ampicillin, chloramphenicol, and ceftriaxone, can treat the infection.

PREVENTION AND OUTCOMES

Several surveillance data conclude that immunization with a meningococcal vaccine offers the best intervention strategy. Routine vaccination is also recommended for high-risk groups, including college freshmen living in dormitories, travelers, populations experiencing outbreaks of meningococcal disease, and persons with increased susceptibility.

There are three types of effective and safe vaccines for preventing MM: meningococcal polysaccharide vaccines, as either bivalent (groups A and C), trivalent (groups A, C, and W), or tetravalent (groups A, C, Y, and W-135); outer membrane proteins against serogroup B; and meningococcal conjugate vaccines against group C and a tetravalent A, C, Y, and W-135 conjugate vaccine.

Oladayo Oyelola, Ph.D., SC(ASCP)

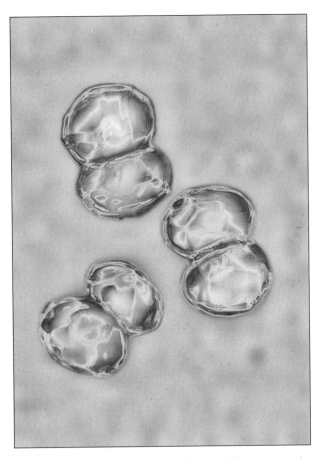

The bacterium Neisseria meningitidis, *which causes meningococcal meningitis.*

World Health Organization. *Control of Epidemic Meningococcal Disease.* 2d ed. Geneva: Author, 1998.

WEB SITES OF INTEREST

Centers for Disease Control and Prevention
http://www/cdc.gov

Meningitis Foundation of America
http://www.musa.org

National Institute of Neurological Disorders and Stroke
http://www.ninds.nih.gov

See also: Bacterial infections; Bacterial meningitis; Inflammation; Meningococcal vaccine; *Neisseria*; Neisserial infections; Respiratory route of transmission; Viral meningitis.

FURTHER READING

Centers for Disease Control and Prevention. "Meningococcal Disease." Available at http://www.cdc.gov.

Klein, D. L., and R. W. Ellis. "Conjugate Vaccines Against *Streptococcus pneumoniae*." In *New Generation Vaccines*, edited by M. M. Levine at al. 2d ed. New York: Marcel Dekker, 1997.

Kvalsvig, A. J., and D. J. Unsworth. "The Immunopathogenesis of Meningococcal Disease." *Journal of Clinical Pathology* 56 (2003): 417-422.

Pollard, A. J. "Global Epidemiology of Meningococcal Disease and Vaccine Efficacy." *Pediatric Infectious Disease Journal* 23 (2004): S274-S279.

Meningococcal vaccine

CATEGORY: Prevention
ALSO KNOWN AS: *Neisseria meningitidis* vaccine

DEFINITION

The meningococcal vaccine protects against disease caused by *Neisseria meningitidis*. This bacterium is a very serious cause of bacterial meningitis and is most virulent in areas where many people live together in close contact, such as in dormitories or military barracks. Meningococcal meningitis can present with headache, stiff neck, and fever and can progress rapidly to bloodstream infection (meningococcemia), shock, and death.

MECHANISM OF ACTION

The vaccine is made by taking the shell, or polysaccharide coating, of the *N. meningitidis* bacterium and linking it to another protein. Injection of this safe combination incites the body to produce an immune response against this bacterial coating without actually causing the disease, thus protecting against future infection.

Complicating matters, however, is that there are five different types of this bacterium. To be an effective vaccine, each different polysaccharide coating from each type of bacterium needs to be isolated and incorporated into the vaccine. To date, only four of the five types have been isolated and included in the vaccine.

VACCINE HISTORY

The first meningococcal vaccine was licensed in 1974 and provided protection against only one type of *N. meningitidis*. The vaccine was further improved by adding protection against more types of meningococcal bacteria. The final form of the vaccine was licensed in 2005 and includes protection against four of the five known types, A, C, Y, and W-135.

VACCINE ADMINISTRATION

Medical experts recommend that the meningococcal vaccine be given to all children once they reach eleven years of age. It is usually administered at the standard preadolescent visit to the family doctor or other health care provider.

IMPACT

N. meningitidis is a particularly dangerous cause of bacterial meningitis, with an estimated mortality rate of 10 percent despite prompt and appropriate antibiotic treatment. Likewise, fulminant meningococcemia carries an estimated mortality rate of 50 percent in spite of antibiotics. Without treatment, both of these diseases are fatal. The meningococcal vaccine has dramatically reduced the morbidity and mortality attributed to these diseases. It is important to note that other bacterial causes of meningitis still exist, but the incidence of meningitis overall has dramatically declined since the meningococcal vaccine was added to the routine immunization schedule.

Jennifer Birkhauser, M.D.

FURTHER READING

Behrman, Richard E., Robert M. Kliegman, and Hal B. Jenson, eds. *Nelson Textbook of Pediatrics.* 18th ed. Philadelphia: Saunders/Elsevier, 2007.

EBSCO Publishing. *Health Library: Meningococcal Vaccine.* Available through http://www.ebscohost.com.

Ferreiros, C. *Emerging Strategies in the Fight Against Meningitis.* New York: Garland Science, 2002.

Harvey, Richard A., Pamela C. Champe, and Bruce D. Fisher. *Lippincott's Illustrated Reviews: Microbiology.* 2d ed. Philadelphia: Lippincott Williams and Wilkins, 2006.

Loehr, Jamie. *The Vaccine Answer Book: Two Hundred Essential Answers to Help You Make the Right Decisions for Your Child.* Naperville, Ill.: Sourcebooks, 2010.

Pollard, A. J. "Global Epidemiology of Meningococcal Disease and Vaccine Efficacy." *Pediatric Infectious Disease Journal* 23 (2004): S274-S279.

World Health Organization. *Control of Epidemic Meningococcal Disease.* 2d ed. Geneva: Author, 1998.

WEB SITES OF INTEREST

Centers for Disease Control and Prevention, Vaccine Information
http://www.cdc.gov/vaccines/pubs/vis

Children's Hospital of Philadelphia, Vaccine Education Center
http://www.chop.edu/service/vaccine-education-center

MedlinePlus Medical Encyclopedia
http://www.nlm.nih.gov/medlineplus/druginfo/
meds/a607020.html

Meningitis Foundation of America
http://www.musa.org

National Institute of Neurological Disorders and Stroke
http://www.ninds.nih.gov

See also: Bacterial infections; Bacterial meningitis; Meningococcal meningitis; *Neisseria*; Neisserial infections; Respiratory route of transmission; Vaccines: Types; Viral meningitis.

Metapneumovirus infection

CATEGORY: Diseases and conditions
ANATOMY OR SYSTEM AFFECTED: Respiratory system
ALSO KNOWN AS: Human metapneumovirus infection

DEFINITION

Metapneumovirus infection is a respiratory infection with the human metapneumovirus (hMPV). The virus infects about 50 percent of children by age two years and virtually all children by age five years, but reinfection occurs throughout a person's life. As a cause of serious pediatric respiratory infection, hMPV is exceeded only by influenza and respiratory syncytial virus (RSV). Most adult infections are asymptomatic or mild, but serious lower respiratory tract disease may result if the person is elderly or immunocompromised.

CAUSES

The virus hMPV is a single-stranded, negative-sense ribonucleic acid (RNA) virus and a member of the paramyxovirus family. It is closely related to RSV and avian pneumovirus (APV). Serologic studies have shown that hMPV has infected humans since the mid-twentieth century or earlier. While the origin of hMPV is uncertain, its similarities to APV suggests that it may have come from birds. The virus remained unidentified until 2001 because it causes nondistinctive respiratory disease and is very difficult to culture. hMPV is present worldwide, and infections are seen in the late winter and early spring in the Northern Hemisphere.

The virus targets the bronchiolar epithelial cells. In fatal cases there is diffuse alveolar damage.

RISK FACTORS

Exacerbations of asthma may be seen when hMPV infects children younger than three years of age. Adults with chronic heart or lung diseases who become infected with hMPV are at risk of developing more severe respiratory disease requiring hospitalization. Outbreaks have occurred among the elderly residents of nursing homes. Persons with human immunodeficiency virus infection or who have had transplants, and persons on chemotherapy, often experience more severe infection; some transplant recipients have had organ rejection.

SYMPTOMS

Fever, cough, and rhinorrhea are present in most children infected with hMPV after an incubation period of three to six days. Wheezing and febrile seizures are common. Acute otitis media accompanies the infection in more than one-half of the infected children three years of age and younger. In healthy adults, infection with hMPV is often asymptomatic but may cause an illness resembling influenza or the common cold. Adults with underlying cardiopulmonary disease may have worsening of asthma or chronic obstructive pulmonary disease (COPD) or may develop pneumonia or heart failure as a consequence of infection. Immunocompromised persons can develop diffuse pneumonia accompanied by life-threatening respiratory failure.

SCREENING AND DIAGNOSIS

The most sensitive tests employ molecular methods with a variety of polymerase chain reaction (PCR) assays. Infection with hMPV may be identified in respiratory secretions using immunofluorescent antibody, which is only slightly less sensitive (85 percent) than the more complicated PCR methods. Viral culture may be used but requires the repeated passage of the virus in tissue culture with observation for twenty-one days. Serology may be used, but seroconversion or a fourfold rise in antibody titer are necessary for the diagnosis of acute infection.

TREATMENT AND THERAPY

Treatment is supportive because no specific antiviral or antibody therapy is available for the infection.

PREVENTION AND OUTCOMES

Handwashing and disinfection of contaminated surfaces and objects are the best forms of prevention, as transmission of hMPV is thought to occur through contact with infectious secretions, fomites (inanimate objects), and aerosols. Viral shedding may continue for as long as three weeks. No effective vaccine is available.

H. Bradford Hawley, M.D.

FURTHER READING

Falsey, Ann R. "Human Metapneumovirus." In *Mandell, Douglas, and Bennett's Principles and Practice of Infectious Diseases*, edited by Gerald L. Mandell, John F. Bennett, and Raphael Dolin. 7th ed. New York: Churchill Livingstone/Elsevier, 2010.

Kahn, Jeffrey S. "Epidemiology of Human Metapneumovirus." *Clinical Microbiology Reviews* 19 (2006): 546-557.

Williams, John V. "The Clinical Presentation and Outcomes of Children Infected with Newly Identified Respiratory Tract Viruses." *Infectious Disease Clinics of North America* 19 (2005): 569-584.

WEB SITES OF INTEREST

American Lung Association
http://www.lungusa.org

KidsHealth
http://kidshealth.org

See also: Birds and infectious disease; Children and infectious disease; Paramyxoviridae; Respiratory syncytial virus infections; Viral infections.

Methicillin-resistant staph infection

CATEGORY: Diseases and conditions
ANATOMY OR SYSTEM AFFECTED: Blood, bones, circulatory system, lungs, respiratory system, skin
ALSO KNOWN AS: CA-MRSA, HA-MRSA, health-care-associated MRSA, methicillin-resistant *Staphylococcus aureus* community-acquired MRSA, methicillin-resistant *Staphylococcus aureus* infection, methicillin-resistant *Staphylococcus aureus* nosocomial MRSA

DEFINITION

A methicillin-resistant staph (MRSA) infection is caused by the bacterium *Staphylococcus aureus*. The bacterium can affect the skin, blood, bones, or lungs. A person can be infected or colonized with MRSA. When a person is infected, the bacterium produces symptoms. A person colonized also has the bacterium, but the bacterium may not cause any symptoms.

There are two types of MRSA infection: community acquired and nosocomial. People who have community-acquired MRSA infection were infected outside a hospital setting (such as a dormitory). Nosocomial MRSA infections occur in hospital settings.

CAUSES

An MRSA infection can spread through several mechanisms, including from contaminated surfaces, from person to person, and from one area of the body to another.

RISK FACTORS

The following factors increase the chance of community acquired infection: impaired immunity, sharing crowded spaces (such as dormitories and locker rooms), using intravenous drugs, serious illness, exposure to animals (as pet owners, veterinarians, and pig farmers, for example), using antibiotics, having a chronic skin disorder, and past MRSA infection. Also at higher risk are young children, athletes, prisoners, and military personnel.

For nosocomial infection, the risk factors are impaired immunity, exposure to hospital or clinical settings, advanced age, chronic illness, using antibiotics, having a wound, living in a long-term-care center, and having an indwelling medical device (such as a feeding tube or intravenous catheter). Also, men are at higher risk.

SYMPTOMS

The symptoms of MRSA include folliculitis (infection of hair follicles), boils (a skin infection that may drain pus, blood, or an amber-colored liquid), scalded skin syndrome (a skin infection characterized by a fever, rash, and sometimes blisters), impetigo (large blisters on the skin), toxic shock syndrome (a rare but serious bacterial infection whose primary symptoms are a rash and high fever), cellulitis (a skin infection characterized by a swollen, red area that spreads quickly), and an abscess.

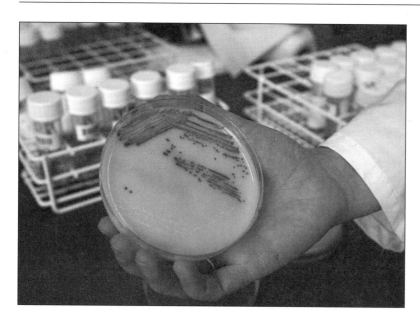

A culture plate with methicillin-resistant Staphylococcus aureus. *(AP/Wide World Photos)*

SCREENING AND DIAGNOSIS

A doctor will ask about symptoms and medical history and will perform a physical exam. Tests may include cultures, blood tests, urine tests, and a skin biopsy (removal of a sample of skin to test for infection).

TREATMENT AND THERAPY

Treatment options include medications such as antibiotics, prescribed to kill the bacteria, and incision and drainage of an abscess, in which the doctor (but not the patient) opens the abscess and allows the fluid to drain. Another treatment is cleansing the skin. To treat the infection and to keep it from spreading, one should wash skin with an antibacterial cleanser, apply an antibiotic, and cover skin with a sterile dressing.

PREVENTION AND OUTCOMES

To help reduce the chance of getting an MRSA infection, one should thoroughly wash hands with soap and water, keep cuts and wounds clean and covered until healed, and avoid contact with other people's wounds and with materials contaminated by wounds. Hospitalized persons' visitors, and health care workers, may be required to wear special clothing and gloves to prevent spreading the infection to others.

Krisha McCoy, M.S.;
reviewed by David L. Horn, M.D., FACP

FURTHER READING

Archer, G. L. "Staphylococcal Infections." In *Andreoli and Carpenter's Cecil Essentials of Medicine,* edited by Thomas E. Andreoli et al. 8th ed. Philadelphia: Saunders/Elsevier, 2010.

Centers for Disease Control and Prevention. "Seasonal Flu and Staph Infection." Available at http://www.cdc.gov/flu/about/qa/flustaph.htm.

Crossley, Kent B., Kimberly K. Jefferson, and Gordon L. Archer, eds. *Staphylococci in Human Disease.* Hoboken, N.J.: John Wiley & Sons, 2009.

EBSCO Publishing. *DynaMed: Community-Acquired Methicillin-Resistant "Staphylococcus aureus" (MRSA) Infection.* Available through http://www.ebscohost.com/dynamed.

_____. *DynaMed: Nosocomial Methicillin-Resistant "Staphylococcus aureus" (MRSA) Infection.* Available through http://www.ebscohost.com/dynamed.

Laibl, V. R., et al. "Clinical Presentation of Community-Acquired Methicillin-Resistant *Staphylococcus aureus* in Pregnancy." *Obstetrics and Gynecology* 106 (2005): 461-465.

WEB SITES OF INTEREST

American Academy of Dermatology
http://www.aad.org

Centers for Disease Control and Prevention
http://www.cdc.gov

National Institute of Allergy and Infectious Diseases
http://www.niaid.nih.gov

Public Health Agency of Canada
http://www.phac-aspc.gc.ca

See also: Abscesses; Anal abscess; Antibiotic resistance; Antibiotics: Types; Bacterial infections; Cellulitis; Contagious diseases; Drug resistance; Hospitals and infectious disease; Iatrogenic infections; Impetigo; Pilonidal cyst; Schools and infectious disease; Skin infections; Staphylococcal infections; *Staphylococcus.*

Microbiology

CATEGORY: Epidemiology

DEFINITION

"Microbiology," a term derived from Greek words essentially meaning "examination of small life," is the study of microorganisms, a large and diverse group of microscopic organisms existing as single cells or cell clusters. Of note, viruses are also studied in microbiology, although they are not considered to be cellular. Microbes are distinct from animal and plant cells because they can, mostly, carry out their life processes (such as growth and reproduction) and survive independent of other cells or a host (with the exception of viruses).

In general, microorganisms can be divided into prokaryotes (organisms such as bacteria that lack a cell nucleus and other membrane-bound organelles), eukaryotes (organisms such as algae, fungi, and protists that have a cell nucleus), and viruses (noncellular organisms that rely on host cells for achievement of life processes and survival). Of note, in modern classification systems, prokaryotes are commonly further divided into the domains Bacteria and Archaea, whereby the latter domain represents microbes that are phylogenetically related to the former domain, but that have many structural, genetic, and biochemical distinctions. In general, eukaryotes are larger than prokaryotes, which are larger than viruses, although the range of each of these groups can vary widely.

HISTORY AND MODERN PROGRESS

Scientists hypothesized the existence of microorganisms for many centuries before they were actually discovered, although these early claims were not based on observation or data. Robert Hooke is credited with publishing the first report of the fruiting bodies of molds in 1665, and he is notable for coining the term "cell" to refer to the basic unit of life. However, microbes were directly observed for the first time more than three hundred years ago, when Antoni van Leeuwenhoek designed a single-lens microscope for research purposes and reported the observation of bacteria and other microorganisms in 1676.

Louis Pasteur and Robert Koch are considered the founders of microbiology and medical microbiology, respectively. Pasteur is well known for his experiments disproving the theory of spontaneous generation,

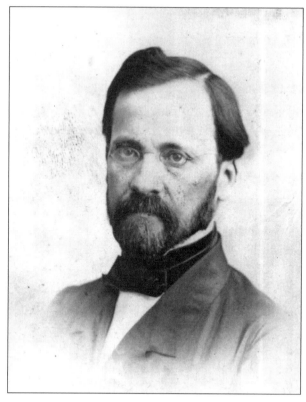

Louis Pasteur. (Library of Congress)

giving microbiological studies a basis. Koch is best known for his contributions to the germ theory of disease, which proved that diseases were indeed caused by specific microbes called pathogens, or harmful microbes.

Since the early years of microbiological studies, the field has evolved tremendously. In particular, a few significant advances that have stemmed from microbiology include the development of antibiotics, vaccines, and bioremediation agents. However, because microbiology (and its various subdisciplines) is a relatively new field, it is still considered to be in its infancy, especially when compared with long-established disciplines such as botany and zoology.

SUBDISCIPLINES

The field of microbiology is tremendously broad, in that it includes a number of general areas, including bacteriology (the study of bacteria), mycology (the study of fungi), parasitology (the study of parasites), and virology (the study of viruses and, more recently,

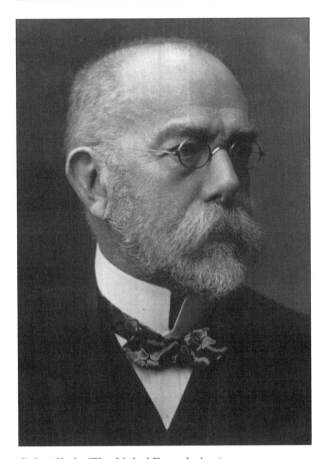

Robert Koch. (The Nobel Foundation)

virus-like agents, including prions, viroids, and satellites). These areas can be further divided into a variety of subtopics. For example, a virologist can focus on deoxyribonucleic acid (DNA) viruses only. A microbiologist can, by definition, study any or all of these topics, although microbiology researchers typically specialize and practice in either of several scientific fields: human medicine, veterinary medicine, environmental studies, agricultural studies, food science, pharmaceuticals, and biotechnology and bioengineering, among many others. Furthermore, a researcher may also focus on a particular aspect of a certain microorganism or group or organisms, such as microbial growth, structure, metabolism, genetics, and evolution.

Because the immune system typically interacts with and influences microbes (especially pathogens), immunology is often coupled with the study of microbiology. Although immunology can be studied independently of microbiology (or in the context of other disciplines), these two fields are often coupled because much of the pertinent information intersects. Thus, many academic institutions offer joint programs in the study of both disciplines.

With modern advances in research, medicine, and technology, new subdisciplines of microbiology continue to emerge. For instance, nanomicrobiology and industrial microbiology are two fairly novel fields that study microbes at the nanoscale (nanomicrobiology) and study the use of microorganisms for the production of food or industrial products (industrial microbiology).

IMPACT

Harmful microbes (pathogens) make up a small fraction of the total population of microorganisms on Earth, yet they play a particularly powerful role in human life. Given the significance of these harmful microbes, microbiology is critical to the fields of health and medicine. In addition, because microbes contribute to the pathogenesis of many diseases that affect nonhuman animals, plants, water, and soil, for example, microbiology also plays a critical role in the environmental and agricultural sciences.

Even more, microbiology studies the microbes that are responsible for a number of beneficial processes, including antibody production (for treating humans, animals, and plants), fermentation (producing dairy products, alcohol, and other consumables), and a variety of other biotechnological applications in research and medicine (producing useful enzymes and amino acids).

Several agencies monitor and regulate the various aspects of infectious diseases associated with microbiological organisms. These agencies include the World Health Organization, the Centers for Disease Control and Prevention, the U.S. Food and Drug Administration, and the U.S. Environmental Protection Agency. With scientific researchers, clinicians, industry professionals, support organizations, and other contributors, these agencies work to advance knowledge of microbes, both good and bad.

Brandy Weidow, M.S.

FURTHER READING

Gladwin, Mark, and Bill Trattler. *Clinical Microbiology Made Ridiculously Simple.* 4th ed. Miami: MedMaster, 2007.

Madigan, Michael T., and John M. Martinko. *Brock Biology of Microorganisms*. 12th ed. Upper Saddle River, N.J.: Pearson/Prentice Hall, 2010.

Ryan, Kenneth J., and C. George Ray, eds. *Sherris Medical Microbiology: An Introduction to Infectious Diseases*. 5th ed. New York: McGraw-Hill, 2010.

Through the Microscope: A Look at All Things Small. Available at http://www.microbiologytext.com.

Tortora, Gerard J., Berdell R. Funke, and Christine L. Case. *Microbiology: An Introduction.* 10th ed. San Francisco: Benjamin Cummings, 2010.

WEB SITES OF INTEREST

American Society for Microbiology
http://www.asm.org

Microbiology and Immunology On-line
http://pathmicro.med.sc.edu/book/welcome.htm

Microbiology Information Portal
http://www.microbes.info

Mycology Online
http://www.mycology.adelaide.edu.au

Todar's Online Textbook of Bacteriology
http://www.textbookofbacteriology.net

U.S. Environmental Protection Agency
http://www.epa.gov/nerlcwww

Virology.net
http://www.virology.net

See also: Bacteria: Classification and types; Bacteria: Structure and growth; Bacterial infections; Bacteriology; Centers for Disease Control and Prevention (CDC); Epidemiology; Fungal infections; Fungi: Classification and types; Fungi: Structure and growth; Koch's postulates; Microscopy; Parasites: Classification and types; Parasitic diseases; Pathogenicity; Pathogens; Prion diseases; Protozoan diseases; Serology; Viral infections; Virology; Virulence; Viruses: Types; World Health Organization (WHO).

Microscopy

CATEGORY: Diagnosis

DEFINITION

The word "microscopy" defines the technique wherein microscopes are used to study organisms and cells that are too small to be seen by the unaided eye. When first invented, microscopes comprised simply a series of magnifying lenses that made the object or specimen under study appear much bigger than its actual size. Moreover, these early inventions relied on sunlight as the source of illumination, a feature that has been modified over the years and now includes microscopes with a diverse collection of illuminators, from visible light and ultraviolet light and laser to sound waves, electron beams, and thin metal probes. The spectrum of microscopy also has changed since the technique that began with two-dimensional images of protists now offers, for example, three-dimensional colored imaging that can be used to study molecular processes in atomic detail.

HISTORICAL BACKGROUND

As early as the first century, the Romans, while experimenting with different kinds of glass and their ability to enhance the visibility of objects seen through them, discovered lenses. In the late sixteenth century, Dutch spectacle makerZaccharias Jansen created the world's first compound microscope by placing several lenses inside a tube. Encouraged by their findings, Galileo started building his own microscope. The word "microscope," though, was coined by Giovanni Faber in the seventeenth century to describe his friend Galileo's invention. "Microscope" was derived from two Greek words, *micron*, meaning "small," and *skopein*, meaning "to look at."

Soon thereafter, in the mid-seventeenth century, British scientist Robert Hooke made several important contributions in the field of microscopy and documented them in his famous book *Micrographia* (1665). Hooke was studying sections of cork tissue and discovered tiny chambers in the tissue that he called "cells."

In the late seventeenth and early eighteenth centuries, several pioneering discoveries (influenced by Hooke) in the field of biology were made using microscopes made by a Dutch tradesman, Antoni van Leeuwenhoek. Leeuwenhoek, despite a lack of formal training as a scientist, discovered bacteria, protists, and many other microbes, thus opening up the field of microbiology. He often is regarded as the founder of microscopy, which now includes microscopes such as the scanning probe and atomic probe, which allows one to visualize structures at the atomic and molecular levels.

THE PROCESS OF MICROSCOPY

In all kinds of microscopy, a major goal is to enhance the contrast between the specimen that is being studied and the medium (also called the background). This is done to provide a sharp and detailed image, because most cells and organisms have very slight coloration, if any. Common methods to enhance contrast include stains, dyes, and alternative sources of illumination, such as ultraviolet and laser.

The process of staining will be discussed here as it applies to the widely used compound light microscope. There are two broad categories of stains: acidic stain, wherein the chromophore (coloring unit) is an anion, and basic stain, wherein the chromophore is a cation. Stains also are classified as simple or differential. Simple stains will color all microbes in a nonspecific manner; thus, they are typically helpful for studying cell shapes, morphology, and arrangements. Differential stains are specific and, therefore, will stain only certain cells; they often are used in microbial identification.

The staining process typically starts with the creation of a smear, composed of simply two to three drops of the bacterial suspension spread out on a clean glass slide. The next step is fixing, which helps attach the specimen to the glass slide. Typically, bacterial specimens are fixed by quickly passing the air-dried smear over a flame. Once the specimen has been fixed, the actual staining process begins. It typically involves adding the stain or dye, then waiting a few minutes before washing off the stain, adding a mordant (color enhancer) if required, and counterstaining (with the secondary stain).

Once the staining process is finished, depending upon the specimen size, the slide is covered with a square piece of thin glass called the cover slip and then observed under the microscope. If greater magnification is required with the brightfield microscope (a compound light microscope that is commonly used), a drop of immersion oil is placed over the specimen and the specimen is then viewed using a special objective called the immersion lens.

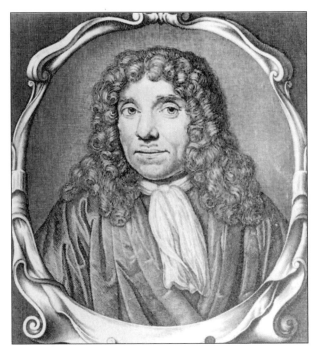

Antoni van Leeuwenhoek. (Library of Congress)

IMPACT

With the evolution of microscopy and with ongoing advances in the field, microscopy is now an integral part of clinical diagnostics. For instance, several imaging tools, such as confocal, multiphoton, and wide-field microscopes, have been integrated to allow studies of tumor cell migration. Such imaging allows one to see intricate details, such as how the tumor cells interact with the extracellular matrix and if there is any likelihood of metastasis. These microscopic studies, which provide insight into the molecular basis of tumor cell migration, can in the long run help scientists develop anticancer therapies.

Another more recent advance is diagnosing malaria. Malaria is an infectious disease prevalent primarily in the tropical regions. According to the World Health Organization, each year it causes more than one million deaths worldwide. Traditionally, the standard method to confirm the presence of the malarial parasite in red blood cells relied on manual microscopy, which, in addition to being error-prone, is tedious. Scientists now combine computer vision with imaging tools to allow for malarial parasite diagnosis in thin blood smears, a feature that will allow clinicians to treat malaria in the early stages.

Furthermore, the development of super resolution microscopes, such as those that incorporate multiphoton techniques in fiber optic microscopy and automated image analysis for high throughput screens, have allowed scientists and the pharmaceutical industry not only to improve current drug assays but also to equip them with newer and better disease models. Microscopy and imaging tools thus continue to play a critical role not only in traditional cell biology but also in more recent clinical diagnosis and drug discovery.

Sibani Sengupta, Ph.D.

FURTHER READING

Boray Tek, F., A. G. Dempster, and I. Kale. "Computer Vision for Microscopy Diagnosis of Malaria." *Malaria Journal* 8 (2009):153. This article offers details of computerized imaging for malaria diagnosis.

Croft, William J. *Under the Microscope: A Brief History of Microscopy.* Hackensack, N.J.: World Scientific, 2006. A straightforward history of microscopy.

Le Dévédec, S. E., et al. "Systems Microscopy Approaches to Understand Cancer Cell Migration and Metastasis." *Cellular and Molecular Life Sciences* 67 (2010): 3219-3240. This article reviews recent imaging tools that can be used to study cancer cell migration.

Tortora, Gerard J., Berdell R. Funke, and Christine L. Case. *Microbiology: An Introduction.* 10th ed. San Francisco: Benjamin Cummings, 2010. A good introductory work that covers the basics of microscopy.

WEB SITES OF INTEREST

Microscopy Society of America
http://www.microscopy.org

Optical Society
http://www.osa.org

Protocolpedia
http://www.protocolpedia.com

See also: Acid-fastness; Bacteria: Classification and types; Bacteria: Structure and growth; Bacteriology; Biochemical tests; Biostatistics; Diagnosis of bacterial infections; Diagnosis of viral infections; Gram staining; Immunoassay; Microbiology; Parasites: Classification and types; Pathogens; Polymerase chain reaction (PCR) method; Pulsed-field gel electrophoresis; Serology; Virology; Viruses: Types.

Microsporum

CATEGORY: Pathogen
TRANSMISSION ROUTE: Inhalation

DEFINITION

Microsporum is a genus of fungus that causes infections of the skin, hair, and nails.

**Taxonomic Classification
for *Microsporum***

Kingdom: Fungi
Phylum: Ascomyta
Order: Onygenales
Family: Arthrodermataceae
Genus: *Microsporum*
Species:
M. audouinii
M. canis
M. ferrugineum
M. gypseum

NATURAL HABITAT AND FEATURES

Microsporum species are widely distributed throughout the world, although some have restricted geographic distribution. Their natural habitat may be soil (geophilic species), animals (zoophilic species), or humans (anthropophilic species). Among soil species are *cookei* (also isolated from cat, dog, and rodent hair) and *gypseum* (also isolated from rodent fur). *Nanum* is found both in soil and on animals (swine). Animal species include *canis* (cats and dogs), *gallinae* (fowl), and *persicolor* (field rodents). Species with humans as the natural host include *audouinii* and *ferrugineum.*

Microsporum is the asexual (mitosporic) phase of the fungus. The sexual (teleomorphic) phase is assigned to the genus *Arthroderma. Microsporum* are molds with septate hyphae, that is, filaments with partitioned cavities. Conidia, asexual sporelike reproductive bodies, may be borne directly on the hyphae or on conidiospores, branching structures designed to bear conidia. Microconidia are one-celled, solitary, and oval- to club-shaped. Macroconidia are multicellular, spindle-shaped (fusiform), and have spiny (echinulate) or rough transparent (hyaline) walls. *Microsporum* grow on Sabouraud's dextrose agar at 77° Fahrenheit (25° Celsius). After seven days of incubation, the colony varies between 1 and 6 centimeters. The color of the colony varies depending on the species.

PATHOGENICITY AND CLINICAL SIGNIFICANCE

Microsporum is a dermatophyte, a fungus that causes dermatophytosis, a superficial infection of the skin, hair, or nails. *Epidermophyton* and *Trichophyton* are two other genera of fungi with species that cause dermatophytosis. Most pathogenic *Microsporum* species infect the skin and hair. In the United States, *canis*, transmitted to humans from pet dogs and cats, is the most common cause of skin and hair fungal infections. It is also often the cause of mild tinea capitis (scalp and hair infections) and tinea corporis (trunk, leg, and arm infections). Less frequently, *canis* and *gypseum* are implicated in tinea manuum (ringworm of the hands). The anthropophilic species *audouinii* and *ferrugineum* can cause contagious tinea capitis, especially in children. *Persicolor* only infects the skin. Nail infections (onychomycosis) caused by *Microsporum* species are rare. Most nail infections are caused by *Tricophytoses*, *Candida*, or other fungal species.

Overall, the risk of infection with *Microsporum* species is low. However, pathogenic fungi can be introduced by contact with contaminated soil or infected animals, such as household pets, or with infected persons or with objects (such as a shared comb or towel) that have been used by infected persons. Barber shops, hair and nail salons, and gyms are public locations where a person may come into contact with contaminated items.

Pathogens colonize the surface of the body by destroying keratin, the major protein found in skin, hair, and nails. Infections spread laterally, with sharp, advancing margins. They do not become invasive. As the infection was thought to look like the burrows of worms, the common name for *Microsporum* infections, in general, became "ringworm." The root name in Latin for many forms of *Microsporum* infections is *tinea*, which means "worm."

Many cases of infection with *Microsporum* are asymptomatic. Other, mild cases may be self-limiting or they can be managed with nonprescription topical agents. Persistent, recurring, or severe cases require directed medical treatment.

DRUG SUSCEPTIBILITY

Griseofulvin was once the drug of choice for treatment of infections caused by *Microsporum* species and other dermatophytes. One of this drug's main drawbacks was that it often took several months to effect a cure, particularly in cases of tinea capitis. Monthly drug monitoring was required too.

More convenient, safer, and more effective agents are now available and preferred. Topical formulations of azoles (imidazole, clotrimazole, miconazole, and sulconazole) may be sufficient treatment for mild, localized cases. Using them avoids the risk of side effects that can accompany the use of oral medications. For persistent, recurring, or more virulent infections, oral therapy with itraconazole or terbinafine is now the drug of first choice.

Standardized in vitro susceptibility tests for antifungal agents used to treat infections caused by *Microsporum* have not been established. Nonstandardized in vitro comparison studies of the three major oral agents have been carried out with selected *Trichophyton* species. Griseofulvin yielded higher minimum inhibitory concentrations (MICs) than did itraconazole, which had higher MICs than did terbinafine. However, the meaning and clinical significance of these data require further investigation and might not hold if tested against *Microsporum* species. In limited clinical studies, itraconazole and terbinafine appeared to show greater efficacy against fungal skin infections than did griseofulvin. Depending on the study, itracanozole and terbinafine were comparable in efficacy, or terbinafine was superior.

Ernest Kohlmetz, M.A.

FURTHER READING

Richardson, Malcolm D., and David W. Warnock. *Fungal Infection: Diagnosis and Management.* New ed. Malden, Mass.: Wiley-Blackwell, 2010.

Ryan, Kenneth J., and C. George Ray, eds. *Sherris Medical Microbiology: An Introduction to Infectious Diseases.* 5th ed. New York: McGraw-Hill, 2010.

White, Gary M., and Neil H. Cox. *Diseases of the Skin: A Color Atlas and Text.* 2d ed. Philadelphia: Mosby/Elsevier, 2006.

See also: Antifungal drugs: Types; *Candida*; Chromoblastomycosis; Dermatomycosis; Dermatophytosis; *Epidermophyton*; Fungi: Classification and types; *Malassezia*; Mycoses; Onychomycosis; Skin infections; Soilborne illness and disease; *Trichophyton*.

Middle-ear infection

Category: Diseases and conditions
Anatomy or system affected: Auditory system, ears
Also known as: Acute otitis, otitis media

Definition

An infection of the middle ear occurs when the middle ear, which is located behind the eardrum, becomes infected and inflamed.

Causes

A middle-ear infection is caused by bacteria such as *Streptococcus pneumoniae* (most common), *Haemophilus influenzae*, *Moraxella* (*Branhamella*) *catarrhalis*, and *S. pyogenes* (less common). Viruses that cause middle-ear infections include those associated with the common cold.

Risk Factors

The factors that increase the chance of developing a middle-ear infection include a recent viral infection (such as a cold); recent sinusitis; day care attendance; medical conditions that cause abnormalities of the eustachian tubes, such as cleft palate; Down syndrome; history of allergies (environmental allergies and food allergies); gastroesophageal reflux disease (GERD); and exposure to secondhand smoke from cigarettes, cooking, and burning wood. Also at higher risk are infants and toddlers, infants whose mothers drank alcohol while pregnant, and infants who are formula-fed. Middle-ear infections are most common in the winter months.

Key Terms: Middle-Ear Infections

- *Cholesteatoma.* A tumor-like mass of cells that usually results from chronic middle-ear infection.

- *Eardrum.* The membrane separating the outer ear canal from the middle ear that changes sound waves into movements of the ossicles; also called the tympanic membrane.

- *Eustachian tube.* The tube connecting the middle ear to the back of the throat; air exchange through this tube equalizes air pressure in the middle ear with outside air pressure.

- *Labyrinth.* A structure consisting of three fluid-filled, semicircular canals at right angles to one another in the inner ear; they monitor the position and movement of the head.

- *Middle ear.* The air-filled cavity in which vibrations are transmitted from the eardrum to the inner ear via the ossicles.

- *Ossicles.* Three small bones in the middle ear that transmit vibrations from the eardrum to the fluid of the inner ear.

- *Otoscope.* An instrument for viewing the ear canal and the eardrum.

- *Tympanic membrane.* Another term for the eardrum.

Infants and toddlers. Three-quarters of children will experience an ear infection before their third birthday, and nearly one-half of these children will have three or more infections by age three years. Although adults can get ear infections, children between the ages of six months and six years are the most prone to ear infections. The risk of ear infections is higher in children because their immune systems have had less exposure to common viruses. Virus infections are, most likely, the direct or indirect cause of most middle-ear infections. Moreover, children's shorter eustachian tubes (the small channels that let air pass from the nose into the middle ear) make it easier for bacteria to gain access to the middle ear. Larger adenoids in some children also contribute to the development of ear infections. Boys are probably more likely to get otitis, especially chronic otitis media, than are girls.

Day care attendance. Children in day care or in nursery schools are more likely to get ear infections because they are exposed to more upper respiratory infections that can subsequently infect the middle ear. While day care is a necessary fact of life for many children, it is also one of the strongest risk factors for ear infection.

Exposure to cigarette smoke. Children who live with adults who smoke cigarettes are more likely to develop ear infections.

Poverty. While ear infections are common in persons from all levels of income, they tend to be more frequent and more prolonged in poor children, who often lack adequate health care.

Breast-feeding. Infants who are breast-fed, especially for four to six months or longer, have fewer and shorter ear infections than do bottle-fed infants.

Other infections. Children are more likely to get an ear infection if they have a cold, sore throat, or eye infection. Although ear infections are not themselves contagious, colds, sore throats, and other respiratory infections are readily passed from person to person.

Allergies and asthma. People with allergies or asthma are more likely to develop ear infections. The reasons for this increased risk remain incompletely understood.

Immune suppression. Children with immune disorders, including acquired immunodeficiency syndrome (AIDS), and those receiving immunosuppressive therapy are more likely to develop ear infections because their bodies fight bacteria and viruses less effectively. The occurrence of an ear infection, or even multiple ear infections, is not itself an indication of AIDS or another immune disorder.

Congenital conditions. Medical conditions that cause abnormalities of the eustachian tubes, such as cleft palate, increase the risk of developing ear infections.

Drinking from a bottle while lying down. Children who drink from a bottle while lying on their backs are more likely to develop ear infections, possibly because fluid is allowed to accumulate in the eustachian tubes.

Pacifier use. Children who use pacifiers continually may be at greater risk for developing ear infections than children who use them less frequently or not at all.

Family history. A strong family history of ear infections, especially in older brothers or sisters, also increases risk.

SYMPTOMS

Ear infections frequently develop during or shortly after another infection, such as a cold or sore throat.

Symptoms include ear pain (children who can talk may say that their ear hurts, while babies may tug or rub at the ear or face or become irritable); drainage from the ear, which may appear as blood, clear fluid, pus, or dry crust on the outer portion of the ear after sleeping; hearing loss, which resolves with appropriate treatment; fever; irritability; decreased appetite or difficulty feeding; disturbed sleep; difficulty with balance, frequent falling, or sensations of dizziness; nausea, vomiting, or diarrhea; malaise (a feeling of general illness); chills; and inattentiveness.

Some children with ear infection, particularly chronic otitis, have no symptoms. Their condition may be discovered on examination for some other problem.

SCREENING AND DIAGNOSIS

When there is ear pain or drainage from the ear, then infection is likely present. If a child is too young to report pain, the doctor or nurse practitioner must rely solely on looking into the child's ear with a special lighted instrument (an otoscope). A small tube and bulb (insufflator) may be attached to the otoscope so that a light puff of air can be blown into the ear. This helps the health care provider see if the eardrum is moving normally. When infection is present the eardrum is often stiffened by the presence of fluid behind it and does not move. The eardrum may also be red and bulge outward because the fluid behind it is under pressure. A red, bulging drum that does not move with an air puff is a good sign that acute otitis is present.

It is often difficult to see the eardrum in young children, and ear wax frequently makes getting a good view of the drum difficult. Even in the absence of wax, the accurate diagnosis of middle-ear infection using an otoscope is not easy. Most studies suggest that even experienced doctors may overdiagnose acute ear infections, especially if an air puff insufflator is not used. Doctors may have a particularly difficult time distinguishing between children with chronic otitis (who frequently do not need antibiotics) and those with acute otitis (for whom antibiotics are often helpful). The use of a microscope to examine the ear may also help.

Other tests may also be performed, especially if the parent or child has had repeated ear infections. Tests may include the following:

Tympanocentesis. A needle is used to withdraw fluid

or pus from the middle ear under local or general anesthesia. This fluid can then be cultured to determine if bacteria are present in the fluid. Once the bacteria are cultured, the lab can determine what drugs are best for treatment. However, the fluid does not always have bacteria.

Tympanometry. A soft plug is inserted into the opening of the ear canal. The plug contains a speaker, a microphone, and a device that is able to alter the air pressure in the ear canal. This allows several different measures of the middle ear and eardrum and provides important information about the condition of the ear, but it is not a hearing test.

Hearing test. A hearing test may be ordered for persons with repeated ear infections or with signs of hearing impairment, such as speaking in a louder voice, sitting closer to a television, or turning up the volume of a television or stereo.

TREATMENT AND THERAPY

Treatments include antibiotics that are commonly used to treat ear infections. These include amoxicillin (Amoxil, Polymox) and clavulanate (Augmentin). Other medications are cephalosporins (cefprozil, cefdinir, cefpodoxime, and ceftriaxone) and sulfa drugs (such as Septra, Bactrim, and Pediazole).

Because bacteria develop a resistance to antibiotics, doctors may take a "wait and see" approach before writing a prescription. In some cases, the doctor may prescribe an antibiotic for children and ask the parent to administer the medication if the pain or fever lasts for a certain number of days. This approach has been effective. Some ear infections are caused by a virus and thus cannot be treated with antibiotics. Most middle-ear infections (including bacterial infections) tend to improve on their own in two to three days.

Over-the-counter pain relievers, which can help reduce pain, fever, and irritability, include acetaminophen, ibuprofen, and aspirin. Aspirin is not recommended for children or teens with a current or recent viral infection because of the risk of Reye's syndrome. One should consult the doctor about medicines that are safe for children. Decongestants and antihistamines are not recommended to treat an ear infection.

In children, ear drops that have a local anaesthetic (such as ametocaine, benzocaine, or lidocaine) can help decrease pain, especially when the drops are used with oral pain relievers. If there is a chance that the eardrum has ruptured, one should avoid using ear drops. Another treatment option is myringotomy, surgery to open the eardrum. A tiny cut is made in the eardrum to drain fluid and pus.

PREVENTION AND OUTCOMES

To reduce the chance of getting an ear infection, one should avoid exposure to smoke and should breast-feed for the first six months or so of an infant's life and should try to avoid giving the infant a pacifier. If the infant is bottle-fed, his or her head should be propped up as much as possible. One should not leave a bottle in the crib with the infant.

Other preventive measures include getting tested for allergies, treating conditions such as GERD, practicing good hygiene, and ensuring children's vaccinations are up to date. The pneumococcal vaccine and the flu vaccine can prevent middle-ear infections. If the child has a history of ear infections, one should consult the doctor about long-term antibiotic use. Another option for the child is the use of tympanostomy tubes, which help equalize pressure behind the eardrum. Large adenoids can interfere with the eustachian tubes. The child's doctor should be consulted about having the adenoids removed.

Alayne Ronnenberg, Sc.D., and Rosalyn Carson-DeWitt, M.D.; reviewed by Elie Edmond Rebeiz, M.D., FACS

FURTHER READING

Coleman, C., and M. Moore. "Decongestants and Antihistamines for Acute Otitis Media in Children." *Cochrane Database of Systematic Reviews* (2008): CD001727. Available through *EBSCO DynaMed Systematic Literature Surveillance* at http://www.ebscohost.com/dynamed. A survey of certain medications for use in children with middle-ear infection.

EBSCO Publishing. *DynaMed: Acute Otitis Media.* Available through http://www.ebscohost.com/dynamed. A brief, online discussion of middle-ear infection.

Ferrari, Mario. *PDxMD Ear, Nose, and Throat Disorders.* Philadelphia: PDxMD, 2003. A clinical yet accessible reference text that provides a comprehensive list of disorders, with a summary of the condition, background, diagnosis, treatment, outcomes, prevention, and resources.

Foxlee, R., et al. "Topical Analgesia for Acute Otitis Media." *Cochrane Database of Systematic Reviews* (2009): CD005657. Available through *EBSCO DynaMed Systematic Literature Surveillance* at http://

www.ebscohost.com/dynamed. Presents a review of topical medications for relief of middle-ear infection pain.

Roush, Jackson, ed. *Screening for Hearing Loss and Otitis Media in Children*. San Diego, Calif.: Singular, 2001. Although clinical in nature, this book describes myriad hearing tests in great detail.

St. Sauven, J., et al. "Risk Factors for Otitis Media and Carriage of Multiple Strains of *Haemophilus influenzae* and *Streptococcus pneumoniae*." *Emerging Infectious Diseases* 6, no. 6 (2000): 622-630. Examines the combined effects on persons of having a middle-ear infection caused by infective viruses and bacteria.

WEB SITES OF INTEREST

American Academy of Otolaryngology—Head and Neck Surgery
http://www.entnet.org

American Academy of Pediatrics
http://www.healthychildren.org

National Institute on Deafness and Other Communication Disorders
http://www.nidcd.nih.gov

See also: Bacterial infections; Children and infectious disease; Common cold; Influenza vaccine; Labyrinthitis; Nasopharyngeal infections; Pharyngitis and tonsillopharyngitis; Pneumococcal infections; Pneumococcal vaccine; Schools and infectious disease; Sinusitis; Viral infections; Viral pharyngitis.

Mites and chiggers and infectious disease

CATEGORY: Transmission

DEFINITION

Mites are small-to-microscopic arachnids. They have a body without a constriction between the cephalothorax and abdomen, mandibles adapted for piercing, and, usually, four pairs of short legs in the adult and three in the juvenile form (larvae). The scabies mite, *Sarcoptes scabiei*, is a member of a family of parasitic mites that cause scabies in humans. Chiggers are the larvae of a certain type of mite of the family Trombiculidae. These very small, reddish mites feed on humans and other animals only when they are in the larval stage.

MITES

S. scabiei var. *hominis*, the human itch-mite that causes scabies, is in the arthropod class Arachnida, subclass Acari, family Sarcoptidae. Mites are among the most diverse and successful of all the invertebrate groups. An estimated 48,200 species have been identified and described. They have exploited an incredible array of habitats, and because of their small size (most are microscopic), they go largely unnoticed. Many live freely in the soil or water, but many species live as parasites on plants and animals.

Disease signs and symptoms. The scabies mite, *S. scabiei*, causes scabies in humans. Persons with scabies usually have no symptoms during the first two to six weeks of infestation; however, infected persons can spread scabies during this time. Severe itching, especially at night, and a pimple-like, itchy rash are the earliest and most common symptoms of scabies. These symptoms are caused by sensitization to the proteins and feces of the parasite. The itching and rash may affect much of the body or be limited to common sites such as the wrist, elbow, armpit, webbing between the fingers, nipples, penis, waist, belt line, and buttocks. The rash also can include tiny blisters and scales. Scratching the rash can cause skin sores, which can become infected with bacteria.

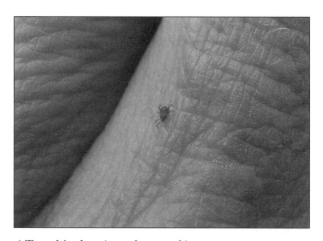

A Trombicula *mite on human skin.*

Transmission route. The microscopic scabies mite burrows into the upper layer of the skin, where it lives and lays its eggs. The burrows appear as tiny raised serpentine lines that are grayish or skin-colored and are a centimeter or more in length. Scabies is usually spread by direct, prolonged, skin-to-skin contact with a person who already has scabies. It is spread easily to sexual partners and to persons in the same household. Scabies is sometimes spread indirectly by sharing the clothing, towels, or bedding used by an infested person. Animals do not spread human scabies.

Diagnosis and treatment. Diagnosis of a scabies infestation is usually made based on the customary appearance and distribution of the rash and the presence of burrows. Whenever possible, the diagnosis should be confirmed by identifying the mite, mite eggs, or mite fecal matter. This can be done by carefully removing a mite from the end of its burrow using the tip of a needle or by obtaining a skin scraping for microscopic examination.

Products used to treat scabies are called scabicides because they kill scabies mites; some also kill eggs. Scabicide creams or lotions are prescription medications that should be applied to all areas of the body. Following treatment, the infected person should wear clean clothes. Treatment also is recommended for household members and sexual contacts.

CHIGGERS

Chiggers are the juvenile form of a certain type of mite of the family Trombiculidae. These very small mites feed on humans and other animals only when they are in the larval stage. Chiggers are classified in the phylum that includes the arachnids and are in the order of Acari and the suborder Prostigmata. The scientific name for the chigger is *Eutrombicula alfreddugesi.*

Chiggers are invertebrates with four pairs of legs. They are less than 1/150th of an inch long and are reddish-brown. The juvenile forms have six legs, although the harmless adult mites have eight legs. Chiggers reproduce by laying eggs. They are found from Central Mexico to Canada and are commonly encountered in woodlands, along the periphery of swamps, in shrub thickets, and in grass that has not been mowed.

Transmission route. Chiggers are parasites that rely on blood from a host for food, and humans are especially vulnerable. Unlike scabies mites, chiggers do not burrow into the skin. They feed at the base of a hair follicle or in a skin pore. They are well known for the rash they cause in humans upon attachment.

A common myth about chiggers is that they burrow into and remain inside the skin. Chiggers insert their feeding structures into the skin and inject enzymes that cause the destruction of host tissue. Hardening of the surrounding skin results in the formation of a feeding tube called a stylostome, which works like a straw for the feeding chigger and also irritates the surrounding skin, producing intense itching because of the body's reaction to the stylostome and the chigger's saliva. A species of chigger in the Pacific Islands and in East Asia is a vector for Japanese river fever.

Disease signs and symptoms. A chigger bite is not noticeable, but the bite becomes annoying and itchy after a few hours because of the injection of digestive enzymes into the skin. Intense itching within one or two days of the bite is the most common symptom. The bite area may become red and raised, resembling a blister. The itching persists for several days, and complete resolution of the skin lesions can take up to two weeks. Chigger bites do not produce any long-term complications.

Diagnosis and treatment. A chigger bite is diagnosed from symptoms. The chigger's feeding tube that creates many of the symptoms cannot be removed from the person's skin. However, the person's body will eventually break down the skin tissue that forms the tube; healing then begins in a process that can take from ten days to three weeks. Relief from the itching may be found with topical hydrocortisone cream, Benadryl ointment, or calamine lotion. Prolonged scratching may lead to skin wounds that may become infected with bacteria.

IMPACT

Globally, mites are important nuisance pests. The biting and bloodsucking behavior of the scabies mite, for example, causes considerable discomfort, and a few species also cause serious allergic reactions, such as asthma. Scabies occurs worldwide and affects people of all races and social classes. It can spread rapidly under crowded conditions where close body contact is frequent. Institutions such as nursing homes, extended-care facilities, and prisons are often sites of scabies outbreaks.

Dermatologists estimate that more than three hundred million cases of scabies occur worldwide every year, and there are one million cases in the United

States annually. With better detection methods and treatments, however, having a scabies infection can amount to nothing more than temporary distress.

Chigger bites do not produce any long-term complications. However, because of the intense itching it causes, prolonged scratching of the itches may lead to skin wounds that may become infected by bacteria.

Gerald W. Keister, M.A.

FURTHER READING

Atkinson, P. W., ed. *Vector Biology, Ecology, and Control.* New York: Springer Science, 2010. A good source for the reader needing a detailed study of vectors and the latest methods for effective vector control.

Chosidow, O. "Clinical Practices: Scabies." *New England Journal of Medicine* 354 (2006): 1718-1727. An informative guide to the identification, causes, symptoms, and treatment of scabies.

Maguire, J. H., R. J. Pollack, and A. Spielman. "Ectoparasite Infestations and Arthropod Bites and Stings." In *Harrison's Principles of Internal Medicine,* edited by Joan Butterton. 17th ed. New York: McGraw-Hill, 2008. A detailed presentation of the epidemiology of ectoparasite infestations and the identification and treatment of arthropod bites and stings.

Wilson, B. B., and M. E. Mathieu. "Mites (Including Chiggers)." In *Mandell, Douglas, and Bennett's Principles and Practice of Infectious Diseases,* edited by Gerald L. Mandell, John F. Bennett, and Raphael Dolin. 7th ed. New York: Churchill Livingstone/Elsevier, 2010. This chapter in a standard medical textbook features a detailed discussion of mites and chiggers and their taxonomic classifications, natural habitats, and pathogenicity.

WEB SITES OF INTEREST

Centers for Disease Control and Prevention, Division of Vector Borne Infectious Diseases
http://www.cdc.gov//ncidod/dvbid

Microbiology and Immunology On-line: Parasitology
http://pathmicro.med.sc.edu/book/parasit-sta.htm

See also: Arthropod-borne illness and disease; Bloodborne illness and disease; Body lice; Crab lice; Fleas and infectious disease; Flies and infectious disease; Head lice; Impetigo; Insect-borne illness and disease; Mosquitoes and infectious disease; Parasites: Classification and types; Parasitic diseases; Parasitology; Plague; Saliva and infectious disease; Scabies; Sexually transmitted diseases (STDs); Skin infections; Ticks and infectious disease; Transmission routes; Vectors and vector control.

MMR vaccine

CATEGORY: Prevention

The MMR vaccine combines immunizations for three diseases (measles, mumps, and rubella) into a single series of injections. Each of these childhood diseases is caused by a different virus. Measles leads to rash, fever, cough, and irritated eyes, and it may lead to pneumonia, seizures, and (in severe cases) brain damage and death. Mumps results in characteristic swollen glands in the neck, accompanied by a fever and headaches. Mumps may lead to meningitis, deafness, painful and damaging swelling of the testes, and (in severe cases) death. Rubella, or German measles, causes a rash with a mild fever and arthritis. Rubella infection in pregnant women can cause miscarriage or birth defects and disorders.

BENEFITS OF VACCINATION

The combined MMR vaccine protects children and adults against these three diseases. Before the vaccine was developed, these highly contagious diseases were prevalent, and virtually all children became infected. Outbreaks of measles, mumps, and rubella occur in areas with clusters of nonimmunized children, such as in religious communities that avoid immunization or in families in which a parent or parents fear that the MMR vaccine has harmful side effects and has a link to autism.

MMR vaccine and autism. A controversial study published in 1998 by the journal *The Lancet* suggested a link between the MMR vaccine and rising rates of autism. The article soon led to widespread fear among parents of the safety of the vaccine, and some parents refused the vaccine for their children. Pockets of nonimmunized children contributed to outbreaks of measles, mumps, and rubella in the United States and in the United Kingdom and other European countries. The original study, however, was flawed, and *The Lancet* officially retracted the report in February, 2010. The

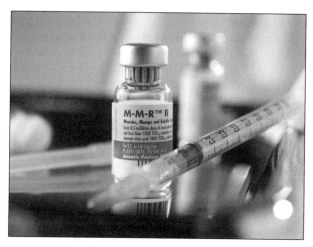

The MMR vaccine.

article, authored by the discredited British researcher Andrew Wakefield and coauthors, had erroneous conclusions. Additional research attempting to replicate Wakefield's findings did not support his results. Rather, further study found no evidence of a link between the MMR vaccine and autism, supporting the safety of vaccination.

Side effects. The MMR vaccine is associated with mild side effects that include fever, mild rash, and swollen glands. Less common side effects include seizure and temporary joint pain. Rarely, allergic reactions or serious side effects such as deafness, long-term seizures, and brain damage may occur.

IMPACT

The MMR vaccine has reduced the incidence of these diseases by more than 99 percent, according to the Centers for Disease Control and Prevention. The success of the vaccine in dramatically reducing the spread of these diseases has enabled the U.S. government's Childhood Immunization Initiative to set a goal of eradicating native measles, mumps, and rubella in the United States. This goal acknowledges that the viruses may be brought to the United States by people who were infected in other countries.

The vaccine leads to lifelong immunity. Children receive the dose between twelve and fifteen months of age and get a booster shot between four and six years of age. After two doses, the vaccine protects 99 percent of the children immunized.

Cheryl Pokalo Jones

FURTHER READING

Centers for Disease Control and Prevention. "Vaccine Safety: Measles, Mumps, and Rubella (MMR) Vaccine." Available at http://www.cdc.gov/vaccinesafety.

Editors of *The Lancet.* "Retraction: Ileal-Lymphoid-Nodular Hyperplasia, Non-specific Colitis, and Pervasive Developmental Disorder in Children." *The Lancet* 375 (2010): 445.

Griffin, Diane E., and Michael B. A. Oldstone, eds. *Measles: History and Basic Biology.* New York: Springer, 2009.

Hawkins, Trisha. *Everything You Need to Know About Measles and Rubella.* New York: Rosen, 2001.

Institute of Medicine. *Immunization Safety Review: Vaccines and Autism.* Washington, D.C.: National Academies Press, 2004.

WEB SITES OF INTEREST

Centers for Disease Control and Prevention
http://www.cdc.gov/mmwr

College of Physicians of Philadelphia, History of Vaccines
http://www.historyofvaccines.org

Vaccine Research Center
http://www.niaid.nih.gov/about/organization/vrc

See also: Children and infectious disease; DTaP vaccine; Immunization; Measles; Mumps; Rubella; Vaccines: Types; Viral infections.

Mold infections

CATEGORY: Diseases and conditions
ANATOMY OR SYSTEM AFFECTED: All
ALSO KNOWN AS: Fungal infection, mycosis

DEFINITION

A mold infection, or mycosis, is the growth of mold or fungi in the body. Molds are fungi that grow in a filamentous form. Generally, an infection implies active growth and not merely presence in a particular body site.

CAUSES

Mold infections are caused by fungi. Fungi (the plural of fungus) are eukaryotic and nonphotosynthetic, and they (usually) contain the chemical compound chitin in their cell walls. All of these features distinguish fungi from other classes of infectious agents such as bacteria, viruses, and parasites.

Fungi are divided into yeasts and molds. Molds grow by branching and longitudinal extension (adding cells to the end of filament), while yeasts grow by budding or by binary cell division. Molds are composed of long, thin hyphae that aggregate to form a mycelium. The mycelium (plural mycelia) is the mass formed when hyphae grow extensively around and on top other hyphae.

Although there are thousands of species of molds, most do not cause disease in healthy people. However, almost all fungi have the potential to colonize humans, especially people with severely compromised immune systems. Molds are acquired from an environmental source and not through person-to-person contact.

RISK FACTORS

Healthy people generally have the ability to combat the fungi they encounter. Accordingly, the most important risk factor for developing mycoses is the health of the host. Deficiencies in the immune system, such as human immunodeficiency virus (HIV) infection, acquired immunodeficiency syndrome (AIDS), and neutropenia, and deficiencies caused by immunosuppressive therapy and even old age, substantially increase the risk of mycoses. Other risk factors include poor lung function from other conditions such as chronic obstructive pulmonary disease, bronchiectasis, tuberculosis, sarcoidosis, and asthma.

Molds thrive in soil and moist environments, so people exposed long-term to soil, dust, and dirt are at greater risk of developing mold infections. Also, environments with poor ventilation can allow mold growth and spore formation, resulting in a higher risk of mold infections.

SYMPTOMS

The symptoms of mold infection depend on the nature of the fungus and the body site affected. Mold can cause disease in humans in three ways: by ingestion or inhalation of toxins, by infection (mycosis), or by triggering allergic responses. For example, *Stachybotrys* (also called black mold) in buildings causes an allergic response triggered by environmental exposure.

The most common sites of infection are the respiratory tract (especially the lungs) and the skin and nails.

Fungi that are invasive, especially in immunocompromised persons, can infect the internal organs, including the kidneys. It also can infect the central nervous system, the urogenital tract, and the lymphatic system.

Infections of the skin and nails, while serious to the person affected, almost never proceed to more serious invasive or systemic infections. These infections are usually caused by fungi capable of degrading keratin. Skin infections are often called ringworm, while nail infections are called ringworm of the nail. Infection of the toenails or fingernails is more formally called onychomycosis, a common affliction of persons with poor circulation, especially the elderly. The most common fungi causing these infections are dermatophytes, principally of the genera *Epidermophyton, Microsporum,* and *Trichophyton.*

The most serious fungal infections are often transmitted through the respiratory tract, that is, through inhalation of airborne spores. Symptoms of respiratory mold infections are often nonspecific and can include fever, cough, headache, rash, muscle aches, night sweats, and hemoptysis (coughing up blood).

SCREENING AND DIAGNOSIS

The diagnosis of fungal infections generally involves an examination, or clinical observation, to check for particular symptoms. Also, diagnosis may include a laboratory fungal culture from affected body sites, serological tests for antibodies to a specific fungi, and radiologic imaging. Definitive diagnosis usually requires laboratory culture of the fungus and identification based on morphological characteristics. Histologic examination of biopsy material is often used to suggest the existence of a mold infection.

The more recent use of molecular identification tests (tests for specific genes of a fungus) has led to more rapid identification and to avoiding the need for identification based on sporulation. An example of a molecular test is the polymerase chain reaction (PCR), which can rapidly identify an organism both from culture and from affected clinical material (tissue or fluids).

TREATMENT AND THERAPY

Historically, mold infections, especially invasive infections, have been difficult to treat. Molds are not susceptible to antibiotics. Antifungal drugs have not usually matched antibiotics for convenience, efficacy, or safety. The most effective antifungal for serious or systemic fungal infections for many years was amphotericin B. However, while effective, amphotericin B has many deleterious side effects and must be administered intravenously. After being injected, many people experience high fever, hypotension, vomiting, headache, and nausea; these side effects subside within several hours.

Newer antifungals or new formulations of older antifungals have been approved for human use. Liposomal formulations of amphotericin B have significantly less toxicity, but they are still effective against many invasive fungi. Liposomal formulations of amphotericin B are not effective against dermatophyte fungi.

New drugs in the azole class of antifungals have been developed and may be of use both in systemic and in other fungal infections. These triazoles include itraconazole, voriconazole, ravuconazole, and posaconazole. An entirely new class of antifungals, the echinocandins, has recently been developed. These compounds act by inhibiting a specific step in the synthesis of fungal cell-wall components. They are effective at preventing fungal growth but have minimal toxicity to humans. Caspofungin was the first of the echinocandins to receive approval from the U.S. Food and Drug Administration. Other echinocandins available are micafungin and anidulafungin.

PREVENTION AND OUTCOMES

Most mold infections are very difficult, if not impossible, to prevent. Fungi are present in all environments. Generally, mold infections begin with airborne spores, which makes it impossible to avoid infection.

For persons who are immunocompromised, some measures that may be helpful include the avoidance of dusty environments and activities where dust exposure is likely (such as construction zones), the wearing of respirators when in or near dusty environments, and the avoidance of activities that disturb dirt or soil (such as gardening and yard work). In health care settings, air quality measures, such as high-efficiency particulate air (HEPA) filtration, should be followed.

David M. Faguy, Ph.D.

FURTHER READING

Midgley G., Yvonne M. Clayton, and Roderick J. Hay. *Diagnosis in Color: Medical Mycology.* Chicago: Mosby-Wolfe, 1997. A medical mycology textbook with many color images. Includes detailed descriptions of common mycoses and the organisms that cause them.

Patterson, Thomas F. "Fungal Infections." *Infectious Disease Clinics of North America* 20 (2006): 485-734. This special journal issue covers fungal infections and includes many useful articles on specific fungal diseases, emerging fungi, diagnosis, and therapy.

Richardson, Malcolm D., and Elizabeth M. Johnson. *Pocket Guide to Fungal Infection.* 2d ed. Malden, Mass.: Blackwell, 2006. A handy guide, with much visual information for both the nonexpert and the specialist. Includes clinical presentation, diagnosis, and treatment for the major fungal diseases of humans.

Zumla, Alimudin, Wing-Wai Yew, and David S. C. Hui, eds. *Emerging Respiratory Infections in the Twenty-first Century.* Philadelphia: Saunders/Elsevier, 2010. A comprehensive work that includes discussion of the relationship between respiratory infection and molds and yeasts.

WEB SITES OF INTEREST

American Lung Association
http://www.lungusa.org

Centers for Disease Control and Prevention, Division of Foodborne, Bacterial, and Mycotic Diseases
http://www.cdc.gov/nczved/divisions/dfbmd

Environmental Protection Agency: Mold and Moisture
http://www.epa.gov/mold

Microbiology and Immunology On-line: Mycology
http://pathmicro.med.sc.edu/book/mycol-sta.htm

See also: Allergic bronchopulmonary aspergillosis; Antifungal drugs: Mechanisms of action; Antifungal drugs: Types; Aspergillosis; Blastomycosis; Coccidiosis; Diagnosis of fungal infections; *Epidermophyton*; Fungal infections; Fungi: Classification and types; *Fusarium*; Histoplasmosis; *Microsporum*; Mycoses; Paracoccidioidomycosis; Respiratory route of transmission; Soilborne illness and disease; Treatment of fungal infections; *Trichophyton*.

Molluscum contagiosum

CATEGORY: Diseases and conditions
ANATOMY OR SYSTEM AFFECTED: Genitalia, skin

DEFINITION

Molluscum contagiosum is an infection of the skin. It is caused by the molluscum virus. In children, the most common areas affected are the face, neck, arms, and hands. In adults, molluscum contagiosum is a sexually transmitted disease. In these cases the genitals and surrounding skin are most commonly affected.

CAUSES

Contact with the virus causes this skin infection. This can occur with skin to skin contact.

RISK FACTORS

Having skin-to-skin contact with an infected person is the main risk factor. Other risk factors include indirect contact with an infected person through a swimming pool or bath or by sharing towels or clothing, sexual contact with an infected person, and having a weakened immune system (such as human immunodeficiency virus infection and acquired immunodeficiency syndrome). Broken skin increases the risk for getting the disease and causes more severe symptoms.

SYMPTOMS

Skin lesions are the main symptom. A person who experiences a similar skin lesion should not assume it is caused by this condition. These lesions may be caused by other health conditions.

Molluscum contagiosum skin lesions usually are small, dome-shaped bumps with dimpling in center; are painless, but may be itchy or tender; first appear translucent, pearly, or flesh-colored and later may turn gray and drain; and have a white or waxy substance in the center of the lesion. Multiple lesions usually are in groups. Common sites in children are the face, trunk, arms, and legs; in adults, common sites are the genitals, abdomen, and inner thigh. The lesions can last from several weeks to several years.

SCREENING AND DIAGNOSIS

Diagnosis is usually made based on the lesions. Sometimes a biopsy will be taken. The sample will be looked at under a microscope. The examining doctor may refer the patient to a dermatologist, a specialist who focuses on skin conditions.

TREATMENT AND THERAPY

Left untreated, molluscum contagiosum usually resolves within six months. If untreated in people with human immunodeficiency virus infection, the lesions usually persist and spread indefinitely. The doctor may recommend removal of the lesions to prevent spreading and to avoid infecting others.

Treatment options include surgical removal of the lesions, which can be removed by cutting them off the surface of the skin. With chemical treatment, chemicals are placed directly on the lesions to remove them. Common chemical treatments include podophyllin, cantharidin, phenol, silver nitrate, trichloracetic acid, and iodine. Other treatments include cryotherapy, which uses cold to freeze the lesions off of the skin (liquid nitrogen may be used for this treatment), and retinoid or imiquimod cream, separately or in combination.

PREVENTION AND OUTCOMES

Molluscum contagiosum is contagious. To reduce the risk of exposure to the virus, one should avoid contact with an infected person (this includes not sharing towels, clothing, baths, and pools) and avoid sexual contact with an infected person. To reduce the risk of spreading the disease, one should not touch the lesions (nor scratch them) and should wash hands promptly if he or she contacts the lesions.

Patricia Griffin Kellicker, B.S.N.;
reviewed by Ross Zeltser, M.D., FAAD

FURTHER READING

Dohil, M. A., et al. "The Epidemiology of Molluscum Contagiosum in Children." *Journal of the American Academy of Dermatology* 54, no. 1 (2006): 47-54.

Hanson, D., and D. G. Diven. "Molluscum Contagiosum." *Dermatology Online Journal* 9, no. 2 (2003). Available at http://dermatology.cdlib.org/92/reviews/molluscum/diven.html.

Theos, A. U., et al. "Effectiveness of Imiquimod Cream 5 Percent for Treating Childhood Molluscum Contagiosum in a Double-Blind, Randomized Pilot Trial." *Cutis* 74, no. 2 (2004): 134-138, 141-142.

See also: Chickenpox; Children and infectious disease; Contagious diseases; Erythema infectiosum; Erythema nodosum; HIV; Impetigo; Measles; Pityriasis rosea; Poxvirus infections; Rubella; Scarlet fever; Sexually transmitted diseases (STDs); Skin infections; Viral infections; Warts.

Monkeypox

CATEGORY: Diseases and conditions
ANATOMY OR SYSTEM AFFECTED: Lymph nodes, lymphatic system, skin

DEFINITION

Monkeypox is a rare viral infection caused by the monkeypox virus. It is endemic to rodents and monkeys in the rainforests of Central Africa and West Africa. Monkeypox, similar to smallpox, is a systemic illness characterized by a vesicular rash consisting of small blisters on the skin.

CAUSES

The monkeypox virus is an orthopoxvirus similar to *Variola* (smallpox), vaccinia (used for smallpox vaccine), and cowpox viruses. Monkeypox is a zoonotic disease transmitted to humans from infected rodents, pets, and primates. Transmission of the disease occurs through contact with infected skin lesions, blood, or bodily fluids, or through ingestion or an animal bite. Although monkeypox is less infectious than smallpox, human to human transmission of the disease can occur.

RISK FACTORS

All ages may be affected by the disease, but the disease affects children most often. Public health officials and laboratory, animal, and health care workers are most vulnerable to the disease. People having received the smallpox vaccine may be at a reduced risk of contracting monkeypox.

SYMPTOMS

Monkeypox has clinical symptoms similar to that of smallpox but milder and with lymphadenopathy, swelling of the lymph nodes. Symptoms begin with fever, headache, muscle and back pain, respiratory problems, and lymph node swelling. A blister-like or ulcerated skin rash follows and spreads over the body. The eruptions develop through various stages: crust, scab, and "fall off." Monkeypox typically lasts several weeks.

SCREENING AND DIAGNOSIS

Monkeypox is difficult to distinguish from smallpox. Primary care physicians should consult with an infectious disease specialist and the Centers for Disease Control and Prevention (CDC) for appropriate treatment and diagnosis. Diagnostic tests include deoxyribonucleic acid (DNA)-based tests, such as polymerase chain reaction, immunochemistry, and electron microscopy. Definitive diagnosis of monkeypox requires the isolation, culture, and confirmation of the monkeypox virus from infected specimens.

TREATMENT AND THERAPY

There is no treatment for monkeypox; however, the smallpox vaccine has been shown to help prevent and reduce the severity of the disease. The CDC recommends the smallpox vaccine (within four to fourteen days of exposure) be administered to laboratory, animal, and health care workers who are in close contact with infected hosts and specimens. However, organ transplant recipients and persons with weakened immune systems, autoimmune disorders, or allergies should not receive the vaccine. Treatment of severe illness with vaccinia immunoglobulin or with cidofovir, a broad spectrum antiviral drug, may be considered.

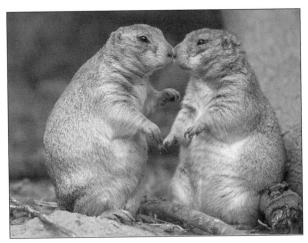

Certain pet prairie dogs in the United States, who were likely infected with the monkeypox virus by the giant Gambian rat in 2003, passed the virus to humans. (AP/Wide World Photos)

PREVENTION AND OUTCOMES

The smallpox vaccine is the best prevention against monkeypox. In high-risk areas, people should limit exposure to wild animals. Any suspected cases of monkeypox should be reported to state or local health agencies to help prevent a global health outbreak. The CDC has established prevention and infection-control guidelines to limit the spread of the disease and to identify the cause of any outbreak.

Rose Ciulla-Bohling, Ph.D.

FURTHER READING

Damon, Inger K. "Smallpox, Monkeypox, and Other Poxvirus Infections." In *Cecil Medicine*, edited by Lee Goldman and Dennis Arthur Ausiello. 23d ed. Philadelphia: Saunders/Elsevier, 2008.

Hoff, Brent H., and Carter Smith III. *Mapping Epidemics: A Historical Atlas of Disease.* New York: Franklin Watts, 2000.

Reed, Kurt D. "Monkeypox and Other Emerging Orthopoxvirus Infections." In *Emerging Infectious Diseases: Trends and Issues,* edited by Felissa R. Lashley and Jerry D. Durham. 2d ed. New York: Springer, 2007.

WEB SITES OF INTEREST

Centers for Disease Control and Prevention
http://www.cdc.gov/ncidod/monkeypox

PathInfo Project
http://ci.vbi.vt.edu/pathinfo

See also: Children and infectious disease; Hantavirus infection; Poxvirus infections; Primates and infectious disease; Rodents and infectious disease; Smallpox; Viral infections; Zoonotic diseases.

Mononucleosis

CATEGORY: Diseases and conditions
ANATOMY OR SYSTEM AFFECTED: All
ALSO KNOWN AS: Epstein-Barr virus, glandular fever, infectious mononucleosis, kissing disease, mono

DEFINITION

Mononucleosis is a disease caused by either the Epstein-Barr virus (EBV) or the cytomegalovirus, both of which are related to the herpesvirus.

CAUSES

EBV causes infection in the throat and mucous membranes. The immune system reacts to this infection by raising the body's temperature, usually to about 103° Fahrenheit but sometimes as high as 105° F. The virus is transmitted through saliva, which is why mononucleosis is often referred to as the kissing disease. Most adults have an immunity to the virus that causes mononucleosis, but adolescents, in whom the disease is most frequently found, often lack such an immunity. Once in the body, the virus builds rapidly in the white blood cells that are part of the body's protective system. As these cells, called lymphocytes, multiply, they cause swollen glands and an extremely sore throat.

RISK FACTORS

Risk factors that increase the likelihood that EBV will develop into mononucleosis include contracting EBV after the age of ten years; a lowered immune resistance because of other illnesses, stress, or fatigue; and living in close quarters with many people, such as in a college or university dormitory. One episode of mononucleosis usually produces permanent immunity.

SYMPTOMS

Mononucleosis most often begins with a fever accompanied by a headache. In the early stages, the symptoms may be mistaken for a cold or influenza. As the disease progresses, infected persons experience swollen lymph glands in the neck and, in some cases, in the armpits and groin. Infected persons then get an acute sore throat and may also develop tonsillitis. The tonsils may become so enlarged that swallowing is excruciating and, in some cases, may interfere with breathing.

Some sufferers of mononucleosis experience liver damage, which results in jaundice within a few days of the disease's onset. An enlarged spleen, in the upper left section of the abdomen, may accompany the disease and can be detected manually; it is sometimes apparent visually. The greatest danger associated with mononucleosis is a ruptured spleen, which causes excessive internal bleeding. If a swollen spleen is detected, it is essential that patients not lift heavy objects and that they avoid hard pressure to the spleen.

Persons with mononucleosis usually experience extreme fatigue, often to the point that they will doze off during the day or will be unable to stand without danger of falling. The fatigue that accompanies the disease is usually so extreme that it makes normal activities impossible. Those suffering from mononucleosis require considerable bed rest.

Mononucleosis results in death in less that 1 percent of those suffering from the disease. Most of these deaths are caused not by the mononucleosis virus but by related complications of the disease. Still, mononucleosis is a disabling disease during the four to six weeks it usually takes to run its course.

SCREENING AND DIAGNOSIS

Because mononucleosis in its early stages resembles influenza or the common cold, it is easy to misdiagnose the disease at its onset. As the illness develops, however, the extreme fatigue that accompanies it differentiates it from influenza or the common cold. Usually a blood smear is examined for the presence of atypical lymphocytes.

The heterophil antibodies test, designed specifically to detect mononucleosis by identifying antibodies in blood samples, involves mixing a human blood sample with blood from sheep or horses that will clump if mono antibodies are present. The results of these tests are available quickly, and they clearly point to the presence of the mononucleosis virus in persons tested.

TREATMENT AND THERAPY

There is no cure for mononucleosis. Although the disease is disabling, it generally runs its course in four to six weeks. Infected persons can return gradually to their normal activities. Medications usually are not required, although corticosteroid drugs are sometimes prescribed when breathing is obstructed by swollen tonsils.

To relieve the pain of the sore throat that accompanies mononucleosis, infected persons are urged to gargle regularly with warm water that includes a tablespoon of dissolved salt. Some persons respond well to drinking smoothies (blended fruit drinks) or other cooling substances that may reduce the throat pain.

Pain relievers such as acetaminophen and ibuprofen may be recommended to reduce the muscle pains and headaches that often occur with mono. Children and adolescents should not take aspirin, however, because doing so risks the development of Reye's syndrome, which can lead to dangerous swelling of the brain and organ failure.

Throughout the course of this disease, infected persons should eat healthy, balanced meals. Healthy food will help the body build the resources it needs to fight the infection. One also should drink substantial quantities of fluids, particularly water and fruit juices, to prevent dehydration, and should rest extensively and not attempt to resume normal activities too soon. The body needs time to rebuild.

PREVENTION AND OUTCOMES

No medications prevent the disease, although the spread of mononucleosis can be controlled, especially in communities of adolescents, such as in schools and dormitories, by limiting contact with saliva. One should ensure that commonly used eating utensils (such as dishes, drinking glasses, and bottles) are carefully washed in hot water.

R. Baird Shuman, Ph.D.

FURTHER READING

Cohen, J. I. "Epstein-Barr Virus Infections, Including Infectious Mononucleosis." In *Harrison's Principles of Internal Medicine*, edited by Joan Butterton. 17th ed. New York: McGraw-Hill, 2008.

Daniel, Erno. *Stealth Germs in Your Body*. New York: Union Square Press, 2008.

Decker, Janet, and Alan Hecht. *Mononucleosis*. 2d ed. New York: Chelsea House, 2009.

Fort, G. G., et al. "Mononucleosis." In *Ferri's Clinical Advisor 2011: Instant Diagnosis and Treatment*, edited by Fred F. Ferri. Philadelphia: Mosby/Elsevier, 2011.

Hoffman, Gretchen. *Mononucleosis*. New York: Marshall Cavendish, 2006.

Katz, B. Z. "Epstein-Barr Virus Infections (Mononucleosis and Lymphoproliferative Disorders)." In *Principles and Practice of Pediatric Infectious Diseases*, edited by Sarah S. Long, Larry K. Pickering, and Charles G. Prober. 3d ed. Philadelphia: Churchill Livingstone/Elsevier, 2008.

Klatz, Ronald M., and Robert M. Goldman. *Infection Protection*. New York: HarperResource, 2002.

WEB SITES OF INTEREST

About Kids Health
http://www.aboutkidshealth.ca

American Academy of Family Physicians
http://familydoctor.org

Centers for Disease Control and Prevention
http://www.cdc.gov

National Institute of Allergy and Infectious Diseases
http://www.niaid.nih.gov

See also: Asplenia; Bronchiolitis; Bronchitis; Chickenpox; Children and infectious disease; Chronic fatigue syndrome; Common cold; Croup; Cytomegalovirus infection; Epiglottitis; Epstein-Barr virus infection; Fever; Herpesviridae; Immunity; Inflammation; Influenza; Lymphadenitis; Measles; Mumps; Nasopharyngeal infections; Parotitis; Pharyngitis and tonsillopharyngitis; Pneumonia; Rubella; Saliva and infectious disease; Strep throat; Viral infections; Viral pharyngitis; Viral upper respiratory infections.

Mosquito-borne viral encephalitis

CATEGORY: Diseases and conditions
ANATOMY OR SYSTEM AFFECTED: Brain, central nervous system

DEFINITION

Mosquito-borne viral encephalitis is an infection transmitted by mosquitoes that can lead to encephalitis, or inflammation of the brain. In the United States, there are five main types of mosquito-borne viral encephalitis: eastern equine, western equine, West Nile, St. Louis, and LaCrosse. Outside the United States, the most common types of mosquito-borne viral encephalitis are Japanese and Venezuelan equine. Mosquito-borne viral encephalitis is a potentially serious condition that requires care from a doctor.

CAUSES

Mosquito-borne viral encephalitis is caused by a bite from a mosquito that carries the virus from animals to humans. When mosquitoes bite an infected bird, horse, or other animal, they can pass the infection to humans. It usually takes between four and fifteen days for a person to have any symptoms after he or she has been bitten by an infected mosquito. Rarely, the infection can be passed through organ transplants or blood transfusions.

RISK FACTORS

The factors that increase the chance of developing mosquito-borne viral encephalitis include living in an area where outbreaks of viral encephalitis have occurred, spending much time outdoors for work or play, being fifty years of age and older or less than fifteen years of age, having a weak immune system, and using immunosuppressant drugs.

SYMPTOMS

Most people who become infected with the viruses that can cause encephalitis do not develop any symptoms, and the infection runs its course without being dangerous. Many others develop only mild symptoms, including mild fever, headache, nausea, body ache, and restlessness.

Some who become infected with one of these viruses actually develop encephalitis, which can cause death or brain damage. The more serious symptoms of encephalitis include seizures, high fever, coma, weight loss, weakness, changes in mental state, stiff neck, tremors, paralysis, vision loss, and numbness. These symptoms, however, should not lead one to assume he or she has mosquito-borne viral encephalitis. The symptoms may be caused by other, less serious health conditions.

SCREENING AND DIAGNOSIS

Doctors will ask the patient about symptoms and medical history and perform a physical exam. Questions concern travel to areas that have had mosquito-borne viral encephalitis outbreaks, recent mosquito bites, and exposure to dead animals. Tests may include a neurological exam (a series of tests to measure reflexes, memory, and other brain functions), blood tests to look for signs of infection in the blood; a spinal tap (removal of a small amount of cerebrospinal fluid to check for signs of infection), a magnetic resonance imaging (MRI) scan (a scan that uses radio waves and a powerful magnet to produce detailed computer images), a computed tomography (CT) scan (a detailed X-ray picture that identifies abnormalities of fine tissue structure), and an electroencephalogram (EEG), a test that records the brain's activity by measuring electrical currents through the brain.

TREATMENT AND THERAPY

No drug exists to treat mosquito-borne viral encephalitis, so doctors usually prescribe supportive care, which means treating the symptoms while the immune system fights the disease. Supportive treatment options include intravenous fluids, a respirator to help with breathing, anticonvulsants to treat seizures, sedatives to treat restlessness, pain relievers to treat headache and fever, and corticosteroids (anti-inflammatory drugs) to reduce brain swelling.

PREVENTION AND OUTCOMES

The best way to reduce the chance of getting mosquito-borne viral encephalitis is to avoid being bitten by mosquitoes. One should limit outside activities where mosquitoes are present; wear long sleeve shirts and long pants at dusk and dawn, when mosquitoes are most active; use bug repellent that contains NN-diethyl metatoluamide (DEET); and empty sources of standing water around the home, such as bird baths and gutters, where mosquitoes may breed.

Other prevention tips include avoiding handling dead birds or other animals that can carry the virus and getting vaccinated (for Japanese encephalitis) if planning a long visit (greater than one month) to areas in Asia where outbreaks have occurred.

Nicky Lowney, M.A.;
reviewed by David L. Horn, M.D., FACP

FURTHER READING

Booss, John, Margaret Esiri, and Margaret M. Esin, eds. *Viral Encephalitis in Humans.* Washington, D.C.: ASM Press, 2003.

Centers for Disease Control and Prevention. "Arboviral Encephalitides." Available at http://www.cdc.gov/ncidod/dvbid/arbor.

Goddard, Jerome. *Physician's Guide to Arthropods of Medical Importance.* 4th ed. Boca Raton, Fla.: CRC Press, 2003.

Marquardt, William C., ed. *Biology of Disease Vectors.* 2d ed. New York: Academic Press/Elsevier, 2005.

National Institute of Neurological Disorders and Stroke. "Meningitis and Encephalitis Fact Sheet." Available at http://www.ninds.nih.gov.

Peters, C. J. "Infections Caused by Arthropod- and Rodent-Borne Viruses." In *Harrison's Principles of Internal Medicine,* edited by Anthony Fauci et al. 17th ed. New York: McGraw-Hill, 2008.

WEB SITES OF INTEREST

Centers for Disease Control and Prevention, Division of Vector Borne Infectious Diseases
http://www.cdc.gov/ncidod/dvbid

Encephalitis Society
http://www.encephalitis.info

National Institute of Neurological Disorders and Stroke
http://www.ninds.nih.gov

Public Health Agency of Canada, Travel Health
http://www.phac-aspc.gc.ca/tmp-pmv

See also: Arthropod-borne illness and disease; Bacterial meningitis; Blood-borne illness and disease; Chikungunya; Dengue fever; Eastern equine encephalitis; Encephalitis; Encephalitis vaccine; Fever; Inflammation; Insect-borne illness and disease; Japanese encephalitis; Malaria; Mosquitoes and infectious disease; Sleeping nets; Sleeping sickness; Subacute sclerosing panencephalitis; Vectors and vector control; Viral infections; Viral meningitis; West Nile virus; Yellow fever.

Mosquitoes and infectious disease

CATEGORY: Transmission

DEFINITION

Mosquito-borne infectious diseases are diseases transmitted through the bites of infected mosquitoes. Mosquitoes act as biological vectors by transmitting pathogens or parasites from one host to another. The most prevalent infectious diseases transmitted by mosquito bites are malaria, yellow fever, dengue fever, Chikungunya, West Nile fever, various types of encephalitis, and Oroya fever, a bacterial disease.

CAUSES

Mosquito-borne infectious diseases are caused by the presence of the transmitted virus or *Plasmodium* parasites in the blood of human and nonhuman animals. More than one hundred types of viruses and parasites are transmitted to humans and animals through mosquito bites. Malaria is caused by infection with *Plasmodium falciparum* or *P. vivax* parasites. These parasites develop in the mosquito's body and are then passed on when the mosquito injects saliva during feeding (biting).

West Nile fever results from the transfer of the West Nile virus (WNV) from infected birds to humans by the *Culex* mosquito. After multiplication in the human blood, WNV is transported to the brain, where it causes inflammation of the brain tissue.

Dengue fever is caused by the dengue virus, one of the four viruses common to tropical and subtropical climates. It is spread from one infected person to another by the *Aedes* mosquito. As the dengue virus multiplies and damages cells, an infected person begins to show symptoms similar to those of other mosquito-borne infections.

Chikungunya fever is caused by an arbovirus infection transmitted primarily through *A. aegypti* and *A. albopictus* mosquitoes. The mosquitoes feed on an infected person during the viremic period of that person's infection (that is, within five days from the onset of the mosquito bite and symptoms) and then transmit the virus to other humans.

RISK FACTORS

Causal risk factors for mosquito-borne infectious diseases include mosquito bites; living in habitats with stagnant water, which are ideal environments for mosquito breeding; international travel to mosquito-endemic areas; habitation in areas with large mosquito populations; occupations involving exposure to woodlands and forests; having a suppressed immune system; and receiving a blood transfusion with infected blood product.

SYMPTOMS

The common symptoms associated with mosquito-borne infectious diseases are high fever, back and joint pain, rash, eye pain, chills, headache, malaise, muscle weakness, flulike symptoms, hypotension, and fatigue. There are additional physiological and clinical symptoms specific to each disease type. The additional symptoms of the various forms of encephalitis include brain inflammation, brain damage, and coma; death can follow.

Yellow fever is associated with additional symptoms, including "furry" tongue, irritability, slowed pulse, decreased urine volume, bloodshot eyes, constipation, facial flushing and proteinuria, and hepatic coagu-

Mosquito-Borne Diseases

Mosquito	Habits	Features	Diseases
Aedes	Day biter, urban or rural	Head bent, body parallel to surface, black and white in color	Dengue, yellow fever, viral encephalitis
Anopheles	Night biter, mainly rural	Head and body in line, at angle to surface	Malaria filariasis
Culex	Day biter, urban or rural	Shaped like *Aedes* but brown; whines in flight	Viral encephalitis filariasis

lopathy that produces hemorrhagic symptoms such as black vomit, nose bleeds, gum bleeds, and bruising. In the late stages of yellow fever, infected persons develop hypotension, shock, metabolic acidosis, acute tubular necrosis, myocardial dysfunction, cardiac arrhythmia, seizure, and coma. Recovery from yellow fever generally confers long-lasting immunity against subsequent infection.

Malaria is characterized by high fever, shaking, and chills in its early stages. If untreated, these symptoms are followed by nausea and vomiting, high fever, dizziness, delirium, headache, and pain, and symptoms such as splenomegaly, decreased body temperature, hepatomegaly, sweating, fever and chills, fatigue, shortness of breath, anemia, pale skin, and extreme exhaustion in its final stages.

Symptoms of dengue fever also include swollen lymph nodes, rash, pain behind the eyes, decreased heart rate, severe muscle pain, severe weakness, headaches, and enlarged lymph nodes (in children).

Symptoms of Chikungunya fever usually manifest after an incubation period of three to seven days after a mosquito bite. Symptoms include sudden fever, joint pain with or without swelling, chills, headache, nausea, vomiting, lower back pain, and rash.

SCREENING AND DIAGNOSIS

The presence of a mosquito-transmitted disease is often diagnosed after observing an associated fever that is common with all infectious disease types. Biological fluids such as saliva and urine are screened for the presence of a virus or parasites.

Symptomatic diagnosis is based on the history of subjective fever and on a rectal temperature and a splenomegaly. These methods are often used in parts of the world with limited laboratory facilities. Microscopic examination of blood films provide the most reliable diagnosis of the presence of the virus. Other tests include antigen tests (using venous blood) and molecular methods-based tests.

TREATMENT AND THERAPY

Treatment for a mosquito-borne infectious disease is designed to eliminate the viral and plasmodium parasite loads that cause the illness. For malaria, treatment and therapy involves one or more antimalarial prophylactic drugs, such as mefloquine, doxycycline, and the combination atovaquone and proguanil hydrochloride. In malaria-endemic areas, the drug treatment regime of choice is artemisinin combination therapy.

Yellow fever is treated using vaccines. The vaccine is an attenuated live-virus vaccine that has been used for several decades. A single dose confers immunity for ten years or more.

Antibiotics and antiviral medications are effective upon diagnosis of viral encephalitis. Corticosteroids and medications for fever are administered to reduce brain swelling and inflammation and to decrease the fever or treat headaches. Additional supportive treatment includes drinking extra fluids for hydration and bed rest.

PREVENTION AND OUTCOMES

Mosquito control and eradication with chemical and biological agents is the key, first-line defense against mosquitoes and mosquito-borne infectious diseases. Insecticides (such as Malathion and permethrin) and repellants (such as NN-diethyl metatoluamide, or DEET) are common chemical control agents. Some garden plants, including lemon thyme and rosemary, are known mosquito repellants. Biological agents, such as predatory fish (mosquitofish) and dragonflies, feed on mosquito larva and adult mosquitoes. Other preventive measures include behavioral and physical modifications, such as staying indoors at night and using insecticide-treated sleeping nets and permethrin-treated clothing to cover as much of the body as possible.

Yellow fever vaccine, a live attenuated vaccine, is commonly used as a preventive agent. A single dose of the vaccine confers immunity for up to ten years in adults.

Olalekan E. Odeleye, Ph.D.

FURTHER READING

Goddard, Jerome. *Infectious Diseases and Arthropods.* Totowa, N.J.: Humana Press, 2008. Summarizes the biological, entomological, and clinical aspects of mosquito-borne and other arthropod-related diseases. Each disease has a description of the involved vector, notes on its biology and ecology, distribution maps, and general clinical guidelines for treatment and control.

Marquardt, William C., ed. *Biology of Disease Vectors.* 2d ed. New York: Academic Press/Elsevier, 2005. This textbook on the biology of disease vectors, including mosquitoes, is geared to graduate students and researchers, but most of the information is accessible to general readers.

Tolle, Michael A. "Mosquito-Borne Diseases." *Current Problems in Pediatric and Adolescent Health Care* 39 (2009): 97-140. A thorough review of the life cycles of insects, including mosquitoes, as disease agents. Includes discussion of the diagnoses, treatments, and vaccines for several mosquito-borne diseases.

WEB SITES OF INTEREST

American Society of Tropical Medicine and Hygiene
http://www.astmh.org

Centers for Disease Control and Prevention, Division of Vector Borne Infectious Diseases
http://www.cdc.gov/ncidod/dvbid

Malaria Foundation International
http://www.malaria.org

National Institute of Allergy and Infectious Diseases
http://www.niaid.nih.gov/topics/vector

See also: Arthropod-borne illness and disease; *Bartonella* infections; Birds and infectious disease; Blood-borne illness and disease; Carriers; Chikungunya; Dengue fever; Developing countries and infectious disease; Encephalitis; Hosts; Insect-borne illness and disease; Malaria; Mosquito-borne viral encephalitis; Parasitic diseases; Parasitology; Ticks and infectious disease; Transmission routes; Tropical medicine; Vectors and vector control; West Nile virus; Yellow fever.

Mouth infections

CATEGORY: Diseases and conditions
ANATOMY OR SYSTEM AFFECTED: Lips, mouth, tissue, tongue

DEFINITION

Infections of the mouth can range from minor to severe to life-threatening. They occur when the natural protective mechanisms of the oral cavity are breached. Organisms that cause mouth infections are those that normally reside in the oral cavity and those that have been introduced from other sources.

The healthiness of a person's immune system, the integrity of natural barriers, and the infectious capacity of the organism determine if an infection will occur. Resident and foreign mouth microorganisms can infect the tongue, gums, the roof of the mouth, tooth-supporting structures, and the inner lining of the cheeks and lips (buccal mucosa). These infections are most often localized to the mouth but can also spread to other areas of the body, including the heart. Mouth infections are classified as fungal, viral, or bacterial.

CAUSES

Fungal infections of the mouth include the infections listed here.

Superficial oral infections. The most common fungus to cause mouth infections is the *Candida* species. This fungus normally resides in the mouth and invades the protective barriers when opportunities arise. The most common species are *C. albicans, C. galbrata,* and *C. tropicalis.* The resulting fungal infection, thrush or pseudomembranous candidiasis, appears as cream-colored patches on the tongue, buccal mucosa, or palate. Wiped-off patches reveal surface redness. Hyperplastic candidiasis is a chronic superficial infection that cannot be easily wiped away. Erythematous candidiasis appears as red patches most commonly found on the roof of the mouth or under the tongue. Angular cheilitis (perleche) affects the corners of the mouth, causing redness and cracking of the skin.

Noncandidal fungal infections. These fungal infections tend to deeply penetrate the mucosal layers of the mouth. They have the potential of causing damage to oral tissue, and their presence typically indicates that the body has other infections. Aspergillosis is the second most common fungal mouth infection; it is caused by the *Aspergillus* group of fungus. Aspergillosis is evidenced by ulcers on the roof of the mouth. The most common species of *Aspergillus* that cause mouth disease are *A. flavus, A. terreus,* and *A. fumigates.* Histoplasmosis (*Histoplasma capsulatum*), cryptococcosis (*Cryptococcus neoformans*), blastomycosis (*Blastomyces dermatitidis*), zygomycosis (*Rhizopus*), geotrichosis (*Geotrichum capitatum*), and coccidioidomycosis (*Coccidioides immitis*) are rare fungi that cause infections in the deep layers of the mouth. These fungi can cause life-threatening illnesses. All but geotrichosis appear as ulcers or nodules on the interior walls of the cheek, tongue, or roof of the mouth. Much like

Candida, geotrichosis infections appear as cream-colored patches.

Bacterial mouth infections include the infections listed here.

Oral mucosal infections. Although hundreds of types of bacterial organisms can potentially cause oral mucosal infections, there are several that are most common. *Streptococcus, Bacteroides, Peptostreptococcus,* oral anaerobic bacteria, and gram-negative bacilli are the most common organisms that cause oral mucosal infections.

Gangrenous stomatitis. Gangrenous stomatitis, also known as noma, is a rapidly spreading infection of oral and facial tissues typically found in the presence of debilitating illnesses. Caused by multiple bacteria, this infection begins as a small vesicle found on the gum. Ulceration of the deeper layers causes eventual destruction of the mouth, facial tissues, and bones. Several types of bacteria can cause this polymicrobial disease, but the most commonly isolated organisms are *Fusobacterium nucleatum, Borrelia vincentii,* and *Prevotella melaninogenica.*

Oral syphilis. Syphilis is a sexually transmitted disease caused by the bacterium *Treponema pallidum.* Oral lesions are a manifestation of this systemic disease. In the primary form of the disease, ulcers of the lips and tongue develop. Secondary syphilis rarely produces oral ulcerations and is most likely to manifest as flat or raised red patches on the roof of the mouth or tongue. Nodular lesions are rare and can be mistaken for oral cancer. Tertiary syphilis can gives rise to a rare mouth lesion called gumma. Gumma is a painless mass that is surrounded by inflamed tissue and forms on the tongue or on roof of the mouth. Uncommonly, gumma may erode into oral blood vessels.

Oral tuberculosis. Caused by *Mycobacteria tuberculosis,* oral tuberculous lesions are rare. They may present as single ulcers or as a small mass on the gums or tongue. Difficult to diagnose, oral tuberculosis may invade and cause destruction to the bones of the face.

Bacterial salivary gland infections (sialadenitis). Located in the cheeks at the angle of the jaw and under the tongue, the salivary glands may become infected with bacteria, causing pain and swelling. Although dozens of bacteria can cause salivary gland infections, the most common are *Staphylococcus aureus, Prevotella, Porphyromonas, Fusobacterium,* and *Peptostreptococcus.*

Bacterial gingivitis. Gingivitis is a common gum infection caused by poor oral hygiene. Most commonly caused by *Streptococccus* and *Actinomyces,* bacterial gingivitis causes discoloration and thickening of the gums. A more severe form of gingivitis known as acute necrotizing ulcerative gingivitis, or Vincent's angina, causes erosive lesions of the gums. *Prevotella, Fusobacterium, Tannerella,* and *Treponema* are the most common varieties of bacteria that cause this form of gingivitis.

Bacterial periondontitis, periodontal abscess, and pericoronitis. Like gingivitis, poor oral hygiene can lead to bacterial infections of the deep supporting structures of the teeth. Although periodontitis is typically an inflammatory disease, a more destructive form of periodontitis caused by bacteria infiltration can develop, causing breakdown of the supporting structures of the teeth and, ultimately, tooth loss. Pericoronitis is an infection under the gum flaps of wisdom teeth or nonerupted teeth. Bacteria can become trapped under the gums and cause local infection or an abscess. The most common bacteria causing bacterial periodontitis and pericoronitis are *Actinobacillus, Treponema, Prevotella, Porphyromona,* and *Tannerella.*

Viral mouth infections include the infections listed here.

Human herpes viral infections. Herpetic gingivostomatitis (oral herpes) is the classic cold sore caused by human herpetic virus 1 (HHV-1). Presenting as small vesicles on lips, gums, or the roof of the mouth, HHV-1 can be isolated in about 80 percent of adults. Recurrent infections are triggered by emotional stress, sunlight, and systemic illnesses. Herpetic stomatitis is a condition in young children that likely represents the initial herpes simplex infection, causing fever and blisters on the tongue or cheeks. Genital herpes (HHV-2) causes lesions similar to HHV-1, although it is less commonly found in the oral cavity.

Chickenpox and shingles are a result of HHV-3. This vesicular rash occurs primarily in children age three to six years who have not been vaccinated for the varicella virus and who are at risk for chickenpox. Shingles or herpes zoster is the reactivation of the disease in adults, especially persons age sixty years and older. Herpes zoster rarely occurs in those vaccinated with the varicella vaccine. The vesicular lesions of shingles occur unilaterally and localize in an area of the skin corresponding to a spinal nerve.

Mononucleosis is an infectious disease caused by Epstein-Barr virus or HHV-4. It infects the salivary glands, causing pain and swelling. Occasionally, red spots (petechiae) on the roof of the mouth are seen.

Oral hairy leukoplakia is also caused by HHV-4. This disease manifests as white patches on the sides of the tongue.

Cytomegalovirus infection caused by HHV-5 is typically found in immunosuppressed persons. Although most commonly asymptomatic, cytomegalovirus infection can cause swelling of the salivary glands and ulcerative lesions of the oral mucosa. Oral Kaposi's sarcoma (KS) shows raised, purple-colored tumors and is caused by HHV-8.

Human papilloma virus (HPV). Condyloma acuminate is primarily caused by human papilloma virus (HPV)-6 and HPV-11. Condyloma, which causes clusters of warty, pink, or whitish lesions on the tongue, roof of the mouth, and gums, is seen primarily in the genital area. Focal epithelial hyperplasia, or Heck disease, is caused by HPV-13 and HPV-32. These contagious lesions manifest as multiple, smooth nodules and are found most often on the buccal mucosa. Verruca vulgaris is caused by a variety of HPVs, but HPV-16 is the most common cause. These contagious lesions manifest as hard, rough, pointy clusters of white lesions and are found on the tongue, gums, and the roof of the mouth.

Coxsackie virus causes two primary types of disorders in the mouth, namely hand, foot, and mouth disease and herpangina. Hand, foot, and mouth disease manifests as multiple vesicles surrounded by a red base and are found on the cheeks, tongue, and the roof of the mouth. Herpangina initially appears as painful small red lesions, which then become vesicles and, eventually, ulcers. They are found primarily on the cheeks.

Caused by the *Rubulavirus* genus, mumps are a viral infection of the salivary glands of the cheek (parotid glands). It is seen primarily in unvaccinated or "failed" vaccinated children age five to nine years. Infected children have the characteristic chipmunk appearance because of swollen parotid glands. Caused by the *Morbillivirus* genus, measles is a highly infectious disease typically seen in unvaccinated or failed vaccinated children less than five years of age. Koplik spots are small, white lesions found on the buccal mucosa during the initial stages of measles infection. Rubella is caused by the *Rubivirus* genus. This contagious disease rarely causes mouth infections. There are, however, cases reported in the literature in which children have developed red spots on the buccal mucosa.

RISK FACTORS

Oral fungus infections are opportunistic diseases that mainly occur because of compromised defense mechanisms. Medications such as corticosteroids, broad-spectrum antibiotics, tricyclic antidepressants, and immunosuppressive agents (chemotherapy) can cause superficial oral infections. Additionally, a high carbohydrate diet, iron deficiency anemia, and ill-fitting dentures have been implicated in causing oral candida. The noncandidal infections that cause deeper mouth infections usually occur because of systemic diseases that cause compromised immune systems. Systemic diseases such as diabetes, thyroid disease, leukemia, advanced-stage cancer, and acquired immunodeficiency syndrome (AIDS) allow fungi to grow in the oral cavity. The elderly, pregnant women, and infants are also at risk of oral fungal infections because of compromised or inadequate immune responses.

Bacterial oral mucosal and salivary gland infections, like fungal infections, generally arise because of defective immune systems. The most common cases involve persons who are undergoing chemotherapy or radiation therapy. Inflammation of the mucosal surfaces (mucositis) causes a breakdown of the protective surfaces, opening the door for oral bacteria. Because of compromised systemic defenses in these diseases, bacterial infections develop. Malnutrition, dehydration, and unsanitary conditions have been shown to contribute to these infections.

Gum and periodontal infections arise because of poor oral hygiene. Immunosuppressive drugs, smoking, and systemic diseases such as diabetes, kidney failure, and cancer increase the severity of disease.

Viral mouth infections can be contracted from person to person through saliva droplets. Although any person may be at risk for contracting a virus, the susceptibility and severity of the disease is largely dictated by the health of a person's immune system. Chronic disease and medications resulting in diminished immunity may increase the prevalence and severity of the infection. Although there are several forms noted worldwide, Kaposi's sarcoma (KS) is mostly seen in persons infected with the human immunodeficiency virus (HIV) in the United States. Organ transplant recipients are also known to develop KS.

SYMPTOMS

Infections of the mouth may cause mucosal redness, ulcerations, bad breath, oral bleeding, altered taste sensation, and facial swelling. More severe symptoms include mouth pain, difficulty swallowing, swollen lymph nodes of the neck, fever, fatigue, and destruction of facial tissue. Respiratory, gastrointestinal, urinary, and cardiac symptoms can result from the spread of bacteria to internal organs.

Screening and Diagnosis

The superficial fungal infections such as those caused by *Candida* usually can be diagnosed through examination by a health care provider. Observation is typically enough to make the diagnosis. In unclear cases, a swab of the lesions can be sent to a laboratory for identification. Deep infections should be checked through biopsy. A culture of fungal lesions helps to direct treatment because antifungal sensitivities are established through this mechanism.

Diagnosis of a mucosal bacterial mouth infection is achieved by a swab or biopsy of the lesions. Bacterial and viral infections of the salivary glands, gums, or periodontal structures are typically made by observation. Imaging studies such as a computed tomography (CT) scan, magnetic resonance imaging (MRI), or ultrasound may be needed to determine the location of infected structures or of abscesses. In severe infections, rapid determination of the type and location of infection is critical to affective treatment.

Most viral mouth infections can be diagnosed by observation, but a biopsy or smear of the lesion may be required to identify the virus. Also, antibody levels in the blood may assist in confirming the diagnosis of some viral infections.

Treatment and Therapy

Given that mouth infections can be quite painful, symptomatic relief is important. Analgesics such as acetaminophen and ibuprofen are used for mild to moderate pain. Narcotic pain medication may be needed for severe pain. Oral topical anaesthetics such as dyconine and lidocaine can provide temporary relief of pain.

Superficial oral candidal infections are treated with topical antifungal medications. Nystatin and clotrimazole lozenges, mouth rinses, and creams are typically sufficient. Severe or resistant cases of oral candidiasis are treated with intravenous antiviral medications. Fluconazole, amphotercin B, myconazole, and itraconazole were the first antifungal medications

available. Newer antifungal medications such as caspofungin, flucytosine, posaconazole, and voriconazole cause less side effects and more specificity of action against fungal species. Most important in treating fungal infections is treatment of underlying diseases.

Treatment of uncomplicated bacterial infections of the oral mucosa, salivary glands, gums, and periodontal structures is primarily directed at symptomatic relief. Mouth rinses containing antiseptic solutions or anesthetics are helpful in reducing pain and healing time. Complicated infections are treated with the removal of infected or damaged tissues and with antibiotics that are specific to the organism causing infection.

Although most viral oral lesions resolve without treatment, a few exceptions exist. Genital herpes, shingles, and cytomegalovirus are treated with antiviral agents. Oral hairy leukoplakia and condyloma can be treated with topical gels that break down the lesions. Large condyloma, epithelial hyperplasia, and Verruca vulgaris are treated by excision. KS is treated by correction of the underlying immunosuppression with highly active antiretroviral therapy (HAART). Many infected persons, however, need radiation or chemotherapy.

Prevention and Outcomes

The prevention of all mouth infections is achieved largely through the implementation of adequate oral hygiene and sanitary practices, especially when systemic disease is present. One should brush teeth and tongue twice daily; floss once a day; use antiseptic mouthwash once a day; rinse mouth after using antibiotics or other oral medications; visit a dentist for examinations and teeth cleaning twice yearly; wash hands frequently, especially after coming into contact with dirty objects and surfaces; avoid close contact with persons with communicable diseases; avoid or limit alcohol and sugar intake; stop smoking; consider the use of preventive antifungal, antibacterial, or antiviral treatments (persons with compromised immune systems); and complete vaccinations recommended by a physician.

Marie President, M.D.

Further Reading

Chow, Anthony W. "Infections of the Oral Cavity, Head, and Neck." In *Mandell, Douglas, and Bennett's*

Principles and Practice of Infectious Diseases, edited by Gerald L. Mandell, John F. Bennett, and Raphael Dolin. 7th ed. New York: Churchill Livingstone/Elsevier, 2010. A comprehensive guide to the features, diagnosis, and treatment of infections of the mouth, head, and neck

Epstein, Joel B. "Mucositis in the Cancer Patient and Immunosuppressed Host." *Infectious Disease Clinics of North America* 21 (2007): 503-522. A study discussing the prevention, diagnosis, and treatment of mouth disease in persons with compromised immunity.

Gordon, Sara C., et al. "Viral Infections of the Mouth." Available at http://emedicine.medscape.com/article/1079920-overview. A comprehensive review article discussing the pathophysiology, diagnosis, and treatment of viral mouth infections.

Scully, Crispian, and Maria R. Sposto. "Noncandidal Fungal Infections of the Mouth." Available at http://emedicine.medscape.com/article/1077685-overview. The candida group is the most common type of fungal mouth infection. A review article describing the pathophysiology, diagnosis, and treatment of noncandidal mouth infections.

WEB SITES OF INTEREST

American Dental Association
http://www.ada.org

American Dental Hygienists' Association
http://www.adha.org/oralhealth

Centers for Disease Control and Prevention
http://www.cdc.gov

See also: Abscesses; Actinomycosis; Acute necrotizing ulcerative gingivitis; Candidiasis; Cold sores; *Eikenella* infections; Gingivitis; Herpes simplex infection; Herpesviridae; Herpesvirus infections; Hygiene; Oral transmission; Parotitis; Saliva and infectious disease; Sexually transmitted diseases (STDs); Syphilis; Tetanus; Thrush; Tooth abscess; Vincent's angina.

MRSA infection. *See* Methicillin-resistant staph infection.

Mucormycosis

CATEGORY: Diseases and conditions
ANATOMY OR SYSTEM AFFECTED: Brain, central nervous system, lungs, respiratory system
ALSO KNOWN AS: Zygomycosis

DEFINITION

Mucormycosis is a serious infection caused by a fungus that affects the sinuses, brain, and lungs. The infection occurs most often in people who have a compromised immune system. The prognosis is usually poor, even with treatment.

CAUSES

The fungus is often found in soil and in decaying plants. It will not make most people sick. People are more likely to get the infection if they have a weakened immune system.

RISK FACTORS

The factors that increase the chance of developing mucormycosis include having a weakened immune system caused by diabetes, acquired immunodeficiency syndrome, leukemia, or lymphoma; recently receiving an organ transplant; long-term steroid use; treatment with deferoxamine (an antidote to iron poisoning); metabolic acidosis (too much acid in the blood); having a sinus infection or pneumonia; and having mucormycosis of the gastrointestinal tract, skin, or kidneys.

SYMPTOMS

Symptoms of mucormycosis depend on the location of the infection. Infections of the sinuses and the brain (rhinocerebral mucormycosis) include acute sinusitis, fever, swollen or protruding eyes, dark nasal scabs, and redness of the skin over the sinuses. Symptoms of infections of the lungs (pulmonary mucormycosis) include fever, cough, coughing up blood, and shortness of breath. Symptoms of infections of the gastrointestinal tract (gastrointestinal mucormycosis) include abdominal pain and vomiting blood. Symptoms of infections in the kidneys (renal mucormycosis) include fever and pain in the side between the upper abdomen and the back.

SCREENING AND DIAGNOSIS

A doctor will ask about symptoms and medical history and will perform a physical exam. Tests might include a magnetic resonance imaging (MRI) scan (a scan that uses radio waves and a powerful magnet to produce detailed computer images), a computed tomography (CT) scan (a detailed X-ray picture that identifies abnormalities of fine tissue structure), and an analysis of a tissue sample.

TREATMENT AND THERAPY

Treatment options for mucormycosis include aggressive surgery to remove all the dead or infected tissue; early surgery may improve the prognosis. Another treatment is antifungal therapy, in which IV antifungal medications are used to kill the fungus throughout the body; even with this treatment, however, the prognosis is usually poor.

PREVENTION AND OUTCOMES

The fungus that causes mucormycosis is found in many places, so avoiding contact with it is difficult. The best prevention is to control or prevent the conditions related to this infection.

Diana Kohnle; reviewed by David L. Horn, M.D., FACP

FURTHER READING

Alcamo, I. Edward. *Microbes and Society: An Introduction to Microbiology.* 2d ed. Sudbury, Mass.: Jones and Bartlett, 2008.

Murray, Patrick R., Ken S. Rosenthal, and Michael A. Pfaller. *Medical Microbiology.* 6th ed. Philadelphia: Mosby/Elsevier, 2009.

Radha, S., et al. "Gastric Zygomycosis (Mucormycosis)." *Internet Journal of Pathology* 5, no. 2 (2007).

Roden, M. M., et al. "Epidemiology and Outcome of Mucormycosis: A Review of 929 Reported Cases." *Clinical Infectious Diseases* 41, no. 5 (September, 2005): 634-653.

Sugar, A. M. "Agents of Mucormycosis and Related Species." In *Mandell, Douglas, and Bennett's Principles and Practice of Infectious Diseases,* edited by Gerald L. Mandell, John F. Bennett, and Raphael Dolin. 7th ed. New York: Churchill Livingstone/Elsevier, 2010.

WEB SITES OF INTEREST

Canadian Lung Association
http://www.lung.ca

Centers for Disease Control and Prevention
http://www.cdc.gov

National Foundation for Infectious Diseases
http://www.nfid.org

See also: Allergic bronchopulmonary aspergillosis; Antifungal drugs: Types; Aspergillosis; *Aspergillus*; Blastomycosis; Coccidiosis; Diagnosis of fungal infections; Fungal infections; Fungi: Classification and types; *Fusarium*; Histoplasmosis; Mycoses; Paracoccidioidomycosis; Respiratory route of transmission; *Rhizopus*; Soil-borne illness and disease; Zygomycosis.

Mumps

CATEGORY: Diseases and conditions
ANATOMY OR SYSTEM AFFECTED: All

DEFINITION

Mumps is an acute, systemic, communicable viral infection caused by a single-stranded paramyxovirus whose virion consists of ribonucleic acid (RNA) and seven proteins. The RNA of the virus is surrounded by two surface glycoproteins, the hemagglutinin-neuraminidase and a hemolysis cell fusion antigen. Mumps is a benign and self-limited disease, and up to one-third of persons contracting the disease have a subclinical infection. As is the case with many viral infec-

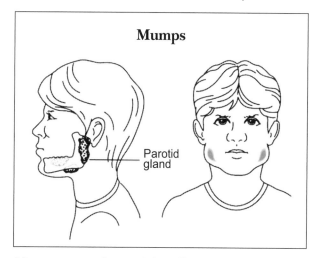

Mumps causes a characteristic swelling of the parotid, or salivary, glands.

tions, mumps is commonly more severe in people past puberty than it is in younger children.

CAUSES

The mumps virus produces an acute generalized infection that mostly occurs in children of school age, including adolescents. It is transmitted by droplets of saliva and by inanimate objects (fomites) that, when contaminated with the virus, can transfer the pathogen to a host. The virus multiplies in the epithelium of the upper respiratory tract, after which the viral particles enter the bloodstream. This is followed by the infection of one or both of the parotid glands, the largest of the salivary glands. This infection is known as parotitis.

Infection of other salivary glands and the meninges, pancreas, and gonads is also often seen, but it is not as common. Orchitis, an infection of the testis, is a common (about one in four cases) complication associated with mumps. In rare but severe cases, orchitis may result in sterility. Affected glands show edema and lymphocyte infiltration. Long-term immunity is produced with immunization, and one attack of mumps usually produces lifelong immunity.

RISK FACTORS

Lack of immunization, international travel, and immune deficiencies can make a child more prone to infection by paramyxovirus. Because the virus is present throughout the world, the risk of exposure to mumps outside the United States may be high, as mumps vaccine is used in only 57 percent of countries that are members of the World Health Organization.

The primary risk factor for contracting mumps is failure to immunize young children. Following the introduction of mumps vaccine in 1967, the incidence of mumps declined significantly in the United States. At that time, the Advisory Committee on Immunization Practices of the Centers for Disease Control and Prevention recommended that children approaching puberty, and adolescents and adults, be vaccinated. The use of mumps vaccine in young children was ex-

In the News: Mumps Outbreak in the United States

In December, 2005, several students at an unnamed college in eastern Iowa displayed symptoms of illness that included glandular swelling in the salivary region. Antibody testing indicated that the students had active cases of mumps. Several weeks later, an additional case was diagnosed. In the following months, additional cases were reported in the surrounding states of Illinois, Kansas, Minnesota, and Nebraska. Serotyping of isolated viruses indicated that all cases originated from a similar or identical strain. Because not all the cases were directly linked–that is, not all involved known contact–the suspicion among health workers was that portions of the outbreak were maintained through unnoticed infections.

The source of the illness remains unclear, but the initial case may have been contracted in Great Britain. In 2005, some 56,000 cases were diagnosed there, and the strain that first appeared in Iowa appears to be identical. It is likely that a student had either traveled to Great Britain during the outbreak or had contact with someone who had.

By the time the infection had run its course in the summer of 2006, more than 4,700 persons had been diagnosed with mumps, with cases reported in California. Approximately 25 percent of the cases involved college students. Mumps is generally a benign infection, and while there were no fatalities, pregnant women and persons with compromised immune systems, such as those who are HIV-positive, may be at risk for severe illness.

An unusual feature of the outbreak was that more than two-thirds of infected persons had already received the recommended two doses of the MMR (measles, mumps, and rubella) vaccine, calling into question the long-term effectiveness of current immunization practices. In the light of the outbreak, health authorities recommended that all students be sure of prior immunization against mumps, or that they receive an additional two doses of the vaccine.

Richard Adler, Ph.D.

pedited by the introduction and extensive use of the measles, mumps, rubella (MMR) vaccine beginning in 1977.

SYMPTOMS

Parotitis is the classic syndrome of mumps and is evidenced by swelling and inflammation of one or both of the salivary (parotid) glands. Symptoms include low-grade fever, headache, malaise, and anorexia. The incubation period for the disease is fourteen to twenty-one days, and it is communicable from six days before to nine days after facial swelling becomes apparent. However, in 30 percent of infections, no symptoms are observed.

Within twenty-four hours, infected persons experience ear pain near the lobe of the ear; this pain is made more severe by a chewing movement of the jaw. Acidic foods may exacerbate pain in the parotid gland. After the onset of the disease, one or both parotid glands begin to enlarge; in 70 to 80 percent of cases, the enlargement is bilateral. Pain with pressure is present over the parotid gland. Ordinarily, the parotid gland is not discernible to the touch, but in persons with mumps, it quickly swells during a period of several days. Fever diminishes within one week and disappears before swelling of the parotid gland ceases, which may take up to ten days.

Orchitis, or inflammation of the testis, is the second most common manifestation of mumps. It develops in 20 to 30 percent of postpubertal males who have the mumps and is bilateral in one to six of those with testicular involvement. It is uncommon in boys younger than ten years of age. Onset is abrupt, and symptoms include a fever from 102° to 105° Fahrenheit (39° to 41° Celsius), chills, headache, vomiting, and testicular pain. Fever and gonadal swelling usually resolve in one week, but tenderness may persist. The anxiety caused by mumps orchitis is difficult to ease, but the psychological fears of sexual impotence and sterility far outweigh the potential debility from testicular atrophy. Sterility is rare even with bilateral involvement.

SCREENING AND DIAGNOSIS

In most cases, the diagnosis of mumps is made utilizing a history of exposure and evidence of swelling and tenderness of the parotid glands and other classic symptoms of the disease. Although the definitive diagnosis of mumps is dependent on serologic studies or viral isolation, laboratory confirmation of typical mumps is unnecessary.

TREATMENT AND THERAPY

A person with mumps should drink plenty of fluids to promote adequate hydration. Foods and liquids that contain acid, such as tomatoes or orange juice, may cause difficulty in swallowing. Analgesics, such as ibuprofen, aspirin, or acetaminophen, can relieve headache or the discomfort of parotitis and can reduce fever. In orchitis, stronger analgesics may be needed.

Topical application of warm or cold packs to the parotid glands may relieve discomfort.

Administration of an antiviral agent is not indicated for mumps, as the disease is self-limited. Bed rest is recommended to promote a more rapid recovery.

PREVENTION AND OUTCOMES

The most effective way to prevent mumps is to vaccinate susceptible children, adolescents, and adults. This is best achieved in children with the administration of the MMR vaccine. For children, the typical recommended two-dose schedule is administered at age twelve to fifteen months for the first dose and age four to six years for the second dose.

Among the recommendations for the management of mumps once the disease has been contracted is to isolate the infected person until the parotid swelling has disappeared. After swelling of the parotid gland is detected, children should be kept out of school or day-care centers for nine days. If an outbreak in these settings should occur, all children involved should be vaccinated. Isolation, however, may be of little value, especially in closed environments such as schools or day-care centers. The virus is present in saliva for several days before parotitis develops and because children with asymptomatic infection can still shed the virus.

Gerald W. Keister, M.A.

FURTHER READING

Arumugam, V., et al. "Mumps." In *Ferri's Clinical Advisor 2011: Instant Diagnosis and Treatment*, edited by Fred F. Ferri. Philadelphia: Mosby/Elsevier, 2011. Provides recommendations on clinical treatments for mumps.

Gershon, Anne. "Mumps." In *Harrison's Principles of Internal Medicine*, edited by Joan Butterton. 17th ed. New York: McGraw-Hill, 2008. A chapter on mumps in a respected text on internal medicine.

Gutierrez, K. M. "Mumps Virus." In *Principles and Practice of Pediatric Infectious Diseases*, edited by Sarah S. Long, Larry K. Pickering, and Charles G. Prober. 3d ed. Philadelphia: Churchill Livingstone/Elsevier, 2008. An excellent text focusing on children and infectious diseases and conditions, including mumps.

Hviid, A., S. Rubin, and K. Mühlemann. "Mumps." *The Lancet* 371 (March, 2008): 932-944. An extensive study of mumps in a respected medical journal.

Litman, Nathan, and Stephen G. Baum. "Mumps Virus." In *Mandell, Douglas, and Bennett's Principles and Practice of Infectious Diseases*, edited by Gerald L. Mandell, John F. Bennett, and Raphael Dolin. 7th ed. New York: Churchill Livingstone/Elsevier, 2010. Infectious disease textbook with referenced discussion of the mumps and the mumps virus, including disease epidemiology, life cycle, clinical manifestations, diagnosis, and treatment.

Peltola, H., et al. "Mumps Outbreaks in Canada and the United States: Time for New Thinking on Mumps Vaccines." *Clinical Infectious Diseases* 45 (August, 2007): 459-466. A review of mumps vaccines in light of recent outbreaks in North America.

WEB SITES OF INTEREST

About Kids Health
http://www.aboutkidshealth.ca

American Academy of Family Physicians
http://familydoctor.org

Centers for Disease Control and Prevention
http://www.cdc.gov

See also: Children and infectious disease; Contagious diseases; Encephalitis; Epididymitis; Immunity; Inflammation; Measles; MMR vaccine; Mononucleosis; Paramyxoviridae; Parotitis; Respiratory route of transmission; Rubella; Saliva and infectious disease; Vaccines: Types; Viral infections; Viral meningitis.

Mutation of pathogens

CATEGORY: Transmission

DEFINITION

A mutation is any change in genetic material that is passed from one generation to another. If the mutation occurs in a disease-causing (pathogenic) microorganism, such as a bacterium of virus, and if the change enhances the pathogenicity of that bacterium or virus, then the mutation can be problematic.

MUTATION TYPES AND MECHANISMS

Mutations have a genetic basis. A change in the sequence of nucleotides, the building blocks of a gene,

can affect the production (more or less product produced) or the structure of the encoded product. An alteration in the sequence of nucleotides, but not in the number of nucleotides, is a nucleotide substitution.

Two types of nucleotide substitution mutations exist. A missense mutation is a change in only one nucleotide, which results in the substitution of one amino acid for another in the protein product. A nonsense mutation is also a single nucleotide change, but the alteration halts the transcription of the gene, which results in a shortened, dysfunctional protein product.

Other mutations do change the number of nucleotides. An increase is caused by the insertion of more nucleotides and is termed an "insertion mutation." Accordingly, a "deletion mutation" involves the removal of nucleotides. Removing or adding nucleotides produces a frameshift, in which the normal sequence with which the genetic material is interpreted is altered. The alteration causes the gene to code for a different sequence of amino acids in the protein product than would normally be produced. The result is a protein that functions differently (better or worse, depending on the mutation) or not all, as compared to the normally encoded version.

Gene transfer between bacteria can occur even between species that are unrelated. This horizontal gene transfer occurs in nature. It can be important in infectious disease, for example, in the acquisition of a gene that determines antibiotic resistance.

The transfer of genes between bacteria can occur in several ways. A gene in the genome of the donor microbe can be transferred to the recipient bacterium through a tube that transiently connects the two cells. The recipient is then able to express the encoded product. Bacterial genes also can reside on more readily mobile structures called plasmids. Plasmids are more easily transferable between bacteria.

Another genetic mechanism of bacterial evolution involves bacteriophages, viruses that specifically infect a particular type of bacteria (for example, various types of coliphages infect various strains of *Escherichia coli*). When a bacteriophage infects a bacterium, the viral genetic material can insert into the host's genetic material. When the viral material is excised, some of the host's genetic material can be removed as well, to become part of the genome of the bacteriophage. A subsequent infection of another bacterium can transfer genes from the first bacterium to the second bacterial host. If the new gene confers an advantage to the second bacterium, it will be retained and passed on to subsequent generations of bacteria.

PATHOGENS AND MUTATION

Mutations are an important driver of the development of pathogens. A good example is the influenza virus. Three types of orthomyxoviruses cause illness in humans and animals: types A, B, and C. Type A influenza has produced several epidemics, in which large numbers of people become infected during a short period of time, and pandemics, in which the illness can extend globally. The influenza epidemic of 1918 killed more people than the just-ended World War I. Mutated versions of this virus were responsible for epidemics that occurred in 1957, 1968, and 1977.

Type A viruses infect both humans and animals and usually originate in the Far East, where a large population of ducks and swine incubate the virus and pass it to humans. The passage of virus in the duck or swine populations promotes the formation of mutants. While some of the mutants will confer no advantage, others will. From these, new infections can emerge.

In 1997, a new strain of influenza A jumped from the poultry population in Hong Kong to the human population. The strain of virus, which was dubbed H5N1 (and was dubbed avian flu), produces a severe and sometimes fatal infection in humans. Beginning in 2004, avian flu began to display signs of acquiring the genetic ability to pass directly from person to person. As of 2006, only a few such cases had been reported. Thereafter, the disease gained strength. According to figures from the World Health Organization, by the end of 2010, 510 human cases had been officially recorded, with 303 of these cases resulting in death (a death rate of 59 percent).

Experts fear that further mutations of the H5N1 virus will increase the efficiency of bird-to-human transmission, enhance the ease of human-to-human transmission, and increase the already high death rate. The result could be a pandemic that dwarfs the casualties of the 1918 epidemic.

Because of the small amount of ribonucleic acid (RNA) genetic material within influenza viruses, mutation of the genetic material is very common. The result of this frequent mutation is that each flu virus is different, and people who have become immune to one variety of influenza virus are not necessarily immune to other influenza viruses. The ability to mutate

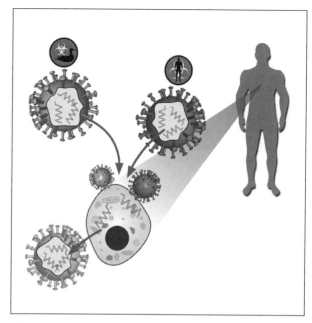

The cycle of two viruses, avian (top left) and human influenza (top right), mutate to form a new viral strain (bottom).

frequently therefore allows these viruses to cause frequent outbreaks. Annual flu shots are recommended because protection conferred by the vaccine from the previous year is not guaranteed to be effective again.

EMERGING INFECTIONS

Pathogen mutations also play a role in emerging infectious diseases, those human diseases of microbial origin that have increased in prevalence since the 1970's or have threatened to become more widespread.

Emergence may be genuine. In this case, a mutation has occurred that changes the character of a once-innocuous microbe. An example is *E. coli* O157:H7, which acquired a gene that encodes a destructive toxin. Without the gene, the organism is a normal (commensal) resident of the intestinal tract, where it may even confer some benefits to the host. With the toxin gene, the bacterium can cause a serious disease that can permanently damage the kidneys and can be lethal. Other mutation-related changes can make bacteria or viruses more capable of infecting a host, better able to survive in the external environment (and better able to be transferred from person-to-person), or resistant to antibacterial agents.

In the era of rapid worldwide travel, diseases can quickly spread globally. This was exemplified by the 2003 outbreak of severe acute respiratory syndrome (SARS), which spread within days from Taiwan to North America, causing 229 deaths. While another SARS outbreak has not occurred, the 2003 incident underscored how quickly a mutated organism can spread worldwide. An outbreak that occurs in a remote area of the globe is no guarantee that people far away from the site of original infection are safe.

IMPACT

The ability of disease-causing organisms (pathogens) to change (mutate) is vital to their ability to cause disease. An important example is bacterial antibiotic resistance. Some pathogenic bacteria have developed resistance to nearly all known antibiotics and, for one species, all antibiotics.

Brian Hoyle, Ph.D.

FURTHER READING

Drlica, Karl, and David S. Perlin. *Antibiotic Resistance: Understanding and Responding to an Emerging Crisis.* Upper Saddle River, N.J.: FT Press, 2011. Details the development of antibiotic resistance, which critically depends on mutations.

Kuijper, E. J., et al. "*Clostridium difficile*: Changing Epidemiology and New Treatment Options." *Current Opinions in Infectious Disease* 20 (2007): 376-383. Chronicles the increased prevalence of drug-resistant *Clostridium difficile* and the increasing threat posed by the pathogen in hospital-acquired (nosocomial) infections.

Madigan, Michael T., and John M. Martinko. *Brock Biology of Microorganisms.* 12th ed. Upper Saddle River, N.J.: Pearson/Prentice Hall, 2010. An introductory microbiology textbook for students of medicine and microbiology, with simplified descriptions of pathogenic organisms.

Miller, A. A., and P. F. Miller. *Emerging Trends in Antibacterial Discovery: Answering the Call to Arms.* Norwich, England: Caister Academic Press, 2011. Describes the development of compounds that kill bacteria, including bacterial pathogens that have arisen from mutations.

Schnayerson, Michael, and Mark J. Plotkin. *The Killers Within: The Deadly Rise of Drug-Resistant Bacteria.* Boston: Back Bay Books, 2003. Clearly describes how the overuse of antibiotics in agriculture and medicine has spawned the development of drug-resistant bacteria.

WEB SITES OF INTEREST

Emerging and Reemerging Infectious Diseases Resource Center
http://www.medscape.com/resource/infections

Microbiology Information Portal
http://www.microbes.info

Todar's Online Textbook of Bacteriology
http://www.textbookofbacteriology.net

Viral Zone
http://www.expasy.org/viralzone

See also: Antibiotic resistance; Antibiotics: Types; Bacteria: Classification and types; Bacteria: Structure and growth; Bacteriology; Drug resistance; Emerging and reemerging infectious diseases; Epidemics and pandemics: Causes and management; Epidemiology; Fungi: Classification and types; Fungi: Structure and growth; Hosts; Microbiology; Outbreaks; Parasites: Classification and types; Parasitic diseases; Pathogenicity; Pathogens; Prion diseases; Protozoan diseases; Public health; Transmission routes; Virology; Virulence; Viruses: Types.

Mycetoma

CATEGORY: Diseases and conditions
ANATOMY OR SYSTEM AFFECTED: Respiratory system, skin
ALSO KNOWN AS: Actinomycetoma, aspergilloma, eumycetoma, Madura foot

DEFINITION

A mycetoma is a mass or abscess caused by fungi or actinomycete bacteria. The mass often resembles a tumor, hence the form of the name meaning "fungal tumor." There are two distinct mycetoma diseases: One occurs in the respiratory tract (as an aspergilloma) and the other occurs on or in the skin or subcutaneously in the foot, hand, or back (as Madura foot).

CAUSES

Pulmonary mycetoma is most often caused by species of the fungus *Aspergillus* (and is often called an aspergilloma), but other respiratory fungal pathogens can also form pulmonary mycetomas. Pulmonary mycetomas often form in preexisting lung cavities.

Subcutaneous mycetomas can be caused by both fungi (eumycetoma) and filamentous actinomycete bacteria (actinomycetoma). Fungi of the genera *Madurella* and *Scedosporium* are commonly implicated, but other fungi are also known to cause mycetomas. Actinomycetes, although they are bacteria, not fungi, resemble fungi in both microbiological and clinical ways. *Actinomadura* sp., *Streptomyces* sp., and *Nocardia* sp. are the most commonly implicated actinomycetes in subcutaneous mycetomas. Cutaneous and subcutaneous mycetomas are often acquired when organisms enter the skin after local trauma.

RISK FACTORS

Pulmonary mycetomas have a predisposition to occur in preexisting lung cavities. These cavities are frequently caused by tuberculosis, coccidioidomycosis, histoplasmosis, lung neoplasms, sarcoidosis, bronchiectasis, and lung abscesses. Mycetomas may occur in up to 15 percent of persons with cavitating lung diseases caused by tuberculosis.

Cutaneous mycetoma occurs mainly in tropical or subtropical areas, especially in Africa and South Asia. Madura foot is named after the region of India where this form of the disease was first described medically. A strong risk factor is outdoor work, especially in underdeveloped countries.

SYMPTOMS

For pulmonary mycetoma, most persons are asymptomatic. When symptoms occur, the most common are cough, chest pain, and hemoptysis.

Subcutaneous mycetomas progress slowly over months or years, with little or no initial symptoms. After years, the affected area can have extensive swelling, induration, skin rupture, and sinus formation. The infection can destroy nearby muscle, tendon, bone, and other tissue, eventually causing severe deformity and tissue destruction.

SCREENING AND DIAGNOSIS

Pulmonary mycetoma is most often diagnosed after lung imaging, often when looking for other conditions, such as tuberculosis or lung neoplasia. Subcutaneous mycetoma often goes undiagnosed for many years until the mycetoma erupts. Exudates of the sinus tracts have grains of the causative agent. The cause is usually confirmed by a culture of exudates.

TREATMENT AND THERAPY

Because the nature of pulmonary mycetoma is highly variable, most infected persons are kept under observation without therapy. However, if persons develop hemoptysis (coughing up blood), then antifungal therapy is usually initiated. The primary antifungal drugs used are itraconazole, voriconazole, and amphotericin B. In severe cases, surgical resection of the affected lung or arterial embolization may be necessary.

For subcutaneous mycetoma, treatment includes antimicrobials specific to the causative organism or organisms, surgical debridement, and, sometimes, amputation. Bacterial secondary infections may lead to sepsis, and if untreated, may result in death.

David M. Faguy, Ph.D.

FURTHER READING

Ameen, M. "Managing Mycetomas." *Tropical Doctor* 30 (2009): 66-68.

Bustamante, B., and P. E. Campos. "Eumycetoma." In *Clinical Mycology*, edited by William E. Dismukes, Peter G. Pappas, and Jack D. Sobel. New York: Oxford University Press, 2003.

Riscili, B. P., and K. L. Wood. "Noninvasive Pulmonary Aspergillus Infections." *Clinics in Chest Medicine* 30 (2009): 315-335.

WEB SITES OF INTEREST

American Lung Association
http://www.lungusa.org

British Mycological Society
http://fungionline.org.uk

See also: Abscesses; Airborne illness and disease; Allergic bronchopulmonary aspergillosis; Antifungal drugs: Types; Aspergillosis; *Aspergillus*; Bacterial infections; Chromoblastomycosis; Coccidiosis; Diagnosis of fungal infections; Fungal infections; Fungi: Classification and types; *Fusarium*; Histoplasmosis; Melioidosis; Mold infections; Mucormycosis; Mycoses; Paracoccidioidomycosis; Respiratory route of transmission; Sarcoidosis; Skin infections.

Mycobacterial infections

CATEGORY: Diseases and conditions
ANATOMY OR SYSTEM AFFECTED: All

DEFINITION

Mycobacterial infections are chronic or acute systemic infections that are spread by a common type of bacteria in the environment, especially aquatic environments. Mycobacterial infections include tuberculosis; atypical mycobacterial infections include those of the skin, bone, soft tissue, lymph nodes, and gastrointestinal tract; they also include lung disease and septic arthritis.

CAUSES

Mycobacterial infections are caused by one of the species within the gram-positive, aerobic bacteria family called Mycobacteriaceae, which belongs to the Actinomycetales order. Specifically, *Mycobacterium tuberculosis* causes tuberculosis, *M. kansasii* causes lung disease, and *M. ulcerans* and *M. marinum* cause skin infections. *M. avium* subspecies *intracellulare* causes lung disease but primarily affects the lungs of those with acquired immunodeficiency syndrome; *M. avium* subspecies *intracellulare* also causes ulcers, diarrhea, fever, pustules, nodules, lesions, and swollen lymph nodes.

RISK FACTORS

Exposure to contaminated water sources is a major risk factor for mycobacterial infection. Other risk factors are having a preexisting lung disease, having an impaired immune system, undergoing surgery, and having an organ transplant. Also at higher risk are persons with human immunodeficiency virus (HIV) infection and persons living in unsanitary conditions.

SYMPTOMS

Persons with HIV who have a mycobacterial infection often show a cough, weight loss, chest pain, breathlessness, hemoptysis, night sweats, chills, and fever. Persons with a mycobacterial skin infection will often have reddish raised nodules on the elbows, feet, knees, and hands. Pain in the joints, tendons, and bones can be signs of tenosynovitis and of infections that could lead to arthritis and osteomyelitis. Enlarged lymph nodes are often a symptom of persons with mycobacterial infection of the lymph nodes. Signs of tuberculosis include fever and chills, rapid breathing, night sweats, pale skin, prolonged coughing that produces bloody sputum, weight loss, loss of appetite, and pleurisy.

SCREENING AND DIAGNOSIS

Screening methods include blood, bone marrow, lymph node, sputum, and stool cultures. Traditional methods of bacteria analysis, including growth rate and pigmentation studies and acid-fast staining, confirm the identity of the bacteria. A bacterial-species-specific polymerase chain reaction analysis for screening assays has been developed. Deoxyribonucleic acid (DNA) fingerprinting and DNA sequencing techniques are often used for bacteria identification. A tissue biopsy is useful for diagnosis, and X rays or computed tomography scans may be used to detect internal infection sites.

TREATMENT AND THERAPY

Antibiotics including rifampicin, streptomycin, and tetracyclines have been helpful for preventing the spread of the bacteria. The use of these antibiotics for two weeks to eighteen months can decrease the

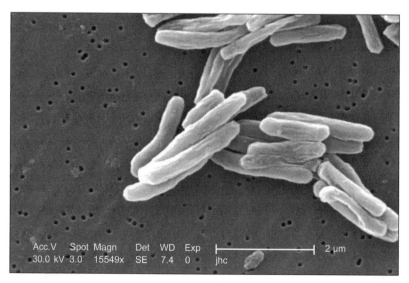

Mycobacterium tuberculosis, *which causes the human disease tuberculosis.* (CDC)

growth of the bacteria enough to prevent an infection that could lead to lung disease, skin disease, or tuberculosis. If the antibiotics have not been effective enough, then surgery, debridement of the infected tissues, or amputation of infected limbs may be needed to remove the bacteria.

PREVENTION AND OUTCOMES

To decrease the chance of getting a mycobacterial infection, one should avoid stagnant aquatic environments and should avoid contact with fish and cattle. Chlorination of swimming pools is also an effective method of prevention because chlorine kills the bacteria that can cause these infections.

Jeanne L. Kuhler, Ph.D.

FURTHER READING

Heifets, Leonid, ed. *Drug Susceptibility in the Chemotherapy of Mycobacterial Infections.* Boca Raton, Fla.: CRC Press, 1991.

LaBombardi, Vincent J. "The Genus *Mycobacteria.*" In *Practical Handbook of Microbiology*, edited by Emanuel Goldman and Lorrence H. Green. 2d ed. Boca Raton, Fla.: CRC Press, 2009.

Madigan, Michael T., and John M. Martinko. *Brock Biology of Microorganisms.* 12th ed. Upper Saddle River, N.J.: Pearson/Prentice Hall, 2010.

Schlossberg, David, ed. *Tuberculosis and Nontuberculous Mycobacterial Infections.* 5th ed. New York: McGraw-Hill Professional, 2006.

WEB SITES OF INTEREST

American Lung Association
http://www.lungusa.org

Centers for Disease Control and Prevention, Division of Foodborne, Bacterial, and Mycotic Diseases
http://www.cdc.gov/nczved/divisions/dfbmd

Virtual Museum of Bacteria
http://www.bacteriamuseum.org

See also: Intestinal and stomach infections; Leprosy; Lymphadenitis; *Mycobacterium*; Septic arthritis; Skin infections; Tuberculosis (TB); Waterborne illness and disease.

Mycobacterium

CATEGORY: Pathogen
TRANSMISSION ROUTE: Ingestion, inhalation

DEFINITION

Members of the bacterial genus *Mycobacterium* are widely distributed in nature. Mycobacteria, which cause noteworthy diseases such as tuberculosis and leprosy, affect healthy humans, nonhuman animals, and persons with compromised immune systems.

Taxonomic Classification for *Mycobacterium*

Kingdom: Bacteria
Phylum: Actinobacteria
Order: Actinomycetales
Family: Mycobacteriaceae
Genus: *Mycobacterium*
Species:
M. tuberculosis
M. bovis
M. africanum
M. canetti
M. caprae
M. microti
M. pinnipedii
M. avium
M. kansasii
M. terrae
M. ulcerans
M. malmoense
M. leprae
M. intercellare
M. marinum
M. intermedium

NATURAL HABITAT AND FEATURES

Members of the genus *Mycobacterium* are widely distributed, rod-shaped bacteria. Many are free-living and are found in soil, water, and marshes and in association with various animal species; a few can live only in or on animals. In culture, mycobacteria cells can vary from spherical (cocci) to ovoid (coccobacilli) to rods (bacilli) to branched rods to long cordlike rods. They are nonmotile, with the exception of *marinum*.

When grown on artificial media, mycobacteria form flat, dry, scaly colonies. Some *Mycobacterium* spp.

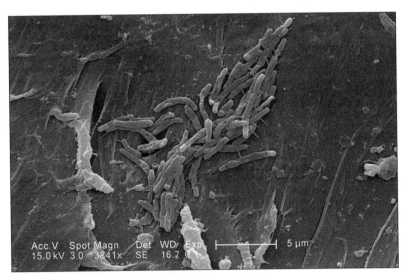

Acc.V Spot Magn   Det WD Exp
15.0 kV 3.0 3841x   SE 16.7 0

5 μm

A micrograph of Mycobacterium fortuitum. (CDC)

are pigmented. Photochromogens, such as *kansasii, marinum,* and *simae,* form pigmented colonies only when grown in the light. Scotochomogens, such as *scrofulaceum, gordonae,* and *szulgai,* form yellow to orange colonies when grown in the dark or in the light. *Tuberculosis, bovis, ulcerans,* and *fortuitum* nonchromogens produce dull-colored colonies that are white or cream-colored, pale yellow, or tan if grown in the light or in the dark.

The growth rates of mycobacteria differ wildly. Those mycobacteria that can form colonies within seven days are classified as rapid growing, and those that require more time to form colonies are called slow growing.

All members of the genus *Mycobacterium* are surrounded by a rather thick cell wall that is waxy. Bacteria typically contain a cell wall composed of a polymer called peptidoglycan, but mycobacteria have a modified peptidoglycan layer that is cross-linked to polysaccharides called arabinogalactans and unusual lipids known as mycolic acids. These mycolic acids form a waxy layer outside the peptidoglycan layer with a poorly characterized outer lipid layer. Mycobacteria do not stain when subjected to a Gram's stain, but are, instead, successfully stained by an acid-fast stain that uses carbolfuschin, which stains members of the *Mycobacterium* red.

Mycobacteria were formerly identified by biochemical tests, but methods of identification, now more rapid, include the separation of cell-wall mycolic acids,

in which mycolic acids from mycobacterial cell walls are separated by high performance liquid chromatography and compared with a database of known standards to identify specific *Mycobacterium* spp. Another way to identify members is through nucleic acid sequencing, which uses gene sequencing systems to sequence the 16S ribosomal ribonucleic acid (RNA) genes and compare them with published sequences to rapidly identify mycobacterial isolates.

PATHOGENICITY AND CLINICAL SIGNIFICANCE

The most clinically significant disease caused by mycobacteria is tuberculosis. *Tuberculosis* causes the vast majority of tuberculosis cases, but members of the *tuberculosis* complex, which include *bovis, africanum, canetti, caprae,* and *microti,* can also cause tuberculosis, or tuberculosis-like diseases, especially in persons whose immune systems are compromised.

When tuberculosis-causing mycobacteria are inhaled, they settle deep within the lungs and are engulfed by a lung-based white blood cell called an alveolar macrophage. The organisms can survive and divide within the macrophages. Other uninfected macrophages surround the infected cell, fuse, and then engulf the cell to deprive the bacterial cells of oxygen. This type of response is called a granuloma, which produces a bump or tubercle in the lung. These tubercles can last the remainder of a person's life; they constitute pulmonary tuberculosis.

Many cases of pulmonary tuberculosis cause no visible symptoms, and so are asymptomatic, but one system that does commonly appear is a cough. Additional symptoms include trouble breathing (dyspnea) and coughing up blood (hemoptysis). Chest X rays show middle and lower lung infiltrates. The tuberculin skin test is the most reliable way to diagnose tuberculosis.

If the infected person becomes weakened, these tubercles can break open, and the mycobacterial cells can disseminate to any organ of the body. This represents disseminated or extrapulmonary tuberculosis. The main sites of dissemination are the lymphatic system and the pleural membranes of the lungs, but the organism can spread to other organs as well. The wasting caused by disseminated tuberculosis is popularly known as consumption.

Leprosy (Hansen's disease), a chronic, progressive disease that can permanently damage the nerves, skin, eyes, and limbs, is caused by *leprae* and *lepromatosis*. This disease results from granulomas of the peripheral nerves and mucosae of the upper respiratory tract. The primary external sign of this disease is a skin lesion.

Nontuberculous mycobacteria (NTM) or environmental or atypical mycobacteria, cause neither tuberculosis nor leprosy. NTM cause lung diseases, lymph node infections (lymphadenitis), skin and soft tissue infections, and disseminated disease in persons with acquired immunodeficiency syndrome (AIDS).

DRUG SUSCEPTIBILITY

Combination drug treatments are the rule when treating mycobacterial infections. Because mycobacteria are resistant to antibiotics typically used to treat bacterial infections, separate groups of antibiotics have been designed especially for these infections.

First-line treatment for pulmonary tuberculosis consists of daily isoniazid, rifampin, ethambutol, and pyrazinamide for two months followed by four months of isoniazid and rifampin three times per week. Alternative treatment regimes exist, and if first-line drugs do not work or are not tolerated, available second-line drugs include cycloserine, ethionamide, fluoroquinolones (levofloxacin, moxifloxacin, and gatifloxacin), p-aminosalicyclic acid, aminoglycosides (streptomycin, kanamycin, and amikacin), and capreomycin.

Treatment of extrapulmonary tuberculosis extends the second phase of treatment for seven months, but treatment of tuberculosis of the central nervous system extends the second phase of treatment for ten months. Steroid drugs are also given to reduce the swelling and inflammation associated with extrapulmonary tuberculosis.

Mycobacteria that are resistant to isoniazid and rifampicin are termed multi-drug-resistant (MDR). Those mycobacteria that are resistant to isoniazid, rifampin, fluoroquinolone, kanamycin, capreomycin, or amikacin are designated as extensively drug-resistant (XDR). To treat MDR- or XDR-tuberculosis, the infecting *Mycobacterium* is isolated from the infected person and are laboratory tested for drug sensitivities, after which the infected person is given a combina-

tion of five drugs, against which the infecting *Mycobacterium* is sensitive for at least eighteen months.

Leprosy is treated with a combination of rifampin, dapsone (a sulfa drug), and clofazimine for twelve months. NTM infections require a combination of macrolides, ethambutol, and rifamycin for up to one year.

Michael A. Buratovich, Ph.D.

FURTHER READING

Dormandy, Thomas. *The White Death: A History of Tuberculosis.* London: Hambledon & London, 2001. A pathologist traces the impression left by tuberculosis on human history, examines the suffering the disease has caused, and discusses how Western countries mitigated its effects.

Gandy, Matthew, and Alimuddin Zumia, eds. *The Return of the White Plague: Global Poverty and the "New" Tuberculosis.* New York: Verso, 2003. An engrossing analysis of the social and economic impacts of multi-drug-resistant tuberculosis.

Hopewell, Philip C., and Robert M. Jasmer. "Overview of Clinical Tuberculosis." In *Tuberculosis and the Tubercle Bacillus,* edited by Steward T. Cole et al. Washington, D.C.: ASM Press, 2005. A clear and magisterial treatment of the clinical features of tuberculosis.

LaBombardi, Vincent J. "The Genus *Mycobacteria.*" In *Practical Handbook of Microbiology,* edited by Emanuel Goldman and Lorrence H. Green. 2d ed. Boca Raton, Fla.: CRC Press, 2009. A brief, informative summary of the clinical aspects of the genus *Mycobacterium* in a standard medical microbiology reference book.

Madigan, Michael T., and John M. Martinko. *Brock Biology of Microorganisms.* 12th ed. Upper Saddle River, N.J.: Pearson/Prentice Hall, 2010. This text outlines many common bacteria and describes their natural history, pathogenicity, and other characteristics.

WEB SITES OF INTEREST

American Lung Association
http://www.lungusa.org

Centers for Disease Control and Prevention, Division of Foodborne, Bacterial, and Mycotic Diseases
http://www.cdc.gov/nczved/divisions/dfbmd

Emerging and Reemerging Infectious Diseases Resource Center
http://www.medscape.com/resource/infections

Virtual Museum of Bacteria
http://www.bacteriamuseum.org

See also: Bacteria: Classification and types; Bacterial infections; Emerging and reemerging infectious diseases; Leprosy; Lymphadenitis; Mycobacterial infections; Septic arthritis; Tuberculosis (TB); Waterborne illness and disease.

Mycoplasma

CATEGORY: Pathogen
TRANSMISSION ROUTE: Blood, inhalation

DEFINITION

Mycoplasma is a bacterial genus belonging to the class Mollicutes. A number of *Mycoplasma* species have been established as human pathogens, including *pneumoniae, hominis,* and *genitalium.*

NATURAL HABITAT AND FEATURES

Mycoplasma has been isolated from humans and animals including cows, dogs, cats, pigs, horses, poultry, sheep, goats, and small rodents. *Mycoplasma* is the smallest bacteria that can live independently. It has a small genome size that is in the lower limit of complexity necessary for self-replicating organisms. *Mycoplasma* can survive in the presence or absence of oxygen.

Mycoplasma lacks a cell wall, so it does not react in a Gram's stain and is not susceptible to antibiotics that target cell walls. It has a specialized organelle, or tip, that provides motility and mediates bacterial interactions with its host cells. Adherence proteins allow *Mycoplasma* attachment to cells lining the respiratory and genitourinary tracts, acting like a parasite on the surface of its host cells and using their precursors for production of its genetic material. Some species (*pneumoniae, genitalium, fermentans, penetrans,* and *gallisepticum,* a poultry pathogen) can invade host cells and live intracellularly.

Mycoplasma produces hydrogen peroxide and superoxide, substances that cause injuries to the mucosal surface; the activation of inflammatory mediators is

Taxonomic Classification for *Mycoplasma*

Kingdom: Bacteria
Phylum: Firmicutes
Class: Mollicutes
Order: Mycoplasmatales
Family: Mycoplasmataceae
Genus: *Mycoplasma*
Species:
M. fermentans
M. genitalium
M. hominis
M. penetrans
M. pneumoniae

The inclusion of some *Mycoplasma* species in other genera within the class of Mollicutes raises a challenge in the taxonomic classification of *Mycoplasma.* Another taxonomic challenge is the use of the term "mycoplasma" to refer to organisms belonging to different genera within the class of Mollicutes, such as *Ureaplasma* species.

The family of Mycoplasmataceae has two genera, *Mycoplasma* and *Ureaplasma.* It is significant that both genera have species in the normal flora of the lower genitourinary tract and can cause urogenital and extragenital infections. These species include M. *hominis, M. genitalium, U. urealyticum,* and *U. parvum.* The two *Ureaplasma* species are generally not distinguished from each other for clinical purposes and are referred to as the *Ureaplasma* species.

associated with its infectious process. *Mycoplasma* is challenging to grow in culture; thus, bacterial identification mainly depends on molecular-biochemical techniques.

PATHOGENICITY AND CLINICAL SIGNIFICANCE

Although there are seven *Mycoplasma* species detected in the human sgenitourinary tract, only three species (*genitalium, hominis,* and *Ureaplasma* species) are associated with urogenital disease. Nonchlamydial nongonococcal urethritis in men may result from *genitalium* and *Ureaplasma* species. *Genitalium* has also been isolated from the urogenital tract of women with cervicitis and pelvic inflammatory disease. *Genitalium* and *Ureaplasma* species have also been implicated in extragenital infections.

Hominis and *Ureaplasma* species have been implicated in chorioamnionitis, endometritis, pyelonephritis, postpartum or postabortum fevers, neonatal meningitis, pneumonia, bacteremia, and arthritis (specifically, *hominis* in postpartum women and *Ureaplasma* species in sexually acquired reactive arthritis).

Hominis has been related to extragenital infections, including sepsis, hematoma infection, vascular and catheter-related infections, sternal wound infections following thoracic surgery, prosthetic valve endocarditis, brain abscesses, and pneumonia. These infections occurred mainly through the spread of bacteria in the bloodstream and mostly in immunocompromised persons who had injuries of anatomical barriers and had polytrauma.

Pneumoniae causes lung infections, often called atypical pneumonia or walking pneumonia. It is transmitted through respiratory droplets between persons. At highest risk for infection are those persons who are in close contact with others, including those who live, work, or perform activities in crowded places such as schools, homeless shelters, hospitals, prisons, and dormitories. Other risk factors for *Mycoplasma* respiratory infection include smoking and lower levels of preexisting immunoglobulin G levels. *Mycoplasma* pneumonia has pulmonary manifestations (such as nonproductive cough) and extrapulmonary manifestations (such as cardiologic, neurologic, and dermatologic symptoms). There is no age or gender predilection for the disease. Although people of all ages are at risk, infection rarely occurs in children younger than five years of age.

DRUG SUSCEPTIBILITY

Hominis is treated with tetracycline, the drug of choice, usually for seven days, but the duration of treatment is based on observations of symptom resolution and clinical judgment. Resistant strains have been reported, and alternate choices of antibiotics include clindamycin and fluoroquinolones (such as gatifloxacin and moxifloxacin).

Ureaplasma infections are treated with tetracycline or erythromycin, the drugs of choice. A seven day course of doxycycline can be used for treatment of urethritis caused by *Ureaplasma* species. Alternative antimicrobials for *Ureaplasma* include fluoroquinolones (such as levofloxacin and ofloxacin) and chloramphenicol. Clinical observations are important in considering treatment duration.

Neonatal meningitis caused by *hominis* and *Ureaplasma* species is often treated with tetracyclines, despite contraindications for use in children. Alternative medications for use in children include chloramphenicol for both bacteria, clindamycin for *hominis*, and erythromycin for *Ureaplasma* species. Lower respiratory infections in newborns can be treated with azithromycin or erythromycin. The suggested duration of treatment for *Mycoplasma* infections in newborns is ten to fourteen days.

Genitalium and *pneumonia* are treated with macrolides (such as azithromycin, clarithromycin, and erythromycin), fluoroquinolones (such as levofloxacin and moxifloxacin), and tetracyclines (such as doxycycline). The duration of treatment ranges from five to fourteen days, depending on what antibiotic is used.

*Miriam E. Schwartz, M.D., Ph.D.,
and Shawkat Dhanani, M.D., M.P.H.*

FURTHER READING

Blanchard, Alain, and Cecile M. Bebear. "Mycoplasmas of Humans." In *Molecular Biology and Pathogenicity of Mycoplasmas*, edited by Shmuel Razin and Richard Herrmann. New York: Kluwer Academic, 2002.

Johannson, Karl-Erik, and Bertil Petterrson. "Taxonomy of Mollicutes." In *Molecular Biology and Pathogenicity of Mycoplasmas*, edited by Shmuel Razin and Richard Herrmann. New York: Kluwer Academic, 2002.

Mandell, Lionel A., et al. "Infectious Diseases Society of America/American Thoracic Society Consensus Guidelines on the Management of Community Acquired Pneumonia in Adults." *Clinical Infectious Diseases* 44 (2007): S27-S72.

Ryan, Kenneth J. "*Mycoplasma* and *Ureaplasma*." In *Sherris Medical Microbiology*, edited by Kenneth J. Ryan and C. George Ray. 5th ed. New York: McGraw-Hill, 2010.

WEB SITES OF INTEREST

Todar's Online Textbook of Bacteriology
http://www.textbookofbacteriology.net

Virtual Museum of Bacteriology
http://www.bacteriamuseum.org

See also: Atypical pneumonia; Bacteria: Classification and types; *Mycoplasma* pneumonia; Pelvic inflammatory disease; Prostatitis; Urethritis.

Mycoplasma pneumonia

CATEGORY: Diseases and conditions
ANATOMY OR SYSTEM AFFECTED: Lungs, respiratory system
ALSO KNOWN AS: Atypical pneumonia, walking pneumonia

DEFINITION

Mycoplasma pneumonia is a bacterial infection of the lungs. The infection is considered an atypical pneumonia.

CAUSES

The etiologic agent is *Mycoplasma pneumoniae*, a bacterial species found to be widespread in the environment. This bacterium, which has no cell wall, can survive alone in the presence or absence of oxygen. It has a specialized tip (organelle) that provides motility and mediates bacterial interactions with its host cells. Moreover, adherence proteins allow *M. pneumoniae* to attach to the lining of the respiratory tract (from the nasal passage to the lungs), acting like a parasite on the surface of its host cells. The bacteria produce hydrogen peroxide and superoxide, substances that injure the respiratory lining.

RISK FACTORS

M. pneumoniae is transmitted through respiratory droplets between people. Persons who are in close contact are at highest risk for this infection and include those who live, work, or perform activities in crowded places, such as schools, homeless shelters, prisons, dormitories, military facilities, and hospitals. Other associated risk factors for *Mycoplasma* respiratory infection include smoking and lower levels of preexisting immunoglobulin G levels. There is no age or gender predilection for the disease.

SYMPTOMS

The symptoms of *Mycoplasma* pneumonia gradually appear from one to three weeks after infection. Symptoms may be divided into those of the respiratory tract (pulmonary) versus those that have extrapulmonary manifestations (cardiologic, neurologic, dermatologic, and others). The general symptoms include malaise, fever, chills, and excessive sweating, which may precede the onset of illness. The common pulmonary symptoms include nonproductive cough, runny nose, and sore throat. Extrapulmonary symptoms may include chest pain, headache, eye pain, muscle aches, joint stiffness, skin rash, and a breakdown of red blood cells. Central nervous system involvement may manifest as encephalitis and meningitis.

SCREENING AND DIAGNOSIS

A physician will obtain a medical history, perform a physical examination, and evaluate the list of symptoms. A chest X ray will be ordered along with laboratory studies (complete blood count and basic electrolytes). Other diagnostic tests include blood cultures, sputum cultures, a urine test, and a throat swab. Serology tests may also be obtained to evaluate the presence and levels of antibodies against *Mycoplasma* antigens. Other nonroutine tests include detection of *Mycoplasma* genetic material, *Mycoplasma* antigens, or cold agglutinins. Depending on the severity of the clinical presentation, a computed tomography (CT) scan of the chest and bronchoscopy (in which a thin fiberoptic scope is used to view the respiratory tract and the lungs) may be performed. Open lung biopsy is done only in very serious illnesses when the diagnosis is uncertain or the person's symptoms are not resolving.

TREATMENT AND THERAPY

Antibiotic options against *M. pneumoniae* include macrolides (such as azithromycin, clarithromycin, and erythromycin), fluoroquinolones (such as levofloxacin and moxifloxacin), and tetracyclines (such as doxycycline). Adjunct therapies may be necessary if extrapulmonary symptoms are present. For example, steroids have shown benefit in treating children with neurologic disease.

PREVENTION AND OUTCOMES

Antibiotic prophylaxis with azithromycin has been shown to prevent outbreaks of *Mycoplasma* pneumonia and to decrease the occurrence of respiratory infections. Another preventive measure is minimizing the transfer of respiratory droplets from infected persons to others.

Miriam E. Schwartz, M.D., Ph.D.,
and Shawkat Dhanani, M.D., M.P.H.

FURTHER READING

Brooks, Geo F., et al. "*Mycoplasma* and Cell Wall Defective Bacteria." In *Jawetz, Melnick, and Adelberg's*

Medical Microbiology. 25th ed. New York: McGraw-Hill Medical, 2010.

Mandell, Lionel A., et al. "Infectious Diseases Society of America/American Thoracic Society Consensus Guidelines on the Management of Community Acquired Pneumonia in Adults." *Clinical Infectious Diseases* 44 (2007): S27-S72.

Ryan, Kenneth J. "*Mycoplasma* and *Ureaplasma.*" In *Sherris Medical Microbiology*, edited by Kenneth J. Ryan and C. George Ray. 5th ed. New York: McGraw-Hill, 2010.

Web Sites of Interest

Centers for Disease Control and Prevention, Division of Foodborne, Bacterial, and Mycotic Diseases
http://www.cdc.gov/nczved/divisions/dfbmd

Todar's Online Textbook of Bacteriology
http://www.textbookofbacteriology.net

See also: Airborne illness and disease; Atypical pneumonia; Bacteria: Classification and types; Bacterial infections; *Mycoplasma*; Pneumonia; Respiratory route of transmission.

Mycoses

Category: Diseases and conditions
Anatomy or system affected: Hair, lungs, nails, respiratory system, scalp, skin
Also known as: Fungal infections

Definition

Mycoses (singular "mycosis") are infections caused by molds (filamentous fungi).

Causes

Mycoses are caused by filamentous fungi or molds. There are thousands of species of molds, but most do not cause disease in healthy people. Molds are acquired from an environmental source and not through person-to-person contact. The most serious mycoses (such as aspergillosis, caused by *Aspergillus* sp., and coccidioidomycosis, caused by *Coccidioides*) are those that begin in the lungs and may invade other tissues.

Risk Factors

Healthy people generally have the ability to combat the fungi they encounter. Deficiencies in the immune system, such as human immunodeficiency virus (HIV) infection, acquired immunodeficiency syndrome (AIDS), and neutropenia, and deficiencies caused by immunosuppressive therapy and even old age, substantially increase the risk of mycoses. Other risk factors include poor lung function from other conditions such as chronic obstructive pulmonary disease, bronchiectasis, tuberculosis, sarcoidosis, and asthma.

Molds thrive in soil and moist environments. People who have prolonged exposure to soil, dust, and dirt are at greater risk of developing mold infections. Also, environments with poor ventilation can allow mold growth and spore formation, resulting in a higher risk of mold infections.

Symptoms

The symptoms of mycoses depend on the mold causing the infection and on the body site of the infection. Mycoses can be superficial-cutaneous or respiratory-systemic. Many mycoses are confined to the skin, hair, and nails. These superficial infections rarely penetrate or become a serious health concern, although with injury to the skin they can become subcutaneous. Infection of the toenails or fingernails is called onychomycosis. More serious are respiratory mycoses, which can often spread to other organs and sites. Symptoms of respiratory mold infections are often nonspecific and can include fever, cough, headache, rash, muscle aches, night sweats, and hemoptysis (coughing up blood).

Screening and Diagnosis

The diagnosis of fungal infections generally involves an examination, or clinical observation, to check for particular symptoms. Also, diagnosis may include a laboratory fungal culture from affected body sites, histologic examination of clinical material, serological tests for antibodies to a specific fungi, and radiologic imaging. Definitive diagnosis usually requires laboratory culture of the fungus and identification based on morphological characteristics.

Treatment and Therapy

In many cases, no treatment is required for superficial or cutaneous mycoses. If the onychomycosis is serious, topical and oral therapies are available. Topical agents include amorolfine, ciclopirox olamine, and bifonazole/urea. Newer antifungal agents, such as itraconazole (Sporanox), fluconazole (Diflucan), and terbinafine (Lamisil and Terbinex), have been used to treat onychomycosis.

For systemic or otherwise more serious mycoses, the most effective antifungal for many years was amphotericin B. Liposomal formulations of amphotericin B have been developed with significantly less toxicity, but they remain effective against many invasive fungi.

New drugs in the azole class, such as itraconazole, voriconazole, ravuconazole, and posaconazole, are often used. An entirely new class of antifungals, the echinocandins, has also recently been developed.

PREVENTION AND OUTCOMES

Most mold infections are very difficult, if not impossible, to prevent. Fungi are present in all environments. Generally, mold infections begin with airborne spores, which makes it impossible to avoid infection.

David M. Faguy, Ph.D.

FURTHER READING

Midgley G., Yvonne M. Clayton, and Roderick J. Hay. *Diagnosis in Color: Medical Mycology.* Chicago: Mosby-Wolfe, 1997.

Patterson, Thomas F., ed. "Fungal Infections." *Infectious Disease Clinics of North America* 20 (2006): 485-734.

Richardson, Malcolm D., and Elizabeth M. Johnson. *Pocket Guide to Fungal Infection.* 2d ed. Malden, Mass.: Wiley-Blackwell, 2006.

Weitzman, I., and A. A. Padhye. "Dermatophytes: Gross and Microscopic." *Dermatologic Clinics* 14 (1996): 9-22.

WEB SITES OF INTEREST

American Lung Association
http://www.lungusa.org

Centers for Disease Control and Prevention, Division of Foodborne, Bacterial, and Mycotic Diseases
http://www.cdc.gov/nczved/divisions/dfbmd

Microbiology and Immunology On-line: Mycology
http://pathmicro.med.sc.edu/book/mycol-sta.htm

See also: Allergic bronchopulmonary aspergillosis; Antifungal drugs: Types; Aspergillosis; Blastomycosis; Coccidiosis; Cryptococcosis; Diagnosis of fungal infections; Fungal infections; Fungi: Classification and types; Histoplasmosis; Mold infections; Mucormycosis; Respiratory route of transmission; Sarcoidosis; Soilborne illness and disease.

Mycotic aneurysm

CATEGORY: Diseases and conditions
ANATOMY OR SYSTEM AFFECTED: Arteries, blood, cardiovascular system, circulatory system, heart

DEFINITION

A mycotic aneurysm is a rare condition in which bacteria infect the wall of an artery and cause dilation of the artery and a mass of infectious material. Pieces of this mass can break off and travel to other parts of the body, where they can colonize a new site or interfere with blood flow. A mycotic aneurysm is more likely in an artery. It can occur in any artery in the body, although it is most common in the femoral artery and the abdominal aorta. In rare instances, a mycotic aneurysm is preceded by infective endocarditis or valvular heart disease.

CAUSES

Although the term "mycotic" implies a fungal infection, most mycotic aneurysms are caused by bacteria. Some of the organisms that can cause a mycotic aneurysm are *Streptococcus pneumoniae, S. viridans, Staphylococcus aureus,* and *Salmonella* species. Often, the mycotic aneurysm develops at a tear in an artery caused by atherosclerosis.

RISK FACTORS

Persons with existing health issues are more likely to develop a mycotic aneurysm. These health issues include cancer, liver cirrhosis, systemic lupus erythematosus, acquired immunodeficiency syndrome, inflammatory bowel disease, and diabetes. Higher risk is associated also with old age, immunosuppressive therapy or glucocorticoid therapy, and intravenous drug abuse.

SYMPTOMS

The symptoms of a mycotic aneurysm vary according to their size and their site. If the site of the mycotic aneurysm is bleeding, there will be additional symptoms. The symptoms include fever; abdominal, thigh, neck, or arm pain; palpable mass; nausea; weakness; and fatigue. If the mycotic aneurysm is in the arteries of the brain, the symptoms will be headache, seizures, bleeding into the brain, and nausea and vomiting.

SCREENING AND DIAGNOSIS

There is no routine screening for a mycotic aneurysm. The diagnosis is based on the symptoms, on increased white blood cells, and on diagnostic imaging. Testing includes blood cell count (CBC), transesophageal echocardiography, color Doppler echocardiography, angiography, computed tomography (CT) scan, and magnetic resonance imaging (MRI). The imaging focuses on the area that is painful or where there is a mass.

TREATMENT AND THERAPY

The treatment for mycotic aneurysm is antibiotics and surgery. The antibiotics used will depend on the bacteria involved. If the bacterium has not been identified, antibiotics will be chosen based on the likely bacteria. A brain mycotic aneurysm sometimes requires that the aneurysm be blocked off with tiny metal coils to prevent rupture.

Mycotic aneurysms require surgery to remove the infective debris and to replace or bypass the damaged artery. Sometimes, cardiac valve replacement is required too.

PREVENTION AND OUTCOMES

There is no way to prevent a mycotic aneurysm. It is thought that avoiding *Salmonella* infections of the gastrointestinal tract can decrease the likelihood of contracting a *Salmonella* infection, including a mycotic aneurysm, in other parts of the body. *Salmonella* infections are contracted by contact with infected chickens, pigs, and eggs.

Christine M. Carroll, R.N.

FURTHER READING

Ahsan, Humera, et al. "Cerebral Fungal Infection with Mycotic Aneurysm of Basilar Artery and Subarachnoid Haemorrhage." *Singapore Medical Journal* 50 (2009): 22-25.

Erdogan, Hasan Basri, et al. "Endovascular Treatment of Intercerebral Mycotic Aneuryms Before Surgical Treatment of Infective Endocarditis." *Texas Heart Institute Journal* 31 (2004): 165-167. Also available at http://www.ncbi.nlm.nih.gov/pmc/articles/pmc427378.

Hoffman, Gary S., and Cornelia M. Weyland, eds. *Inflammatory Diseases of Blood Vessels.* New York: Marcel Dekker, 2002.

WEB SITES OF INTEREST

National Heart, Lung, and Blood Institute
http://www.nhlbi.nih.gov

National Organization for Rare Disorders
http://www.rarediseases.org

See also: Bacterial endocarditis; Bacterial infections; Behçet's syndrome; Endocarditis; Infection; Inflammation; Myocarditis; Pericarditis.

Myocarditis

CATEGORY: Diseases and conditions
ANATOMY OR SYSTEM AFFECTED: Cardiovascular system, heart

DEFINITION

Myocarditis is an inflammation of the heart's muscular wall, the myocardium. Although rare, it can be devastating. Myocarditis can occur with no symptoms and can remain undiagnosed.

CAUSES

Many cases of myocarditis have no identifiable cause and are called idiopathic myocarditis. When a cause is identified, the myocarditis falls into one of three categories: infectious, toxic, and immune-mediated.

Infectious myocarditis is caused by either a viral infection from viruses such as measles, rabies, or human immunodeficiency virus (HIV); a bacterial infection from bacteria such as diphtheria or *Mycobacterium*; or a fungal infection from *Aspergillus* or *Candida*.

Toxic myocarditis is caused by drugs such as chemotherapeutic drugs, lithium, or cocaine; by heavy metals such as copper, iron, or lead; by toxic substances such as arsenic, carbon monoxide, or other inhalants; and by physical agents such as electric shock or radiation.

Immune-mediated myocarditis is caused by an allergic reaction to penicillin or streptomycin; by alloantigens, including heart transplant rejection; and by autoantigens, including Chagas' disease, scleroderma, or lupus.

RISK FACTORS

There are no known risk factors for developing myocarditis.

SYMPTOMS

The symptoms of myocarditis vary from person to person depending on the cause and the severity. Furthermore, some people have no symptoms and are thus asymptomatic. The following symptoms may appear slowly or suddenly: flulike complaints, including fever, fatigue, muscle pain, vomiting, diarrhea, and weakness; a rapid heart rate; chest pain; shortness of breath and respiratory distress; and a loss of consciousness. Sudden, intense myocarditis can lead to congestive heart failure and death.

SCREENING AND DIAGNOSIS

The diagnosis of myocarditis is often difficult. There is no specific test for it. Many other causes of heart problems must be ruled out. To do this, a doctor will ask the patient about symptoms and medical history and will perform a physical exam. Tests may include an electrocardiogram (ECG), which records the heart's activity by measuring electrical currents through the heart muscle; a chest X ray, which uses radiation to take pictures of structures inside the body; a cardiac enzyme blood test (because, in some cases, certain enzymes are elevated); an echocardiogram, which uses high-frequency sound waves, or ultrasound, to examine the size, shape, and motion of the heart; a biopsy (the removal of a sample of heart tissue to test for infection); and cardiovascular magnetic resonance imaging (the use of magnetic waves to take pictures of structures inside the body).

TREATMENT AND THERAPY

The universally recommended therapy for myocarditis is bed rest, no physical activity, and supplemental oxygen. Corticosteroids may be given to help inflammation, and the patient will most likely be admitted to a hospital.

Specific treatment is directed at the underlying cause, if possible. For instance, if the cause is a bacte-

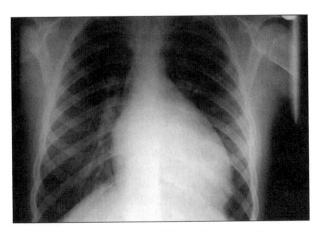

Chest X ray of a sixteen-year-old boy with myocarditis.

rial infection, the doctor will prescribe antibiotics; if the cause is viral, the doctor will prescribe antiviral agents. Immunosuppressive therapy may be used if the myocarditis is caused by an autoimmune disorder such as lupus or scleroderma.

If heart failure symptoms are present, the doctor will prescribe medications to support the function of the heart. These medications include diuretics, ACE-inhibitors, beta-blockers, and antiarrhythmic agents. Additionally, a defibrillator, which helps maintain the normal rhythm of the heart, may be implanted into the patient's chest. Severe cases may require a cardiac transplant.

PREVENTION AND OUTCOMES

Myocarditis is difficult to prevent. To help reduce the chance of getting myocarditis, one should reduce exposure to identified causes. Some examples of prevention include practicing good hygiene to avoid the spread of infection (for example, washing one's hands regularly), always using latex condoms during sexual intercourse, having monogamous sex, and avoiding illegal drugs.

Mary Calvagna, M.S.;
reviewed by David N. Smith, M.D.

FURTHER READING

Brady, W. J., et al. "Myocarditis: Emergency Department Recognition and Management. *Emergency Medicine Clinics of North America* 22, no. 4 (2004): 865-885.

Crawford, Michael, ed. *Current Diagnosis and Treatment—Cardiology.* 3d ed. New York: McGraw-Hill Medical, 2009.

Feldman, A. M., and D. McNamara. "Myocarditis." *New England Journal of Medicine* 343, no. 19 (2000): 1388-1398.

Felker, G. M., et al. "Underlying Causes and Long-Term Survival in Patients with Initially Unexplained Cardiomyopathy." *New England Journal of Medicine* 342 (2000): 1077.

Zipes, Douglas P., et al., eds. *Braunwald's Heart Disease: A Textbook of Cardiovascular Medicine.* 8th ed. Philadelphia: Saunders/Elsevier, 2008.

Web Sites of Interest

American Heart Association
http://www.heart.org

National Heart, Lung, and Blood Institute
http://www.nhlbi.nih.gov

See also: Bacterial endocarditis; Bacterial infections; Diagnosis of fungal infections; Endocarditis; Immune response to fungal infections; Inflammation; Myositis; Pericarditis; Rheumatic fever; Viral infections.

Myositis

CATEGORY: Diseases and conditions
ANATOMY OR SYSTEM AFFECTED: Muscles, musculoskeletal system
ALSO KNOWN AS: Idiopathic inflammatory myopathy, inflammatory myopathy

DEFINITION

Myositis is a general term for a group of rare chronic conditions characterized by inflammation of the skeletal muscles. This inflammation can cause muscle weakness. Myositis refers to the inflammatory myopathies, including polymyositis, dermatomyositis, inclusion-body myositis, and juvenile myositis. It is thought that all these disorders are autoimmune diseases. Inflammatory myopathies can also be caused by certain medications or by exposure to a toxic substance; these myopathies are usually not chronic and resolve once the harmful substance is removed.

CAUSES

It is not known what causes myositis. It is believed that an environmental factor, such as a viral infection, triggers myositis in people who might be genetically predisposed to the condition. The damage in myositis is caused by the body's own immune system, as white blood cells and antibodies attack the muscle and, in some cases, the skin.

RISK FACTORS

Generally, women are affected more often than men, although inclusion-body myositis affects twice as many men as women. Polymyositis is observed in persons between twenty and sixty years of age, whereas inclusion-body myositis is more common after age fifty years. Children can develop dermatomyositis. African Americans are at higher risk for myositis, while the lowest rates of myositis are reported in persons of Japanese origin.

SYMPTOMS

Common symptoms of the inflammatory myopathies include muscle weakness, sometimes with muscle pain, that lasts for more than a few weeks; general tiredness and fatigue; difficulty climbing stairs, standing up from a seated position, or reaching up; and difficulty swallowing. Additional symptoms for the various myopathies include a variety of skin symptoms (such as a rash or scaly, dry, and rough skin) in dermatomyositis; and hardened lumps of calcium (calcinosis) under the skin in juvenile dermatomyositis. Unlike other inflammatory myopathies, the muscle weakness in inclusion-body myositis is often asymmetrical.

SCREENING AND DIAGNOSIS

Myositis varies from person to person and can often resemble other diseases, such as scleroderma or lupus. Tests used to help confirm a diagnosis include a physical exam; tests of muscle strength; magnetic resonance imaging (MRI) scan; an electromyogram (EMG); blood tests, including erythrocyte sedimentation rate, creatinine kinase, and antinuclear antibodies; and muscle and skin biopsies.

TREATMENT AND THERAPY

Treatment for myositis generally includes rest, physical therapy, and the use of anti-inflammatories (corticosteroids as first-line therapy and methotrexate, hydroxychloroquine, and azathioprine), and intravenous immunoglobulin. If left untreated, inflammatory myopathy can cause permanent damage.

PREVENTION AND OUTCOMES

Because the cause of myositis is unknown, there is no known way to prevent the condition. To lessen the severity of dermatomyositis, however, persons with the condition should avoid excessive exposure to the sun, which can worsen any dermatomyositis-associated skin rashes.

Anita P. Kuan, Ph.D.

FURTHER READING

Isenberg, D. A., et al. "International Consensus Outcome Measures for Patients with Idiopathic Inflammatory Myopathies: Development and Initial Validation of Myositis Activity and Damage Indices in Patients with Adult Onset Disease." *Rheumatology* 43, no. 1 (January, 2004): 49-54.

Kagen, Lawrence J., ed. *The Inflammatory Myopathies.* Totowa, N.J.: Humana Press, 2009.

Marieb, Elaine N. *Essentials of Human Anatomy and Physiology.* 8th ed. San Francisco: Pearson/Benjamin Cummings, 2006.

Murphy, Kenneth, Paul Travers, and Mark Walport. *Janeway's Immunobiology.* 7th ed. New York: Garland Science, 2008.

Parker, James N., and Philip M. Parker, eds. *Myositis: A Medical Dictionary, Bibliography, and Annotated Research Guide to Internet References.* San Diego, Calif.: ICON Health, 2004.

WEB SITES OF INTEREST

American Autoimmune Related Diseases Association
http://www.aarda.org

Myositis Association
http://www.myositis.org

National Institute of Neurological Disorders and Stroke
http://www.ninds.nih.gov/disorders

National Organization for Rare Disorders
http://www.rarediseases.org

See also: Acute cerebellar ataxia; Autoimmune disorders; Bacterial endocarditis; Bell's palsy; Creutzfeldt-Jakob disease; Endocarditis; Gerstmann-Sträussler-Scheinker syndrome; Guillain-Barré syndrome; Inflammation; Meningococcal meningitis; Myocarditis; Pericarditis; Rheumatic fever; Sarcosporidiosis; Tetanus.

N

Nasopharyngeal infections

CATEGORY: Diseases and conditions
ANATOMY OR SYSTEM AFFECTED: Nose, pharynx, upper respiratory tract, throat
ALSO KNOWN AS: Upper respiratory tract infections

DEFINITION

Nasopharyngeal infections are upper respiratory infections (URIs) caused by bacteria or viruses growing in the nasopharynx, the back of the throat, the top of the soft palate, and the nasal passages.

CAUSES

Nasopharyngeal infections result from direct contact with discharge or droplets from the mouth or nose of infected persons through coughing or sneezing. The most frequent illnesses from organisms in the nasopharynx include the common cold and influenza. Some two hundred viruses cause the common cold, including retrovirus, coronaviruses, adenovirus, enterovirus, respiratory syncytial virus (RSV), and influenza A and B viruses. Retrovirus accounts for about 53 percent of colds.

About 5 to 15 percent of URIs are caused by group A streptococcal bacteria, including *Streptococcus pyogenes*. *Bordetella pertussis* and *Corynebacterium diphtheriae*, sometimes found in the nasopharynx, cause severe upper respiratory infections but are infrequent in the United States because of immunizations.

Asymptomatic carriers of nasopharyngeal organisms such as *Staphylococcus aureus*, *Streptococcus pneumonia*, and *Neisseria meningitidis* spread these organisms through nasal secretions. *S. aureus* and *S. pneumonia* can cause pneumonia and *N. meningitidis* can result in meningitis.

The incubation period for URIs varies with causative organisms. Cold viruses can show symptoms within sixteen hours of contact with infected persons; an average incubation period is twenty-four to forty-eight hours, with a duration of seven to ten days.

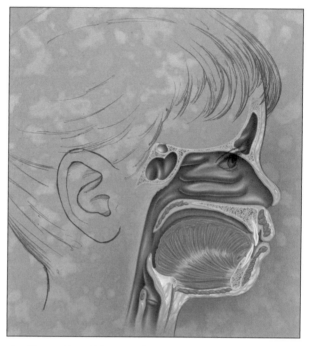

An illustration of the nasopharynx of a child.

RISK FACTORS

Nasopharyngeal infections are the most common infectious diseases in the United States. More than one billion people contract colds each year. Incidence varies by age, with greatest risk for children younger than age five years. The prevalence of the cold for children attending school or day care is between three and eight per year. Older youth and adults contract colds two to four times yearly, while those older than age sixty experience yearly colds.

Persons with influenza usually experience URI symptoms in the early stages of disease. Some 5 to 15 percent of Americans experience flu annually. Influenza outbreaks are risky to public health.

URIs occur anytime of the year, but mostly in the fall to early spring. In cold weather, people tend to gather indoors at work or school in close, less ventilated environments, increasing exposure to infected persons. Humidity levels are often lower in winter too; URI viruses thrive in low humidity with cold temperatures. Persons with suppressed immune systems or who are under acute or chronic stress are at risk for URIs. When normal defenses of the nasopharynx are compromised, URIs may occur.

SYMPTOMS

Nasopharyngeal infections produce typical URI symptoms. Cold symptoms include nasal congestion, runny nose, and sneezing. Additional symptoms include sore throat, post nasal drip, cough, mild headache, muscle aches, malaise, watery eyes, hoarseness, mild fever (less than 101° Farhenheit), and decreased appetite. Mucus secretions may change from thin to thick and from clear to yellow or green. However, symptoms of flu include high fever (102° to 104° F) in a three-to-four-day period, prominent headaches, severe aches, chest congestion, and fatigue or exhaustion.

SCREENING AND DIAGNOSIS

Health care providers take medical histories and perform physical examinations to diagnose URIs. They review self-report complaints. Diagnosis is made on assessment of physical symptoms of the suspected URI, ranging from scratchy, nasal stuffiness with reddened pharynx to marked redness of the pharynx and fever. If clinical symptoms indicate a common cold, no further tests are done.

Viral cultures may be needed to diagnose serious URIs, such as influenza with potential complications like pneumonia. A throat or nasal culture guides treatment. A nasopharyngeal culture may be appropriate for infants, the elderly, or for debilitated persons. The culture results will determine the course of therapy.

TREATMENT AND THERAPY

Treatment of nasopharyngeal infections depends on the causative agent and course of the illness. The common cold has no prescribed therapy and can be treated in diverse ways. Some $2.5 billion is spent annually treating colds, including with many over-the-counter medications. Treatment of URIs includes antiviral medications, interferon nasal spray, zinc gluconate lozenges, and high doses of vitamin C. Most people manage their common cold symptomatically, with acetaminophen or ibuprofen used for relief of pain, fever, and muscle aches. Antihistamines, decongestants, and cough syrups or mucolytics address symptoms. One should maintain adequate fluid intake and get plenty of rest.

Antibiotics are not prescribed for the common cold or flu because they are ineffective against viruses. They may treat bacterial complications such as bronchitis, acute otitis media, or pneumonia. Patient comorbidities, including asthma, kidney disease, diabetes, and cardiac concerns, are considered when diagnosing and treating persons with URIs.

PREVENTION AND OUTCOMES

The common cold causes the greatest loss of work and school days in the United States. Some 23 million days of work and 26 million school days are missed annually with colds. Common cold translates to $25 billion in lost productivity. Up to 15 percent of persons in the United States contracts influenza. URIs, combined, cost industry $71 to $167 billion each year.

Primary prevention of URIs depends on a healthy nasopharynx to trap foreign organisms. Precautions include covering the mouth when sneezing or coughing, frequent handwashing, and minimizing touching of the face with hands. Lifestyle changes include exercise, a nutritious diet, and sufficient rest, all of which promote a healthy immune system. Adequate hydration keeps mucus membranes moist so the natural defenses in the nasal passages can function best. Complementary therapies may help boost the immune system to decrease URIs.

Influenza vaccinations are encouraged each fall for healthy people but especially for the most vulnerable, including the young, old, debilitated, or immunosuppressed. Health care workers are at risk of exposure and may benefit from vaccinations.

Marylane Wade Koch, M.S.N., R.N.

FURTHER READING

Brammer, Lynette, et al. "Influenza." *Manual for the Surveillance of Vaccine Preventable-Disease.* 4th ed. Atlanta: Centers for Disease Control and Prevention, 2008. Available online at http://www.cdc.gov/vaccines/pubs/surv-manual/default.htm. Details the surveillance of influenza symptoms, vaccination options, and possible complications.

"Common Cold." MedlinePlus. Available at http://www.nlm.nih.gov/medlineplus/ency/article/000678.htm. Easy-to-read introductory information on the common cold.

Helms, Richard A., et al., eds. *Textbook of Therapeutics: Drug and Disease Management.* 8th ed. Philadelphia: Lippincott Williams & Wilkins, 2006. Provides a comprehensive review of disease and medication management for major body systems, including management of the common cold and flu.

Pettigrew, Melinda M., et al. "Microbial Interactions During Upper Respiratory Tract Infections." *Emerging Infectious Disease* 10 (2008): 1584-1591. Discusses how bacteria can colonize the nasopharynx of children with susceptibility after a URI and with vaccination, and also examines antimicrobial strategies.

WEB SITES OF INTEREST

Centers for Disease Control and Prevention, Flu Vaccinations
http://www.cdc.gov/vaccines/vpd-vac/flu/default.htm

World Health Organization, Fact Sheet on Influenza
http://www.who.int/mediacentre/factsheets/2003/fs211

See also:: Adenovirus infections; Bacterial infections; Bronchiolitis; Bronchitis; Children and infectious disease; Common cold; Coronavirus infections; Enterovirus infections; Epiglottitis; Epstein-Barr virus infection; Fever; Influenza; Mononucleosis; Parotitis; Pharyngitis and tonsillopharyngitis; Pneumonia; Respiratory syncytial virus infections; Retroviral infections; Strep throat; Viral infections; Viral pharyngitis; Viral upper respiratory infections.

National Institute of Allergy and Infectious Diseases

CATEGORY: Epidemiology

DEFINITION

The National Institute of Allergy and Infectious Diseases (NIAID) is one of twenty-seven U.S. government institutes under the umbrella of the National Institutes of Health (NIH), located in Bethesda, Maryland. NIAID conducts and supports basic, translational, and clinical research to better understand, treat, and prevent immunological and infectious diseases. To protect public health, NIAID is in the forefront of disease knowledge, expertise, and response, especially the response to emerging threats. NIAID has identified the following diseases as research priorities for the institute: the human immunodeficiency virus (HIV), acquired immunodeficiency syndrome (AIDS), emerging and reemerging infectious diseases, and bioterrorism.

HISTORY

The beginnings of NIAID can be traced to the Marine Hospital on Staten Island, New York, in 1887, and a young Marine Hospital Service physician named Joseph Kinyoun. As Kinyoun and others began to realize, immigrants arriving on the shores of the United States often brought with them infectious diseases, such as cholera and yellow fever. Kinyoun, who had seen science research centers in Europe, had also learned about the new science of bacteriology and put its principles to use by screening newly arrived immigrants at the bacteriological laboratory he founded on Staten Island. In 1891, Kinyoun's laboratory was moved to Washington, D.C., and was tasked by the U.S. Congress to study infectious diseases and to protect the public health. In 1930, the then-called Hygienic Laboratory was moved to Bethesda, Maryland. The lab became the National Institute of Health in 1938. In 1948, several public health laboratories and divisions within the NIH were combined to form the National Microbiological Institute, and in 1955, Congress changed the name to NIAID to recognize the related scientific disciplines of immunology and the study of allergies.

ACTIVITIES

NIAID operates with an annual budget of nearly $5 billion. Because diseases are not confined to a country's borders, NIAID develops and supports a national and international network of cooperative biomedical research institutions and trains scientists around the world. Through grants and directed research, NIAID ensures the existence of a research infrastructure, directs the research that will fill gaps in knowledge in priority areas, and provides the scientific expertise to assist in applying that knowledge to the development of vaccines, diagnostics, and other therapies. NIAID also communicates research findings to the scientific community, to policymakers, and to the general public.

IMPACT

The swine flu pandemic of 2009 is evidence of the global nature of infectious disease, and NIAID played a crucial role in the national and international response to the pandemic. NIAID remains a necessary globally focused institution whether the health threats it responds to are biological (as in pandemics and drug resistance) or are human made (as in bioterrorism).

Linda J. Miwa, M.P.H.

FURTHER READING

Eberhart-Philips, Jason. *Outbreak Alert: Responding to the Increasing Threat of Infectious Diseases.* Oakland, Calif.: New Harbinger, 2000.

Hannaway, Caroline, ed. *Biomedicine in the Twentieth Century: Practices, Policies, and Politics.* Washington, D.C.: IOS Press, 2008.

National Institute of Allergy and Infectious Diseases. *The Edge of Discovery: A Portrait of the National Institute of Allergy and Infectious Diseases.* Bethesda, Md.: National Institutes of Health, 2009. Also available at http://www.niaid.nih.gov/about/whoweare/documents/niaidedge.pdf.

_____. *NIAID Planning for the Twenty-first Century: 2008 Update.* Bethesda, Md.: National Institutes of Health, 2008. Also available at http://www.niaid.nih.gov/about/whoweare/documents/niaidstrategicplan2008.pdf.

National Research Council, Committee on the Organizational Structure of the National Institutes of Health. *Enhancing the Vitality of the National Institutes of Health.* Washington, D.C.: National Academy Press, 2003.

St. Georgiev, Vassil. *Impact on Global Health.* Vol. 2 in *National Institute of Allergy and Infectious Diseases, NIH,* edited by Vassil St. Georgiev, K. A. Western, and J. J. McGowan. Totowa, N.J.: Humana Press, 2009.

WEB SITES OF INTEREST

Emerging and Reemerging Infectious Diseases Resource Center
http://www.medscape.com/resource/infections

National Institute of Allergy and Infectious Diseases
http://www.niaid.nih.gov

National Institutes of Health
http://history.nih.gov/exhibits/history

See also: Biosurveillance; Bioterrorism; Centers for Disease Control and Prevention (CDC); Developing countries and infectious disease; Disease eradication campaigns; Emerging and reemerging infectious diseases; Emerging Infections Network; Epidemics and pandemics: Causes and management; Epidemiology; Infectious disease specialists; National Institutes of Health; Outbreaks; Public health; Social effects of infectious disease; U.S. Army Medical Research Institute of Infectious Diseases; World Health Organization (WHO).

National Institutes of Health

CATEGORY: Epidemiology

DEFINITION

The National Institutes of Health (NIH) is a United States government agency comprising twenty-seven institutes and centers. Together, the institutes are focused on reducing illness and enhancing health. The NIH also administers the National Library of Medicine (NLM).

HISTORY

The NIH began as a small Marine Hospital Service laboratory on Staten Island, New York, in 1887, with a physician, Joseph Kinyoun, as its only employee. Rather than simply depend on symptoms for diagnostic purposes, Kinyoun discovered that culturing cholera bacteria was a reliable way to determine if immigrants to the United States had cholera. The Hygienic Laboratory, as it was then called, was moved to Washington, D.C., in the late nineteenth century, and the U.S. Congress authorized construction for a lab to investigate infectious diseases. Infectious diseases had only recently been found to be caused by germs.

The name of the lab became the National Institute of Health in 1930, the same year that fellowships were started there. At this point, research was still intramural; in the 1940's, extramural grant funding to researchers at other institutions was established, and the agency grew tremendously during this period. In 1948, the agency became known as the National Institutes (plural) of Health, and specialty areas were split into institutes, which have increased in number since and which are now located in Bethesda, Maryland.

Centers and Institutes of the National Institutes of Health

Center for Information Technology
Center for Scientific Review
Eunice Kennedy Shriver National Institute of Child
   Health and Human Development
John E. Fogarty International Center for Advanced
   Study in the Health Sciences
National Cancer Institute
National Center for Complementary and Alternative
   Medicine
National Center for Research Resources
National Center on Minority Health and Health
   Disparities
National Eye Institute
National Heart, Lung, and Blood Institute
National Human Genome Research Institute
National Institute of Allergy and Infectious Diseases
National Institute of Arthritis and Musculoskeletal and
   Skin Diseases

National Institute of Biomedical Imaging and
   Bioengineering
National Institute of Dental and Craniofacial Research
National Institute of Diabetes and Digestive and Kidney
   Diseases
National Institute of Environmental Health Sciences
National Institute of General Medical Sciences
National Institute of Mental Health
National Institute of Neurological Disorders and Stroke
National Institute of Nursing Research
National Institute on Aging
National Institute on Alcohol Abuse and Alcoholism
National Institute on Deafness and Other
   Communication Disorders
National Institute on Drug Abuse
National Library of Medicine
NIH Clinical Center

The NLM, the world's largest medical library, was founded in 1836 as the library of the surgeon general of the Army; it became part of the NIH in 1968.

The NIH allocates funding for training programs and for intramural and extramural research studies through competitive grant mechanisms. The NIH also provides a wide range of information on published and ongoing research, on clinical trials seeking participants, and on research priorities. All this information is available on the Web sites of the NIH and the NLM.

NATIONAL INSTITUTE OF ALLERGY AND INFECTIOUS DISEASES (NIAID)

NIAID is one of the most highly funded institutes of the NIH, primarily because of the major public health concerns of human immunodeficiency virus (HIV) infection and other global infectious diseases, and of bioterrorism with infectious biological agents. Because infectious disease was the initial focus of research for what would become the NIH, NIAID can trace its roots to the very start of the one-room lab in New York in 1887.

NIAID was officially founded in 1948 with the mission of understanding, preventing, and treating infectious, immunologic, and allergic diseases. NIAID research focuses on diagnostic tests and the creation of vaccines and therapeutic treatments. Research study topics include avian flu, HIV and acquired immuno-

deficiency syndrome (AIDS), antivirals for influenza viruses, malaria, immunomodulation, *Mycobacterium tuberculosis*, and genetic susceptibility to infectious diseases.

NIAID's labs are located at NIH headquarters in Bethesda and at the Rocky Mountain Laboratories in Hamilton, Montana.

MAJOR CONTRIBUTIONS

There are far too many discoveries and advances supported by the NIH in infectious disease research to list, so only a brief sampling is provided here. For example, in one critical case, NIAID had funded an initiative for the discovery of HIV protease inhibitors that ultimately led to the use of combination therapy and to a longer life expectancy for those infected with HIV. Other research has found a vulnerable area on the virus, a finding that could lead to the development of a vaccine. A major initiative for development of drug treatments for tuberculosis is ongoing, leading to the identification of some promising drugs to treat the disease. (Clinical trials can begin when thorough safety data has been obtained.)

NIAID researchers also have developed a technique to rapidly detect influenza strains to determine appropriate treatment, which will limit the spread of a potential flu pandemic. A vaccine was developed in the 1990's for *Streptococcus pneumonia*, an infection that still threatens the lives of children worldwide. Genome sequences of viruses and bacteria, such as *Plasmodium*, which causes malaria, are currently being utilized to develop better vaccines.

About 10 percent of the funds allocated by the NIH for NIAID research is for studies taking place abroad. NIAID collaborates with the World Health Organization and with the United Nations to try to reduce the burden of infectious diseases worldwide. International Centers of Excellence in Research are considered a crucial part of the NIAID research portfolio. Collaborations are forged between established researchers in the United States and scientists in other countries in an effort to foster long-term relationships and to set up infrastructure and training programs in countries that otherwise would not obtain them.

IMPACT

The NIH has had a tremendous impact on the health of U.S. citizens and people throughout the world. The vaccines and treatments for illness discovered through NIH-funded research, particularly by the NIAID, and all future discoveries, will continue to make a difference, especially for the developing world.

Dawn M. Bielawski, Ph.D.

FURTHER READING

Eberhart-Philips, Jason. *Outbreak Alert: Responding to the Increasing Threat of Infectious Diseases.* Oakland, Calif.: New Harbinger, 2000.

Hannaway, Caroline, ed. *Biomedicine in the Twentieth Century: Practices, Policies, and Politics.* Washington, D.C.: IOS Press, 2008.

Kastor, John. A. *The National Institutes of Health, 1991-2008.* New York: Oxford University Press, 2010.

Miles, Wyndham D. *A History of the National Library of Medicine, the Nation's Treasury of Medical Knowledge.* Reprint. Washington, D.C.: Government Printing Office, 1985.

National Institute of Allergy and Infectious Diseases. *The Edge of Discovery: A Portrait of the National Institute of Allergy and Infectious Diseases.* Bethesda, Md.: National Institutes of Health, 2009. Also available at http://www.niaid.nih.gov/about/whoweare/documents/niaidedge.pdf.

National Institutes of Health, Office of Research on Women's Health. *Women in Science at the National Institutes of Health, 2007-2008.* Bethesda, Md.: Author, 2008.

National Research Council, Committee on the Organizational Structure of the National Institutes of Health. *Enhancing the Vitality of the National Institutes of Health.* Washington, D.C.: National Academy Press, 2003.

Potts, John T., Jr. "The Early Days at the National Institutes of Health." *Annals of the New York Academy of Sciences* 1192 (2010): 1-4.

St. Georgiev, Vassil. *Frontiers in Research.* Vol. 1 in *National Institute of Allergy and Infectious Diseases, NIH*, edited by Vassil St. Georgiev, K. A. Western, and J. J. McGowan. Totowa, N.J.: Humana Press, 2008

WEB SITES OF INTEREST

National Institute of Allergy and Infectious Diseases
http://www.niaid.nih.gov

National Institutes of Health
http://history.nih.gov

See also:: Biosurveillance; Bioterrorism; Centers for Disease Control and Prevention (CDC); Developing countries and infectious disease; Disease eradication campaigns; Emerging and reemerging infectious diseases; Emerging Infections Network; Epidemics and pandemics: Causes and management; Epidemiology; Infectious disease specialists; Koch's postulates; National Institute of Allergy and Infectious Diseases; Outbreaks; Public health; Social effects of infectious disease; U.S. Army Medical Research Institute of Infectious Diseases; World Health Organization (WHO).

Natural remedies and therapies. *See* Alternative therapies.

Necrotizing fasciitis

CATEGORY: Diseases and conditions
ANATOMY OR SYSTEM AFFECTED: Skin, tissue
ALSO KNOWN AS: Flesh-eating bacteria, streptococcal gangrene

DEFINITION

Necrotizing fasciitis is a rapidly progressive and aggressive rare infection of fascia and soft tissue that can follow minor trauma or surgery or may occur without any known cause. The term "necrotizing fasciitis" was first used in 1952 to describe a quickly spreading soft tissue infection. The disease has likely existed for centuries and was well documented during the American Civil War.

Although often caused by group A beta-hemolytic streptococci bacteria, the disease, which leads to decaying (gangrenous) skin, can also be caused by many other bacteria and is usually caused by mixed bacterial infection. Prompt diagnosis guided by a high index of suspicion is the key to successful treatment.

CAUSES

Group A streptococcal infection also causes impetigo and strep throat, which are less serious than necrotizing fasciitis. M-protein serotypes of these bacteria may be responsible for the more aggressive necrotizing fasciitis. In most cases, necrotizing fasciitis is caused by a mixed bacterial infection involving aerobic and anaerobic species. Common identified bacterial species include methicillin-resistant *Staphylococcus aureus*, *Escherichia coli*, *Pseudomonas*, *Clostridium*, *Klebsiella*, *Proteus*, *Vibrio*, and *Bacteroides.*

Bacteria may spread to the body from direct contact with an infected person or may already be present on a person's skin. Entry into the body may occur from trauma as minor as a scratch, insect bite, burn, or needle puncture. Surgical procedures are another common cause of entry. Once in the subcutaneous tissue, the infection spreads along facial plains and move deeper into soft tissues to involve muscle and fat. Enzymes and toxins produced by the bacteria may cause vascular occlusion, resulting in a loss of oxygen, tissue necrosis, and toxic shock.

RISK FACTORS

Any person at any age can be affected by necrotizing fasciitis, but persons with compromised immune systems or with certain underlying conditions are at

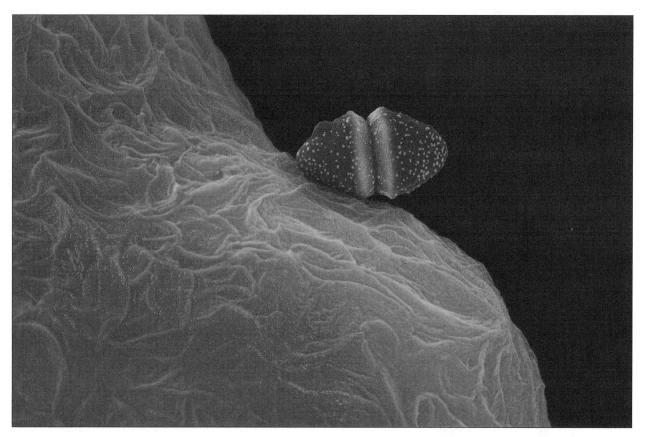

A Streptococcus *bacterium divides into two daughter cells.* S. pyogenes *can cause necrotizing fasciitis, or flesh-eating bacteria.*

higher risk. These risk factors include intravenous drug use, alcoholism, human immunodeficiency virus infection, diabetes, peripheral vascular disease, cancer, renal failure, liver disease, and treatment with chemotherapy or corticosteroids.

SYMPTOMS

Early symptoms of necrotizing fasciitis include an unusual amount of pain in an area of a recent injury. Pain may be like that of a pulled muscle. Symptoms of generalized illness, such as fever, nausea, and weakness, may soon follow.

Within a few days, signs of infection occur. These signs include redness, warmth, and swelling. A blistering rash or dark purple discoloration of the skin may appear. Severe pain may give way to numbness. A cracking noise or sensation beneath the skin (crepitus) may be present. The wound area may begin to open and drain. Signs of toxic shock may include a rapid drop in blood pressure and loss of consciousness.

SCREENING AND DIAGNOSIS

A doctor will ask about symptoms and medical history and will perform a physical exam. Although laboratory studies, tissue cultures, biopsy results, and imaging studies may aid in the diagnosis of necrotizing fasciitis, a presumptive diagnosis may need to be made on history and physical examination alone. The absolute necessity of prompt treatment precludes the need to wait for results of supporting diagnostic tests. Early signs and symptoms can be deceptive, so a high index of suspicion is the key to diagnosis.

Laboratory testing may include a complete blood count that shows elevated white blood cells. Blood cultures may show bacterial growth. Tissue cultures and biopsy are often critical to identifying the infection's pathogens. Helpful imaging studies include a computed tomography scan, magnetic resonance imaging, and an ultrasound.

TREATMENT AND THERAPY

Necrotizing fasciitis is a medical emergency and may require treatment in an intensive care setting. Initial treatment is aimed at stabilizing blood pressure and breathing. Intravenous fluid administration, medication to control blood pressure, oxygen, cardiac monitoring, and intubation may all be necessary in a person presenting with toxic shock.

Broad-spectrum antibiotics should be started without waiting for the results of blood or tissue cultures. Some commonly used antibiotics for this infection are penicillin, clindamycin, vancomycin, and cephalosporins.

The primary and most critical treatment is surgical debridement of all necrotic tissue as soon as the person is stable enough for surgery. A wide surgical field may be needed to remove all diseased tissue until normal tissue is found. Debridement may need to be repeated as necessary until healing of healthy tissue begins. Surgical wounds are often left open and then closed at a later time with skin grafts and reconstructive surgery. In cases where necrotizing fasciitis involves fingers, toes, or other limbs, amputation may be necessary.

Two adjunctive treatments that may be helpful are hyperbaric oxygen therapy and intravenous immunoglobulin. Hyperbaric oxygen may inhibit the growth of anaerobic bacteria and may speed healing. Intravenous immunoglobulin has been shown to neutralize toxins that are produced by streptococcal bacteria.

PREVENTION AND OUTCOMES

Necrotizing fasciitis cannot be completely prevented. Up to 30 percent of persons are asymptomatic carriers of group A streptococcal bacteria. Although the incidence of necrotizing fasciitis has increased in past decades, it is still a very rare disease. The best prevention is to practice good personal hygiene, treat all wounds antiseptically, and seek prompt medical attention for any symptoms of wound infection. Hospitals can help prevent necrotizing fasciitis by maintaining strict surgical, barrier, and isolation techniques. Both patients and caregivers should wash their hands frequently.

Christopher Iliades, M.D.

FURTHER READING

Doer, Steven E. "Necrotizing Fasciitis." Available at http://www.emedicinehealth.com/necrotizing_fasciitis/article_em.htm.

Elliott, D., J. A. Kufera, and R. A. Myers. "The Microbiology of Necrotizing Soft Tissue Infections." *American Journal of Surgery* 179 (2000): 361-366.

Morgan, M. S. "Diagnosis and Management of Necrotizing Fasciitis: A Multiparametric Approach." *Journal of Hospital Infection* 75 (2010): 249-257.

Schwartz, Robert A., and Rajendra Kapila. "Necrotizing Fasciitis." Available at http://emedicine.medscape.com/article/1054438-overview.

WEB SITES OF INTEREST

Centers for Disease Control and Prevention
http://www.cdc.gov

National Necrotizing Fasciitis Foundation
http://www.nnff.org

See also:: Bacterial infections; Cellulitis; Fasciitis; Gangrene; Group A streptococcal infection; Hospitals and infectious disease; Hyperbaric oxygen; Iatrogenic infections; Impetigo; Osteomyelitis; Skin infections; Streptococcal infections; Wound infections.

Neglected tropical diseases. *See* Developing countries and infectious disease; Emerging and reemerging infectious diseases; Tropical medicine; World Health Organization (WHO).

Neisseria

CATEGORY: Pathogen
TRANSMISSION ROUTE: Direct contact, inhalation

DEFINITION

Neisseria is a gram-negative, nonmotile, non-sporeforming, aerobic coccus often found in pairs. The bacterium was named for Albert Neisser, who discovered *N. gonorrhoeae*. Many *Neisseria* are normal flora in the nasopharynx of humans and other animals, but some are human pathogens.

NATURAL HABITAT AND FEATURES

Most *Neisseria* spp. are commensal organisms of the upper respiratory mucosa in humans and other animals. Some species show pathogenicity in humans but pathogenicity has not been reported in other animals. *N. meningitidis* is the most pathogenic of the respiratory species. Of the other respiratory *Neisseria* spp., some are opportunistic pathogens that cause infections in people who are immune compromised or who are otherwise debilitated, while other species are nonpathogenic.

N. gonorrhoeae is an obligate human parasite of the urogenital mucosa. In the laboratory, *Neisseria* spp.

Taxonomic Classification for *Neisseria*

Kingdom: Bacteria
Phylum: Proteobacteria
Class: Betaproteobacteria
Order: Neisseriales
Family: Neisseriaceae
Genus: *Neisseria*
Species:
N. canis
N. cinerea
N. cuniculi
N. elongata
N. gonorrhoeae
N. lactamica
N. macacae
N. meningitidis
N. ovis
N. pharyngis
N. sicca

---

grow best on media that have been enriched with the coenzyme nicotinamide adenine dinucleotide (NAD) and with blood and yeast extract. Incubation is best at 98.6° Fahrenheit (37° Celsius) in a moist chamber enriched with carbon dioxide. *N. meningitidis* strains are especially sensitive to temperature fluctuations and media must be warmed to 98.6° F before inoculation. *Neisseria* spp. are also subject to drying and to ultraviolet light and rarely survive long when away from mucous membranes. Most species appear under the microscope as paired cocci that are somewhat flattened at the junction. *N. elongata* appears as a short rod.

N. gonorrhoeae, also called gonococcus, is the only *Neisseria* sp. that is always parasitic and never commensal, and humans are its only known host. It is the causative agent of both gonorrhea and neonatal ophthalmia and has been associated with meningitis and other systemic infections. Although this species is nonencapsulated, it is still able to evade the human immune system. Immunity is rare and reinfection is common, in part because of the extreme variability and changeability of the surface antigens of *N. gonorrhoeae*.

The bacteria can be transmitted by sexual contact or during the birthing process. Gonorrhea is a common sexually transmitted disease, and it is estimated that more than 700,000 persons are infected in United

States each year. About one-half of the women infected are asymptomatic, while other women show varying degrees of symptoms, including vulvovaginitis, urethritis, and pelvic inflammatory disease. Infected men are usually symptomatic and most commonly show urethritis. Systemic infection is quite rare, but can occur in both genders.

The usual antibiotic treatment for gonorrhea includes third generation cephalosporins such as cefexaime or ceftriaxone, which have replaced penicillins and quinolines because *N. gonorrhoeae* strains that are resistant to these antibiotics have become more common. Azithromycin, an antichlamidial, is often also given in conjunction with cephalosporins because many persons with gonorrhea are also infected with *Chlamydia* spp. An infected female can pass *N. gonorrhoeae* to her fetus during the birthing process. The most common consequence is neonatal ophthalmia, but systemic infections can occur. In the United States, neonatal ophthalmia is usually treated with antibiotic ointment containing erythromycin, neomycin, or tetracycline. Silver nitrate used to be the preferred treatment, but its use has been discontinued as better treatments emerged. Outside the United States, providone-iodine is the preferred treatment because it is less irritating and is a broader-spectrum bacteriocide. No effective vaccine against *N. gonorrhoeae* has been developed, which is not surprising because natural immunity rarely, if ever, develops.

N. meningitidis, also called meningococcus, the most pathogenic of the respiratory *Neisseria*, is host specific to humans, as is gonococcus. It is biochemically and structurally identical to *N. gonorrhoeae* except for its polysaccharide capsule, which it uses to evade the immune system. *N. meningitidis* is subdivided into twelve groups, each defined by capsular antigens. In the United States, group B meningococci are most commonly seen. Other major human pathogenic strains fall into groups A, C, Y, and W. Humans exposed to meningococcus can develop natural immunity to the capsular antigens. The immunity is group specific, but there is some overlap. About 30 percent of people infected with *N. meningitidis* become asymptomatic carriers. The rest develop pharyngitis or other upper respiratory infections. In a small percentage, systemic infection ensues; the most serious of these is meningitis. Although considered a respiratory organism, *N. meningitidis* strains have been found in the urogenital mucosa associated with gonorrhea. Meningococcal

infections are most often spread in schools, barracks, or other places where groups of children or young adults, who have less chance of having developed immunity, congregate.

Although strains resistant to penicillin have emerged, penicillin G is still the preferred treatment. Cephalosporins are also commonly used, especially if penicillin resistance is suspected. When an *N. meningitidis* infection is discovered, all of the infected person's contacts are given prophylactic antibiotic treatment. Vaccines against group B strains have been developed and are commonly administered in the United States. In sub-Saharan Africa, a region known as the meningitis belt, group A strains are the most common pathogenic strains. Although group B vaccines have some effect on group A and other strains, work is underway to develop better broad-spectrum vaccines that will be effective against all groups of *N. meningitidis*.

Among the other *Neisseria* spp., *N. lactamica* and *N. cinerea* are common opportunistic human pathogens. Some human commensals, such as *N. elongata* and *N. subflava*, have occasionally been seen in pathogenic infections. Other species are species-specific nonpathogenic commensals in humans and other animals: *N. canis* in dogs, *N. cuniculus* in rabbits, and *N. macacae* in Rhesus monkeys.

Richard W. Cheney, Jr., Ph.D.

FURTHER READING

Brogden, K., et al. *Virulence Mechanisms of Bacterial Pathogens.* 4th ed. Washington, D.C.: ASM Press, 2007. An overview of the mechanisms used by bacterial pathogens to cause disease. Includes proven strategies for overcoming these mechanisms.

Garrity, George M., ed. *The Proteobacteria.* Vol. 2 in *Bergey's Manual of Systematic Bacteriology.* 2d ed. New York: Springer, 2005. This volume describes the Proteobacteria in detail.

Madigan, Michael T., and John M. Martinko. *Brock Biology of Microorganisms.* 12th ed. Upper Saddle River, N.J.: Pearson/Prentice Hall, 2010. This text outlines many common bacteria and describes their natural history, pathogenicity, and other characteristics.

Shmaefsky, Brian. *Meningitis.* Rev. ed. Philadelphia: Chelsea House, 2010. An updated discussion of meningitis.

Workowski, Kimberly A., Stuart M. Berman, and John

M. Douglas, Jr. "Emerging Antimicrobial Resistance in *Neisseria gonorrhea*: Urgent Need to Strengthen Prevention Strategies." *Annals of Internal Medicine* 148 (2008): 606-613. Discusses the problems associated with antibiotic resistance in treating *N. gonorrhoeae* infections.

Web Sites of Interest

American Social Health Association
http://www.ashastd.org

Centers for Disease Control and Prevention
http://www.cdc.gov

See also:: Bacterial infections; Bacterial meningitis; Conjunctivitis; Eye infections; Gonorrhea; Guillain-Barré syndrome; Meningococcal meningitis; Meningococcal vaccine; Neisserial infections; Sexually transmitted diseases (STDs); Urethritis.

Neisserial infections

Category: Diseases and conditions
Anatomy or system affected: Brain, central nervous system, eyes, genitourinary tract, spinal cord, throat, tissue, vision
Also known as: Bacterial meningitis, clap, gonococcus, gonorrhea, meningococcus, spinal meningitis

Definition

Neisseria is a gram-negative, bean-shaped cocci that grows in pairs, or diplococci. The bacterium infects the genitourinary tract, rectum, throat, conjunctiva, and the tissue covering the brain and spinal cord.

Causes

Most meningococci are grouped based on the composition of their polysaccharide capsule. Meningococci in groups A, B, C, W135, and Y cause meningitis. However, *N. meningitidis* commonly inhabits the human throat without causing disease. Disease begins when meningococci invade a person's bloodstream. From the blood, the bacteria penetrate the tissue covering the brain and spinal cord and infect the cerebrospinal fluid. Excessive production of endotoxin can lead to tissue destruction, amputations, and death in 85 percent of untreated cases.

N. gonorrhoeae causes the sexually transmitted disease gonorrhea. The genitourinary tract, throat, and rectum are infected through sexual contact. The conjunctiva of a newborn can be infected during childbirth in cases in which the pregnant woman is infected.

Risk Factors

N. meningitidis is transmitted in droplets caused by coughing, so persons in close contact, such as dormitory residents or personnel in military barracks, are at risk for transmission. It is hypothesized that tobacco smokers are more susceptible. *N. gonorrhoeae* is transmitted through sexual contact; failing to use condoms is the greatest risk.

Symptoms

Meningococcal meningitis is characterized by a rapidly rising fever followed by coma. Common symptoms are a stiff neck disallowing the infected person from touching chin to chest and a spotty rash that does not "bleach" when pressed with a clear glass.

Men with gonorrhea have pain with urination and have a pus-filled discharge. These symptoms usually develop less than one week after sexual contact with an infected partner. If untreated, the gonococci can infect the prostate gland. Sterility results if the sperm ducts are blocked with scar tissue.

The symptoms of gonorrhea are less pronounced in women. Gonococci enter the vagina and then move into the cervix, uterus, and Fallopian tubes. The only symptom of infection is a pus-filled discharge. Sterility, a long-term consequence of gonorrhea in women, occurs when scar tissue is deposited and blocks the Fallopian tubes. Pelvic inflammatory disease caused by *N. gonorrhoeae* also can lead to loss of fertility.

Screening and Diagnosis

Definitive diagnosis of meningococcal meningitis is performed by identifying the bacterium in the cerebrospinal fluid, which is retrieved by a spinal tap. In the laboratory, clinical specimens are applied to a glass slide and stained using the Gram-staining procedure. Gram-negative, bean-shaped diplococci that are visible under the microscope indicate infection. Especially in females, the Gram's stain can yield a false-negative result. Analysis to detect bacterial deoxyribonucleic acid (DNA) is performed in many labs too.

TREATMENT AND THERAPY

Rifampin is used to prevent the development of meningitis in asymptomatic persons exposed to infected persons. Erythromycin and chloramphenicol are used to treat meningitis in persons who are sensitive to penicillin and ampicillin. Triple antibiotic therapy with doxycycline, ciprofloxacin, and metronidazole is recommended for gonorrhea.

PREVENTION AND OUTCOMES

Meningitis caused by four groups is preventable with a tetravalent glycoconjugate vaccine. Group B meningococcal infection is not vaccine preventable because the capsular polysaccharide shares the same structure with fetal brain tissue and is, therefore, non-immunogenic. Suspicion of meningococcal meningitis will cause public health officials to recommend immediate initiation of antibiotic treatment for all close contacts of the infected person. Gonorrhea is preventable through the use of condoms or through abstinence.

Kimberly A. Napoli, M.S.

FURTHER READING

Handsfield, H. H., et al. "*Neisseria gonorrhoeae.*" In *Mandell, Douglas, and Bennett's Principles and Practice of Infectious Diseases*, edited by Gerald L. Mandell, John F. Bennett, and Raphael Dolin. 7th ed. New York: Churchill Livingstone/Elsevier, 2010.

Schrier, Robert W., ed. *Diseases of the Kidney and Urinary Tract.* 8th ed. Philadelphia: Wolters Kluwer Health/Lippincott Williams & Wilkins, 2007.

Shmaefsky, Brian. *Meningitis.* Rev. ed. Philadelphia: Chelsea House, 2010.

WEB SITES OF INTEREST

American Social Health Association
http://www.ashastd.org

Centers for Disease Control and Prevention
http://www/cdc.gov

Meningitis Foundation of America
http://www.musa.org

National Institute of Neurological Disorders and Stroke
http://www.ninds.nih.gov

See also:: Bacterial infections; Bacterial meningitis; Conjunctivitis; Eye infections; Gonorrhea; Guillain-Barré syndrome; Meningococcal meningitis; Meningococcal vaccine; *Neisseria*; Sexually transmitted diseases (STDs); Urethritis.

Neonatal sepsis

CATEGORY: Diseases and conditions
ANATOMY OR SYSTEM AFFECTED: Blood, reproductive system

DEFINITION

Neonatal sepsis, a bacterial infection in the blood that may become a serious condition, is sometimes found in infants during the first month of life.

CAUSES

Neonatal sepsis is caused when the fetus or baby is exposed to bacteria. Early-onset sepsis that develops within the first week of birth comes from the pregnant woman (through the placenta or from passing through the birth canal). Late-onset sepsis that develops one week after birth comes from the caregiving environment. Intrapartum antibiotics have prevented early-onset bacterial sepsis.

Some factors related to a woman's pregnancy or health also add to the chance that the fetus or newborn can get this condition. These factors include labor complications resulting in traumatic or premature delivery, the breaking of the woman's "water" more than eighteen hours before giving birth, a fever or other infection while in labor, and the long-term need for a catheter while pregnant.

RISK FACTORS

In addition to the foregoing risk factors, the following increase a fetus's or a newborn's chance of developing neonatal sepsis: the baby is born more than three weeks before the due date (it is premature); the woman goes into labor more than three weeks before the due date; the fetus is in distress before being born; the newborn has a low birth weight; the fetus has a bowel movement before being born and the uterus contains fetal stool; and the amniotic fluid that surrounds the baby has a bad smell or the baby has a bad smell at birth. Newborn boys are at greater risk for neonatal sepsis than are newborn girls.

SYMPTOMS

In most cases, symptoms are present within twenty-four hours of birth. In almost all cases, they will be present within forty-eight hours of birth. The following symptoms are not necessarily caused by neonatal sepsis; they may be caused by other, less serious health conditions. However, one should consult a doctor if the baby displays any of the following: a fever or frequent changes in temperature; poor feeding from breast or bottle; decreased or absent urination or a bloated abdomen; vomiting of yellowish material; diarrhea; extreme redness around the belly button; skin rashes; unexplained high or low blood sugar; difficulty waking or unusual sleepiness; jaundiced or overly pale skin; abnormally slow or fast heartbeat; rapid breathing; difficult breathing; periods of no breathing (apnea); bruising or bleeding; seizures; and cool, clammy skin.

SCREENING AND DIAGNOSIS

A doctor will ask about the baby's symptoms and medical history and will perform a physical exam. Tests may include a complete blood count; cultures of the blood, urine, cerebrospinal fluid, and skin lesions; and X rays of the chest or abdomen.

TREATMENT AND THERAPY

One should consult the doctor about the best treatment plan. Treatment depends on the severity of the condition and may last two to twenty-one days. In general, neonates suspected of having sepsis are hospitalized for a minimum of two days to wait for culture results. A well-appearing infant may be monitored without antibiotics. The infant is sent home when cultures are negative. Culture-proven sepsis is treated for seven to twenty-one days, depending on the location of the infection.

The baby may also need to receive antibiotic medication, fluids, glucose, and electrolytes intravenously, or to receive oxygen to help with ventilation (breathing).

PREVENTION AND OUTCOMES

To reduce the chance that a fetus or newborn will get neonatal sepsis, the doctor may prescribe antibi-

otics near the due date for women who have given birth to a baby with neonatal sepsis. The antibiotics will kill dangerous bacteria in the birth canal. The doctor also may test the woman for the bacteria before the due date and prescribe antibiotics, and he or she may recommend breast-feeding, which can help prevent sepsis in some infants.

Julie Rackliffe Lucey, M.S.; reviewed by J. Thomas Megerian, M.D., Ph.D., FAAP

FURTHER READING

Behrman, Richard E., Robert M. Kliegman, and Hal B. Jenson, eds. *Nelson Textbook of Pediatrics.* 18th ed. Philadelphia: Saunders/Elsevier, 2007.

EBSCO Publishing. *DynaMed: Neonatal Sepsis.* Available through http://www.ebscohost.com/dynamed.

Herbst, A., and K. Källén. "Time Between Membrane Rupture and Delivery and Septicemia in Term Neonates." *Obstetrics and Gynecology* 110, no. 3 (September, 2007): 612-618.

Martin, Richard J., Avroy A. Fanaroff, and Michele C. Walsh, eds. *Fanaroff and Martin's Neonatal-Perinatal Medicine: Diseases of the Fetus and Infant.* 2 vols. 8th ed. Philadelphia: Mosby/Elsevier, 2006.

Merenstein, Gerald B., and Sandra L. Gardner, eds. *Merenstein and Gardner's Handbook of Neonatal Intensive Care.* 7th ed. Maryland Heights, Mo.: Mosby/Elsevier, 2011.

WEB SITES OF INTEREST

American Congress of Obstetricians and Gynecologists
http://www.acog.org

Society of Obstetricians and Gynaecologists of Canada
http://www.sogc.org

Women's Health Matters
http://www.womenshealthmatters.ca

See also:: Bloodstream infections; Childbirth and infectious disease; Children and infectious disease; Cytomegalovirus infection; Erythema infectiosum; Group B streptococcal infection; Ophthalmia neonatorum; Pregnancy and infectious disease; Sepsis; Septic arthritis; Vancomycin-resistant enterococci infection; Women and infectious disease.

Neutropenia

CATEGORY: Immune response
ALSO KNOWN AS: Agranulocytosis, granulocytopenia

DEFINITION

Neutropenia occurs when the peripheral blood contains an abnormally low number of circulating neutrophils, a type of white blood cell that helps the body fight bacterial infections. Diagnosis is made when a blood test, the absolute neutrophil count (ANC), is less than 1.5 x 109/liters.

NEUTROPENIA AND THE IMMUNE SYSTEM

Neutrophils are essential to the immune system because they help to destroy bacteria. In homeostasis (physiologic health), the body maintains an equilibrium between neutrophil production and utilization. When this balance is disrupted and more neutrophils are needed than are produced, neutropenia results.

Healthy adults produce about sixty billion neutrophils per day, but only a small percentage is usually expended. Neutrophils, sometimes called granulocytes, are produced in the bone marrow and released through the bloodstream. Neutrophils contain microscopic granules (sacs of enzymes) that help them kill and digest invading microorganisms through a process known as phagocytosis. People with neutropenia cannot rid the body of these foreign organisms and thus become highly susceptible to infection.

SEVERE CHRONIC NEUTROPENIA (SCN)

SCN is characterized by abnormalities in neutrophil production and classified as congenital, cyclic, and chronic idiopathic neutropenia, the causes of which are thought to be a receptor signaling/postreceptor defect, a regulatory defect, and faulty immune mechanisms, respectively. SCNs affect the body's integumentary system and cause infections in the oropharyngeal (throat), respiratory, and gastrointestinal mucosa; the hair follicles; and the skin's glandular structures.

Kostmann's syndrome is an inherited disorder that causes significant fever and infection at birth and throughout life. Newborns typically have little evidence of mature neutrophil production and extremely low ANCs (0.1 x 109/liters). People with cyclic neutropenia have recurring three-to-six-day episodes of neutropenia followed by recovery, and are especially prone to fever and infection during extreme neutropenic periods when ANCs can fall as low as 0.1 x 109/liters. In chronic idiopathic neutropenia, ANCs are normal at birth but become lower in time, thus predisposing patients to infection.

ACQUIRED OR SECONDARY NEUTROPENIA

Autoimmune neutropenia occurs when the immune system attacks the body's own blood neutrophils; diagnosis requires that neutrophil-specific antibodies be present. Many drugs used to treat autoimmune diseases cause bone marrow suppression, compromising blood cell production and increasing the risk for neutropenia.

Chemotherapy-induced neutropenia (CIN) is a serious side effect of cancer treatment. In chemotherapy, cytotoxic agents destroy bone marrow cells and strip the body of its natural defenses against infection. Patients who become very neutropenic may need to halt chemotherapy or have their dosages lowered to prevent infection. CIN is called febrile neutropenia when fever develops in patients with ANCs below 500/cubic millimeters. Fever is the body's response to infection and is especially troubling in these patients because they do not show the usual signs of redness, swelling, and pus associated with infection.

IMPACT

Neutropenia, particularly CIN, results in high morbidity and mortality, increases medical costs, and lowers quality of life. The challenge is to minimize the incidence of infection with the judicious use of therapeutic interventions, such as granulocyte colony stimulating factor (G-CSF) or hematopoietic growth factor, corticosteroids, and broad-spectrum antibiotics.

Barbara Woldin, B.S.

FURTHER READING

"Disorders of Phagocyte Function and Number." In *Hematology: Basic Principles and Practice*, edited by Ronald Hoffman et al. 5th ed. Philadelphia: Churchill Livingstone/Elsevier, 2009.

Hadley, Andrew G., and Peter Soothill, eds. *Alloimmune Disorders of Pregnancy: Anaemia, Thrombocytopenia, and Neutropenia in the Fetus and Newborn.* New York: Cambridge University Press, 2002.

Holland, Steven, et al. "Immunodeficiencies." In *Infectious Diseases*, edited by Jon Cohen, William Powderly, and Steven Opal. Philadelphia: Mosby/Elsevier, 2010.

"Infectious Diseases: Neutropenia (Agranulocytosis; Granulocytopenia)." In *The Merck Manual of Diagnosis and Therapy*, edited by Mark H. Beers et al. 18th ed. Whitehouse Station, N.J.: Merck Research Laboratories, 2006.

Provan, Drew, and John Gribben, eds. *Molecular Haematology*. 2d ed. Malden, Mass.: Blackwell, 2005.

WEB SITES OF INTEREST

Genetic and Rare Diseases Information Center
http://rarediseases.info.nih.gov/gard

Immune Deficiency Foundation
http://www.primaryimmune.org

National Neutropenia Network
http://www.neutropenianet.org

See also:: Agammaglobulinemia; AIDS; Antibiotics: Types; Antibodies; Asplenia; Autoimmune disorders; Bacteria: Classification and types; Bacterial infections; Bloodstream infections; Graft-versus-host disease; HIV; Idiopathic thrombocytopenic purpura; Immune response to bacterial infections; Immune response to fungal infections; Immune response to parasitic diseases; Immune response to viral infections; Immunity; Immunoassay; Immunodeficiency; Seroconversion; T lymphocytes.

Nocardiosis

CATEGORY: Diseases and conditions
ANATOMY OR SYSTEM AFFECTED: Lungs, respiratory system

DEFINITION

Nocardiosis is a respiratory infection caused by the bacterium *Nocardia*, which lives in soil, sand, and water worldwide. Although exposure to *Nocardia* is widespread, infection primarily occurs in people with compromised immunity, such as persons with acquired immunodeficiency syndrome (AIDS).

CAUSES

N. asteroides particularly is the member of the *Nocardia* species that is associated with causing infection in humans. Nocardiosis is believed to occur when air-

borne microbes are inhaled and then colonize the lungs. Infection typically manifests with pneumonia or with the formation of a lung abscess or pus-filled cavity (empyema), or both. Persons who are immunocompromised are susceptible to spread of the infection by way of the bloodstream from the lungs to other organs, such as the heart and adjacent tissues, the brain, skin, bone, and kidneys. In some people, infection is limited to areas outside the lungs (extrapulmonary nocardiosis), while in others, the infection becomes widespread (disseminated nocardiosis).

RISK FACTORS

The risk for nocardiosis is increased by any physical condition that results in an impaired immune system. These conditions include AIDS or human immunodeficiency virus (HIV) infection, lowered immunity from the use of medications (such as corticosteroids and chemotherapy), having undergone organ or bone marrow transplantation, and having a serious chronic illness, such as liver disease or lupus. Chronic lung disease also increases the risk for nocardiosis because the diseased lungs are compromised and unable to fight infection.

SYMPTOMS

Nocardiosis that affects the lungs can result in symptoms that include shortness of breath, a productive cough, weight loss, a fever, and coughing up blood (hemoptysis). Other symptoms depend upon the location of the infection.

SCREENING AND DIAGNOSIS

A complete physical exam and medical history will be completed, together with diagnostic tests that will be used to distinguish the symptoms of nocardiosis from those of other diseases. Tests include bacterial cultures of blood and sputum; chest X ray; computed tomography (CT) scan; magnetic resonance imaging (MRI) scan of involved organs (chest and head); thoracentesis, which involves drainage of fluid from the lung; and, less often, a lumbar puncture, a procedure in which a needle is used to aspirate cerebrospinal fluid for analysis to identify infection of the central nervous system.

TREATMENT AND THERAPY

Treatment may be administered in an intensive care setting, especially for persons with widespread infection. Nocardiosis is treated with an extended course of antibiotic therapy. A class of antibiotics called sulfonamides are effective in eradicating *Nocardia*, but alternative antibiotics may be used. Affected persons may also receive supportive treatments such as medications for fever and pain and supplemental oxygen. Surgical drainage of an abscess may also be necessary.

PREVENTION AND OUTCOMES

Exposure to *Nocardia* cannot be avoided; as such, there is no specific method of prevention of nocardiosis. Nocardiosis, however, is uncommon in people of average or better health.

Carita Caple, M.S.H.S., R.N.

FURTHER READING

Ambrosioni, Juan, Daniel Lew, and Jorge Garbino. "Nocardiosis: Updated Clinical Review and Experience at a Tertiary Center." *Infection* 38, no. 2 (2010): 89-97.

Filice, Gregory A. "Nocardiosis." In *Harrison's Principles of Internal Medicine*, edited by Joan Butterton. 17th ed. New York: McGraw-Hill, 2008.

Martinez, Raquel, Soledad Reyes, and Rosario Menendez. "Pulmonary Nocardiosis: Risk Factors, Clinical Features, Diagnosis, and Prognosis." *Current Opinion in Pulmonary Medicine* 14 (2008): 218-227.

Schwartz, Brian S., and Henry F. Chambers. "Bacterial and Chlamydial Infections." In *Current Medical Diagnosis and Treatment 2011*, edited by Stephen J. McPhee and Maxine A. Papadakis. 50th ed. New York: McGraw-Hill Medical, 2011.

West, John B. *Pulmonary Pathophysiology: The Essentials.* 7th ed. Philadelphia: Wolters Kluwer/Lippincott Williams & Wilkins, 2008.

WEB SITES OF INTEREST

American Lung Association
http://www.lungusa.org

Centers for Disease Control and Prevention
http://www.cdc.gov

See also:: Airborne illness and disease; Atypical pneumonia; Bacterial infections; Bronchiolitis; Bronchitis; Croup; Cryptococcosis; Legionnaires' disease; Opportunistic infections; Pleurisy; Pneumocystis pneumonia; Pneumonia; Respiratory route of transmission; Soilborne illness and disease; Tuberculosis (TB); Waterborne illness and disease; Whooping cough.

Nonprescription drugs. *See* Over-the-counter (OTC) drugs.

Norovirus infection

CATEGORY: Diseases and conditions
ANATOMY OR SYSTEM AFFECTED: All
ALSO KNOWN AS: Acute nonbacterial gastroenteritis, calicivirus infection, Norwalk virus, Norwalk-like virus, small round structure viruses, stomach flu, viral gastroenteritis

DEFINITION

Noroviruses refer to a group of viruses that cause inflammation of the stomach and intestines. This inflammation is called gastroenteritis, or the stomach flu. In the United States, noroviruses are the second leading cause of illness. Outbreaks have occurred in settings such as cruise ships, restaurants, nursing homes, and hospitals, locations where the virus can spread quickly to a large group of people.

CAUSES

The noroviruses are highly contagious. They are spread by fecal to oral contamination of water and food. Infection can occur through contaminated municipal water supplies, recreational lakes, swimming pools, wells, and water stored on cruise ships; by ingesting raw (or improperly steamed) shellfish, especially clams and oysters, and other foods and drinks that are contaminated by infected food handlers; and by touching contaminated surfaces such as door knobs and then touching one's mouth. The viruses can also spread by direct contact with an ill person. This is common in day-care centers and nursing homes.

RISK FACTORS

The following factors increase the chance of developing norovirus infection: exposure to a contaminated water supply, consuming contaminated foods or liquids, touching contaminated surfaces, and taking care of someone who is infected with the virus. A person is contagious from the start of symptoms to a minimum of three days after recovery. A person can sometimes be contagious up to three weeks.

Even if a person had been infected with a norovirus in the past, he or she can become ill again if this new virus is of a different strain or if more than twenty-four months have passed since the last exposure. Norovirus infection is more common in adults and older children than it is in the very young.

SYMPTOMS

Symptoms of norovirus infection include nausea and vomiting (an infected person may vomit often, sometimes violently and without warning, during one day), diarrhea, abdominal pain, headache, low-grade fever, chills, muscle aches, tiredness, and dehydration. Dehydration may require medical attention, especially in children, the elderly, and those with compromised immune systems. One can prevent dehydration by drinking increased amounts of fluids, including water and juice.

After exposure to the virus, symptoms often appear within twenty-four to forty-eight hours. A person may feel ill as early as twelve hours. Symptoms often last about twenty-four to sixty hours.

SCREENING AND DIAGNOSIS

Diagnosis can be made based on a stool specimen. Often, a doctor can determine this illness without ordering laboratory tests.

TREATMENT AND THERAPY

There are no treatments for norovirus infection. Because gastroenteritis is caused by a virus, antibiotics cannot cure it. There are no antiviral medications or vaccines. The illness, however, is often brief, and the only complication would be dehydration caused by vomiting and diarrhea. In certain groups of people, dehydration may require a hospital stay to replenish fluids.

PREVENTION AND OUTCOMES

Noroviruses can survive extreme heat and cold. The viruses also can live in water with chlorine levels of up to ten parts per million. (This is much higher than the levels of public water supplies.) There are ways, though, to limit exposure to the viruses.

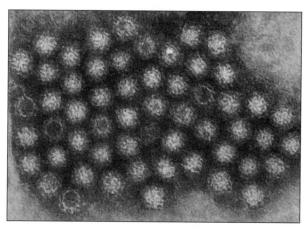

Norovirus virions, or virus particles. (CDC)

To help reduce the chance of getting norovirus infection, one should wash hands thoroughly after using the toilet (or after changing diapers). This is important before handling food or eating. Caregivers should ensure that infected persons thoroughly wash their hands.

Food preparers should wash fruits and vegetables and steam oysters and clams. One should not prepare food if having symptoms and should wait three days after recovery before handling food again. Also, one should throw away contaminated food.

If ill or caring for someone who is ill, the caregiver should immediately clean and disinfect contaminated surfaces using bleach cleaner and should remove and wash soiled linens (using hot water and soap).

Sick persons should not go to work. Staying home will prevent passing the virus to others. If the norovirus-infected person works in a health care facility, sick persons in that facility should be isolated to keep the virus from spreading.

Rebecca J. Stahl, M.A.;
reviewed by David L. Horn, M.D., FACP

FURTHER READING

Centers for Disease Control and Prevention. "Outbreaks of Gastroenteritis Associated with Noroviruses on Cruise Ships–United States, 2002." *Morbidity and Mortality Weekly Report* 51 (2002): 1112-1115.

Dolan, Raphael. "Noroviruses–Challenges to Control." *New England Journal of Medicine* 357 (2007): 1072-1073.

Fankhauser, R. L., S. S. Monroe, J. S. Noel, et al. "Epidemiologic and Molecular Trends of 'Norwalk-Like

Viruses' Associated with Outbreaks of Gastroenteritis in the United States." *Journal of Infectious Disease*, no. 186 (2002): 1-7.

National Institute of Allergies and Infectious Diseases. "Foodborne Diseases: Norovirus Infection." Available at http://www.niaid.nih.gov/topics/norovirus.

"Norwalk Virus Family." In *The Bad Bug Book: Foodborne Pathogenic Microorganisms and Natural Toxins Handbook*. U.S. Food and Drug Administration, Center for Food Safety and Applied Nutrition. Available at http://www.fda.gov/food/foodsafety/foodborneillness.

WEB SITES OF INTEREST

Centers for Disease Control and Prevention
http://www.cdc.gov

National Center for Emerging and Zoonotic Infectious Diseases
http://www.cdc.gov/ncezid

National Institute of Allergy and Infectious Diseases
http://www.niaid.nih.gov

U.S. Food and Drug Administration
http://www.fda.gov

See also:: Adenovirus infections; Antibiotic-associated colitis; Ascariasis; Caliciviridae; Cholera; Contagious diseases; Cryptosporidiosis; Enteritis; Fecal-oral route of transmission; Food-borne illness and disease; Gastritis; Hospitals and infectious disease; Inflammation; Intestinal and stomach infections; Peritonitis; Shigellosis; Viral gastroenteritis; Waterborne illness and disease.

O

Onchocerciasis

CATEGORY: Diseases and conditions
ANATOMY OR SYSTEM AFFECTED: Eyes, lymph nodes, skin, tissue, vision
ALSO KNOWN AS: River blindness

DEFINITION

Onchocerciasis is a parasitic infestation by filarial worms (*Onchocerca volvulus*) that affects persons in Africa, Latin America, and the Arabian Peninsula. Worm larvae enter the body from black-fly bites, causing nodular skin swelling that may progress to a harmful eye disease known as river blindness. Almost one-half of the adult population in the West African savanna has some visual impairment caused by onchocerciasis, the second-leading infectious cause of blindness worldwide.

CAUSES

Black flies (genus *Simulium*) feed on the blood of infected people and ingest microfilariae, the embryos of worms, which then mature into larvae in the gut of the fly within seven days. The larvae are then deposited into other persons through fly saliva. The larvae develop into adult worms then live and reproduce in firm nodules in the subcutaneous and deeper layers of skin. Adult worms produce numerous microfilariae, which travel from the parent nodule and move throughout the skin. The presence of the microfilariae, dead and alive, causes the body to have a powerful immune response, leading to a severe inflammatory reaction that damages surrounding skin and eye tissue.

RISK FACTORS

Persons who live in Africa, Latin America, and the Arabian Peninsula near streams and rivers, the breeding habitat for the black fly, are at the greatest risk for developing onchocerciasis.

SYMPTOMS

Symptoms of onchocerciasis may not appear until three to fifteen months after infection. Early indicators include skin nodules that contain two or more adult worms. The migration of microfilariae causes a severe rash and painful, hot, or swollen skin. Lymph nodes in the neck and groin can become enlarged. Chronic infection may lead to thickened, pigmented, or depigmented skin, often in a lizard or leopard pattern. If the microfilariae migrate to the eye, the body's immune system responds by destroying the eye tissue,

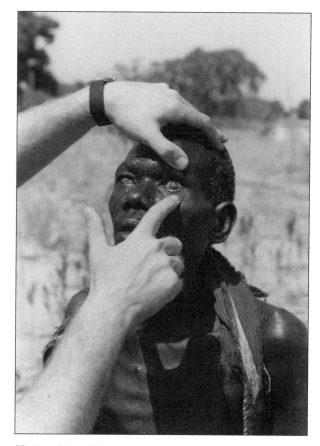

Victim of river blindness.

747

leading to deteriorating vision. People who have been infected with only a few larvae may not experience any noticeable symptoms at all.

SCREENING AND DIAGNOSIS

Diagnosis of onchocerciasis is commonly made by analysis of skin snips that contain microfilariae or by excision of the nodule containing adult worms. A dipstick test for the presence of an antigen in urine or tears has been developed; however, results do not distinguish between current and past infection.

TREATMENT AND THERAPY

In 1986, the World Health Organization (WHO) worked collaboratively with pharmaceutical company Merck to develop ivermectin, the most effective treatment for onchocerciasis. Ivermectin is administered in two doses, six months apart, every three years. Community directed treatment programs have been established to provide treatment at no cost. Damage done to skin and eyes cannot be reversed, but treatment prevents further deterioration by killing the microfilariae. Although treatment does not kill the adult worms, it prevents them from reproducing.

PREVENTION AND OUTCOMES

WHO has initiated the several prevention programs, including the Onchocerciasis Control Programme, the African Programme for Onchocerciasis Control, and the Onchocerciasis Elimination Program for the Americas. Preventive measures by these programs include spraying of insecticides to prevent black-fly breeding in affected areas and distributing ivermectin treatment to persons and communities in need.

April Ingram, B.S.

FURTHER READING

Stingl, Peter. "Onchocerciasis: Developments in Diagnosis, Treatment, and Control." *International Journal of Dermatology* 48 (2009): 393-396.
Taylor, Mark, et al. "Lymphatic Filariasis and Onchocerciasis." *The Lancet* 376 (2010): 1175-1185.
World Health Organization. Special Programme for Research and Training in Tropical Diseases. "Eliminating River Blindness." Available at http://www.who.int/tdrold/publications/publications/elimin_riverblind.htm.

WEB SITES OF INTEREST

Carter Center
http://www.cartercenter.org/health

Centers for Disease Control and Prevention
http://www.cdc.gov/parasites

Global Health Council
http://www.globalhealth.org/infectious_diseases

Partners for Parasite Control
http://www.who.int/wormcontrol

See also: Arthropod-borne illness and disease; Blood-borne illness and disease; Developing countries and infectious disease; Filariasis; Flies and infectious disease; Insect-borne illness and disease; Insecticides and topical repellants; Parasitic diseases; Pathogens; Saliva and infectious disease; Tropical medicine; Vectors and vector control; Worm infections.

Onychomycosis

CATEGORY: Diseases and conditions
ANATOMY OR SYSTEM AFFECTED: Nails, skin
ALSO KNOWN AS: Fungal nail infection, tinea unguium

DEFINITION

Onychomycosis is a nail infection caused by a fungus. The infection occurs more often on toenails than on fingernails.

CAUSES

The fungi that cause onychomycosis thrive in warm, moist environments. Factors that may contribute to onychomycosis include injury to the nail; exposure to warm, moist environments, such as locker rooms; damp socks; tight-fitting shoes; and poor nail care.

RISK FACTORS

Risk factors for onychomycosis include smoking; type 1 or type 2 diabetes; circulatory disorders, such as peripheral vascular disease; and immune system disorders, such as human immunodeficiency virus (HIV) infection. Persons who are sixty years of age or older are at higher risk.

Symptoms

Onychomycosis can affect one or more nails. Symptoms include a thickened nail that is difficult to cut, a brittle or ragged nail, a discolored or unsightly nail, and pain of a finger or toe with ordinary activities.

Screening and Diagnosis

A doctor will ask about symptoms and medical history and will perform a physical exam before possibly referring the patient to a specialist in skin and nail disorders (a dermatologist). The doctor may scrape or clip the nail to send a sample for testing. Tests on the nail sample may include a culture and a microscopic examination.

Treatment and Therapy

Because nails grow slowly, getting a completely clear nail can take up to one year. Onychomycosis can be difficult to treat and may return after treatment. Treatment options include prescription antifungal medications taken by mouth, creams and ointments, and antifungal nail lacquer. Surgery to remove the nail is sometimes performed in severe cases of onychomycosis. A new nail grows in its place.

Prevention and Outcomes

To help reduce the chance of getting onychomycosis, one should keep feet clean and dry them after washing; keep hands dry and wear rubber gloves when cleaning; keep nails short and clean and trimmed straight across; avoid trimming or picking at the skin near nails; take care to avoid injuring toenails; avoid shoes that are too tight; wear absorbent cotton socks and change them if they become damp; avoid walking barefoot around swimming pools, locker rooms, and other public places; choose a reputable salon for manicures and pedicures; avoid artificial nails, which can trap moisture; and stop smoking. For persons with diabetes, the doctor should be consulted about how to better control blood sugar levels.

Reviewed by David L. Horn, M.D., FACP

Further Reading

Haggerty, M. "Don't Let Fungal Nail Infections Get the Upper Hand." *Dermatology Insights* (Spring, 2001). Available at http://www.aad.org/public/conditions/_doc/disspring01.pdf.

Nandedkar-Thomas, M. A., and R. K. Scher. "An Update on Disorders of the Nails." *Journal of the American Academy of Dermatology* 52 (2005): 877-887.

National Library of Medicine. "Fungal Nail Infection." Available at http://www.nlm.nih.gov/medlineplus/ency/article/001330.htm.

Rodgers, P., and M. Bassler. "Treating Onychomycosis." *American Family Physician* 63 (2001): 663-672, 677-678.

Weedon, David. *Skin Pathology.* 3d ed. New York: Churchill Livingstone/Elsevier, 2010.

Wolff, Klaus, and Richard Allen Johnson. *Fitzpatrick's Color Atlas and Synopsis of Clinical Dermatology.* 6th ed. New York: McGraw-Hill Medical, 2009.

Web Sites of Interest

American Academy of Dermatology
http://www.aad.org

American Academy of Family Physicians
http://familydoctor.org

College of Family Physicians of Canada
http://www.cfpc.ca

New Zealand Dermatological Society
http://dermnetnz.org

See also: Antifungal drugs: Types; Athlete's foot; Chromoblastomycosis; Dermatomycosis; Diagnosis of fungal infections; *Epidermophyton*; Fungal infections; Fungi: Classification and types; Jock itch; Plantar warts; Ringworm; Thrush; Tinea capitis; Tinea corporis; Tinea versicolor.

Ophthalmia neonatorum

CATEGORY: Diseases and conditions
ANATOMY OR SYSTEM AFFECTED: Eyes, vision
ALSO KNOWN AS: Neonatal conjunctivitis, newborn conjunctivitis

Definition

Ophthalmia neonatorum is conjunctivitis that occurs in the newborn. Conjunctivitis is inflammation of the surface or covering of the eye from infectious or noninfectious causes. Any eye infection that occurs in the first month of a baby's life can be classified as ophthalmia neonatorum. An infection has the potential to damage the delicate eye of an infant, but there are many ways these infections can be prevented. If an infection does occur, effective treatment is available for infants who develop an eye infection.

CAUSES

The cause of conjunctivitis may be simply an irritation in the eye or a blocked tear duct (dacryocystitis). However, bacteria can also cause an infection in the eye. The most common types of bacteria that cause infection in an infant's eye come from the mother's birth canal and are passed to the infant during delivery. These infections can include sexually transmitted diseases (STDs). The most common bacteria passed to infants during delivery are those from STDs that infect the birth canal. If untreated, many of these infections can cause serious damage to the infant's eye. The STDs that can cause eye damage include chlamydia and gonorrhea; the virus that causes oral and genital herpes; skin bacteria such as *Staphylococcus aureus*; and bacteria from the woman's gastrointestinal tract, such as *Pseudomonas*.

RISK FACTORS

The biggest risk factor for developing ophthalmia neonatorum is a maternal infection or STD at the time of delivery. With some infections, however, the woman may not have any symptoms during delivery and may still be able to transmit the infection. If pregnant, one should discuss any STD infections, past or present, with a doctor.

SYMPTOMS

The most common symptom is redness and swelling of the conjunctiva in the newborn. If the baby has this or any of the following symptoms, one should consult the baby's pediatrician. Other symptoms of ophthalmia neonatorum include drainage and discharge from the eye (which may be watery or thick and pus-like) and swollen eyelids.

SCREENING AND DIAGNOSIS

If the baby's pediatrician suspects ophthalmia neonatorum, he or she will order an eye examination to check for eye irritants and eye damage. The doctor also may look at the baby's tear ducts to see if they are blocked and may also take a sample of any discharge

to determine what type of bacteria or virus is causing the infection.

TREATMENT AND THERAPY

Because the potential for serious eye damage to the infant is so great, it is standard treatment in hospitals in the United States to give infants antibiotic eye drops or ointment immediately following their delivery. The eye drops help prevent the development of an eye infection, even if the mother shows no symptoms of infection.

In cases where conjunctivitis does develop, the treatment of ophthalmia neonatorum depends on the cause. If caused by a blocked tear duct, the treatment may include warm compresses and gentle massage to the area to help unclog the duct. If caused by bacterial irritation, the treatment includes antibiotics after delivery. These antibiotics may be given as topical drops or ointments, orally, or as an injection. In addition, the eye may be irrigated to remove the discharge. Silver nitrate, which was often used in the past to prevent eye infection, can cause irritation in the baby's eye, so hospitals now use other types of antibiotics to avoid this irritation.

Because hospitals have such effective prevention measures, bacterial cases of ophthalmia neonatorum are rare, and when they do occur, they are usually identified quickly. Antibiotic treatment is effective and, generally, the infection resolves rapidly. If a person suspects that an infant may have an eye infection, he or she should consult the baby's doctor to receive prompt treatment.

PREVENTION AND OUTCOMES

The best prevention of ophthalmia neonatorum is treatment of any STDs in the pregnant woman before labor and delivery. In most cases, effective treatment before the time of delivery can prevent the transmission of infection to the newborn. For women with active genital herpes lesions at the time of delivery, a cesarean section can prevent neonatal infection.

Maria Borowski, M.A.;
reviewed by Christopher Cheyer, M.D.

FURTHER READING

Akera, C., and S. Ro. "Medical Concerns in the Neonatal Period." *Clinics in Family Practice* 5, no. 2 (200): 265-292.

Behrman, Richard E., Robert M. Kliegman, and Hal

B. Jenson, eds. *Nelson Textbook of Pediatrics.* 18th ed. Philadelphia: Saunders/Elsevier, 2007.

Cassel, Gary H., Michael D. Billig, and Harry G. Randall. *The Eye Book: A Complete Guide to Eye Disorders and Health.* Baltimore: Johns Hopkins University Press, 2001.

Johnson, Gordon J., et al., eds. *The Epidemiology of Eye Disease.* 2d ed. New York: Oxford University Press, 2003.

Koby, M. "Conjunctivitis." In *Ferri's Clinical Advisor 2011: Instant Diagnosis and Treatment*, edited by Fred F. Ferri. Philadelphia: Mosby/Elsevier, 2011.

The Merck Manuals, Online Medical Library. "Neonatal Infections." Available at http://www.merck.com/mmhe.

Olitzky, S. E., et al. "Disorders of the Conjunctiva." In *Nelson Textbook of Pediatrics*, edited by Richard E. Behrman, Robert M. Kliegman, and Hal B. Jenson. 18th ed. Philadelphia: Saunders/Elsevier, 2007.

Riordan-Eva, Paul, and John P. Whitcher. *Vaughan and Asbury's General Ophthalmology.* 17th ed. New York: Lange Medical Books/McGraw-Hill, 2007.

Rubenstein, J. B., and S. L. Jick. "Disorders of the Conjunctiva and Limbus." In *Ophthalmology.* 2d ed. New York: Mosby, 2004.

WEB SITES OF INTEREST

American Academy of Family Physicians
http://familydoctor.org

American Academy of Ophthalmology
http://www.aao.org

American Academy of Pediatrics
http://www.healthychildren.org

American Association for Pediatric Ophthalmology and Strabismus
http://www.aapos.org

American Optometric Association
http://www.aoanet.org

Canadian Ophthalmological Society
http://www.eyesite.ca

Caring for Kids
http://www.caringforkids.cps.ca

See also: Bacterial infections; Childbirth and infectious disease; Children and infectious disease; Conjunctivitis; Contagious diseases; Dacryocystitis; Eye infections; Genital herpes; Herpesviridae; Hordeola; Inflammation; Keratitis; Neonatal sepsis; Pregnancy and infectious disease; *Pseudomonas*; *Pseudomonas* infections; Sexually transmitted diseases (STDs); *Staphylococcus*; Trachoma; Women and infectious disease.

Opportunistic infections

CATEGORY: Transmission

DEFINITION

An opportunistic infection is an infection that is caused by bacteria, viruses, fungi, or protozoa that, in a healthy person, are not usually harmful. These microorganisms, however, can cause disease in persons whose immune systems are not operating efficiently, and who are, therefore, immunocompromised. Compromised immunity can occur in infants whose immune system is still maturing; in the elderly, whose immune system is deteriorating with age; in people who are very sick, such as those with acquired immunodeficiency syndrome (AIDS); and in people whose immune system has been deliberately suppressed, such as for organ transplantation. In effect, microbes can cause disease if given the opportunity.

NOSOCOMIAL INFECTIONS

Many opportunistic infections occur in the hospital environment. These infections are referred to as nosocomial. Opportunistic infections have been a fact of hospital life for as long as there have been hospitals. The connection between the high death rate of hospitalized persons and infection was first described in the mid-nineteenth century by Hungarian physician Ignaz Semmelweis. Semmelweis also noted that enforcing handwashing among attending physicians dramatically lowered the death rate.

Despite this long history of the benefits of handwashing, compliance remains a challenge for hospital staff and visitors. Indeed, the chances of acquiring an opportunistic infection during hospitalization averages about 10 percent and can increase depending on the length of the hospital stay or the severity of the illness (specifically, whether or not the immune system is compromised).

BACTERIAL INFECTIONS

Opportunistic infections are most often caused by bacteria. Both gram-positive bacteria (bacteria that have a single membrane surrounding the cell) and gram-negative bacteria (which have two membranes) can be opportunistic pathogens. (A pathogen is an organism that can cause disease.) Prominent gram-negative bacteria include *Escherichia coli*, *Proteus mirabilis*, many species of *Salmonella*, and other members of the Enterobacteriaceae family. These bacteria normally reside in the intestinal tract. They are spread by the fecal contamination of people or surfaces. Other gram-negative bacteria that are significant opportunistic pathogens include members of the genera *Pseudomonas* and *Acinetobacter*. *Pseudomonas* can cause infections in persons with burns and with other open wounds who are receiving hydrotherapy. *Acinetobacter*, which is a common resident of soil, can cause serious, even life-threatening, infections in ill people. Increased illness from *A. acidocaldarius*, which has mutated and is now resistant to many antibiotics, has been reported in U.S. military personnel stationed in the Middle East for the conflicts in Iraq and Afghanistan.

Gram-positive bacteria, especially *Staphylococcus aureus*, frequently cause infections by entering the bloodstream through wounds or incisions. This bacterium is a normal resident on the surface of the skin, so this route of entry can easily occur if precautions such as sterilizing the area around a wound or incision have not be properly done.

As with *Acinetobacter*, an important factor in opportunistic infections is the development of bacterial resistance to antibiotics. The resistance of the bacteria is an example of evolutionary change in response to a survival challenge. Those bacteria that are better able to withstand antibiotics will survive better, and so will be "selected." Bacteria that are susceptible to antibiotics will diminish with time. Types of *S. aureus* and *Clostridium perfringens* that are resistant to all but a few antibiotics have appeared and have become prevalent globally since the 1970's.

Tuberculosis (TB) is another opportunistic infection. It is caused by the bacterium *Mycobacterium tuberculosis*. While opportunistic, this infection is widespread, with an estimated 30 percent of the world's population afflicted. Poor health, which can often affect the immune system, is a driver for the disease. Tuberculosis is prominent in developing countries, where the standard of health is below that of developed countries. However, developed nations, including the United States, are not spared. Indeed, the prevalence of TB in the United States has been gradually increasing since the 1970's. The reason for this is not clear, but it may reflect economic disparity and an inaccessible health care system for the working poor and for those living in poverty.

AIDS

Persons who have AIDS or cancer, and those whose immune system has been deliberately compromised to prevent rejection of transplanted organs or to lessen the body's response to an illness, are especially prone to opportunistic infections; the viruses that cause AIDS and cancer, for example, attack and disable components of the immune system.

Opportunistic pathogens of note for those with AIDS include the following: *Pneumocystis jirovecii*, a fungus that causes pneumocystis pneumonia; *Candida albicans*, a fungus that can infect the mouth and gastrointestinal tract; several types of a fungus called *Histoplasma*, which can cause histoplasmosis, a lung infection that can spread to other parts of the body; JC virus, which causes progressive multifocal leukoencephalopathy, in which brain tissue is affected; cytomegalovirus, which is related to herpesvirus and which can cause a life-threatening infection; herpesvirus 8, which can cause a type of cancer known as Kaposi's sarcoma in persons with AIDS; *Toxoplasma gondii*, a protozoan that is common in cats and which can be transferred to humans (the resulting infection can be fatal for the fetus of a pregnant woman); and *Cryptococcus neoformans*, a yeast commonly found in soil that, if inhaled, can cause a serious lung infection called cryptococcosis.

COSTS AND PREVENTION

The exact economic and social costs of opportunistic infections are impossible to determine, yet the cost of caring for those involved and the cost of lost work time are in the billions of dollars for the United States alone. In addition, the social costs exacted by opportunistic infections, costs such as the demands placed on families and others as caregivers, are enormous.

Dealing with opportunistic infections is a matter of recognizing the conditions under which the infections can arise, and then attempting to control those conditions. These steps can include the observance of exemplary hygiene in the hospital environment and the segregation of immunocompromised patients from the general patient population. Also, health experts should control the development of antibiotic resistance in opportunistic bacterial pathogens.

IMPACT

The ability of some microorganisms to cause infection in a host when the host immune defenses are compromised is a significant cause of infection in infants, the elderly, and those with compromised immune systems. Opportunistic infections are especially serious in hospital environments and in the aftermath of natural disasters.

Brian Hoyle, Ph.D.

FURTHER READING

Clark, David P. *Germs, Genes, and Civilization: How Epidemics Shaped Who We Are Today.* Upper Saddle River, N.J.: FT Press, 2010. A consideration of the effect of infectious diseases, including epidemics of opportunistic infections, on human history.

Galanda, Claudia D., ed. *AIDS-Related Opportunistic Infections.* New York: Nova Biomedical Books, 2009. Discusses the various infections that can occur opportunistically in those with acquired immunodeficiency syndrome and the causes of the infections.

Mayer, Kenneth H., and Hank. F. Pizer. *The AIDS Epidemic: Impact on Science and Society.* New York: Academic Press, 2005. A series of essays that considers the impact of AIDS from the individual level to the global level.

Sompayrac, Lauren M. *How the Immune System Works.* 3d ed. Hoboken, N.J.: Wiley-Blackwell, 2008. A helpful introductory text on the workings of the immune system.

St. Georgiev, Vassil. *Opportunistic Infections: Treatment and Prophylaxis.* Totowa, N.J.: Humana Press, 2003. Examines opportunistic infections from a clinical perspective. Covers prevention and treatment.

WEB SITES OF INTEREST

AIDSinfo
http://aidsinfo.nih.gov

Centers for Disease Control and Prevention
http://www.cdc.gov

National Institute of Allergy and Infectious Diseases
http://www.niaid.nig.gov

World Health Organization
http://www.who.int

See also: Aging and infectious disease; AIDS; Antibiotic resistance; Bacterial infections; Contagious diseases; Drug resistance; Epidemiology; Fungal infections; Fungi: Classification and types; Herpesvirus infections; HIV; Hospitals and infectious disease; Iatrogenic infections; Immunity; Immunodeficiency; Infection; Methicillin-resistant staph infection; Public health; Superbacteria; Vancomycin-resistant enterococci infection; Viral infections; Wound infections.

Oral transmission

CATEGORY: Transmission

DEFINITION

Oral transmission is the acquisition of bacteria, viruses, fungi, and parasites through the mouth, either by ingestion or by absorption through the oral mucosa.

FECAL-ORAL TRANSMISSION

Escherichia coli and other enteric bacteria, viruses, and parasites are transmitted when the feces of a person or animal are inadvertently swallowed. This may occur when hands are not washed after using a toilet, after changing a diaper, after working in dirt or soil, after petting animals, and after cleaning up after animals. Surfaces in day-care centers and in public restrooms may be invisibly covered with such microbes unless they are frequently disinfected.

Fecal-oral transmission may also occur when raw fruits and vegetables that are grown in or are otherwise in contact with soil fertilized with manure are not thoroughly washed before they are eaten. Similar foods may also become contaminated when harvesters or food preparers handle them with unwashed, stool-contaminated hands. Food handlers should keep their hands clean by washing with soap and warm water. Cooking food at a high temperature for a sufficient length of time kills these bacteria and parasites.

Fecal-oral transmission may also result from swallowing swimming pool water that has not been sufficiently chlorinated. Similarly, lake or river water may be contaminated with animal feces and should not be ingested. To ensure safe drinking water when camping or in other outdoor situations, water may be boiled, filtered, or chemically treated.

FOOD-BORNE TRANSMISSION

Uncooked meat typically contains bacteria; poultry is known to harbor *Salmonella*. Fish and shellfish that were caught from contaminated water sources may transmit disease. Handling raw meat and neglecting to wash one's hands and the food preparation surface afterward may lead to the contamination of other foods and subsequent bacterial ingestion. Meat should always be stored at the proper temperature before cooking and frozen meat should be thawed in the refrigerator rather than on the kitchen counter to discourage the multiplication of bacteria. Surfaces that come in contact with raw meat juices should be thoroughly disinfected.

A dental cavity is an infectious disease, and studies have shown that parents and caregivers inadvertently infect infants and toddlers with cavity-causing bacteria when they sample the child's food to check the food's temperature. An indigenous Alaskan cultural practice is to chew solid foods before feeding these foods to infants, incidentally transmitting cavity-causing bacteria and other oral pathogens. Persons who engage in this practice should use a chlorhexidine mouthwash before each feeding.

Sharing beverages is another means of oral transmission. Bacteria, viruses, and fungi that live in the mucous lining of the mouth, tongue, and throat may be shed in saliva that is washed back into a beverage after drinking, thus contaminating the beverage for the next drinker. For this reason, beverages that come in containers should be poured into individual cups for serving more than one person.

OBJECTS AND SURFACES

Meningococcal disease caused by *Neisseria meningitidis* may be transmitted by sharing contaminated objects (fomites), such as eating utensils, drinking glasses, drinking straws, and water bottles. These bacteria live in the mucous lining of the throat and are

shed in liquids and on surfaces where they may be immediately picked up by other people. Similarly, viruses such as the influenza virus may be transmitted by sharing toothbrushes and drinking glasses. Dental caries may be transmitted from an adult to a child when the adult puts a pacifier in his or her mouth to clean or moisten it before giving it to an infant or toddler. Thus, personal items should not be shared.

PERSON-TO-PERSON TRANSMISSION

Herpes simplex virus types 1 and 2 may be transmitted through the oral mucous membranes by kissing. Infectious mononucleosis and meningococcal disease may also be passed by kissing. The human immunodeficiency virus (HIV) may be transmitted through the oral mucosa by oral sexual acts involving infected semen or blood.

DENTAL PROCEDURES

Infective endocarditis develops in some people following dental procedures. Oral surgery, such as tooth extraction and root canal therapy, creates access by which bacteria that typically live in the mouth get into the bloodstream. Nonsurgical procedures such as dental prophylaxis, with or without periodontal therapy, may disturb areas of inflammation, increase blood flow, and increase the amount of bacteria; when sharp instruments remove epithelium and the calculus, the oral mucosa barrier is compromised and bacteria enter the circulatory system. Persons who have had heart surgery, particularly valve replacement, or who have abnormal heart valves are most at risk of infective endocarditis and must take a prophylactic antibiotic one hour before undergoing dental treatment.

OTHER MODES OF TRANSMISSION

Hepatitis B, C, D, and G may be transmitted through piercing of the tongue, lip, or cheek, which compromises the oral mucosa barrier.

IMPACT

Food-borne, orally transmitted, disease accounts for 76 million illnesses, 300,000 hospitalizations, and 5,000 deaths annually in the United States. One negligent food handler may be responsible for a disease outbreak requiring costly public health intervention. Meningococcal disease has an annual incidence of 25,000 cases requiring hospitalization and 850 deaths in the United States. Outbreaks have occurred in college dormitories and other close living quarters. To minimize oral transmission, hands should be washed thoroughly with an antibacterial soap not only when visibly soiled but also and especially when preparing and eating food.

Bethany Thivierge, M.P.H.

FURTHER READING

Harrison, Lee H., et al. "Invasive Meningococcal Disease in Adolescents and Young Adults." *Journal of the American Medical Association* 286 (2001): 694-699. Report of a major study on the emergence of meningococcal disease in young people that was conducted during the 1990's in Maryland.

Mandell, Gerald L., John E. Bennett, and Raphael Dolin, eds. *Mandell, Douglas, and Bennett's Principles and Practice of Infectious Diseases.* 7th ed. New York: Churchill Livingstone/Elsevier, 2010. A complete and practical reference book with a worldwide perspective and information about new and emerging infectious diseases.

Tanzer, Jason M. "Dental Caries Is a Transmissible Infectious Disease: The Keyes and Fitzgerald Revolution." *Journal of Dental Research* 74 (1995): 1536-1542. A literature review and synthesis of research regarding dental caries.

Younai, Fariba S. "Oral HIV Transmission." *Journal of the California Dental Association*, February, 2001. A thorough literature review, including case studies and an analysis of risk factors.

WEB SITES OF INTEREST

American Dental Association
http://www.ada.org

Centers for Disease Control and Prevention
http://www.cdc.gov

National Institute of Dental and Craniofacial Research
http://www.nidcr.nih.gov

U.S. Department of Agriculture, Food Safety Information Center
http://foodsafety.nal.usda.gov

See also: Bacterial endocarditis; Fecal-oral route of transmission; Food-borne illness and disease; Meningococcal meningitis; Mouth infections; Neisserial infections; Saliva and infectious disease; Transmission routes.

Ornithosis

CATEGORY: Diseases and conditions
ANATOMY OR SYSTEM AFFECTED: Lungs, respiratory system
ALSO KNOWN AS: Parrot disease, parrot fever, psittacosis

DEFINITION

Ornithosis is an infectious disease spread by birds to humans through the bacterium *Chlamydophila psittaci*, resulting in flulike symptoms, pneumonia, and, rarely, death.

CAUSES

Ornithosis is primarily spread through bird droppings, although a bird's secretions, feathers, and eggs also carry the disease. Bird droppings remain infectious for weeks and, especially after desiccation, become airborne and are easily inhaled by humans. Handling diseased birds, ingesting their eggs, or breathing the dust particles of bird feces all cause the spread of ornithosis.

RISK FACTORS

Persons such as breeders or pet store workers who raise parrots, cockatiels, and parakeets as pets are most at risk of contracting ornithosis. Veterinarians and veterinarian staff are also highly vulnerable. Because chickens, turkeys, gulls, pigeons, and a wide variety of other birds may be carriers of ornithosis, poultry workers, farmers, and bird slaughterhouse workers are also at risk for exposure to the disease. Persons who have a weakened immune system also are at greater risk of contracting ornithosis.

SYMPTOMS

The symptoms of ornithosis include a cough, rash, fever, chills, headache, fatigue, muscle aches, weight loss, congestion, breathlessness, and pneumonia. (In birds, the symptoms are discharge from eyes and nose, loss of appetite, wasting, diarrhea, and ruffled and unkempt coats and feathers.)

SCREENING AND DIAGNOSIS

A physical examination, blood test, sputum culture, chest X ray, and computed tomography scan of the chest are all used to correctly diagnose ornithosis. Further screening may be carried out by isolating specific contact with birds in the weeks before onset of illness because the incubation period of ornithosis is one to four weeks. Most often, symptoms manifest within ten days of infection.

TREATMENT AND THERAPY

The antibiotics doxycycline and tetracycline are primarily prescribed for ornithosis, although rifampin, azithromycin, and erythromycin may also be prescribed, the latter especially for pregnant women and for children under the age of nine years. Most cases of ornithosis are treated successfully with oral antibiotics, but severe cases require antibiotics administered intravenously. It is essential that elderly persons in particular begin treatment as soon as possible. Rare cases of ornithosis, less than 1 percent, result in death.

PREVENTION AND OUTCOMES

For pet-bird owners, the best prevention is to keep birdcages clean so that no bird droppings can accumulate, dry, and become inhaled. Additionally, tetracycline should be administered to imported birds as pets for a minimum of forty-five consecutive days to reduce the likelihood of infection. Veterinarians, laboratory technicians, and anyone exposed to infected birds should always wear gloves and a mask to avoid secretions and airborne bacteria.

Mary E. Markland, M.A.

FURTHER READING

Fryden, Aril, et al. "A Clinical and Epidemiological Study of 'Ornithosis' Caused by *Chlamydia psittacia* and *Chlamydia pneumoniae* (Strain TWAR)." *Scandinavian Journal of Infectious Diseases* 21 (1989): 681-691.

Hall, C., et al. "An Epidemic of Ornithosis in Texas Turkeys in 1974." *Southwestern Veterinarian* 28 (1975): 19-21.

Irons, J., Thelma Sullivan, and Joyce Rowen. "Outbreak of Psittacosis (Ornithosis) from Working with Turkeys or Chickens." *American Journal of Public Health* 41 (1951): 931-937.

National Association of State Public Health Veterinarians. "Compendium of Measures to Control *Chlamydophila psittaci* Infection Among Humans (Psittacosis) and Pet Birds (Avian Chlamydiosis)." 2010. Available at http://www.nasphv.org/documents/psittacosis.pdf.

Schlossberg, D. "*Chlamydia psittaci* (Psittacosis)." In *Mandell, Douglas, and Bennett's Principles and Practice of Infectious Diseases*, edited by Gerald L. Mandell, John F. Bennett, and Raphael Dolin. 7th ed. New York: Churchill Livingstone/Elsevier, 2010.

WEB SITES OF INTEREST

American Veterinary Medicine Association
http://www.avma.org

Centers for Disease Control and Prevention: Healthy Pets Healthy People
http://www.cdc.gov/healthypets

See also: Airborne illness and disease; Avian influenza; Bacterial infections; Birds and infectious disease; *Chlamydophila*; Eastern equine encephalitis; Histoplasmosis; Psittacosis; Respiratory route of transmission; Zoonotic diseases.

Osteomyelitis

CATEGORY: Diseases and conditions
ANATOMY OR SYSTEM AFFECTED: Blood, bones, musculoskeletal system, tissue

DEFINITION

Osteomyelitis is an acute or chronic bone infection that is usually produced by bacteria; occasionally, it is caused by fungi. When the bone becomes infected, the bone marrow often swells, which compresses the blood vessels within. This can cut off the blood supply to the bone and cause parts of the bone to die. The infection can then spread to adjacent soft tissues.

CAUSES

Bacteria such as *Staphylococcus aureus* and some types of fungi cause osteomyelitis by invading and infecting the bone. Invasion paths include through the bloodstream, from adjacent soft tissues, or by direct invasion of the bone. Fungal spores or bacteria may

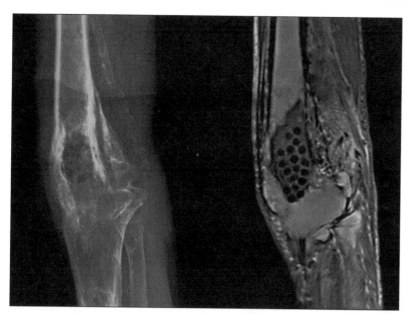

Destruction of bone in a knee caused by osteomyelitis, seen in an X ray, left, and in an MRI scan.

infect the bone at the site where an artificial joint was attached or where metal rods have been used to repair bone fractures. Infections may spread to the bone from tissues damaged by chemotherapy or radiation therapy, from skin ulcers caused by poor circulation, or from other existing infections in the body.

RISK FACTORS

Factors increasing the risk of osteomyelitis include age (the very young and the elderly), past injuries or surgeries that affect bone structure, and other diseases that compromise the immune system, including cancer and diabetes. Sinus, gum, or tooth infections may spread into the skull bones. Although osteomyelitis occurs most often in young children and older people, all age groups are at risk.

SYMPTOMS

The most common symptoms associated with osteomyelitis are bone pain, fever, general discomfort, nausea, and swelling, redness, and warmth above the local area of the infected bone. Abscesses may form in surrounding tissue. In children, the ends of leg and arm bones are usually infected, whereas spinal vertebrate are most commonly infected in adults.

SCREENING AND DIAGNOSIS

A physical examination will reveal bone tenderness and, possibly, swelling and redness. Blood samples, joint fluid samples, and bone biopsies are often taken to identify the source of infection. Elevated erythrocyte sedimentation rate or of C-reactive protein are typically associated with osteomyelitis. Bone X rays, computed tomography (CT) scans, and magnetic resonance imaging (MRI) may identify infected areas. White-blood-cell counts can help distinguish between infection and other bone disorders.

TREATMENT AND THERAPY

Antibiotics are administered from four to eight weeks to destroy causative bacteria. Sometimes more than one antibiotic may be prescribed. Fungal infections are treated with antifungal medications. Surgery may be necessary to remove any dead bone tissue. Voids left from bone removal may be filled with bone grafts to promote the growth of new bone tissue.

PREVENTION AND OUTCOMES

All infections should be quickly and properly treated. Also, persons with an artificial joint or metal component attached to a bone should take antibiotics before any surgical or dental procedure.

Alvin K. Benson, Ph.D.

FURTHER READING

Ballard, Carol. *Bones*. Chicago: Heinemann Library, 2002.

Icon Health. *Osteomyelitis: A Medical Dictionary, Bibliography, and Annotated Research Guide to Internet References*. San Diego, Calif.: Author, 2004.

Meislin, H. W., et al. "Soft Tissue Infections." In *Rosen's Emergency Medicine: Concepts and Clinical Practice*, edited by J. A. Marx et al. 6th ed. St. Louis, Mo.: Mosby, 2006.

Schnettler, Reinhard, and Hans-Ulrich Steinau. *Septic Bone and Joint Surgery*. New York: Thieme Medical, 2010.

Seibel, M. J., P. Robin Simon, and John P. Bilezikian, eds. *Dynamics of Bone and Cartilage Metabolism.* 2d ed. San Diego, Calif.: Academic Press, 2006.

WEB SITES OF INTEREST

Arthritis Foundation
http://www.arthritis.org

National Arthritis and Musculoskeletal and Skin Diseases Information Clearinghouse
http://www.niams.nih.gov

See also: Aging and infectious disease; Bloodstream infections; Gangrene; Graft-versus-host disease; Prosthetic joint infections; Sepsis; *Staphylococcus.*

OTC drugs. *See* Over-the-counter (OTC) drugs.

Outbreaks

CATEGORY: Epidemiology

DEFINITION

The term "outbreak" denotes a larger-than-expected occurrence of a specific disease or infection during a particular time and in a certain place. In other words, an outbreak is present when disease levels are greater than what would be typical or expected in a given community. Such a community could be as small as a school or restaurant or as large as a nation or continent. Outbreaks also can occur globally.

CLASSIFICATION

Although some variation exists on the precise definition of "outbreak" and its patterns of occurrence, the following is a general guide to the various types of outbreaks.

Endemic. An outbreak is considered to be endemic when there is continual presence of a disease or infection within a specific geographic area or among a particular subpopulation. For example, malaria is endemic to certain parts of Africa.

Epidemic. An epidemic is the sudden and severe occurrence of a disease or infection within a particular region or subpopulation. Epidemics usually spread very rapidly. An example of an epidemic is acquired

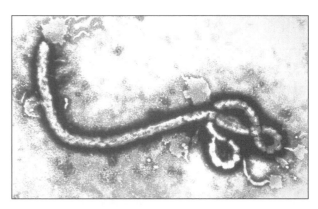

The Ebola virus has caused several deadly disease outbreaks in Africa. (Digital Stock)

immune deficiency syndrome (AIDS) among users of intravenous drugs.

Pandemic. As with an epidemic, a pandemic involves the sudden and severe occurrence of a disease or infection that spreads rapidly. However, a pandemic affects a much larger geographic area (several countries or more) and a sizable proportion of the population. Although a pandemic is the most serious type of outbreak, it is relatively uncommon, having occurred just three or four times per century. Examples include the great influenza (Spanish flu), the Hong Kong flu, and influenza A (H1N1) (also known as swine flu).

DETERMINING THE EXISTENCE OF AN OUTBREAK

To establish whether or not an outbreak truly exists, it is essential to know the expected number of cases for a particular area during a given period of time. This may be done by comparing the current number of cases with the incidence rates in recent months or years. Sources of such information include health department surveillance records, disease registries, and hospital discharge records.

Even if the current number of cases appears to exceed the expected number, the excess may not necessarily indicate an outbreak. Variations in reporting procedures can impact these numbers, as can sudden changes in population size. Such factors must be considered when determining whether the increased number of cases would constitute an outbreak.

IMPLEMENTING MEASURES OF CONTROL AND PREVENTION

Once an outbreak has been confirmed, measures of control and prevention should be implemented immediately. Control methods can be undertaken quickly if the source of the outbreak is known. For instance, if an outbreak is food-borne, a control technique would be to destroy or recall the contaminated products.

Control measures also can be directed at interrupting disease transmission and minimizing exposure to causative agents. Immunizations are helpful for reducing the susceptibility to disease. However, it can take time to develop effective vaccinations. Regardless of the methods used, educating the public is a major component of controlling and preventing outbreaks.

RECENT OUTBREAKS

Listed here are examples of recent outbreaks, mostly in the Western Hemisphere.

Cholera in Haiti (October, 2010). Before this outbreak, cholera had not occurred in Haiti for several decades.

Salmonella (August, 2010). Millions of eggs were recalled after thousands of people in the United States became ill from *Salmonella enteritidis.*

Escherichia coli (July, 2009). This outbreak, involving *E. coli* infection and beef products, occurred in the United States.

E. coli (June, 2009). This outbreak of *E. coli* infection in the United States was linked to the consumption of raw, refrigerated, and prepackaged cookie dough.

Swine flu (April, 2009). Cases of the swine flu were confirmed in the United States and internationally.

IMPACT

The overall impact of a disease outbreak is enormous. In addition to the negative effects on people's health and well being, and its causing death, outbreaks pose tremendous burdens for health care facilities and systems, often draining their resources. Control, prevention, and education must be further developed and implemented. Such efforts require substantial time, energy, financial resources, and collaboration among policymakers and other community groups. Outbreaks can impact productivity in schools and the workplace too, and they create extreme burdens for society as a whole.

Lynda A. Seminara, B.A.

FURTHER READING

Buckeridge, David L., et al. "Predicting Outbreak Detection in Public Health Surveillance: Quantitative Analysis to Enable Evidence-Based Method Selection." *AMIA Annual Symposium Proceedings* 2008 (2008): 76-80.

Chao, D. L., M. E. Halloran, and I. M. Longini, Jr. "School Opening Dates Predict Pandemic Influenza A (H1N2) Outbreaks in the United States." *Journal of Infectious Diseases* 202 (2010): 877-880.

Christakis, N. A., and J. H. Fowler. "Social Network Sensors for Early Detection of Contagious Outbreaks." *PLoS One* 5 (2010): e12948.

Dworkin, Mark S., ed. *Outbreak Investigations Around the World: Case Studies in Infectious Disease Field Epidemiology.* Sudbury, Mass.: Jones and Bartlett, 2010.

Meehan Arias, Kathleen. *Outbreak Investigation and Control in Health Care Settings: Critical Issues for Patient Safety.* 2d ed. Sudbury, Mass.: Jones and Bartlett, 2009.

Sherman, Irwin W. *Twelve Diseases That Changed Our World.* Washington, D.C.: ASM Press, 2007.

Srinivasan, A. "Influential Outbreaks of Healthcare-Associated Infections in the Past Decade." *Infection Control and Hospital Epidemiology* 31, suppl. 1 (2010): S70-S72.

WEB SITES OF INTEREST

Association for Professionals in Infection Control and Epidemiology
http://www.knowledgeisinfectious.org

Centers for Disease Control and Prevention, Emergency Preparedness and Response
http://emergency.cdc.gov

Emerging and Reemerging Infectious Diseases Resource Center
http://www.medscape.com/resource/infections

World Health Organization: Global Alert and Response
http://www.who.int/csr/don

See also: Developing countries and infectious disease; Disease eradication campaigns; Emerging and reemerging infectious diseases; Endemic infections; Epidemics and pandemics: Causes and management; Epidemiology; Globalization and infectious disease; H1N1 influenza; Infectious disease specialists; Koch's postulates; Pathogenicity; Public health; Social effects of infectious disease.

Over-the-counter (OTC) drugs

CATEGORY: Treatment

ALSO KNOWN AS: Nonprescription drugs

DEFINITION

Over-the-counter (OTC) drugs are medications that can be purchased and used without a doctor's prescription. Some OTC medications, however, are restricted and require proof of age or a consultation with a registered pharmacist before purchase.

TYPES

OTCs are drugs or health-care-related preparations that are considered both effective and safe for use by consumers without a doctor's prescription. As of 2010, more than 100,000 OTCs were available in the United States and Canada, according to the Consumer Healthcare Products Association (CHPA). Most OTCs are used to maintain good nutrition or to treat minor illnesses or conditions that do not require a doctor's attention. These nonprescription drugs can be grouped into the following categories:

Nutritional aids. These OTCs include vitamin and mineral supplements and, sometimes, herbal teas, capsules, and similar products considered nutrition-related OTCs because they are sold without a prescription. Unlike vitamins and mineral supplements, however, herbal products are not regulated by the U.S. Food and Drug Administration (FDA).

Digestive aids. OTCs in this category include antiemetic preparations to relieve nausea and vomiting, laxatives to treat constipation, antidiarrheal preparations to stop diarrhea, antacids to relieve acid indigestion by neutralizing stomach acid, and acid reducers that work to relieve heartburn or acid reflux by lowering the amount of acid produced by the stomach. Some preparations in this category can serve more than one function. For example, bismuth subsalicylate, a liquid preparation sold under the trade name Pepto-Bismol, can be used to treat nausea, heartburn, and diarrhea.

Relief of upper respiratory infections and allergies. OTCs can treat coughing, sneezing, and watery eyes associated with colds and seasonal allergies. OTC cough medicines, such as expectorants, are designed to help a person cough up mucus; others, such as antitussives, are designed to stop coughing. Some cough medicines contain both types of ingredients. Allergy medi-

---

Over-the-Counter

The U.S. Food and Drug Administration mandates that all over-the-counter, nonprescription drugs and therapies must be labeled with certain facts and information for consumers. The label is standardized and must display the facts in the following order:

- *Product name*

- *Active ingredient* (therapeutic substance or substances in the product, including the amount in each dosage unit)

- *Purpose* (product category, such as antihistamine, antacid, or cough suppressant)

- *Uses* (symptoms or diseases the product treats or prevents)

- *Warnings* (when not to use the product, when to stop taking it, when to see a doctor, and possible side effects)

- *Directions* (when, how, and how often to take the product)

- *Other information* (for example, how to best store the product)

- *Inactive ingredients* (substances such as binders, colors, or flavoring; helps avoid allergic reactions)

Source: Adapted from the U.S. Food and Drug Administration

---

cations and cold medications contain antihistamines to stop sneezing and decongestants to clear stuffy nasal passages. Decongestants are also available as nasal sprays. Some cold medications also include aspirin or another pain reliever to treat the muscle aches and low-grade fever associated with colds.

Pain relief. OTCs can help to relieve mild pain from such conditions as muscle or menstrual cramping, toothache, arthritis, colds, and tension headache. There are two major categories of pain relievers: those containing acetaminophen (Tylenol) and nonsteroidal anti-inflammatory drugs, or NSAIDs. NSAIDs include such drugs as aspirin, ibuprofen (Advil), and naproxen (Aleve). Acetaminophen is an OTC pain reliever that should be used with caution because it can cause liver damage in high doses.

Topical medications. Topical OTCs, which are products applied to the skin and other surface tissues of the body (such as the eyes or lining of the mouth), include such medications as moisturizing or redness-relieving eye drops; anti-itch creams or lotions to relieve discomfort from sunburn, poison ivy, or other minor skin irritations; soaps and cleansers for treating acne; liniments and gels to relieve the pain of arthritis; local anesthetic gels or liquids to treat mouth ulcers; rubbing alcohol and hydrogen peroxide solutions to cleanse and disinfect minor cuts and scrapes; and anti-cavity, dental sensitivity, tartar control, and tooth-whitening toothpastes.

REGULATION AND ADVERTISING

In the United States, OTCs have been regulated by the FDA since Congress passed the Federal Food, Drug, and Cosmetic Act (FFDCA) of 1938. This legislation was introduced after a tragic mass poisoning in the fall of 1937, in which more than one hundred people died after taking a sulfanilamide medication that had been made with diethylene glycol, a solvent that is poisonous to humans. The then-new medication had not been tested on animals before being sold, even though diethylene glycol was known at the time to be poisonous. The FFDCA replaced the Pure Food and Drug Act of 1906, which did not require companies to submit safety data to the FDA before marketing and selling their products.

Manufacturers of drugs seeking FDA approval for sale as nonprescription items must follow one of two main paths. The first path is to state that the OTC complies with an existing FDA monograph (set of rules) for a specific category of OTC. According to the FDA, these monographs, which are published in the *Federal Register,* "state [the] requirements for categories of non-prescription drugs, such as what ingredients may be used and for what intended use." Examples of OTCs covered by FDA monographs include sunscreen, acne soap and cream, and dandruff shampoo. FDA monographs also cover OTCs that were in use long enough before the 1938 passage of the FFDCA to be considered "generally recognized as safe and effective" when used as directed. This phrase, taken from the FFDCA, is abbreviated as GRAS or GRAS/E. Aspirin is an example of an OTC that is considered GRAS/E.

The other path to FDA approval for an OTC is obtaining a new drug application, or NDA. The manufacturer or sponsor of the proposed drug must show that it is safe and effective and that its benefits outweigh any risks. An NDA must be obtained if the product does not fit within any of the existing FDA monographs for OTCs.

The NDA system is also used to move drugs that were first approved as prescription-only into the OTC category. In addition to determining that OTCs are safe and effective when consumers use them according to package directions, the FDA has the authority to decide that drugs formerly available only with a prescription can be safely sold to consumers as an OTC. This change, which the FDA calls an Rx-to-OTC ("Rx" meaning "prescription") switch, has made available about seven hundred new drugs as OTCs since 1980. Acid reducers and antihistamines are recent examples of the Rx-to-OTC switch.

The major difference between FDA oversight of prescription drugs and its oversight of OTCs is a matter of advertising. In the case of prescription drugs, the FDA regulates advertising and approval for use. Advertising of nonprescription drugs, however, is regulated by the Federal Trade Commission.

An important aspect of FDA regulation of OTCs is labeling. Each OTC approved for sale in the United States must carry a "Drug Facts" label on the product or its package. The label has a standard format and must be clearly and simply written. It has the following parts: product name, active ingredient or ingredients, purpose, uses, warnings, directions, inactive ingredients, and other information.

SAFETY

Although the FDA's definition of OTCs includes the assurance that OTCs are "safe and effective," this assurance assumes that the medications are used correctly by consumers. There are several steps consumers should follow to make sure that they are using nonprescription medications correctly. These steps include the following:

Read the Drug Facts label carefully. It is especially important to note the active ingredients in the medicine, particularly when using two or more OTCs to treat the same condition or illness, such as the common cold. It is possible to take an accidental overdose of the active ingredients in cough and cold medicines because many of these preparations contain several active ingredients. The Drug Facts label will also contain important warnings about drug interactions (particularly interactions with alcohol), activities to avoid while taking the medicine (usually driving and operating heavy equipment), and dosage instructions.

Persons should never take more than the recommended dosage or take the medicine more often than recommended. If one's symptoms do not improve within a few days, that person should see a doctor. Persons should also consult a doctor or pharmacist if they have any questions about the medication, particularly its possible side effects or possible interactions with other drugs.

Check for tampering. Before purchase, one should check the tamper-evident packaging (TEP) features, such as internal plastic seals or blister packaging, to ensure the medication has not been tampered with. TEPs are safety features that were mandated by the FDA in 1983 following a still-unsolved crime in which seven people in Chicago died after taking a pain reliever that had been poisoned with potassium cyanide. If the package or the contents look suspicious in any

way, the consumer should return the OTC to the store or pharmacy where it was purchased.

Store medication in a childproof cabinet or medicine chest. Also, one should keep all medicines away from children. OTCs should never be left on counter tops or tables where curious children can open and use them. Medications should always be kept in their original containers so that no one in the household can take the wrong drug by accident. Expiration dates should be checked periodically; medicines with expired dates should be discarded safely.

OTC ABUSE

The purchase of some OTCs is restricted in the United States because these medications have been abused or have been used illegally. The purchaser may be required to show proof of age before buying the product or may have to ask a registered pharmacist for the product.

The two major types of OTCs in this category are

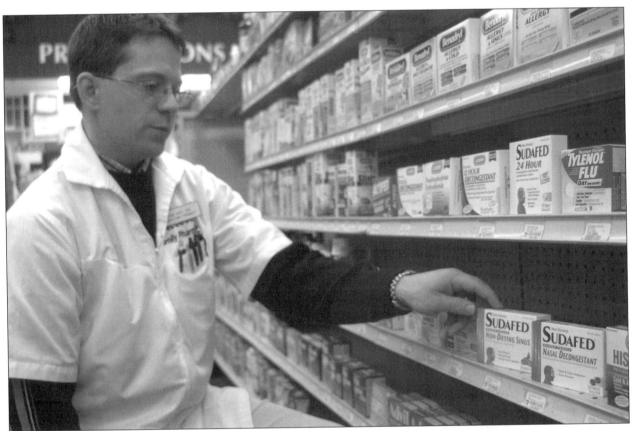

Sudafed, a decongestant, is one of many OTC drugs available to treat common cold symptoms. (AP/Wide World Photos)

cold and allergy medications containing ephedrine or pseudoephedrine, which are decongestants, and cough medicines containing dextromethorphan (DMX), a cough suppressant. Ephedrine and pseudoephedrine can be used to make methamphetamine, a dangerous drug of abuse. To prevent the illicit production of methamphetamine from OTCs, the U.S. Congress passed the Combat Methamphetamine Epidemic Act, or CMEA, in 2005. The CMEA sets monthly limits on the amount of these products that consumers can purchase and requires that consumers show proof of identity to a pharmacist before purchase.

Cough medicines containing DMX have been abused by teenagers and others who consume large amounts of the preparations to get intoxicated. According to the CHPA, about 6 percent of teenagers in the United States abuse cough syrups containing DMX. Although there is no federal legislation controlling the sale of medications containing DMX, some states require proof that a would-be purchaser is eighteen years of age or older at the time of sale.

IMPACT

Over-the-counter medications represent a considerable portion of the money spent on health care in the United States. In the first decade of the twenty-first century, sales of OTCs for minor health conditions came to $20 billion per year, with dietary supplements accounting for another $12 billion. Nonprescription drugs are also widely available for purchase on the Web and in supermarkets and other retail outlets that do not have pharmacies. OTCs can be purchased at more than 750,000 locations in the United States.

The widespread availability of nonprescription products and the ongoing transfer of some classes of prescription drugs into the OTC category make it easier for consumers, particularly older adults, to take a more active part in their health care. The FDA notes that increased access to nonprescription drugs is beneficial to people age sixty-five years and older, 80 percent of whom have some type of chronic health problem that can be managed effectively with OTCs. In terms of infectious diseases, however, it is unlikely that many anti-infective drugs will be switched into the OTC category because of concern about the potential overuse of antibiotics, commonly used for bacterial infections, and concern about the risk of developing even more drug-resistant disease organisms.

Rebecca J. Frey, Ph.D.

FURTHER READING

Dlugosz, Cynthia Knapp, ed. *The Practitioner's Quick Reference to Nonprescription Drugs.* Washington, D.C.: American Pharmacists Association, 2009. Intended for health care professionals, this guide organizes its discussion of nonprescription drugs according to the twenty-five most common conditions consumers treat with OTCs, including acne, allergic rhinitis, tooth hypersensitivity, and warts.

Griffith, Henry Winter. *Complete Guide to Prescription and Nonprescription Drugs.* Rev. and updated by Stephen W. Moore. New York: Penguin Books, 2009. This reference work, updated annually, covers more than five thousand OTCs by brand name and eight hundred more by generic name. Written for nonprofessionals, it includes information on side effects, potentially dangerous drug interactions, and FDA changes in drug labeling or classification.

Knowles, Johanna. *Over-the-Counter Drugs.* New York: Chelsea House, 2008. This book is not a reference guide to OTCs but a discussion of the abuse of OTCs by adolescents and the scope of the problem. Also includes advice about where and how to get help.

2011 PDR for Nonprescription Drugs, Dietary Supplements, and Herbs. Toronto, Ont.: Thomson Health Care, 2010. The basic drug reference book for health care professionals, this PDR guide to nonprescription drugs is updated yearly with information about commonly used OTCs, organized alphabetically by manufacturer's name. The book also includes photographs of OTCs to simplify identification.

WEB SITES OF INTEREST

American Academy of Family Physicians
http://familydoctor.org

Consumer Healthcare Products Association
http://www.chpa-info.org

Make up Your Own Mind About Cough Medicine
http://www.dxmstories.com

OTCsafety.org
http://otcsafety.org

U.S. Food and Drug Administration
http://www.fda.gov/drugs

See also: Acne; Antibiotics: Types; Antifungal drugs: Types; Bacterial infections; Cold sores; Common cold; Drug resistance; Fungal infections; Home remedies; Infection; Influenza; Pharyngitis and tonsillopharyngitis; Treatment of bacterial infections; Treatment of fungal infections; Treatment of viral infections.

Oxazolidinone antibiotics

CATEGORY: Treatment

DEFINITION

Oxazolidinone antibiotics disrupt the synthesis of new proteins. In doing so, they inhibit bacterial growth and reproduction.

HISTORY

The first oxazolidinone antibiotic used in human medicine was cycloserine, which was introduced in 1956 as a second-line drug against *Mycobacterium tuberculosis*, the bacterium that causes tuberculosis. In 2000, the company Amersham Pharmacia (now Pfizer) introduced to the market an oxazolidinone called linezolid (Zyvox). Linezolid was the first new class of antibiotic to pass clinical trials successfully in twenty years. It has proven to be extremely effective against multidrug-resistant bacteria. New oxazolidinones that include torezolid (TR-700), posizolid (AZD-2563), and radezolid (RX-1741) are in clinical trials.

MECHANISMS OF ACTION AND BACTERIAL RESISTANCE

Cells synthesize proteins on large protein-ribonucleic acid (RNA) complexes called ribosomes. Oxazolidinone antibiotics bind to ribosomes and disrupt the synthesis of new proteins, inhibiting bacterial growth and reproduction.

Bacterial resistance to linezolid results in one of two different mechanisms. The first mechanism involves mutations that increase production of efflux proteins that actively pump linezolid from the cell. The second mechanism includes mutations that modify ribosomes so that they can still make proteins but bind linezolid much less tightly. The global tracking of linezolid resistance has shown that the frequency of bacterial resistance to linezolid is low (0.03 to 0.3 percent) and stable, but the increased use of this antibiotic will almost certainly increase rates of resistance to it.

SIDE EFFECTS

Inside human cells are vesicles called mitochondria that make the chemical energy for the cell. Mitochondria possess their own deoxyribonucleic acid (DNA) chromosomes and ribosomes that synthesize some of their proteins. Mitochondrial ribosomes have many similarities to bacterial ribosomes, and these structural resemblances render mitochondrial ribosomes susceptible to inhibition by linezolid.

When used for a short time, linezolid causes headache, nausea, vomiting, and rash in a small minority of persons. It can also cause the overgrowth of various bodily surfaces with yeast (antibiotic candidiasis); a few persons show signs of liver damage. Long-term use of linezolid (more than fourteen days), however, can cause bone marrow suppression, peripheral and optical neuropathy, and the accumulation of lactic acid in the blood (lactic acidosis). All of these side effects directly result from the inhibition of mitochondrial ribosomes.

IMPACT

Linezolid has provided new treatment options for some infectious diseases that have, because of bacterial drug resistance, exhausted all previous antibiotic treatment regimes. It is largely active against gram-positive bacteria; gram-positive bacteria have thick cell walls, and gram-negative bacteria have thin cell walls in addition to an outer membrane.

Physicians use linezolid to treat skin and respiratory tract infections caused by methicillin-resistant *Staphylococcus aureus* and *Streptococcus* strains. Linezolid is also effective against vancomycin-resistant bacterial meningitis and vancomycin-resistant strains of *Enterococcus faecium*, which can cause a variety of infections that are difficult to treat. In combination with other drugs, linezolid also has been used to treat multidrug-resistant tuberculosis.

Michael A. Buratovich, Ph.D.

FURTHER READING

Gallagher, Jason. *Antibiotics Simplified*. Sudbury, Mass.: Jones and Bartlett, 2008.

Goldsmith, Connie. *Superbugs Strike Back: When Antibiotics Fail*. Breckenridge, Colo.: Twenty-First Century Books, 2006.

Walsh, Christopher. *Antibiotics: Actions, Origins, Resistance*. Washington, D.C.: ASM Press, 2003.

WEB SITES OF INTEREST

eMedicineHealth: Antibiotics
http://www.emedicinehealth.com/antibiotics

National Institute of Allergy and Infectious Diseases
http://www.niaid.nih.gov/topics/antimicrobialresistance

Todar's Online Textbook of Bacteriology
http://www.textbookofbacteriology.net

See also: Alliance for the Prudent Use of Antibiotics; Aminoglycoside antibiotics; Antibiotic resistance; Antibiotics: Types; Bacteria: Classification and types; Bacterial infections; Cephalosporin antibiotics; Glycopeptide antibiotics; Ketolide antibiotics; Lipopeptide antibiotics; Macrolide antibiotics; Microbiology; Penicillin antibiotics; Prevention of bacterial infections; Quinolone antibiotics; Superbacteria; Tetracycline antibiotics; Treatment of bacterial infections.

Oxygen therapy. *See* Hyperbaric oxygen therapy.

P

Pacemaker infections

CATEGORY: Diseases and conditions
ANATOMY OR SYSTEM AFFECTED: Abdomen, cardiovascular system, chest, heart

DEFINITION

Pacemaker infections are illnesses caused by contamination of the pacemaker, a small device consisting
of a pulse generator and wire leads that is surgically
implanted in the chest or abdomen to help control
abnormal heart rhythms. Pacemaker infections most
commonly occur in the pocket in which the part of
the pacemaker called the generator is placed. Most infections are thought to occur through contamination
of the pacemaker device by standard skin bacteria
(such as staphylococci and corynebacteria) present at
the time of implantation.

Pacemaker infections are more common in people
who have diabetes mellitus, who use steroids, who
have an underlying malignancy, who have an overlying skin disorder, who have a heart hematoma, who
have emergency pacemaker placement, and who have
had frequent generator replacements. There is also
evidence that implantation of the device by an inexperienced surgical team increases infection risk.

CAUSES

Pacemakers, used to treat abnormal heart rhythms,
are common devices in the United States. The device
consists of a small pulse generator connected to the
right chambers of the heart by two pacing leads. To
keep the heart rate in a regular rhythm, the pulse generator's computer chip creates an electrical impulse
to stimulate the heart muscle to contract (squeeze) at
a particular time and in a pattern. Pacemakers are implanted in the chests or abdomens in persons with too
slow heart rates or with blocks in the natural electrical
conduction system of their hearts.

Pacemaker infections most commonly occur in the
area, or pocket, in which the pacemaker's generator is
placed. Most infections are thought to occur from
contamination of the pacemaker device by standard
skin bacteria that are present at the time of implantation. Even though the bacteria are present at the time
of the pacemaker surgery, symptoms of the infection
may not appear immediately. In some persons, symptoms of pacemaker infection may occur more than
two years after surgery. Infection of the pacemaker's
leads and electrodes occurs less frequently than infections of the generator, although an infection in the
generator pocket can spread up the leads to the heart
and electrode tips.

RISK FACTORS

The risk factors for pacemaker infection are related
to the person's health, the conditions of the device implant, and the skill of the surgical team implanting the
device. An increased risk of pacemaker infection exists in persons with diabetes mellitus, in persons with
an underlying malignancy, in persons who use steroids,
and in persons with an overlying skin disorder (particularly disorders such as pustules). Research also has
determined that persons who had urgent placement
of their original pacemaker, who have had frequent replacement of the pacemaker generator, who have hematoma formation, and whose surgical implantation
was performed by an inexperienced team are also at
increased risk for pacemaker infection.

SYMPTOMS

The main symptoms of a pacemaker infection are a
fever and fatigue. Other symptoms include an infection of the heart's inner layer (endocarditis), a new or
changing heart murmur, and abnormal growths on
the tricuspid valves, pacemaker electrodes, or endo-
cardium of the right ventricle or atrium. The infection may also cause blockage of the main artery of the
lung by a clot called a pulmonary embolus.

SCREENING AND DIAGNOSIS

Diagnosis of a pacemaker infection should be considered in persons with pacemakers and unexplained
fever and fatigue. The infection can be confirmed

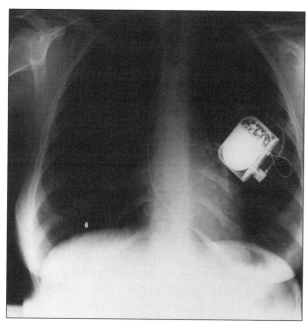

A pacemaker, as it appears on an X-ray image.

through blood cultures that identify specific infection-causing bacteria or pathogens and through an echocardiogram that demonstrates abnormal growths (vegetations) on a pacemaker lead or electrode. Cultures of the blood, the pacemaker pocket, and any wound site should also be used to help confirm a pacemaker infection. Definitive diagnosis of a pacemaker infection can be made upon finding a bacterium or other microorganism infecting the pacemaker pocket or blood.

TREATMENT AND THERAPY

The conservative treatment of a pacemaker infection of the generator or electrode, or both, is a combination therapy using antimicrobial agents tailored to the identified infectious agent and the removal of the pacemaker hardware. A relapse of the infection is usually associated with the failure to remove all hardware.

PREVENTION AND OUTCOMES

The prevention of pacemaker infection is not guaranteed by the use of particular procedures or devices; however, the risk for infection can be decreased. Given identified risk factors, infection risk can be reduced by implantation of the pacemaker by an experi-

enced surgical team using sterile procedures in a scheduled, not urgent, setting. Evidence exists that administering antibiotics, such as levofloxacin, before the procedure decreases the risk for infections. The risk of pacemaker infection can also be decreased through the implantation of drug-eluting devices, or stents, at the time the pacemaker is implanted. Drug-eluting devices emit antimicrobial medications directly at any potential infection site.

Dawn Laney, M.S.

FURTHER READING

Chua, J. D., et al. "Diagnosis and Management of Infections Involving Implantable Electrophysiological Cardiac Devices." *Annals of Internal Medicine* 133 (2000): 604. A review of the diagnosis and medical management of pacemaker infections.

De Oliveira, J. C., et al. "Efficacy of Antibiotic Prophylaxis Before the Implantation of Pacemakers and Cardioverter-Defibrillators." *Circulation: Arrhythmia and Electrophysiology* 2, no. 1 (February, 2009): 29-34. A study describing the benefits of taking antibiotics before pacemaker implantation.

Eggimann, P., and F. Waldvogel. "Pacemaker and Defibrillator Infections." In *Infections Associated with Indwelling Medical Devices*, edited by F. Waldvogel, and A. L. Bisno. Washington, D.C.: ASM Press, 2000. A detailed review of infections involving implanted pacemakers.

Klug, D., et al. "Risk Factors Related to Infections of Implanted Pacemakers and Cardioverter-Defibrillators." *Circulation* 116 (2007): 1349. A study identifying the risk factors for developing pacemaker infections.

Lipsky, Martin S., Marla Mendelson, and Stephen Havas. *American Medical Association Guide to Preventing and Treating Heart Disease*. Hoboken, N.J.: John Wiley & Sons, 2008. Includes an excellent description of the pacemaker device, implantation surgery, and pacemaker infection.

Murphy, Joseph G., and Margaret A. Lloyd, eds. *Mayo Clinic Cardiology: Concise Textbook*. 3d ed. Rochester, Minn.: Mayo Clinic Scientific Press, 2007. Clearly and concisely describes pacemaker infections.

WEB SITES OF INTEREST

American Heart Association
http://www.heart.org

See also: Bacterial infections; Blood-borne illness and disease; Bloodstream infections; *Corynebacterium*; Endocarditis; Hospitals and infectious disease; Iatrogenic infections; Infection; Myocarditis; Prosthetic joint infections; Sepsis; Staphylococcal infections; Wound infections.

Pancreatitis

CATEGORY: Diseases and conditions
ANATOMY OR SYSTEM AFFECTED: Gastrointestinal system, pancreas

DEFINITION

Pancreatitis is inflammation of the pancreas. The acute form typically comes on suddenly, recurs intermittently, and can be mild or severe. Chronic pancreatitis develops over time and results in permanent damage to the organ. Both forms can lead to infection and serious complications involving the blood vessels, heart, lungs, and kidneys.

CAUSES

Although gallstones and alcohol consumption are responsible for most cases of pancreatitis, viral, bacterial, fungal, and parasitic infections can also cause the disease. Viruses linked with pancreatitis include coxsackie, mumps, hepatitis, and echoviruses; linked bacteria include *Salmonella*, *Leptospira*, and *Mycoplasma* species; and linked fungi include *Aspergillus* species. In persons with severe acute pancreatitis, *Escherichia coli*, enterococci, and other organisms can also spread from the intestines and infect the damaged pancreas, increasing the risk of death.

RISK FACTORS

Persons with weakened immune systems are more likely to develop viral forms of pancreatitis. Between 30 and 70 percent of persons with severe pancreatitis will develop a bacterial infection. In general, gallstone disease is associated more often with pancreatitis in women and alcoholism is associated more often with pancreatitis in men. Family history, living with acquired immunodeficiency syndrome (AIDS), and cigarette smoking have also been linked with the disorder. Recurring acute attacks can lead to chronic pancreatitis.

SYMPTOMS

Persons with acute pancreatitis typically have upper abdominal pain that may spread to the back. The pain may be severe and may increase after eating or when lying flat. Nausea and vomiting, fever, rapid pulse, and tenderness and swelling of the abdomen are also seen. In severe cases with internal bleeding, blood pressure levels may drop. Most persons with chronic pancreatitis also experience upper abdominal pain. The pain may come and go, or it may disappear altogether. Nausea and vomiting, foul-smelling diarrhea, and unintended weight loss are also common with this form.

SCREENING AND DIAGNOSIS

Clinicians will review symptoms and also the results from a physical examination and laboratory tests. A viral infection may be identified by antibodies in the blood, whereas a bacterial or fungal infection is diagnosed with blood tests and cultures of pus and other fluids. Computed tomography (CT) scans and ultrasounds of the abdomen and chest can confirm the diagnosis, indicate how severe the disease is, and pinpoint the cause. An endoscopic retrograde cholangiopancreatography may offer a better look at the pancreas and provide tissue samples for analysis.

TREATMENT AND THERAPY

In many cases, infected persons are hospitalized during treatment. Food is withheld to allow the pancreas to recover, and the patient will receive intravenous fluids, pain medications, antibiotics, and tube feedings to treat infections. Antibiotics may also be administered to prevent late infections in severe pancreatitis. Once the patient is stabilized, the cause of pancreatitis can be addressed.

The gallbladder or obstructions in the ducts may need to be removed. In cases of infection, surgery may be necessary to drain fluids or cut away damaged tissue. Persons with chronic pancreatitis may require long-term pain management and also supplemental enzymes. Meditation and yoga may help some patients cope with chronic pain.

PREVENTION AND OUTCOMES

Persons who have had or have pancreatitis are often advised to avoid drinking alcohol and to eat a low-fat diet.

Judy Majewski, M.S.

FURTHER READING

Andris Abby. "Pancreatitis: Understanding the Disease and Implications for Care." *Advanced Critical Care* 21, no. 2 (2010): 195-204.

Beger, Hans G., Seiki Matsuno, and John L. Cameron, eds. *Diseases of the Pancreas: Current Surgical Therapy.* New York: Springer, 2008.

Gloor, B., et al. "Pancreatic Infection in Severe Pancreatitis: The Role of Fungus and Multiresistant Organisms." *Archives of Surgery* 136, no. 5 (2001): 592-596.

Johnson, Leonard R., ed. *Gastrointestinal Physiology.* 7th ed. Philadelphia: Mosby Elsevier, 2007.

Munoz, Abilio, and David A. Katerndahl. "Diagnosis and Management of Acute Pancreatitis." *American Family Physician* 62, no. 1 (July 1, 2000): 164-174.

WEB SITES OF INTEREST

American Gastroenterological Association
http://www.gastro.org

National Digestive Diseases Information Clearinghouse
http://digestive.niddk.nih.gov

Pancreatitis Supporters' Network
http://www.pancreatitis.org.uk

See also: Appendicitis; Cholecystitis; Clonorchiasis; Infection; Inflammation; Intestinal and stomach infections; Kidney infection; Peritonitis.

Pandemics. *See* Epidemics and pandemics.

Paracoccidiodes

CATEGORY: Pathogen
TRANSMISSION ROUTE: Inhalation

DEFINITION

Paracoccidiodes is a genus of dimorphic fungus, with the single species *brasiliensis*. Infection with the fungus leads to paracoccidioidomycosis, a rare disease, primarily, of the lungs. The disease is also known as South American blastomycosis.

**Taxonomic Classification
for *Paracoccidiodes***

Kingdom: Fungi
Phylum: Ascomycota
Subphylum: Ascomycotina
Order: Onygenales
Genus: *Paracoccidiodes*
Species: *P. brasiliensis*

NATURAL HABITAT AND FEATURES

Paracoccidiodes consists of one species, *brasiliensis*. Its natural habitat is Central America and South America, with Brazil the epicenter. The fungus resides in humid soil that is rich in proteins and in subtropical mountain forests. The fungus is the predominant cause of systemic fungal infection in humans in these areas and has also been isolated from fruit bats and armadillos, animals native to these areas.

Paracoccidiodes is a thermally dimorphic fungus. At lower temperatures, as in its natural habitat, it is a mold with many branching hyphae (filaments). At higher temperatures, as in the tissue of an infected host, it becomes a multibudding yeast. It is a mitosporic (asexual) fungus, with no known teleomorphic (sexual) stage.

Mold-to-yeast conversion must be demonstrated to confirm that *brasiliensis* is the fungal pathogen in an infected person. *Brasiliensis* grows as a mold at 77° Fahrenheit (25° Celsius) and as a yeast at 98.6° F (37° C). Mold colonies are filamentous, slow growing, leathery, flat to wrinkled, wooly, and cottony or smooth to velvety. Microscopic observation reveals transparent (hyaline) septate hyphae, that is, hyphae with partitioned cavities. Often, the hyphae are sterile and do not produce conidia, sporelike asexual reproductive bodies. If conidia are present, they are single-cell, oval, and truncated and with a broad base and round apex. They are located along the hyphae. Specialized spores, arthroconidia and chlamydospores, may also be observed. The colony obtains a diameter of 1 to 2 centimeters in two to three weeks. The front color is white cream, tan, or brown. The reverse color is yellowish brown to brown.

Mold-to-yeast conversion requires an enriched medium, such as brain heart infusion agar (or broth). Conversion occurs after ten to twenty days of incubation. The yeast colony is heaped, wrinkled, or folded and white. Microscopic observation reveals multiple buds (blastoconidia) surrounding thick-walled mother yeast cells, similar in shape to a ship pilot's wheel. The buds are attached to the mother cell by a narrow neck portion. Before a bud detaches from the mother cell, secondary buds may form, producing short chains of yeast cells. When only single buds are observed, *brasiliensis* must be differentiated from *Blastomyces dermatitidis*. In contrast to the buds of *brasiliensis*, those of *dermatitidis* are broad-based.

PATHOGENICITY AND CLINICAL SIGNIFICANCE

Brasiliensis causes paracoccidioidomycosis. For the most part, cases of paracoccidioidomycosis are limited to areas where *brasiliensis* is native. Agricultural and forestry workers are particularly prone to infection. Isolated cases occur in persons, including immigrants and migrants, who have traveled to or from endemic regions. The infection is acquired through inhalation of conidia, which are transformed into yeast cells within alveolar macrophages in the lungs. Animal-to-animal and human-to-human transmission have not been demonstrated.

The development and degree of disease depends on the virility of the strain, the general health and immune status of the host, and, in adults, whether the host is a man or a woman. Men are fifteen times as likely as women to develop adult chronic infection. This appears to be so because fungal receptors bind to estrogen, the female sex hormone, but not to androgen, the male sex hormone. This inhibits conversion of the mold phase into the yeast phase.

Diagnosis of infection with *brasiliensis* is often difficult. Infection may not become apparent for several years after exposure. This suggests the possibility of a long latent period. For most infected persons, the first symptom of active disease is mucocutaneous lesions, especially of the mouth, nose, and throat, followed by respiratory symptoms, such as productive cough and shortness of breath.

In addition to causing primary pulmonary infection, *brasiliensis* can also cause acute primary, chronic primary, and disseminated disease. In disseminated disease, the reticuloendothelial system, lymph nodes, and skin and mucous membranes can become involved. Involvement of the reticuloendothelial system can lead to the suppression of the activity of phagocytic monocytes in the spleen, bone marrow, and lymph nodes. Aortitis, inflammation of the aorta, is also a risk. Immunocompromised persons are susceptible to the development of acute pulmonary and disseminated disease. The mortality rate from chronic infection with paracoccidioidomycosis among persons with acquired immunodeficiency syndrome (AIDS) ranges between 30 and 45 percent.

DRUG SUSCEPTIBILITY

In vitro data on the susceptibility profile of *brasiliensis* are limited. A standardized in vitro susceptibility test has not been established. Testing methods that have been used have had varying results, making meaningful comparisons difficult. In general, relatively low minimum inhibitory concentrations (MICs) have been detected for amphotericin B and azoles, including ketoconazole, itraconazole, and fluconazole, when tested against the yeast phase of *brasiliensis*. Higher MICs have been reported for some isolates.

In the past, sulfonamides, amphotericin B, and ketoconazole were used to treat infection caused by *brasiliensis*. Sulfonamides, in particular trimethoprim/sulfamethoxazole (TMP) and sulfadiazine, are still used in Latin America because of their low costs. Paracoccidioidomycosis is the only systemic fungal infection that is treated with sulfonamides. Itraconazole has replaced ketoconazole because it is better tolerated and more effective. It has become the drug of first choice. Amphotericin B is reserved for persons with severe diseases who cannot tolerate oral medications.

Ernest Kohlmetz, M.A.

FURTHER READING

Carlile, Michael J., Sarah C. Watkinson, and Graham W. Gooday. *The Fungi.* 2d ed. San Diego, Calif.: Academic Press, 2005.

Larone, Davise H. *Medically Important Fungi: A Guide to Identification.* 4th ed. Washington, D.C.: ASM Press, 2002.

Restrepo, A., and A. M. Tobon. "*Paracoccidioides brasiliensis.*" In *Mandell, Douglas, and Bennett's Principles and Practice of Infectious Diseases,* edited by Gerald L. Mandell, John F. Bennett, and Raphael Dolin. 7th ed. New York: Churchill Livingstone/Elsevier, 2010.

Webster, John, and Roland Weber. *Introduction to Fungi.* New York: Cambridge University Press, 2007.

WEB SITES OF INTEREST

Centers for Disease Control and Prevention, Division of Foodborne, Bacterial, and Mycotic Diseases
http://www.cdc.gov/nczved/divisions/dfbmd

Microbiology and Immunology On-line: Mycology
http://pathmicro.med.sc.edu/book/mycol-sta.htm

Systematic Mycology and Microbiology Laboratory
http://www.ars.usda.gov

See also: Airborne illness and disease; Antifungal drugs: Types; Aspergillosis; *Aspergillus*; Blastomycosis; Chromoblastomycosis; *Coccidioides*; Coccidiosis; Diagnosis of fungal infections; Fungal infections; Fungi: Classification and types; *Fusarium*; Histoplasmosis; Immune response to fungal infections; Melioidosis; Mucormycosis; Mycetoma; Mycoses; Paracoccidioidomycosis; Respiratory route of transmission; Soilborne illness and disease.

Paracoccidioidomycosis

CATEGORY: Diseases and conditions
ANATOMY OR SYSTEM AFFECTED: Lungs, respiratory system, skin, tissue
ALSO KNOWN AS: South American blastomycosis

DEFINITION

Paracoccidioidomycosis is a rare infection caused by *Paracoccidiodes brasiliensis*, a soil fungus. It is prevalent in the coffee- and tobacco-growing regions of South America and Central America. This type of infection primarily affects the lungs but may spread to other areas of the body and form ulcerations.

CAUSES

Brasiliensis is a dimorphic fungus that exists in mold or yeast form depending on the conditions. In the environment, the fungus exists as a mold that produces spores. Inhalation of the fungal spores causes a pulmonary infection. Once inside the body, the spores transform to yeast and disperse to other areas of the body (mouth, throat, skin, and lymph nodes). Human-to-human transmission of the disease is uncommon.

RISK FACTORS

All ages can be affected by the disease; however, the majority of cases involve healthy males with an outdoor occupation or hobby, especially agricultural workers, coffee and tobacco growers, and hunters. Other factors, such as malnutrition, smoking, and alcoholism, increase the chance of acquiring paracoccidioidomycosis. Younger and immunocompromised persons, including those with acquired immunodeficiency syndrome (AIDS) and human immunodeficiency virus (HIV) infection, are more likely to have acute (severe) disease.

SYMPTOMS

Symptoms of chronic pulmonary paracoccidioidomycosis include cough, difficulty breathing, fever, weight loss, and fatigue. As the disease progresses, mucosal, oral, and cutaneous lesions, usually on the face, appear and may be papular, nodular, ulcerative, or plaque-like. Ulcerations on the gums, tongue, lips, and palate are also common. Persons with a severe infection may have widespread disseminated disease with lesions causing inflammation of the intestines, liver, spleen, lymph nodes, or brain, and adrenal gland destruction and abdominal pain. Some persons can develop paracoccidioidomycosis many years after initial contact with the etiologic agent. Although symptoms can last for years, the disease is rarely fatal.

SCREENING AND DIAGNOSIS

Because paracoccidioidomycosis is rare, primary care physicians should inquire about the previous residence of the person seeking diagnosis. Consultation with a dermatologist for a skin biopsy and with an infectious disease specialist for diagnosis and treatment is recommended. Diagnostic tests may include sputum culture, tissue biopsy, various serological tests to detect antibodies, and chest radiography. Definitive diagnosis requires isolation, culture, and analysis of infected tissue under a microscope to detect *brasiliensis*.

TREATMENT AND THERAPY

Persons with paracoccidioidomycosis should be treated based on the severity of the disease. Infection is susceptible to sulfonamides, amphotericin B, and azole antifungals. Oral itraconazole is the drug of choice because of its availability, effectiveness, and decreased toxicity. Because of side effects, amphotericin B is recommended only for persons with severe disease.

Paracoccidioidomycosis has the potential to be fatal if left untreated or if the infection is severe. However, with early intervention, the prognosis for persons with chronic paracoccidioidomycosis is good.

PREVENTION AND OUTCOMES

Because *brasiliensis* is a microscopic fungus, the best form of prevention is to avoid areas where it is prevalent.

Rose Ciulla-Bohling, Ph.D.

FURTHER READING

Hospenthal, Duane R. "Paracoccidioidomycosis." Available at http://emedicine.medscape.com/article/224628-overview.

Kauffman, Carol A. "Paracoccidioidomycosis." In *Cecil Medicine*, edited by Lee Goldman and Dennis Ausiello. 23d ed. Philadelphia: Saunders/Elsevier, 2008.

Restrepo, A., A. M. Tobon, and C. A. Agudelo. "Paracoccidioidomycosis." In *Diagnosis and Treatment of Human Mycoses*, edited by Duane R. Hospenthal and Michael G. Rinaldi. Totowa, N.J.: Humana Press, 2008.

Richardson, Malcolm D., and Elizabeth M. Johnson. *Pocket Guide to Fungal Infection*. 2d ed. Malden, Mass.: Wiley-Blackwell, 2006.

WEB SITES OF INTEREST

Centers for Disease Control and Prevention, Division of Foodborne, Bacterial, and Mycotic Diseases
http://www.cdc.gov/nczved/divisions/dfbmd

Microbiology and Immunology On-line: Mycology
http://pathmicro.med.sc.edu/book/mycol-sta.htm

Systematic Mycology and Microbiology Laboratory
http://www.ars.usda.gov

See also: Airborne illness and disease; Antifungal drugs: Types; Aspergillosis; *Aspergillus*; Blastomycosis; Chromoblastomycosis; *Coccidioides*; Coccidiosis; Diagnosis of fungal infections; Fungal infections; Fungi: Classification and types; *Fusarium*; Histoplasmosis; Immune response to fungal infections; Melioidosis; Mucormycosis; Mycetoma; Mycoses; *Paracoccidioides*; Respiratory route of transmission; Soilborne illness and disease.

Paramyxoviridae

CATEGORY: Pathogen
TRANSMISSION ROUTE: Direct contact

DEFINITION

The Paramyxoviridae is a virus family containing single-stranded, negative-sense RNA (ribonucleic acid), with a helically symmetrical nucleocapsid. The viruses cause a variety of highly contagious and virulent diseases in mammals and birds. However, several previously unknown paramyxoviruses have emerged to cause fatal disease in humans and nonhuman animals.

**Taxonomic Classification
for Paramyxoviridae**

Order: Monongavirales
Family: Paramyxoviridae
Subfamily: Paramyxovirinae
Genus: *Henipavirus*
Species:
Hendra virus
Nipah virus
Genus: *Morbillivirus*
Species: Measles virus
Genus: *Respirovirus*
Species: Human parainfluenza viruses 1 and 3
Genus: *Rubulavirus*
Species:
Mumps virus
Human parainfluenza viruses 2 and 4
Subfamily: Pneumovirinae
Genus: *Pneumovirus*
Species: Human respiratory syncytial virus
Genus: *Metapneumovirus*
Species: Human metapneumovirus

NATURAL HABITAT AND FEATURES

Viral particles consist of a single helical strand of RNA, contained within a lipoprotein envelope, a nucleocapsid, and a matrix protein. Typically, paramyxoviral particles are spherical to pleomorphic, ranging from 150 to 200 nanometers (nm) in diameter and 1,000 to 10,000 nm in length. The nucleocapsid is between 600 and 1000 nm, depending on the genus. The genome of paramyxoviridae is made up of an RNA molecule between 15,200 and 15,900 nucleotides long, comprising six genes for six proteins.

Viral particles enter the host cell by binding with the cell using a binding hemagglutinin (H) protein. They fuse the viral envelope with the host cell membrane, facilitated by a fusion (F) protein. Viral particles enter the cytoplasm, where negative-sense RNA genes are turned into messenger RNA, then to nucleocapsid proteins. A positive-sense RNA template is then used to produce more viral RNA.

Paramyxoviruses often produce an excess of nucleocapsids that form large inclusion bodies in the host cells. Individual viruses escape the cell by pushing through the cell's membranes to form envelopes from the host cell membrane. Paramyxovirus F proteins fuse host cell membranes, which can cause multiple host cells to fuse and form a large, multinucleated syncytium.

Paramyxoviruses do not remain viable for long in the environment, depending instead upon being spread by direct contact between carriers and susceptible persons. Contact is usually through respiratory droplets, and the viruses attack the respiratory system initially and preferentially. As direct contact between susceptible persons is necessary for the survival of paramyxoviruses in populations, diseases caused by these viruses tend to proliferate in areas that are densely crowded, such as in cities.

PATHOGENICITY AND CLINICAL SIGNIFICANCE

Diseases caused by paramyxoviruses include what were once called the childhood diseases: measles and mumps. In addition, common respiratory illnesses such as respiratory syncytial virus and parainfluenza virus, the cause of childhood croup, are caused by paramyxoviruses. Paramyxoviruses also lead to devastating animal illnesses, such as canine distemper, rinderpest and Newcastle disease; new viruses have emerged to cause fatal infections in humans in Australia, India, Bangladesh, and Malaysia, and to cause massive die-offs of seals and porpoises.

Measles is perhaps the best known of the paramyxoviruses. Measles is considered one of the most highly contagious diseases known, causing disease in more than 90 percent of exposed persons. Measles is usually self-limiting, causing an initial fever, respiratory illness, and a generalized rash, all resolving within fourteen days. Still, as many as 1 in 20 children develops pneumonia, and 1 child in 1,000 contracts encepha-

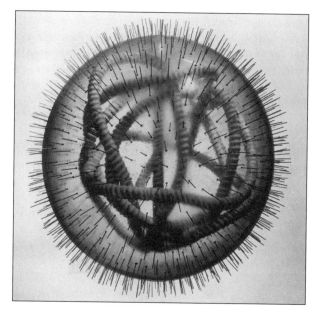

An illustration of the measles virus, part of the Paramxyoviridae family of viruses.

litis, which can lead to permanent deafness, retardation, or death.

Vaccination has made measles rare in developed nations, but malnutrition, particularly vitamin A deficiency, keeps measles a serious threat in developing nations. An estimated 10 million cases of measles occur each year, with 197,000 deaths, mostly among children younger than age five years.

Respiratory syncytial virus is the most common cause of lower respiratory tract disease worldwide, and estimates show that all children will have had RSV infection by their second birthday. Parainfluenza viruses are included among viruses that cause the common cold, and they are second only to RSV in number of infections. Like RSV, parainfluenza viruses can also cause more serious infections in the lower respiratory tract (lungs) and can cause croup in children and in the elderly.

Mumps is a virus that causes a localized swelling of the parotid salivary glands. In some cases, the virus will cause testicular swelling that can lead to infertility, particularly in young men. Two new viruses have emerged in the early twenty-first century to form a new class of paramyxovirus. Hendra virus and nipah virus originated in bats and jumped to domestic animal species and then to humans, causing encephalitis and a high rate of fatalities in affected persons.

DRUG SUSCEPTIBILITY

No antiviral therapy exists that is effective against the paramyxoviruses. Treatment for any paramyxovirus disease is supportive. Vaccination has been shown to be an effective and long-lasting preventive measure for most paramyxoviral diseases.

Cynthia L. Mills, D.V.M.

FURTHER READING

Lamb, Robert A., and Griffith D. Parks. "Paramyxoviridae: The Viruses and Their Replication." In *Fields' Virology*, edited by David M. Knipe and Peter M. Howley. Philadelphia: Wolters Kluwer Health/ Lippincott Williams & Wilkins, 2007.

Schaffer, Kirsten, Alberto M. LaRosa, and Estella Whimbey. "Respiratory Viruses." In *Cohen and Powderly Infectious Diseases*, edited by Jonathan Cohen, Steven M. Opal, and William G. Powderly. 3d ed. Philadelphia: Mosby/Elsevier, 2010.

Strauss, James, and Ellen Strauss. *Viruses and Human Disease*. Burlington, Mass.: Elsevier, 2008.

WEB SITES OF INTEREST

Big Picture Book of Viruses
http://www.virology.net/big_virology

Centers for Disease Control and Prevention
http://www.cdc.gov

Virus Pathogen Database and Analysis Resource
http://www.viprbrc.org/brc

See also: Children and infectious disease; Common cold; Croup; Immunization; Infection; Influenza; Measles; Metapneumovirus infection; Mumps; Primates and infectious disease; Respiratory syncytial virus infections; Viral upper respiratory infections.

Parasites: Classification and types

CATEGORY: Epidemiology

DEFINITION

A parasite is a pathogenic organism that feeds and grows on another organism, known as a host, and causes what are known as parasitic diseases. Some-times, a parasite produces little or no symptoms in the host. Often, however, a parasite is detrimental and even fatal to the host organism. Parasitic diseases are prevalent worldwide, but their incidence is significantly higher in developing nations.

Humans, as hosts, are susceptible to a number of parasites, namely protozoa (single-celled organisms), helminths (worms or wormlike organisms), and ectoparasites (such as fleas, lice, ticks, and mites). Ectoparasites infest the external (cutaneous) body surface (the skin and hair). Protozoa and helminths are endoparasites (parasites that invade the body). Endoparasites can infect the intestinal tract, the bloodstream, and internal organs (such as the brain, eyes, liver, and kidneys).

Some parasites are transmitted by an insect vector, an organism that transmits disease to another organism. For example the *Anopheles* mosquito transmits malaria (*Plasmodium* species) to humans.

Parasites often have a life cycle in which one stage of development exists in another animal or environment. For example, a tapeworm infection begins when a person consumes water that has been contaminated with the eggs or larvae of tapeworms. The eggs hatch in the intestines and develop into larvae. Larvae, which have hatched before or after entering the intestines, develop into adult tapeworms. The adults attach to the intestinal wall, from which they derive nourishment. The adults lay eggs, which pass out in the feces. This fecal material can contaminate the water supply and, thus, complete the life cycle.

CLASSIFICATION

Parasites can be classified a number of ways, such as by the location of the body affected—cutaneous (ectoparasite) or invasive (endoparasite)—and by type of parasite—protozoa, helminth, or ectoparasite. Endoparasites specifically can be further classified by the area of the body that they invade (intestines, brain, or liver).

Ectoparasitic infections, which most often cause skin irritation, are relatively easy to treat. Most endoparasites are protozoa or helminths; some are arachnids. Endoparasitic infections range from asymptomatic to fatal, and virtually every organ in the body is susceptible to more than one type of this infection. Helminths are further subdivided into platyhelminthes (flatworms) and nemathelminthes (roundworms).

IMPACT

Parasitic infections are a major health concern, and the risk of infection is present throughout the globe. However, these infections are of particular concern in subtropical and tropical regions of developing countries. At risk are not only residents of the regions but also travelers to these areas. In many cases, manifestations of the disease do not appear until a traveler has returned home to an area where the disease is not present; thus, a diagnosis may be missed. Parasitic diseases have a far greater impact on residents of endemic areas.

Many parasites cause serious, debilitating, and sometimes fatal illnesses. They affect people of all ages, including infants and children. In fact, some illnesses are more common in children.

Beyond the impact on health, the medical costs for pharmaceuticals, health care professionals, and hospitalization are significant. Many developing nations do not possess adequate resources for the treatment of parasitic infections; thus, they must rely on aid from developed nations and international support groups.

Contaminated water, food, and soil are major contributors to parasitic diseases. The eggs of many parasites are present in feces; thus, fecal-oral transmission is common. International groups, such as the World Health Organization (WHO), expend considerable resources educating people in developing nations about the importance of adequate sanitation and improved personal hygiene.

Some parasitic infections are responsible for significant mortality, while others rarely cause death. Even with this low mortality rate, some parasitic infections significantly effect societies, as they lead to lost wages and time away from schooling.

Parasitic infections that are common in developing nations are rare in the developed world. For example, about forty cases of trichinosis, which is caused by the beef or pork tapeworm, are reported annually in the United States. Malaria, too, is rare in the United States, and most cases are seen in immigrants from endemic countries or from U.S. citizens who have traveled abroad. The Centers for Disease Control and Prevention (CDC) estimates that 300 to 500 million cases of malaria arise each year and that more than 1 million people die from the disease annually.

Malaria. Beginning in the 1940's, the pesticide dichloro-diphenyl-trichloroethane (DDT) was used to spray areas in which the *Anopheles* mosquito was present; this resulted in reduced rates (and even eradication) of malaria in many regions. However, the effect of DDT on wildlife, and its possible carcinogenic effects in humans, led to public outcry. In 1972, DDT was banned in the United States and, subsequently, worldwide. Subsequently, malaria reappeared, resulting in millions of deaths.

Malaria is one parasitic infection responsible for significant loss of life worldwide; there are many others, including elephantiasis (lymphatic filariasis), *Loa loa* filariasis (African eye worm), Chagas' disease, trypanosomiasis (African sleeping sickness), and schistosomiasis.

Schistosomiasis. Schistosomiasis is ranked second behind malaria in terms of public health and socioeconomic significance in endemic areas, which include tropical and subtropical areas of Africa, Asia, and South America. The disease, caused by the parasitic worms of the genus *Schistosoma*, is prevalent in areas in which the local water supplies contain freshwater snails, which carry the parasite. More than 200 million people are infected and more than 600 million people who live in rural and semiurban areas are at risk. Although this disease has a low mortality rate, it causes chronic illnesses involving the intestines, bladder, kidneys, ureters, and lungs.

Elephantiasis. More than 120 million people have elephantiasis, and more than 40 million of them are seriously disfigured and incapacitated. Affected body parts include the arms, legs, genitals, and breasts. Tremendously swollen legs and genitals make walking difficult if not impossible. Kidney damage can cause serious health problems and even death. More than 1 billion people in developing countries are at risk of infection.

Amebiasis. Amebiasis is a gastrointestinal infection caused by *Entamoeba histolytica*. The disease is responsible for about seventy thousand deaths annually. The usual symptom is diarrhea, which ranges from mild to severe. If untreated, the infection can remain in the gastrointestinal tract for years. Asymptomatic persons can infect others through poor hygienic practices. Sometimes, the infection invades the bloodstream and can form liver abscesses.

Loa loa filariasis. Approximately thirteen million people in western and central Africa are infected with *Loa loa* filariasis, which is caused by a bite from the deer fly or mango fly. The nematode invades the subcutaneous layers of the skin and the subconjunctival layers of the eyes, where it can be readily observed. The disease is rarely fatal.

Chagas' disease. Chagas' disease, which is caused by *Trypanosoma cruzi*, is endemic to Latin American countries, where it affects 8 to 10 million people; an additional 300,000 to 400,000 people in nonendemic countries, including Spain and the United States, are affected. Approximately 41,200 new cases occur annually in endemic countries, and more than 14,000 infants are born with congenital Chagas' disease annually. The disease is responsible for approximately 20,000 deaths each year.

Trypanosomiasis. Trypanosomiasis, which is caused by *T. brucei* and transmitted by the tsetse fly, infects between 50,000 and 70,000 people in sub-Saharan Africa. In 2008, the parasite led to about 48,000 deaths. Since the late nineteenth century, four major epidemics have occurred: 1896 through 1906, primarily in Uganda and the Congo Basin; 1920 and 1970, in several African countries; and 2008, in Uganda.

Onchocerciasis. Onchocerciasis, also known as river blindness, is caused by the nematode *Onchocerca volvulus*. Most infections occur in sub-Saharan Africa; however, cases have been reported in Central America, South America, and Yemen. WHO estimates that worldwide, 37 million people are infected with the parasite; of these persons, 270,000 have been blinded and 500,000 have impaired vision. About 90 million people are at risk for becoming infected with the parasite.

Hookworms. Two hookworm species frequently infect humans: *Ancylostoma duodenale*, which is present in India, the Middle East, and North Africa, and *Necator americanus*, which is found in the Americas, China, Indonesia, Southeast Asia, and sub-Saharan Africa. More than 600 million people are believed to be infected worldwide. Although the infection can be asymptomatic for more than one year, it can be extremely harmful to its host. It causes iron deficiency anemia, intestinal blood loss, and malnutrition.

Trichinosis. Worldwide, about eleven million persons are infected with trichinosis. Formerly, it was common in developed and undeveloped nations; however, it now is rare in developed countries. Most infections are caused by *Trichinella spiralis* and arise from eating raw or undercooked pork. Infections are often asymptomatic or produce mild muscular pain, which disappears over time. Occasionally, trichinosis invades the lungs, heart, and brain, resulting in severe illness or in death.

Robin Wulffson, M.D., FACOG

FURTHER READING

Combes, Claude, and Claude Simberloff. *The Art of Being a Parasite.* Chicago: University of Chicago Press, 2005. An extensive collection of stories that illuminate the ecology and evolution of interactions between species.

Fritsche, Thomas, and Rangaraj Selvarangan. "Medical Parasitology." In *Henry's Clinical Diagnosis and Management by Laboratory Methods,* edited by Richard McPherson and Matthew Pincus. 21st ed. Philadelphia: W. B. Saunders, 2007. A detailed discussion of parasitic infections that includes illustrations of the life cycles and characteristics of parasites.

Jong, Elaine C., and Russell McMullen, eds. *Travel and Tropical Medicine Manual.* 4th ed. Philadelphia: Saunders/Elsevier, 2008. A useful reference manual with advice on preventing, evaluating, and managing diseases that can be acquired in tropical environments and countries outside the United States.

Roberts, Larry S., and John Janovy, Jr. *Gerald D. Schmidt and Larry S. Roberts' Foundations of Parasitology.* 8th ed. Boston: McGraw-Hill, 2009. A classic work focusing on the parasites of humans.

WEB SITES OF INTEREST

Centers for Disease Control and Prevention
http://www.cdc.gov/parasites

Emerging and Reemerging Infectious Diseases Resource Center
http://www.medscape.com/resource/infections

Microbiology and Immunology On-line: Parasitology
http://pathmicro.med.sc.edu/book/parasit-sta.htm

Partners for Parasite Control
http://www.who.int/wormcontrol

See also: Antiparasitic drugs: Mechanisms of action; Antiparasitic drugs: Types; Chagas' disease; Children and infectious disease; DDT; Developing countries and infectious disease; Diagnosis of parasitic diseases; Elephantiasis; Emerging and reemerging infectious diseases; Globalization and infectious disease; Hookworms; Hosts; Immune response to parasitic diseases; Malaria; Onchocerciasis; Parasites: Classification and types; Parasitology; Pathogens; Prevention of parasitic diseases; Schistosomiasis; Treatment of parasitic diseases; Tropical medicine; Trypanosomiasis.

Parasitic diseases

CATEGORY: Diseases and conditions
ANATOMY OR SYSTEM AFFECTED: All
ALSO KNOWN AS: Parasitic infections

DEFINITION

Parasites are pathogenic organisms that depend on a host organism for their food source and survival. This relationship does not benefit the host and usually results in either transient or persistent infection. The Centers for Disease Control and Prevention (CDC) lists more than one hundred parasites that establish themselves in humans, carrying and causing disease.

Parasites originate in locations around the world and are endemic to the tropics and subtropics. They are transmitted through contaminated food or water, by insect bites, and sometimes by human contact. Parasites can be intestinal, can be carried in the bloodstream, or can be lodged in the skin, hair, nails, eyes, mouth, or lungs. Entry into the body is usually by way of the mouth or skin.

CAUSES

Parasitic disease can develop from exposure to the following three types of parasites:

Protozoa. Protozoa are groups of single-celled organisms transmitted by infected humans to other humans through feces-contaminated food or water and through mosquito or flea bites. Protozoa occupy the intestines, blood, or tissue, but can also live independently.

Helminths. Helminths are worms or wormlike, multicelled organisms big enough to be seen in their adult form but unable to multiply in humans. Where the helminth lives is determined by the kind of worm it is (flatworm or platyhelminth, such as a tapeworm; roundworm or nematode; fluke or trematode). They live in the gastrointestinal tract, blood, lymph fluid, or under the skin (subcutaneous tissue). Helminths can also live independently.

Ectoparasites. Ectoparasites are fleas, ticks, lice, and mites in the environment that attach themselves to skin or tunnel under it, depositing the diseases they carry; arthropod vectors such as blood-sucking mosquitos are ectoparasites even though they feed externally rather than occupy the body.

Every year, plasmodium, the malaria parasite, accounts for one million deaths around the world. A category of parasitic infections called neglected tropical diseases (NTDs) accounts for another one-half million deaths worldwide from diseases such as elephantiasis (lymphatic filariasis), onchocerciasis (which results in blindness), and trypanosomiasis (African sleeping sickness). *Toxoplasma* (toxoplasmosis), *Trichomonas, Giardia* (giardiasis), *Borrelia burgdorferi* (tick-caused Lyme disease), *Enterobius vermicularis* (pinworm), and *Cryptosporidium* (found in stagnant lakes or ponds) cause a high incidence of parasitic infection in moderate climates, including parts of developed countries such as the United States, Japan, and China, and in Europe. Rural areas of poor countries are most vulnerable to parasitic infections. In addition to enduring a high toll of sickness and death, parasitic disease also affects the rural poor with lost school and work time, reduced cognitive function, and stunted growth in children.

RISK FACTORS

Living in or traveling to tropical and subtropical areas where parasites are prevalent is associated with greatest risk. Poverty is a recognized risk factor within developed countries or in the rural areas of poor or underdeveloped countries with limited access to public health and generally poor hygiene and nutrition. Risk is higher in infants and young children, the elderly, and immunodeficient persons, such as those with human immunodeficiency virus infection or acquired immunodeficiency syndrome.

SYMPTOMS

The symptoms and clinical course of parasitic diseases vary according to the causative organism. First symptoms include high fever, headache, aching limbs (myalgia), diarrhea, abdominal cramps, sleepiness, and malaise. Insect bites may become infected and chancres may develop. Swollen glands (lymphadenopathy) may appear in the neck, under arms, or in the groin. Intestinal worms may lead to nutrient deficiencies and weight loss. With longer duration of

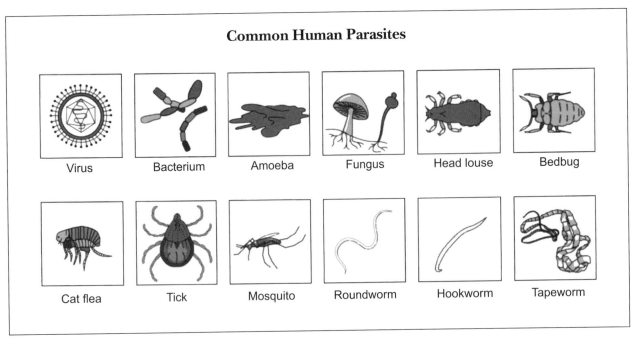

Common Human Parasites

Virus Bacterium Amoeba Fungus Head louse Bedbug

Cat flea Tick Mosquito Roundworm Hookworm Tapeworm

A parasite is any organism that, temporarily or permanently, lives on or in another organism to feed. Parasites often cause infection in the host.

parasitic infection, more serious symptoms may develop, including an enlarged spleen (splenomegaly), renal failure, heart or central nervous system problems, and changes in memory or behavior.

SCREENING AND DIAGNOSIS

Serologic and immunodiagnostic tests that detect immune system factors (antibodies) that are produced in response to the infection, or surface markers on the organisms themselves (antigens), are able to confirm most parasitic infections. Examination of stained peripheral blood smears can detect organisms such as the malaria parasite in blood cells. Examination of multiple stool samples may reveal eggs (ova) of intestinal parasites. Urine or sputum samples may also be tested. A lighted tubular instrument (endoscope) that is passed through the mouth or rectum may also be used to identify parasites within the intestines. Diagnostic imaging (computed tomography scan, ultrasound, and magnetic resonance imaging) may be used to investigate intra-abdominal infection.

TREATMENT AND THERAPY

Receiving the earliest possible treatment for parasitic infection often can reduce the infection's dura-

tion and severity. Sufficient fluid intake may be critical if high fever is present. Drugs are often available for specific parasitic infections. These drugs include melarsoprol and suramin for sleeping sickness and antimalarial quinine-related drugs. Antiparasitic agents (such as fluconazole and azithromycin) are available for gastrointestinal infections and also as topical agents. Sulfonamides (such as sulfadiazine) and diaminopyrimidines (such as pyrimaethamine or iclaprim) and certain antibacterial drugs (such as doxycycline or clindamycin for malaria) may be used too.

PREVENTION AND OUTCOMES

Exposure to parasites cannot always be avoided. Preventive measures include careful planning for travel to tropical and subtropical areas where parasites are prevalent. One should have insect repellants containing DEET (NN-diethyl metatoluamide), should get inoculated, if possible (vaccines are not available for all parasites), and should be prepared to treat drinking water. Eating only well-cooked foods and avoiding public water sources are essential preventive measures when traveling in tropical zones. Avoiding areas where mosquitoes and ticks are abundant helps to prevent bites. Removing outdoor clothing carefully to avoid carrying fleas or ticks indoors, and showering immediately to wash off parasites, are important steps too.

Pets should be brushed outdoors so that they do not bring fleas or ticks indoors; veterinarians offer safe antiflea and antitick medication for pets. Preventing lice infestation means avoiding close contact with other people, their clothing or hats, and especially their combs and brushes. Careful inspection and immediate treatment for bites may help prevent infection.

L. Lee Culvert, B.S., CLS

FURTHER READING

"Approach to Parasitic Infections." In *The Merck Manual of Disease and Prevention*, edited by Mark Beers et al. 18th ed. Whitehouse Station, N.J.: Merck Laboratories, 2007. A general clinical discussion of parasitic infections.

Curtis, Carmelle M., and Peter L. Chiodini. "Parasitic Infections of the Gastrointestinal Tract." In *Cohen and Powderly Infectious Diseases*, edited by Jonathan Cohen, Steven M. Opal, and William G. Powderly. 3d ed. Philadelphia: Mosby/Elsevier, 2010. Examines the connections between parasitic infections and gastrointestinal disorders.

Scrimgeour, Euan M. "Other Parasitic Disease of the Nervous System." In *Cohen and Powderly Infectious Diseases*, edited by Jonathan Cohen, Steven M. Opal, and William G. Powderly. 3d ed. Philadelphia: Mosby/Elsevier, 2010. Examines the connections between parasitic infections and nervous system diseases.

Tortora, Gerard J., Berdell R. Funke, and Christine L. Case. *Microbiology: An Introduction.* 10th ed. San Francisco: Benjamin Cummings, 2010. A good reference for those interested in exploring the microbial world. Provides readers with an appreciation of the pathogenicity and usefulness of microorganisms.

WEB SITES OF INTEREST

Centers for Disease Control and Prevention
http://www.cdc.gov/parasites

Emerging and Reemerging Infectious Diseases Resource Center
http://www.medscape.com/resource/infections

Microbiology and Immunology On-line: Parasitology
http://pathmicro.med.sc.edu/book/parasit-sta.htm

Partners for Parasite Control
http://www.who.int/wormcontrol

See also: Antiparasitic drugs: Mechanisms of action; Antiparasitic drugs: Types; Children and infectious disease; Developing countries and infectious disease; Diagnosis of parasitic diseases; Emerging and re-emerging infectious diseases; Globalization and infectious disease; Hosts; Immune response to parasitic diseases; Parasites: Classification and types; Parasitology; Pathogens; Prevention of parasitic diseases; Treatment of parasitic diseases; Trichinosis; Tropical medicine.

Parasitology

CATEGORY: Epidemiology

DEFINITION

Medical parasitology is the study of parasites and the human diseases caused by these organisms. By definition, parasites are dependent upon their hosts for survival. Numerous species of organisms, ranging from unicellular protozoa to large, physiologically complex helminths, parasitize human hosts. Additionally, several species of arthropods act as parasitic disease vectors. Parasites remain a significant cause of global morbidity and mortality.

INTESTINAL PROTOZOA

Intestinal protozoa are single-celled parasites that commonly infect humans through a person's ingestion of fecal-contaminated water or food. *Entamoeba histolytica* causes amebiasis, also known as amebic dysentery, characterized by abdominal pain and tenderness, bloody diarrhea, and fever. *Giardia intestinalis* (also known as *G. lamblia*) is the most commonly diagnosed intestinal parasite in the United States. Symptoms of giardiasis include abdominal pain, diarrhea, increased flatulence, and steatorrhea. *Cryptosporidium parvum, C. hominis,* and other species of this sporozoan are common intestinal parasites found throughout the world. *Balantidium coli,* a ciliated protozoan, is found predominantly in tropical and subtropical climates.

BLOOD AND VISCERAL PROTOZOA

Diseases caused by blood and visceral protozoa are among the most debilitating and potentially life-threatening of all parasitic infections, including malaria, trypanosomiasis, and leishmaniasis. Malaria, caused by *Plasmodium falciparum, P. vivax, P. ovale, P. malariae,* and *P. knowlesi,* is transmitted by the female *Anopheles* mosquito. The parasite initially infects hepatocytes before spreading to the erythrocytes. Classic symptoms include fever, chills, sweats, head and body aches, nausea, vomiting, and malaise. Malaria is the fifth leading cause of infectious-disease-related deaths worldwide.

Trypanosomes are flagellated protozoans carried by arthropod vectors. African trypanosomiasis (African sleeping sickness), caused by *Trypanosoma brucei gambiense* and *T. b. rhodesiense,* is carried by the tsetse fly. The parasite migrates from the circulatory system to the central nervous system. American trypanosomiasis (Chagas' disease) is caused by *T. cruzi* and is carried by triatomine bugs. Chagas' disease occurs commonly in Central America, South America, and Mexico. Acute signs and symptoms include fever, lymphadenopathy, and hepatosplenomegaly. Potentially fatal complications include meningoencephalitis and myocarditis.

Leishmaniasis describes a group of diseases transmitted by sandflies and caused by *Leishmania* species, including *L. aethiopica, L. amazonensis, L. donovani, L. infantum, L. major, L. mexicana, L. tropica,* and *L. venezuelensis.* With cutaneous leishmaniasis, the parasites infect tissue macrophages, typically leading to localized, painless ulcers. Visceral leishmaniasis, also known as kala-azar, involves diffuse parasitic invasion of the macrophages of the liver, spleen, and other organs. Symptoms and signs include hepatosplenomegaly, malaise, anorexia, and weight loss. Leishmaniasis is most prevalent in India, the Middle East, and parts of South America.

INTESTINAL HELMINTHS

Intestinal helminths are complex organisms that include numerous species of nematodes (roundworms), trematodes (flukes), and cestodes (tapeworms). The World Health Organization estimates that approximately two billion people worldwide are infected with one or more soil-transmitted nematodes, including common roundworms (*Ascaris lumbricoides*), whipworms (*Trichuris trichiura*), and hookworms (*Necator americanus* and *Ancylostoma duodenale*). Other prevalent intestinal nematodes include *Enterobius vermicularis* and *Strongyloides stercoralis. Fasciolopsis buski* and

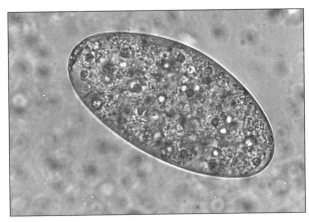

A micrograph shows an egg of an intestinal fluke, a type of worm, in a stool sample. Flukes and other parasites are common causes of infectious disease.

Heterophyes heterophyes are flukes that parasitize the small bowel.

Intestinal tapeworms are typically contracted from the inadvertent ingestion of larvae in raw or undercooked animal meats. The larvae mature into adult worms in the host's gastrointestinal tract. Human intestinal cestodes include *Diphyllobothrium latum* (fish tapeworm), *Taenia saginata* (beef tapeworm), *T. solium* (pork tapeworm), and *Hymenolepis nana* (dwarf tapeworm).

BLOOD AND VISCERAL HELMINTHS

Parasitic blood and tissue nematodes and cestodes cause a variety of human infections, which range in severity from mild to potentially life-threatening. Rare or undercooked meats infested with *Trichinella* larvae cause trichinellosis. Worms mature in the intestine and give rise to larvae, which invade systemically. Larvae-contaminated water is the source of guinea worm (*Dracunculus medinensis*) infections. Adult female worms migrate to the subcutaneous tissues and burrow through the skin surface to discharge larvae. *Onchocerca volvulus, Wuchereria bancrofti, Brugia malayi, B. timori, Loa loa, Mansonella ozzardi,* and *M. perstans* are parasitic blood and tissue nematodes transmitted to humans by arthropod vectors common in tropical and subtropical regions.

Snails are the primary intermediate hosts of several blood and tissue flukes that parasitize humans. The most common human blood flukes include *Schistosoma mansoni, S. japonicum,* and *S. haematobium.* Adult worms reside in the venules of the mesenteric, vesical, and pelvic plexuses. *Clonorchis sinensis, Opisthorchis viverrini, O. felineus, Fasciola hepatica,* and *F. gigantic* are parasitic liver flukes, or flatworms. Potential complications of liver fluke infestation include bile duct obstruction, biliary cirrhosis, cholangitis, cholangiohepatitis, and cholangiocarcinoma.

Lung flukes, including *Paragonimus westermani, P. kellicotti, P. mexicanus,* and *P. africanus,* are contracted from ingesting raw or undercooked fresh-water crustaceans contaminated with metacercariae. The parasites migrate from the intestine to the lungs and mature, potentially causing chronic bronchitis and bronchiectasis. Adult worms may migrate to other body tissues, including the central nervous system.

Invasive larvae from certain tapeworm species cause parasitic cysts in human tissues. Ingestion of *T. solium* eggs causes cysticercosis, characterized by larval cyst formation in various body tissues. Neurocysticercosis may prove life-threatening. Echinococcosis, caused by *Echinococcus granulosus, E. vogeli,* and *E. multilocularis,* most commonly affects the liver or lungs. Less commonly, the brain, bones or heart may be involved.

IMPACT

Although far from eradicated, parasitic diseases cause significantly less morbidity and mortality in wealthy, industrialized nations compared with the developing world. On a global scale, however, parasites continue to exact a significant toll on humankind, adversely affecting quality of life, productivity, and longevity.

Tina M. St. John, M.D.

FURTHER READING

Bogitsh, Burton J., Clint Earl Carter, and Thomas N. Oeltmann. *Human Parasitology.* 3d ed. Boston: Academic Press/Elsevier, 2005. A medical parasitology text with detailed information on the biology, epidemiology, and pathophysiology of human parasites, including protozoans, helminths, and arthropod vectors.

Despommier, Dickson D., et al. *Parasitic Diseases.* 5th ed. New York: Apple Tree, 2005. Provides a list of parasitic diseases of special concern to public health professionals. Also describes the assessment of and treatment options for a variety of these diseases.

Garcia, Lynne Shore. *Diagnostic Medical Parasitology.* 5th ed. Washington, D.C.: ASM Press, 2007. A good reference source on the diagnostic aspects of parasitology.

Gillespie, Stephen H., and Richard D. Pearson, eds. *Principles and Practice of Clinical Parasitology.* New York: John Wiley & Sons, 2001. Reference text that discusses the epidemiology, pathophysiology, and management of the most prevalent human parasitic infections.

Sheorey, Harsha, John Walker, and Beverley-Ann Biggs. *Clinical Parasitology.* Carlton South, Vic.: Melbourne University Press, 2000. Reviews global parasitic diseases and includes information regarding classification and geographical distribution of parasites, details of diagnostic tests, availability and treatment regimens of drugs, and means of obtaining uncommon drugs.

World Health Organization. Expert Committee on the Control of Schistosomiasis. *Prevention and Control of Schistosomiasis and Soil-Transmitted Helminthiasis.* Geneva: Author, 2001. Technical report from the World Health Organization reviews the epidemiology, burden, and management of soil-transmitted parasitic diseases.

WEB SITES OF INTEREST

Centers for Disease Control and Prevention
http://www.cdc.gov/parasites

Microbiology and Immunology On-line: Parasitology
http://pathmicro.med.sc.edu/book/parasit-sta.htm

Neglected Tropical Diseases Coalition
http://www.neglectedtropicaldiseases.org

Partners for Parasite Control
http://www.who.int/wormcontrol

See also: Antiparasitic drugs: Mechanisms of action; Antiparasitic drugs: Types; Blood-borne illness and disease; Developing countries and infectious disease; Diagnosis of parasitic diseases; Epidemiology; Fecal-oral route of transmission; Flukes; Food-borne illness and disease; Hosts; Intestinal and stomach infections; Oral transmission; Parasites: Classification and types; Parasitic diseases; Tropical medicine; Vectors and vector control; Waterborne illness and disease; Worm infections.

Parotitis

CATEGORY: Diseases and conditions
ANATOMY OR SYSTEM AFFECTED: Glands, mouth
ALSO KNOWN AS: Salivary gland infection, sialadenitis

DEFINITION

Parotitis causes swelling in one or both of the parotid glands, the two large salivary glands inside each cheek over the jaw and in front of each ear. Usually, the problem goes away by itself, but some cases require treatment. One should see a doctor if there is swelling or other symptoms on this part of the face.

CAUSES

A variety of factors can lead to an inflamed parotid gland. They include a viral infection such as mumps, which is the main viral cause of parotitis (this virus is rare today because of vaccines), and acquired immunodeficiency syndrome (AIDS).

Another cause of parotitis is a blockage of saliva flow, which can lead to a bacterial infection. Causes of this blockage include a salivary stone in the parotid gland, a mucous plug in a salivary duct, a tumor (usually benign), Sjögren's syndrome (an autoimmune disease), sarcoidosis, malnutrition, and radiation treatment of head and neck cancer.

Other conditions can cause the parotid glands to become enlarged, but not infected. These conditions include diabetes, alcoholism, and bulimia.

RISK FACTORS

The risk factors for parotitis are poor oral hygiene; not being vaccinated against mumps; having human immunodeficiency virus infection; having AIDS, Sjögren's syndrome, or diabetes; malnutrition; alcoholism; and bulimia. Also, persons age sixty-five and older are at higher risk.

SYMPTOMS

People with any of the symptoms should not assume those symptoms are caused by parotitis. These symptoms may be caused by other health conditions. To determine the cause of the following symptoms, one should see a doctor: swelling in front of the ears, below the jaw, or on the floor of the mouth; dry mouth; strange or foul taste in mouth; pus draining into the mouth; mouth or facial pain, especially when eating or when opening the mouth; and fever, chills,

and other signs of infection. If parotitis recurs, it can cause severe swelling into the neck and can destroy the salivary glands.

SCREENING AND DIAGNOSIS

A doctor will ask about symptoms and medical history and will perform a physical exam. This may be enough to make a diagnosis. Tests may include removing fluid from the gland and checking it for signs of infection; X rays (a test that uses radiation to take a picture of structures inside the body, in this case, to look for salivary stones); ultrasound (a test that uses sound waves to take pictures of structures inside the body); and a computed tomography (CT) scan (a detailed X-ray picture that identifies abnormalities of fine tissue structure).

TREATMENT AND THERAPY

Treatment options include good oral hygiene, such as flossing and thorough tooth brushing a minimum of twice a day. Warm salt-water rinses can help keep the mouth moist and quitting smoking also may help.

Antibiotics, which are used to control bacterial infections only, are not effective for viral infections such as parotitis. Other medications, which treat underlying conditions such as Sjögren's syndrome or AIDS, may be prescribed instead. Anti-inflammatory drugs may be recommended to help manage swelling and pain.

A doctor may need to remove a stone, tumor, or other blockage. Increasing saliva flow may be all that is needed to remove a mucous plug.

PREVENTION AND OUTCOMES

To help reduce the chance of getting parotitis, one should get treatment for infections, get regular dental care, drink increased amounts of fluids, and suck on sugarless candy or chew sugarless gum to increase the flow of saliva.

Annie Stuart; reviewed by Bridget Sinnott, M.D., FACE

FURTHER READING

Chitre, V. V., and D. J. Premchandra. "Review: Recurrent Parotitis." *Archives of Disease in Childhood* 77 (1997): 359-363.

Ferrari, Mario. *PDxMD Ear, Nose, and Throat Disorders.* Philadelphia: PDxMD, 2003.

National Library of Medicine. "Salivary Gland Infections." Available at http://www.nlm.nih.gov/medlineplus/ency/article/001041.htm.

Scully, Crispian, and Athanasios Kalantzis. *Oxford Handbook of Dental Patient Care.* 2d ed. New York: Oxford University Press, 2005.

WEB SITES OF INTEREST

Canadian Health Network
http://www.canadian-health-network.ca

Centers for Disease Control and Prevention
http://www.cdc.gov

National Library of Medicine
http://www.nlm.nih.gov

See also: Autoimmune disorders; Bacterial infections; Cellulitis; Epiglottitis; Hygiene; Inflammation; Mononucleosis; Mouth infections; Mumps; Oral transmission; Pharyngitis and tonsillopharyngitis; Saliva and infectious disease; Sarcoidosis; Strep throat; Tooth abscess; Viral infections; Viral pharyngitis.

Parvoviridae

CATEGORY: Pathogen
TRANSMISSION ROUTE: Blood, inhalation

DEFINITION

Smallest of the known mammalian viruses, the viruses of the Parvoviridae family (parvoviruses) each have a linear single-stranded genome that encodes approximately two to three proteins, enclosed within an icosahedral (cuboidal) protein capsid.

Taxonomic Classification for Parvoviridae

Order: Unassigned
Family: Parvoviridae
Subfamily: Parvovirinae
Genera: *Erythrovirus, Dependovirus, Bocavirus*
Species:
Human parvovirus B19
Adeno-associated virus 2
Human bocavirus

NATURAL HABITAT AND FEATURES

Parvoviruses are widespread in nature and are found in birds and in mammals such as humans, dogs, cats, and rodents. Parvovirus infection of cats (feline panleukopenia virus) and dogs (canine parvovirus) can result in potentially life-threatening disease for the animals; vaccines exist for the protection of cats and dogs. Despite the severity of infection in nonhuman animals, the parvoviruses are species-specific, so humans are at no known risk from those strains found in other animals.

Human parvoviruses, however, cause the common childhood disease erythema infectiosum. The reservoir for the human virus is unknown. Infection is so common that it is likely passed easily among susceptible children. The adeno-associated parvoviruses are defective and, as the name indicates, require the presence of respiratory adenoviruses or other helper viruses to replicate.

PATHOGENICITY AND CLINICAL SIGNIFICANCE

The most common strain of human parvovirus is B19, the etiological agent for erythema infectiosum, which is more commonly known as fifth disease because it was historically the fifth rashlike illness of childhood. Although the virus is associated with a variety of diseases, serious illness is found primarily in persons with compromised immune systems. Fifth disease is manifested as a rash displaying a slapped-face appearance, which generally lasts no more than several days. The rash may spread to the infected person's trunk after several days. The virus targets replicating red blood cells in the bone marrow, resulting in the death of red cell progenitors. Inhibition of red cell production for release into the circulation may persist for as long as one week.

Because the life span of circulating erythrocytes is several months, in an otherwise healthy person the temporary suppression of cell replacement should pose no problem. However, the suppression of red cell production can result in severe anemia in immunocompromised persons. In addition to the characteristic rash, persons with fifth disease generally exhibit flulike symptoms such as fever, aching in joints, and chills. A minimum of two additional viral strains (K71 and V9) that are similar to B19 are known, although the clinical importance of these strains is unknown. Infection in adults by B19 may be more severe, with inflammation of joints resembling that in rheumatoid arthritis. Symptoms may persist for years.

B19 infection in pregnant women during the first trimester is rare, but an infection may result in fetal death (hydrops fetalis). Infection of persons with red blood cell abnormalities, such as those with sickle cell anemia, thalassemia, or other forms of anemia, may become severe because red cell depletion is a result of viral infection in the bone marrow.

Another type of parvovirus designated for a new genus, *Bocavirus*, was isolated from children with lower respiratory infections. The significance of the isolate is unclear, but it does not appear to be associated with significant clinical symptoms.

Members of the genus *Dependovirus* are replication defective and require the presence of a helper virus for replication. Members are designated as adeno-associated viruses (AAVs) because, historically, the adenoviruses, etiological agents of respiratory illnesses, were the first-known helper viruses for AAVs. However, other viruses, including the papillomaviruses (warts) and the herpesviruses, have been shown to provide helper functions for AAVs too. The actual helper function provided by these viruses is unclear, and it may involve the activation of cell functions required by AAVs. The AAVs are known to integrate into the host chromosome during these infections. The clinical significance of this is unclear. The widespread presence of antibodies against AAVs among adults suggests infection by these viruses is common.

Ironically, coinfection of cervical cells by AAVs with strains of papillomavirus that are associated with the development of cervical cancer may actually reduce the chances of cancer development. The evidence is indirect. Replication of papillomaviruses is partially suppressed under these conditions of coinfection, although women with cervical cancer show minimal production of antibodies against AAVs.

DRUG SUSCEPTIBILITY

Parvovirus infections commonly occur in children and are generally not medically significant in persons with normal immune systems. Conditions are treated symptomatically. More severe illness in persons with blood cell deficiencies, such as sickle cell anemia or thalassemia, may require replacement transfusions.

Immunocompromised persons may be treated with serum containing antibodies that are directed against parvoviruses such as B19. This treatment would pro-

vide a form of short-lived passive immunity. No vaccines exist for the human strains of parvoviruses.

Richard Adler, Ph.D.

FURTHER READING

Brooks, George, et al. *Jawetz, Melnick, and Adelberg's Medical Microbiology.* 25th ed. New York: McGraw-Hill, 2010. Among the most useful of the medical microbiology texts. Chapters provide overviews without overwhelming the reader with minutiae. The chapter on parvoviruses emphasizes pathogenicity in humans and includes descriptions of fifth disease and illnesses associated with persons who are immunocompromised.

Kerr, Jonathon, et al., eds. *Parvoviruses.* New York: Oxford University Press, 2006. History and pathogenesis of the parvoviruses. Chapters include descriptions of human and nonhuman animal strains and the transmission and clinical significance of disease.

Strauss, James, and Ellen Strauss. *Viruses and Human Disease.* 2d ed. New York: Academic Press/Elsevier, 2008. Extensive summary of the most important human pathogens. Chapters are arranged on the basis of types of genomes and include sections on newly emerging diseases. The parvoviruses are discussed in the chapter on DNA viruses.

Wagner, Edward, and Martinez J. Hewlett. *Basic Virology.* 3d ed. Malden, Mass.: Blackwell Science, 2008. Summary of viral replication and pathogenesis. The parvoviruses are among the human viruses described in this text.

WEB SITES OF INTEREST

International Committee on Taxonomy of Viruses
http://www.ictvonline.org

Universal Virus Database
http://www.ictvdb.org

Viral Zone
http://www.expasy.org/viralzone

See also: Blood-borne illness and disease; Children and infectious disease; Erythema infectiosum; Parvovirus infections; Viral infections.

Parvovirus infections

Category: Diseases and conditions
Anatomy or system affected: All
Also known as: B19 infection, bocavirus infection

Definition

Unknown to scientists until the 1960's, parvoviruses are small, simple eukaryotic viruses that contain single-strand deoxyribonucleic acid (DNA) as their genetic material. There are two parvovirus subfamilies: Densovirinae, which affects insects, and Parvovirinae, which affects vertebrates. No cross-transmission of parvovirus exists between humans and animals.

Infection in humans occurs through four known virus types: adeno-associated viruses (AAV) 1 through 6 (genus *Dependovirus*), B19 virus (genus *Erythrovirus*; the first human virus type that was identified), human bocavirus (HuBoV; genus *Bocavirus*), and Parv4/5 (genus *Parvovirus*). Scientists continue to study the potential role of parvoviruses in human disease, and new parvoviruses are still being discovered.

Causes

Knowledge about the cause of parvovirus infection is limited, because parvoviruses are extremely difficult to grow in culture. Routes of transmission for AAVs, Parv4/5, and HuBoV are currently unknown. AAVs 1-6 are not known to cause any human diseases. Parv4/5 has been isolated in a relatively small population, intravenous drug users who are also infected with the human immunodeficiency virus (HIV). HuBoV has been associated with upper and lower respiratory tract infections and gastroenteritis.

The primary route of transmission for B19, which is highly contagious, is through direct contact with respiratory secretions or through droplet infection. Peak seasonal incidence is during late winter and early spring. More than one-half of all adults are seropositive and immune to the virus possibly because of asymptomatic infection as children or adolescents.

A secondary route of B19 transmission is transplacental, reported to occur in approximately one-third of B19-infected pregnant women. A tertiary route is through blood and blood products.

B19 is associated with transient aplastic crisis in chronic hemolytic anemia, chronic anemia in immunodeficiency syndromes, arthritis, nonimmune hy-

drops fetalis, and, most commonly, erythema infectiosum (EI), a mild illness also called fifth disease (so named because it was one of five common rash-producing childhood illnesses).

For EI, incubation and transmission occurs from four to twenty days after viral exposure. Rash onset, approximately seventeen days after exposure, corresponds to immunoglobulin M (IgM) appearance in serum and signals the clearance of viremia.

Risk Factors

Factors increasing the chance of severe complications are pregnancy, sickle cell anemia, and compromised immunity from AIDS, chemotherapy, congenital or acquired immune disorders, and treatment with immunosuppressive drugs. Screening of persons with these conditions is advisable to determine immunity status.

During pregnancy, B19 infection, especially during the first two trimesters, may cause transplacental transmission and resultant severe fetal anemia and nonimmune hydrops fetalis, a serious condition characterized by possible intrauterine growth retardation, myocarditis, and pleural and pericardial effusions. Intrauterine blood transfusion reduces the rate of fetal death to less than 10 percent. Infection does not result in congenital malformation.

B19 infection may decrease red cell production and result in an anemia crisis in persons with anemia; it also could result in aplastic anemia or severe cytopenias in immunocompromised persons.

Symptoms

Parvovirus infection is frequently asymptomatic. Symptoms, when they do appear, are often nonspecific and indistinguishable from those of the common flu.

HuBoV is associated with the symptoms of upper respiratory tract infection, including acute otitis media (middle-ear infection), conjunctivitis, cough, diarrhea, fever, pharyngitis, rash, rhinorrhea, sinusitis, and vomiting; lower respiratory tract infection symptoms of bronchitis, bronchiolitis, croup, exacerbation of asthma, and pneumonia; and gastroenteritis symptoms of blood in stool, diarrhea, fever, mucus in stool, and vomiting.

B19 is associated with biphasic symptoms, including fever, headache, lethargy, malaise, myalgia, nausea, pharyngitis, and rhinorrhea (five to seven days after infection) and a bright, macular exanthema on the cheeks (termed "slapped cheek") one week later; these symptoms are followed one to four days later by a diffuse, lacy, maculopapular rash that gradually extends to the distal extremities. Rashes usually remit after one week but may reappear cyclically for several weeks in response to exercise, temperature change, sunlight exposure, or emotional stress.

Less common manifestations of B19 infection are erythema multiforme, pruritus on the soles of the feet, and papular-purpuric "gloves-and-socks" syndrome, which is an erythematous exanthema of the hands and feet ending at the wrist and ankle joints that usually occurs in young adults and is preceded by localized and painful erythema and induration. The primary clinical manifestation in adults is transient small joint arthropathy, with time to onset that parallels a rash onset in children. Symptoms usually remit within one to two weeks but may persist for months. Persons with severe anemia from transient aplastic crisis may experience fatigue, pallor, or signs of an aplastic crisis; persons with thrombocytopenia may experience bruising.

SCREENING AND DIAGNOSIS

Screening is done through blood tests to determine viral presence, which would indicate a recent infection; antibody presence in serum, which would indicate a prior infection and therefore immunity; and viral and antibody absence, which would indicate potential susceptibility to infection.

The only known method for diagnosing HuBoV is through polymerase chain reaction and viral deoxyribonucleic acid detection using blood, respiratory secretions, or stool samples. For B19, the best known diagnostic method is the IgM-antibody assay using blood or respiratory secretion samples.

TREATMENT AND THERAPY

Treatment is symptom-specific, because there is no known antiviral therapy. Most infections are self-limited. Normal human immunoglobulin injections can be administered to persons at risk for severe complications. Pregnant women with a documented infection can be monitored through maternal serum a-fetoprotein screening and with ultrasound examinations to determine if the fetus requires intrauterine blood transfusion.

PREVENTION AND OUTCOMES

No vaccine exists for human parvoviruses. Frequent handwashing is the most effective means of prevention.

Cynthia L. De Vine, B.A.

FURTHER READING

Broliden, K., T. Tolfvenstam, and O. Norbeck. "Clinical Aspects of Parvovirus B19 Infection." *Journal of Internal Medicine* 260, no. 4 (October, 2006): 285-304.

Brown, Kevin E. "The Expanding Range of Parvoviruses Which Infect Humans." *Reviews in Medical Virology* 20, no. 4 (July, 2010): 231-244.

Centers for Disease Control and Prevention. "Parvovirus B19 Infection and Pregnancy." Available at http://www.cdc.gov/ncird.

Cherry, James. "Human Parvovirus B19." In *Feigin and Cherry's Textbook of Pediatric Infectious Diseases*, edited by Ralph D. Feigin et al. 6th ed. Philadelphia: Saunders/Elsevier, 2009.

Heegard, Erik D., and Kevin E. Brown. "Human Bocaviruses." *Clinical Microbiology Reviews* 15, no. 3 (July, 2002): 485-505.

Knipe, David M., and Peter M. Howley, eds. *Fields' Virology.* 5th ed. Philadelphia: Wolters Kluwer Health/Lippincott Williams & Wilkins, 2007.

Lunardi, C., et al. "Human Parvovirus B19 Infection and Autoimmunity." *Autoimmunity Reviews* 8, no. 2 (December, 2008): 116-120.

Simmonds, P., et al. "A Third Genotype of the Human Parvovirus PARV4 in Sub-Saharan Africa." *Journal of General Virololgy* 89, part 9 (September, 2008): 2299-2302.

Van Regenmortel, M. H., and B. W. Mahy. "Emerging Issues in Virus Taxonomy." *Emerging Infectious Diseases* 10, no. 1 (2004): 8-13.

WEB SITES OF INTEREST

American Academy of Family Physicians
http://familydoctor.org

Centers for Disease Control and Prevention
http://www.cdc.gov

National Heart, Lung, and Blood Institute
http://www.nhlbi.nih.gov

Organization of Teratology Information Specialists
http://www.otispregnancy.org

See also: Bloodstream infections; Children and infectious disease; Erythema infectiosum; Parvoviridae; Pregnancy and infectious disease; Vertical disease transmission; Viral infections.

Pasteurellosis

CATEGORY: Diseases and conditions
ANATOMY OR SYSTEM AFFECTED: Eyes, heart, joints, lungs, respiratory system, skin, tissue
ALSO KNOWN AS: Shipping fever, snuffles

DEFINITION

Pasteurellosis is an infection caused by the bacterial organism *Pasteurella multocida*, which normally lives in the bodies of domestic pets, livestock, and poultry. Because humans frequently associate with these animal species, most cases of pasteurellosis in humans result from animal contact.

CAUSES

P. multocida commonly lives in the upper respiratory tract of many domesticated animals, and most cases of pasteurellosis are contracted through animal bites or scratches or through an animal licking a person's open wound. Dissemination of such infections can also result in joint, heart, eye, and central nervous system infections. Inhaling bacteria as a result of animal contact can also cause respiratory pasteurellosis in persons with underlying medical conditions.

RISK FACTORS

Children who play roughly with domestic pets are at risk for animal bites. Older persons are also at risk for disseminated disease, as are people with underlying lung conditions such as chronic obstructive pulmonary disease and persons with diabetes, liver disease, or conditions that prevent the immune system from functioning properly.

SYMPTOMS

Pasteurellosis symptoms usually appear one day after receiving an animal bite and include extensive soft-tissue inflammation that is marked by pain, redness, swelling, and the feeling of heat. Later, infected persons develop cellulitis (diffuse inflammation of connective tissue and the lower layers of the skin) and abscesses (pus accumulation). Symptoms also include fever and chills and swelling of the local lymph nodes (lymphangitis). Complications include inflammation of the fluid-filled sheath (synovium) that surrounds tendons (tenosynovitis) and bone infections (osteomyelitis) and invasion of joints by bacteria (septic arthritis).

SCREENING AND DIAGNOSIS

A person's medical history usually reveals routine or recent animal exposure. Also, a Gram's stain of fluid from inflamed tissues or pus will show pink-staining (gram-negative) bacteria that look like nonuniform short rods (coccobacilli). In cases of septic arthritis, aspiration of the affected joint (arthrocentesis) will show gram-negative coccobacilli. Antibiotic susceptibility tests can distinguish between *P. multocida*, which is sensitive to penicillin and cephalosporin antibiotics, and those bacterial species that have a similar appearance.

TREATMENT AND THERAPY

Washing and irrigating wounds reduces the number of bacteria and improves the infected person's prognosis. Heavily infected tissue may require surgical debridement.

Pasteurellosis responds favorably to antibiotic treatment. Infected animal bites tend to contain mixtures of various microbes and, therefore, wide-spectrum agents are used in such cases. These antibiotics include cefuroxime and amoxicillin-clavulanic acid (Augmentin), minocycline, ciprofloxacin, ofloxacin, levofloxacin, moxifloxacin, and trimethoprim-sulfamethoxazole. Milder soft-tissue infections are treated for seven to ten days, and more severe infections usually require treatment for ten to fourteen days. Deep-tissue infections initially require intravenous infusions of antibiotics, followed by oral treatments for four to six weeks.

PREVENTION AND OUTCOMES

Persons who have been bitten or scratched by an animal should gently clean the area around the wound and should seek immediate medical attention as soon as any signs of infection appear. People at high risk, such as those with subfunctional immune systems, rheumatoid arthritis, or prosthetic joints, should seek medical attention immediately after any animal bite or scratch.

Michael A. Buratovich, Ph.D.

FURTHER READING

Gladwin, Mark, and Bill Trattler. *Clinical Microbiology Made Ridiculously Simple.* 4th ed. Miami: MedMaster, 2007.
Lacasse, Alexandre, et al. "*Pasteurella multocida* Infection." Available at http://emedicine.medscape.com/article/224920-overview.
Ryan, Kenneth J., and C. George Ray, eds. *Sherris Medical Microbiology: An Introduction to Infectious Diseases.* 5th ed. New York: McGraw-Hill, 2010.

WEB SITES OF INTEREST

National Center for Emerging and Zoonotic Infectious Diseases
http://www.cdc.gov/ncezid

Todar's Online Textbook of Bacteriology
http://www.textbookofbacteriology.net

See also: Bacterial infections; *Bartonella* infections; Brucellosis; Cat scratch fever; Cats and infectious disease; Cellulitis; Children and infectious disease; Dogs and infectious disease; Inflammation; Osteomyelitis; Rabies; Septic arthritis; Wound infections; Zoonotic diseases.

Pathogenicity

CATEGORY: Transmission

DEFINITION

Pathogenicity is the ability of a disease-causing organism (pathogen) to produce an infection in another organism, including a human being.

ESTABLISHING INFECTION

The pathogenicity of bacteria, viruses, yeast, protozoa, and fungi involves the ability to establish an infection in the face of attempts by the host to destroy the infecting organism. Various strategies are involved in infectivity, and not all organisms exhibit all the

strategies. Pathogenicity is influenced also by the damage that the infecting organism inflicts on the host. Again, there are various mechanisms of host destruction.

Normally, the defense mechanisms of the body's immune system prevent infection. However, the immune system sometimes operates inefficiently. Inefficient immunity affects the very young, the elderly, and the already ill. Inefficient immunity also can be caused by a deliberately compromised immune system. One example of this is drug therapy for persons receiving transplanted tissues or organs (to prevent rejection of the transplant). With compromised immunity, infections are common.

TRANSMISSION OF PATHOGENS

Pathogens can be acquired in several ways. A person can get infected through blood that is contaminated with a virus, such as hepatitis A virus or the human immunodeficiency virus (HIV). A person can get infected by ingesting contaminated food and drinking water. These waterborne viruses, bacteria, and protozoa kill millions of people each year around the world, particularly in undeveloped or developing countries. A person can get infected when a pathogen is transferred from person-to-person or by vectors (animals, insects, or birds). One prominent example of vector-to-human transmission is avian influenza. Another example is malaria, whose transfer to humans by infected mosquitoes leads to millions of infections and deaths annually.

Pathogenicity also can involve the air. Some microorganisms, particularly the very small and light spheres known as spores, which are formed by some bacteria, can be inhaled. Germination of the spores to actively growing and dividing bacteria can cause, for example, a deadly lung infection. The most prominent example is the pulmonary form of anthrax.

BREAKING THE HOST'S DEFENSE

Pathogenicity requires circumventing two lines of host defense. The first defense is the barrier between the inside of the body and the outside world: the skin, mucous membranes in the nose and throat, and tiny hairs in the nose that act to physically block invading organisms. Organisms can be washed from body surfaces by tears, blood, and sweat. This defense has no specificity and involves the physical exclusion or removal of the invader.

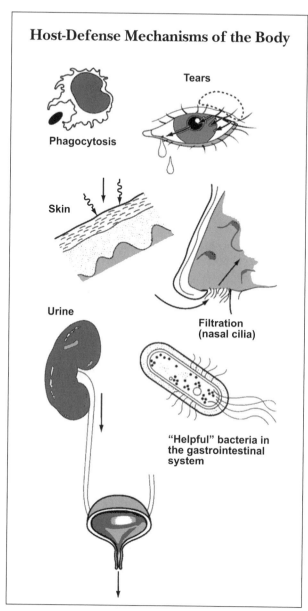

Host-Defense Mechanisms of the Body

Phagocytosis

Tears

Skin

Urine

Filtration
(nasal cilia)

"Helpful" bacteria in
the gastrointestinal
system

For a pathogen to cause infection, it must break through the defense mechanisms of the host. The first line of defense is the barrier between the inside and outside of the host's body. The second line of defense is the host's immune system.

The second line of defense is specific and involves the immune system. The invading organism is recognized and destroyed. This defense can be enhanced by the process of vaccination, which aims to prime the immune system by introducing components of the target pathogen or a living version of the pathogen that has been treated so it is incapable of actually causing the disease. The goal of vaccination is twofold: to protect a person from an existing infection (but one that has not yet affected the vaccinated person) and, for some vaccines, to provide protection against infection that persists for years and even for a lifetime.

RESISTANCE

An increasingly significant method of pathogenicity is bacterial resistance to antibiotics that were once capable of killing the cells. Antibiotic resistance is a major problem worldwide. In 2011, there were several types of bacteria that developed resistance to all known antibiotics.

Antibiotic resistance is caused, in part, by the widespread and sometimes inappropriate use of antibiotics (for example, using antibiotics for viral illnesses and using antibiotics in cattle feed). Bacteria can become antibiotic-resistant by growing as an adherent layer on living and nonliving surfaces. This layer, called a biofilm, was considered a curiosity in the 1970's. Now, it is recognized as a crucial source of pathogenicity. For example, it has been shown that the chronic and often ultimately lethal lung infection that occurs in people with cystic fibrosis is caused by biofilms of *Pseudomonas aeruginosa.*

Bacteria and viruses also can evade destruction by entering host cells and tissues. Once inside the host structures, they are shielded from the immune system and from drugs.

IMPACT

Pathogenicity has become increasingly significant to human and animal health and disease. It is becoming even more important with the evolving ability of certain pathogens to cross species barriers.

Brian Hoyle, Ph.D.

FURTHER READING

Dieckmann, Ulf, et al., eds. *Adaptive Dynamics of Infectious Diseases: In Pursuit of Virulence Management.* New York: Cambridge University Press, 2005. An introductory text for infectious disease researchers.

Drlica, Karl, and David S. Perlin. *Antibiotic Resistance: Understanding and Responding to an Emerging Crisis.* Upper Saddle River, N.J.: FT Press, 2011. Details the development of antibiotic resistance, which critically depends on mutations of pathogens.

Kuijper, E. J., et al. "*Clostridium difficile*: Changing

Epidemiology and New Treatment Options." *Current Opinions in Infectious Disease* 20 (2007): 376-383. Chronicles the increased prevalence of drug-resistant *Clostridium difficile* and the increasing threat posed by the pathogen in hospital-acquired infections.

Miller, A. A., and P. F. Miller. *Emerging Trends in Antibacterial Discovery: Answering the Call to Arms.* Norwich, England: Caister Academic Press, 2011. Describes the development of compounds that kill bacteria, including bacterial pathogens that have arisen due to mutations.

Schnayerson, Michael, and Mark J. Plotkin. *The Killers Within: The Deadly Rise of Drug-Resistant Bacteria.* Boston: Back Bay Books, 2003. Clearly describes how the overuse of antibiotics in agriculture and medicine has spawned the development of drug-resistant bacteria.

Science 321, no. 5887 (July 18, 2008). A special issue devoted to antibiotic resistance, highlighting some particularly difficult infections and discussing issues pertaining to the genetics of antibiotic resistance.

Zabay, Geoffrey. *Agents of Bioterrorism: Pathogens and Their Weaponization.* New York: Columbia University Press, 2008. Discusses how pathogenicity has been harnessed for warfare and terrorism.

WEB SITES OF INTEREST

Centers for Disease Control and Prevention
http://www.cdc.gov/drugresistance

Microbiology Information Portal
http://www.microbes.info

National Institute of Allergy and Infectious Diseases
http://www.niaid.nih.gov/topics/antimicrobialresistance

Virology.net
http://www.virology.net

See also: Alliance for the Prudent Use of Antibiotics; Antibiotics: Types; Bacteria: Classification and types; Bacteria: Structure and growth; Bacterial infections; Drug resistance; Infection; Microbiology; Mutation of pathogens; Parasites: Classification and types; Parasitic diseases; Pathogens; Public health; Secondary infection; Superbacteria; Viral infections; Virulence; Viruses: Types.

Pathogens

CATEGORY: Transmission
ALSO KNOWN AS: Germs, infectious agents

DEFINITION

The term "pathogen," introduced in 1880, is a combination of *patho* ("disease") and *gen*, which indicates a "producer." Hence, the term "pathogen" most commonly refers to any infectious organism that can inflict damage on its host. Pathogens include diverse groups of microorganisms, including bacteria, viruses, fungi, prions, and parasites. The term "pathogen," however, is less commonly used in referring to noninfectious agents of disease, such as chemicals. Furthermore, some organisms classified as pathogens are not negative to their host. That is, they serve as natural or introduced controls to suppress arthropod populations.

Largely, pathogens can best exist in their human, animal, and plant hosts. Harmful microorganisms, however, can be found in abundance in soil, water, air, and on various surfaces for a range of time. Each pathogen has a particular host range or specificity that it can affect. In other words, some pathogens can infect only a particular type (genus and species) of host, such as humans, whereas other pathogens can affect a large number and wide range of hosts. Research has shown, though, that pathogens can evolve because of their interactions with their hosts and other microorganisms in their environment, sometimes leading to a changed or expanded host range. For instance, various strains of the influenza virus can spontaneously arise, leading to the need for regularly altered vaccines to treat annual outbreaks of influenza. The avian influenza virus is an example of a pathogen that was originally found in one host (birds) but can now cause infection in another host (humans).

Many pathogens grow and reproduce preferentially in certain environments and in the presence of certain resources, preferring warm, moist, neutral environments that are representative of the natural physiology of their biological hosts. Many other infectious agents, however, can adapt to and even beat difficult conditions. Most potential hosts have natural defenses against pathogens in the form of immune response, helpful normal flora (in mammals), and other mechanisms; yet, pathogens continue to successfully infect and kill millions of people worldwide annually.

Pathogens prey on persons with weakened immune defenses (caused by diseases such as human immunodeficiency virus infection and acquired immunodeficiency syndrome, and by chemotherapy, malnutrition, and immunosuppression for surgery or pregnancy). Those infections acquired in hospital settings are referred to as nosocomial and can be quite difficult to prevent and control. Furthermore, other pathogens overcome human defense mechanisms by altering their own genetic code and employing other strategies to avoid the defense efforts of the human body. For instance, multi-drug-resistant *Staphylococcus aureus* has acquired resistance to many of the most commonly used and effective antibiotics (including methicillin and penicillin). These superbugs are of constant concern to researchers and clinicians.

TYPES OF PATHOGENS

Pathogens can be divided into five broad classifications: bacterial, viral, fungal, prionic, and other.

Bacterial. A small percentage of bacteria are actually classified as pathogens. In contrast to commensal bacteria, which can be useful or helpful, pathogenic bacteria cause infection and serious disease in humans, nonhuman animals, and plants. The diseases and symptoms caused by pathogenic bacteria are almost as diverse as the biological organisms they infect.

Symptoms of bacterial infection can be minor, such as itchiness or sore throat, to significantly more serious, such as open wounds and sepsis (excessive bacteria in the blood). Certain bacteria have even been linked to certain types of cancer, although this has been shown to occur most commonly in immunocompromised persons.

Some bacterial infections or diseases are caused by a single species or genus, whereas others can result from multiple organismal sources that are either closely related or quite distant in terms of phylogeny. For instance, tetanus, a medical condition sometimes induced by an infected deep cut or wound, is caused only by *Clostridium tetani*. The most common human bacterial disease, tuberculosis, however, can be caused

by many related strains of the *Mycobacterium* genus (*M. tuberculosis*, *M. africanum*, *M. canettii*, *M. caprae*, and *M. microti*). Moreover, pneumonia can be caused by an extremely wide range of bacterial genera, including *Pseudomonas*, *Streptococcus*, *Mycoplasma*, and *Legionella*, rather than by a single organism or closely related organisms. Also, food-borne illnesses and gastrointestinal disorders can be caused by several types of bacteria, including *Salmonellae* spp., *Shigella* spp., *Campylobacter* spp., *Bacillus cereus*, *Clostridium* spp., *Yersinia enterocolitica*, *Cryptosporidium parvum*, *Escherichia coli* (0157:H7), *Listeria monocytogenes*, and *Vibrio* spp.

Conversely, some bacterial species can cause a single ailment, whereas others can lead to several, quite different infections. For example, the microorganism *Salmonella typhi* is known to cause typhoid fever only, whereas the species *Staphylococcus pyogenes* can cause both the commonly diagnosed strep throat, which can be treated with prescription antibiotics, and scarlet or rheumatic fever, which can be chronic and even lead to heart failure.

Other notable ailments caused by bacterial infection include diphtheria (*Corynebacterium diphtheriae*), chlamydia (*Chlamydia trachomatis*), syphilis (*Treponema pallidum*), gonorrhea (*Neisseria gonorrhoeae*), listeriosis (*Listeria monocytogenes*), and various issues affecting the skin, including purulent discharges, boils, blisters, and minor infections (*Staphylococcus aureus*). Bacterial infection also can lead to more serious "flesh-eating" and destructive diseases (*Streptococcus* spp.). Bacteria have also been linked to certain types of cancer. Studies have shown that the organism *Helicobacter pylori*, a bacterial species that can exist in abundance in the stomach, is linked to the formation of ulcers and possibly gastric cancer.

Bacteria also affect agriculture and food-based industries by leading to costly infections, such as fire blight (*Erwinia amylovora*), leaf spot (*Cercopsora* spp. and *Pseudomonas cichorii*), and wilts (*Erwinia tracheiphila*) in commercial crops, and to anthrax (*Bacillus anthracis*), Johne's disease (*M. avium* subspecies *paratuberculosis*), and leptospirosis (*Lectospora* spp.) in livestock.

Viral. Viral pathogens make up the most abundant biological entity, and they can affect various species of animals, plants, and even bacteria through various mechanisms. Examples of common human diseases caused by viral pathogens include the common cold (rhinovirus, coronavirus, and picornavirus), influenza

(Orthomyxoviridae), chickenpox (varicella zoster virus), measles (morbillivirus), mumps (rubulavirus), rubella (rubivirus), cold sores (human papillomavirus types 1 and 2), and mononucleosis. Viral pathogens also cause many serious human diseases, including hepatitis (viruses A, B, C, and D), smallpox (*Variola*), Ebola virus infection (Ebola virus), HIV/AIDS (lentivirus), yellow fever (flavivirus), West Nile virus, SARS-associated coronavirus, and avian influenza.

Many viruses have also been linked to various cancers. Epstein-Barr virus, otherwise known as human herpesvirus-4 (HHV-4), causes not only cold sores and mononucleosis; it has also been linked to Burkitt's lymphoma, nasopharyngeal carcinoma, and central nervous system lymphomas associated with HIV infection. Furthermore, HHV-8 has been linked to Kaposi's sarcoma. HPV is also a causative agent in cervical cancer. Some studies also link viruses to neurological diseases such as multiple sclerosis and chronic fatigue syndrome.

Viruses can also affect animals and agriculture. Some of the commonly found viruses in food, water, and animals include hepatitis virus, rhabdovirus, picornavirus (foot-and-mouth disease), and pararamyxovirus.

Fungal. Fungi are the most common cause of diseases in crops and other plants. Fungal infections also occur in humans, with the majority of advanced infections occurring in immunocompromised persons, particularly on their skin and nails and as yeast infections in body cavities. Some commonly occurring fungal infections include athlete's foot, ringworm (*Trichophyton* and *Microsporum*), and candidiasis (*Candida*).

Prionic. Prions are infectious particles composed primarily of protein that do not, unlike other pathogens, contain nucleic acids. Prions cause a number of diseases in a variety of mammals and have received significant media attention. These prion diseases include bovine spongiform encephalopathy (mad cow disease) in cattle and Creutzfeldt-Jakob disease in humans. All known prion diseases affect brain structure or neural tissue and are untreatable and universally fatal.

Other parasites. Some parasitic eukaryotic organisms, including protists and helminths, also cause disease in humans and animals. Protists in the genus *Plasmodium* are mosquito-borne and cause the highly infectious disease malaria. Other protozoa of the species *Trypanosoma brucei* are transmitted by the tsetse fly and cause African sleeping sickness. *Leishmania* is another genus of protozoa that is carried by sandflies and causes the disease leishmaniasis in many types of mammals. Each of these devastating diseases is endemic to several tropical and subtropical regions of the world, especially in the Americas, Asia, and Africa. Helminths are parasitic wormlike organisms that disrupt their host's digestion and nutrient absorption, causing weakness and disease. These organisms are also more common in developing countries.

TRANSMISSION

In general, the transmission of pathogens largely involves three steps: exit from a primary host, travel or existence in an intermediate location, and infection of a new host. There are, however, several specific routes and mechanisms by which pathogens can reach and colonize their hosts. Collectively, pathogens can essentially affect all facets of anatomy, in mammals and plants alike. The specific pathology and epidemiology of an infection, however, are largely dependent on the pathogen involved.

Scientists typically group transmission into two general categories, direct and indirect contact, which are further divided into several subcategories. Direct transmission refers to those instances when an infected host transmits a pathogen directly to another host. For example, pathogens that cause many sexually transmitted diseases, including gonorrhea, syphilis, and HIV/AIDS, are most commonly passed directly from person to person and cannot survive in environments external to their hosts for any extended time.

In contrast, indirect transmission involves transference of a pathogen from one host to another by way of an intermediate agent, which can be either animate or inanimate. Animate objects include both disease vehicles (including food, water, and air) and disease vectors (including insects, fleas, and rodents). Inanimate objects (or fomites) are those items on which pathogens are deposited and remain; fomites include clothes, bedding, and clinical apparatuses. Many gastrointestinal, respiratory, and blood-borne infections are passed through indirect transmission.

PREVENTION AND OUTCOMES

Because the range of pathogens is great, the ranges of prevention and treatment for infections are similarly broad. Researchers and clinicians have developed many effective strategies for the prevention and treatment of pathogens. It should be noted, however, that many pathogens remain to be understood, preventable, or clinically treatable. Epidemiologists, who study the health and illness of populations, use their knowledge of current trends to predict future behavior and to formulate logical interventions in the interest of public health and preventive medicine. Pathogens are a cornerstone interest to researchers and policymakers alike because they are drivers of disease and death worldwide.

The control of pathogens and related infectious diseases is largely the result of advancements in the comprehensive understanding of disease processes, in improved sanitary and living conditions, and in the discovery of antimicrobial agents and other biotechnological strategies for prevention and treatment. Persons can reduce the incidence of many pathogenic infections by being educated about potential threats, by adopting certain behaviors, and by avoiding other behaviors. In particular, because many pathogens spread indirectly by oral, fecal, genital, and blood-borne routes, good hygiene (such as properly storing and preparing foodstuffs, regularly washing hands and bathing, avoiding intravenous drugs, and avoiding direct sexual contact with infected persons) can prevent many types of infections. At the community level, infectious disease can be prevented by providing uncontaminated water for drinking and agriculture, by educating the public about infectious disease, and by ensuring adequate health care for all.

Vaccination is an effective way of preventing viral infection, which has led to a dramatic decline in morbidity (illness) and mortality (death) associated with infection. Many viral infections have been essentially eradicated (including smallpox, measles, mumps, and rubella) since the introduction of their respective vaccinations.

Treatment

The treatment of pathogens includes using a wide range of compounds and substances collectively known as antimicrobials. Infections caused by bacteria are most commonly treated with prescription antibiotics, which either slow the growth of (bacteriostatic) or kill (bactericidal) certain bacteria. Antibiotics can be naturally derived, synthetic, or semi-synthetic,

and can target either a few or a broad spectrum of organisms.

Some of the most commonly prescribed antibiotics include beta-lactams, sulfonamides, quinolones, and oxazolidinones. Similarly, antifungals are used to treat various fungal infections. Several of these drugs can be purchased without a prescription; others require one. The most commonly prescribed antifungals include those of the azole group. Antiviral drugs are used for treating viral infections. Unlike most antibiotics, antivirals do not destroy their target pathogen; instead, they inhibit their development. In contrast, another group of agents, viricides, destroy virus particles outside the body. Drugs are now available for the management of influenza A and B viruses, HIV, herpesviruses, and hepatitis B and C. Protozoa and other parasites are typically treated with antimicrobial drugs.

Impact

Pathogens make up a very small fraction of all microorganisms, yet they play a particularly powerful role in human life, and in human illness. Several agencies monitor and regulate the control of infectious diseases around the world, including the World Health Organization, the Centers for Disease Control and Prevention in the United States, the U.S. Food and Drug Administration, and the U.S. Environmental Protection Agency.

Despite advancements in the prevention and containment of pathogenic diseases, especially of smallpox, mumps, and plague, some pathogenic diseases, especially HIV, tuberculosis, and influenza, continue to persist in large numbers and to threaten human life. Because the effectiveness of epidemiology directly influences the spread, treatment, and outcome of pathogenic diseases, the developing world, which has limited epidemiological resources, remains unequally affected by diseases that are rarely reported in modern Western nations. There are many reasons for the discrepancy, including a lack of access to infrastructure, education, and funding resources.

Brandy Weidow, M.S.

Further Reading

Black, Jacqueline G. *Microbiology: Principles and Explorations.* 7th ed. Hoboken, N.J.: John Wiley & Sons, 2008. A standard introductory microbiology textbook for allied health students, with detailed descriptions of common infections and the organisms that cause them.

Edwards, R. A., and F. Rohwer. "Viral Metagenomics." *Nature Reviews Microbiology* 3, no. 6 (2005): 504-510. A peer-reviewed literature review on viral metagenomics published in a technical microbiology journal for researchers and students of medicine and microbiology.

Komaroff, A. L. "Is Human Herpesvirus-6 a Trigger for Chronic Fatigue Syndrome?" *Journal of Clinical Virology* 37, suppl. 1 (2006): S39-46. A peer-reviewed study on herpesvirus published in a clinical virology journal that explores the role of viruses in human health.

Madigan, Michael T., and John M. Martinko. *Brock Biology of Microorganisms.* 12th ed. Upper Saddle River, N.J.: Pearson/Prentice Hall, 2010. A standard introductory microbiology textbook for students of medicine and microbiology, with simplified descriptions of common ailments and the organisms that cause them.

Pollack, Andrew. "Rising Threat of Infections Unfazed by Antibiotics" *The New York Times*, February 27, 2010. Discusses the increasing resistance of certain infectious microorganisms to antibiotics.

Prusiner, Stanley B. "Prions." *Proceedings of the National Academy of Sciences* 95, no. 23 (2004): 13363-13383. A peer-reviewed study on the mechanisms and effects of infectious prions published in a high-tier academic journal.

WEB SITES OF INTEREST

Centers for Disease Control and Prevention
http://www.cdc.gov

Microbiology Information Portal
http://www.microbes.info

National Institute of Allergies and Infectious Disease
http://www.niaid.nih.gov

National Institutes of Health
http://www.nih.gov

Todar's Online Textbook of Bacteriology
http://www.textbookofbacteriology.net

U.S. Food and Drug Administration
http://www.fda.gov

Viral Zone
http://www.expasy.org/viralzone

Virtual Museum of Bacteria
http://www.bacteriamuseum.org

See also: Bacteria: Classification and types; Bacteriology; Epidemiology; Fungi: Classification and types; Hosts; Mutation of pathogens; Parasites: Classification and types; Pathogenicity; Prion diseases; Protozoa: Structure and growth; Transmission routes; Virology; Viruses: Types.

Pelvic inflammatory disease

CATEGORY: Diseases and conditions
ANATOMY OR SYSTEM AFFECTED: Reproductive system, uterus
ALSO KNOWN AS: Salpingitis

DEFINITION

Pelvic inflammatory disease (PID) is a serious infection of the female reproductive organs, including the uterus, ovaries, and Fallopian tubes. PID can cause scar tissue to form in the pelvis and Fallopian tubes. This damage may result in infertility, a future tubal pregnancy, or chronic pelvic pain.

CAUSES

PID is caused by bacteria that travel to the reproductive organs. A single type of bacteria or mixture of several types of bacteria may cause the infection. The most common bacteria that initiate PID are gonorrhea and chlamydia.

RISK FACTORS

Risk factors for PID include current or previous sexually transmitted disease (STD), multiple sex partners, sexual intercourse with a partner who has an STD, intercourse without the protection of a condom, and the use of an intrauterine device (IUD) for birth control (this does not increase the risk of getting an STD, but can accelerate the course of PID). Also at higher risk are persons who are between the ages of fifteen and twenty-four years.

SYMPTOMS

Women with PID do not always have symptoms. However, if symptoms do occur, they may include pain in the lower abdomen, vaginal discharge with a foul odor, fatigue, fever, nausea or vomiting, painful intercourse, painful urination, and irregular menstrual bleeding.

SCREENING AND DIAGNOSIS

Because symptoms are often subtle or nonexistent, PID can be difficult to diagnose. There are no specific tests for PID. If PID is suspected, a doctor or other health care provider will ask about symptoms, sexual history, sex partners, and birth control methods. The doctor may perform a general physical exam and a pelvic exam. The pelvic exam is key to making the diagnosis. Samples from the vagina or cervix may be taken to help diagnose the problem. Tests may include cultures of the cervix to test for STD organisms; a blood test to check pregnancy status and to check for infection; ultrasound (a test that uses sound waves to see inside the body); and laparoscopy (insertion of a thin, lighted telescopic tube through a small incision in the abdomen to look at the reproductive organs).

TREATMENT AND THERAPY

The primary treatment for PID is antibiotics. Rest is also an essential part of the treatment. Hospitalization might be required if the diagnosis is uncertain, if there is no improvement, or if symptoms are severe. In the hospital, antibiotics can be given by vein (intravenously). In certain situations, surgery may be required to remove infected or damaged tissue.

PREVENTION AND OUTCOMES

To help prevent PID, women should insist that their sexual partners use a latex condom during intercourse; discuss birth control options with a health care provider; ask what methods may increase or decrease the risk for PID; seek immediate treatment for symptoms, such as unusual vaginal discharge or bleeding; limit the number of one's sexual partners; and have regular screening tests for STDs. If diagnosed with PID or another STD, one should not have sexual intercourse until after treatment is complete and should notify all sexual partners.

Michelle Badash, M.S.;
reviewed by Ganson Purcell, Jr., M.D., FACOG, FACPE

FURTHER READING

Boston Women's Health Collective. *Our Bodies, Ourselves: A New Edition for a New Era.* 35th anniversary ed. New York: Simon & Schuster, 2005.

Carlson, Karen J., Stephanie A. Eisenstat, and Terra Ziporyn. *The New Harvard Guide to Women's Health.* Cambridge, Mass.: Harvard University Press, 2004.

Centers for Disease Control and Prevention. "Pelvic Inflammatory Disease: CDC Fact Sheet." Available at http://www.cdc.gov/std.

EBSCO Publishing. *DynaMed: Pelvic Inflammatory Disease.* Available through http://www.ebscohost.com/dynamed.

Larsen, Laura. *Sexually Transmitted Diseases Sourcebook.* Detroit: Omnigraphics, 2009.

National Institute of Allergy and Infectious Diseases. "Pelvic Inflammatory Disease." Available at http://www.niaid.nih.gov/topics/pelvicinflammatorydisease.

Stewart, Elizabeth Gunther, and Paula Spencer. *The V Book: A Doctor's Guide to Complete Vulvovaginal Health.* New York: Bantam Books, 2002.

Sweet, Richard L., and Harold C. Wiesenfeld, eds. *Pelvic Inflammatory Disease.* New York: Taylor & Francis, 2006.

U.S. Department of Health and Human Services, National Guideline Clearinghouse. "Pelvic Inflammatory Disease: Sexually Transmitted Diseases Treatment Guidelines 2010." Available at http://www.cdc.gov/std/treatment/2010/pid.htm.

WEB SITES OF INTEREST

American Congress of Obstetricians and Gynecologists
http://www.acog.org

National Institute of Allergy and Infectious Diseases
http://www.niaid.nih.gov

National Women's Health Information Center
http://www.womenshealth.gov

Our Bodies Ourselves
http://www.obos.org

Women's Health Matters
http://www.womenshealthmatters.ca

See also: Acute cystitis; Bacterial infections; Bacterial vaginosis; Cervical cancer; Chancroid; Chlamydia;

Chlamydia; Endometritis; Gonorrhea; Herpes simplex infection; Human papillomavirus (HPV) infections; Sexually transmitted diseases (STDs); Trichomonas; Urethritis; Vaginal yeast infection; Women and infectious disease.

Penicillin antibiotics

CATEGORY: Treatment

DEFINITION

Penicillin is a major subclass of beta-lactam antibiotics discovered in 1928 when a culture plate became contaminated with *Penicillium notatum* (now called *P. chrysogenum*). This mold inhibited the *Staphylococcus aureus* that bacteriologist Alexander Fleming was culturing, and eventually the active ingredient, penicillin, was isolated. Subsequent penicillins were derived from either molds or *Streptomyces* spp. bacteria.

Penicillins are highly associated with drug allergy, affecting 6 to 8 percent of the population of the United States. Reactions range from mild rash to cardiovascular collapse, shock, and death. Health care providers should always record a person's allergy history; people who are allergic to other beta-lactam antibiotics, such as cephalosporins, are likely also allergic to penicillins.

MECHANISM OF ACTION

The beta-lactam ring is responsible for the antibacterial actions of the penicillins. Penicillins prevent the formation of peptidoglycan, a substance crucial to the structural stability of bacteria cell walls. The weakened cell walls eventually lyse, or break apart, leading to cell death. Microorganisms that do not have a cell wall, such as *Mycoplasma*, are not susceptible to penicillins.

DRUGS IN THIS CLASS

Several subclasses of penicillins exist. These subclasses are natural penicillins, penicillinase-resistant penicillins, aminopenicillins, and extended spectrum penicillins. Two main factors differentiate the various penicillin products available from each other: resistance to staphylococcal penicillinase and spectrum of activity.

Staphylococcal penicillinase is an enzyme in the beta-lactamase family that inactivates certain beta-

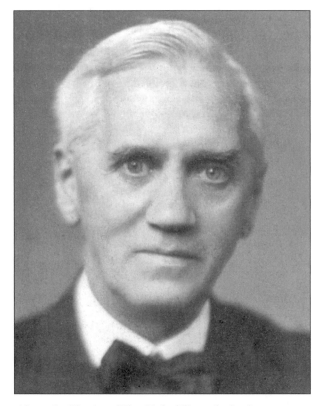

Alexander Fleming. (The Nobel Foundation)

lactam antibiotics. The natural penicillins (penicillins G and V) are narrow-spectrum antibiotics used against a number of gram-positive bacteria such as streptococci. They are not resistant to penicillinase and have only limited activity against staphylococci. Penicillin G (benzylpenicillin) is unstable in stomach acid and must be given as an immediate-action injection. When formulated as insoluble benzathine and procaine salts, it may be given as a long-acting intramuscular injection. Penicillin V (phenoxymethyl penicillin) was the first oral penicillin.

The resistant penicillins (methicillin, nafcillin, oxacillin, and dicloxacillin) retain effectiveness against penicillinase-producing *S. aureus*. They do not, however, have a broad spectrum of activity and are only an improvement on natural penicillins in their activity against staphylococci. Even this advantage is diminishing over time with the development of methicillin-resistant *S. aureus* (MRSA), which refers more broadly to *S. aureus* strains that are resistant to all penicillins; vancomycin is the drug of choice for MRSA. Methicillin itself is no longer clinically relevant.

Aminopenicillins possess a broader spectrum of activity and are effective against some gram-negative bacteria. Ampicillin, the first drug in this category, is effective against a number of gram-negative bacteria, but not against *Pseudomonas*. Amoxicillin is closely related to ampicillin but has better oral absorption; it can cause gastrointestinal upset and drug-induced diarrhea. A combination of amoxicillin with clavulenic acid (Augmentin) lends some protection against penicillinase. These drugs are all available in oral dosage forms.

Subsequent broad-spectrum penicillins for intravenous use (ticarcillin and pipericillin) are active against *Pseudomonas* but are less active against some other gram-negative bacteria. These drugs and the aminopenicillins are as active against gram-positive cocci as are natural penicillins. Ticarcillin is often combined with potassium clavulanate and pipericillin with tazobactam to increase the resistance to penicillinase.

IMPACT

Penicillins remain important antibiotics for a number of conditions. Most are inexpensive and have a reasonably favorable adverse-effect profile. The increased prevalence of MRSA, however, particularly in hospitalized persons, has limited the scope of penicillins in recent years.

Karen M. Nagel, Ph.D.

FURTHER READING

"Antibiotics and Antimicrobial Agents." In *Foye's Principles of Medicinal Chemistry*, edited by Thomas L. Lemke et al. 6th ed. Philadelphia: Lippincott Williams & Wilkins, 2008.

Murray, Patrick R., Ken S. Rosenthal, and Michael A. Pfaller. "Antibacterial Agents." In *Medical Microbiology*. 6th ed. Philadelphia: Mosby/Elsevier, 2009.

Sanford, Jay P., et al. *The Sanford Guide to Antimicrobial Therapy*. 18th ed. Sperryville, Va.: Antimicrobial Therapy, 2010.

Tortora, Gerard J., Berdell R. Funke, and Christine L. Case. "Antimicrobial Drugs." In *Microbiology: An Introduction*. 10th ed. San Francisco: Benjamin Cummings, 2010.

Van Bambeke, Françoise, et al. "Antibiotics That Act on the Cell Wall." In *Cohen and Powderly Infectious Diseases*, edited by Jonathan Cohen, Steven M. Opal, and William G. Powderly. 3d ed. Philadelphia: Mosby/Elsevier, 2010.

WEB SITES OF INTEREST

Alliance for the Prudent Use of Antibiotics
http://www.tufts.edu/med/apua

American Chemical Society: National Historic Chemical Landmarks
http://acswebcontent.acs.org/landmarks/landmarks/penicillin/discover.html

eMedicineHealth: Antibiotics
http://www.emedicinehealth.com/antibiotics

See also: Alliance for the Prudent Use of Antibiotics; Aminoglycoside antibiotics; Antibiotics: Types; Bacteria: Classification and types; Cephalosporin antibiotics; Glycopeptide antibiotics; Ketolide antibiotics; Lipopeptide antibiotics; Macrolide antibiotics; Oxazolidinone antibiotics; Prevention of bacterial infections; Quinolone antibiotics; Reinfection; Secondary infection; Superbacteria; Tetracycline antibiotics; Treatment of bacterial infections.

Penicilliosis

CATEGORY: Diseases and conditions
ANATOMY OR SYSTEM AFFECTED: Blood, lungs, lymphatic system, respiratory system, skin
ALSO KNOWN AS: Penicillosis

DEFINITION

Penicilliosis is the third most common opportunistic infection in persons with human immunodeficiency virus (HIV) infection, namely in the areas of the world in which penicilliosis is endemic. The incidence of penicilliosis, a fungal infection, in endemic areas parallels the incidence of HIV infection.

CAUSES

Penicilliosis is caused by the dimorphic fungus *Penicillium marneffei*, which is either spherical or oval and about 3 to 6 microns long. It is endemic to Southeast Asia, the Guangxi Province of China, Hong Kong, and Taiwan. *P. marneffei* appears in tissue as a unicellular organism that reproduces by planate division. It is a mold at room temperature and converts to the yeast form if incubated at 98.6° Fahrenheit (37° Celsius).

This dimorphism is not found in other members of the genus *Penicillium*.

RISK FACTORS

Compromised immunity and acquired immunodeficiency syndrome (AIDS) render a person susceptible to penicilliosis. Recent exposure to a potential environmental reservoir of organisms is the predominant risk factor. Cases of penicilliosis occasionally are seen outside endemic areas, but most of these cases involve the infected person having a history of travel to an endemic area. The fungus has been isolated from four species of bamboo rats and from soil. Infection seems to be more frequent in the rainy season.

SYMPTOMS

The most common presentation of this disease is disseminated infection, manifested by fever and weight loss (which occur in more than three-fourths of cases), anemia, skin lesions (in approximately two-thirds of cases), generalized lymphadenopathy, and hepatomegaly with or without splenomegaly. Lesions usually appear on the face, trunk, and extremities as papules with central necrotic umbilication; folliculitis and lesions that look like acne also may occur.

Pulmonary symptoms occur in about 50 percent of cases. Chest radiographic abnormalities typically manifest as diffuse reticulonodular infiltrates, though 50 percent of cases have normal chest radiographs. Persons affected by penicilliosis usually have AIDS and low CD4 lymphocyte counts.

SCREENING AND DIAGNOSIS

Diagnosis is usually made by identification of the fungi from clinical specimens. Biopsies of skin lesions, lymph nodes, and bone marrow demonstrate the presence of organisms on histopathology. The elevation of liver enzyme in the blood helps to establish a diagnosis. A specific polymerase chain reaction assay is under evaluation and could be useful as an alternative test for rapid diagnosis.

TREATMENT AND THERAPY

P. marneffei usually demonstrates in vitro susceptibility to multiple antifungal agents, including ketoconazole, itraconazole, miconazole, flucytosine, and amphotericin B. The response to antifungal treatment is good if the treatment is started early; without treatment, the prognosis is poor. Death occurs if the liver fails (that is, it can fail if the fungus releases toxins in the bloodstream). Response rates of up to 97 percent have been reported with amphotericin B therapy for the first two weeks, followed by ten weeks of itraconazole.

After the initial treatment the infected person may need to take an antifungal drug as a secondary prophylaxis for life. Relapse occurs in the absence of prophylaxis in approximately 50 percent of infected persons.

PREVENTION AND OUTCOMES

Primary prophylaxis can prevent the occurrence of penicilliosis. A randomized, placebo-controlled study from Chiang Mai University suggests that primary prophylaxis with itraconazole (200 milligrams daily) can prevent penicilliosis in persons with AIDS and in those with CD4 counts less than 200 cells per microliter. Of 129 persons enrolled in the study, penicilliosis occurred in only one case in the itraconazole group compared with eleven cases in the placebo group, a statistically significant difference. In addition, there were fewer cases of cryptococcosis and candidiasis in the itraconazole group, but no survival difference between groups was detected.

Stephanie Eckenrode, B.A.

FURTHER READING

Dismukes, William E., Peter G. Pappas, and Jack D. Sobel, eds. *Clinical Mycology*. New York: Oxford University Press, 2003.

Galanda, Claudia D., ed. *AIDS-Related Opportunistic Infections*. New York: Nova Biomedical Books, 2009.

St. Georgiev, Vassil. *Opportunistic Infections: Treatment and Prophylaxis*. Totowa, N.J.: Humana Press, 2003.

WEB SITES OF INTEREST

AIDSinfo
http://aidsinfo.nih.gov

Centers for Disease Control and Prevention, Division of Foodborne, Bacterial, and Mycotic Diseases
http://www.cdc.gov/nczved/divisions/dfbmd

Microbiology and Immunology On-line: Mycology
http://pathmicro.med.sc.edu/book/mycol-sta.htm

Mycology Online
http://www.mycology.adelaide.edu.au

See also: AIDS; Antifungal drugs: Types; Autoimmune disorders; Fungal infections; Fungi: Classification and types; HIV; Opportunistic infections; T lymphocytes.

Peptic ulcer

CATEGORY: Diseases and conditions
ANATOMY OR SYSTEM AFFECTED: Abdomen, digestive system, gastrointestinal system, intestines, stomach
ALSO KNOWN AS: Duodenal ulcer, gastric ulcer, ulcer

DEFINITION

Peptic ulcers are eroded areas in the stomach (gastric ulcer) or the first part of the intestine (duodenal ulcer). Ulcers occur in areas where the lining of the stomach or intestine is worn away and irritated, causing pain or bleeding.

CAUSES

Normally, a mucous coating protects the lining of the stomach and the intestine. This coating can be disrupted by a bacterial infection from *Helicobacter pylori* (*H. pylori*) or by stomach-irritating medicines (such as nonsteroidal anti-inflammatory drugs, or NSAIDs). When this mucous coat is disrupted, strong digestive juices can erode the lining underneath it and cause an ulcer.

Lifestyle factors (such as diet and stress) were once thought to be wholly responsible for causing ulcers. They are now known to worsen ulcer conditions, but not to actually cause the erosion. The vast majority of ulcers are caused by *H. pylori* infection or NSAID use.

In addition to creating discomfort, ulcers are serious because they can cause perforation, obstruction, and gastric cancer. An ulcer that eats through the entire wall of the stomach or intestine is called a perforated ulcer. This is a serious and potentially life-threatening condition because the hole allows the contents of the stomach and intestine to leak into the abdominal cavity.

Scarring from ulcers can block flow through the stomach or duodenum, or both. This obstruction can cause repeated vomiting, weight loss, and intense pain. People who have had peptic ulcers have a much higher rate of stomach cancer than others. *H. pylori* is almost certainly a cause of stomach cancer and may account for the excess risk associated with peptic ulcer disease.

Many more people are infected with *H. pylori* than ever develop an ulcer. Researchers do not understand why some people infected with this kind of bacteria develop ulcers and others do not. Researchers also do not know how people become infected with *H. pylori*. The bacterium may be passed in food or water. It also seems to live in the saliva of infected people, allowing the bacteria to be passed through kissing, for example.

RISK FACTORS

It is possible to develop a peptic ulcer with or without the risk factors listed here. Risk factors for peptic ulcers fall into two categories: factors that actually cause peptic ulcers and factors that irritate the stomach or increase acid production, making a person more susceptible to *H. pylori* infection.

Lifestyle factors. Some studies suggest that cigarette smoking can increase the risk of *H. pylori* and can slow the healing of peptic ulcers. Drinking acidic beverages such as fruit juices and consuming caffeine-containing foods and beverages can cause stomach irritation and increase production of stomach acid. This can make a person more susceptible to *H. pylori* infection. Alcohol in large quantities can irritate the stomach, leading to an increased susceptibility to *H. pylori*. Alcohol taken while using NSAIDs can further irritate the stomach, increasing the chance of developing a peptic ulcer.

Even in the absence of alcohol misuse, certain NSAIDs (including aspirin and most other drugs commonly available over the counter or by prescription as "nonsteroidals") can increase the risk of peptic ulcer. These drugs are responsible for at least one-half of all peptic ulcers in elderly persons.

H. pylori infection. Infection with *H. pylori* is the best-defined risk factor for the development of peptic ulcers. A person increases his or her risk of being infected with *H. pylori* by living in crowded or unsanitary conditions; by using certain medications, including NSAIDs, COX-2 inhibitors, and corticosteroid drugs (although this connection is less clear than the others); and by having a history of peptic ulcer disease, Zollinger-Ellison syndrome, recent major surgery or severe injury or burns, head trauma, radiation therapy, congenital malformations of the stomach or duodenum (or both), and specific malignant diseases such as mastocytosis and basophilic leukemia.

Age. Duodenal ulcers are more common in persons

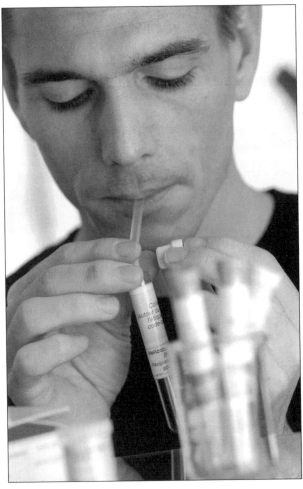

A man blows into a sampling tube during a urea breath test to check for the bacterium Helicobacter pylori, *which can cause a peptic ulcer.*

between the age of thirty and fifty years, while gastric ulcers are more common in people older than the age of sixty years.

Gender. Duodenal ulcers are twice as likely in men, and gastric ulcers are more common in women.

Genetic factors. A person is more likely to develop a peptic ulcer if he or she has other family members who have had ulcers.

Ethnic background. A person has twice the risk of developing a peptic ulcer if he or she is of African American or Hispanic background.

Other risk factors. Stress is no longer believed to cause ulcers. However, many researchers still believe that stress can play a role in exacerbating symptoms

and in the slow healing of preexisting peptic ulcers. Also, a person might have an increased risk of peptic ulcers if he or she has type O blood.

SYMPTOMS

Abdominal pain that may be described in the following ways: as burning, gnawing, feeling worse several hours after eating, improved with eating (duodenal ulcers), stabbing through to the back, coming and going over months, worse in the middle of the night, relieved by taking antacid medicines, bloating of the abdomen, cramping, uncomfortable sensation of fullness, belching, nausea, vomiting (may contain blood or may look like coffee grounds), decreased appetite, weight loss, bloody or tarry black stools, and tired and weak feeling (if anemia is present).

SCREENING AND DIAGNOSIS

The purpose of screening is early diagnosis and treatment. Screening tests are usually administered to people without current symptoms, but who may be at high risk for certain diseases or conditions. For peptic ulcers, however, there are no screening tests or screening guidelines. Because of the relationship between peptic ulcers and the bacterium *H. pylori*, screening for the latter might prove possible. Some data supports screening for bacterial infection, but not specifically for a peptic ulcer.

Peptic ulcers can be diagnosed using both X-ray and endoscopic examinations. Specialized blood, breath, and stool tests are used to identify the presence of *H. pylori*. Rectal examination and stool guaiac test can reveal if a person has a bleeding ulcer. The following exams and tests can be administered:

Barium swallow/upper gastrointestinal (GI) X-ray examination. The person drinks a chalky solution containing barium that coats the digestive tract and helps ensure that X-ray images of the gastrointestinal tract are well-detailed. Multiple X rays are taken before, during, and after barium consumption.

Endoscopy. An examination of the lining of the gastrointestinal tract. After sedation or numbing of the throat, a small tube with a light and camera on the end will be passed into the patient's mouth, into the throat, and into the esophagus, stomach, and duodenum. Other instruments can be passed down through the endoscope to inspect the area, take biopsy samples, and treat any bleeding that is present.

Blood tests. If a peptic ulcer is suspected, a doctor

probably will order a complete blood count to check for anemia. Anemia is common for an untreated bleeding ulcer. Rapid tests in the doctor's office may also be used to identify the presence of *H. pylori*. Blood may also be sent to a laboratory so that more sophisticated tests can be run to confirm or deny the presence of *H. pylori*.

Stool tests. A tiny stool sample might be obtained through a rectal examination and then tested for the presence of *H. pylori*. This is a rapid, on-the-spot test, and can also be used to check for response to antibiotic treatment against *H. pylori*. A stool guaiac uses a small sample obtained through a rectal examination or after a bowel movement. The sample is then smeared onto a little card, and several drops of a chemical are dropped onto the stool sample. This can reveal whether blood is present in the stool, which can be a sign of a bleeding ulcer.

Breath tests. The patient is first given a special drink, a capsule, or a pudding containing urea with carbon, and a special radioactive label. To collect the patient's breath, the health care provider will have the patient inflate a balloon or breathe into a bottle of water. If the breath sample contains the radioactively labeled carbon dioxide, this indicates that the patient has an *H. pylori* infection.

TREATMENT AND THERAPY

The treatment and management of peptic ulcers involves lifestyle changes, medications, alternative and complementary therapies, and surgery. The goals of treatment include eliminating the *H. pylori* infection, treating excess bleeding, promoting healing of the ulcer, relieving pain and discomfort, avoiding the development of complications (such as perforation, obstruction, and gastric cancer), and preventing ulcer recurrence.

Medications for ulcers include antacids (for heartburn relief; they do not heal ulcers); antibiotics (such as amoxicillin, tetracycline, and clarithromycin); a bismuth-containing drug (Pepto-Bismol); proton pump inhibitors (such as omeprazole and lansoprazole); histamine II blockers, to decrease stomach acid production (such as famotidine, ranitidine, cimetidine, and nizatidine); medications to coat the ulcer (such as sucralfate); and medications to protect the stomach against NSAID damage (such as misoprostol).

Surgery and endoscopy may be necessary if the patient has bleeding, a perforation, or an obstruction.

Surgical options include highly elective vagotomy, vagotomy with antrectomy, endoscopy, and vagotomy and drainage. A highly elective vagotomy is a technique in which only part of the vagus nerve is cut and there is no required extra drainage. A vagotomy with antrectomy involves cutting the vagus nerve and removing the lower part of the stomach, or antrum. The antrum makes a chemical that promotes acid production; without that chemical, acid production drops.

An endoscopy involves a thin, lighted tube that is inserted into the throat and to the stomach or intestine. Heat, electricity, epinephrine, or a substance called fibrin glue can then be applied to the area. This should stop the blood flow. In a vagotomy and drainage, the vagotomy cuts parts of the vagus nerve. This procedure can greatly reduce acid production. Cutting the entire nerve can also create further problems with the stomach. In this case, drainage must be created through one of the following procedures: pyloroplasty (widening the opening between the stomach and the duodenum, allowing stomach contents to flow more easily into the intestine); gastroduodenostomy (creating a new opening to connect the stomach and the duodenum); and gastrojejunostomy (creating a new opening to connect the stomach and the jejunum, the second part of the small intestine).

PREVENTION AND OUTCOMES

Because many peptic ulcers are caused by a bacterial infection (*H. pylori*), researchers are hopeful that a vaccine will be found to prevent ulcers. In the meantime, however, the following may provide some benefit:

Practicing good hygiene. Because peptic ulcers are sometimes caused by infection with *H. pylori*, persons should practice good hygiene to decrease their risk of becoming infected. This includes washing one's hands well and regularly and avoiding contact with the vomit or stool of other persons. If cleaning up after another person is necessary, one should wear gloves and then wash hands well.

Stopping smoking. Smokers are urged to quit because smoking has been associated with the development of peptic ulcers. Furthermore, ulcers that do form are slower to heal in persons who smoke.

Decreasing or stopping alcohol consumption. Overuse of alcohol, especially in combination with NSAID use, is thought to increase the risk of peptic ulcers. NSAIDs are proven causes of ulcers, but the causal role of alcohol remains somewhat uncertain, especially in combination with smoking. However, alcohol misuse is a serious health problem regardless of its relationship to ulcer disease.

Reducing intake of caffeine and acidic foods. Some research suggests that foods and drinks high in caffeine (such as coffee) and acid (such as orange juice and tomato products) may cause increased stomach acid, which will increase a person's susceptibility to peptic ulcers caused by *H. pylori.*

Practicing stress management. Although most researchers do not think that stress increases the risk of peptic ulcer, others think that stress can increase stomach acid production. This may make one more susceptible to the effects of *H. pylori* infection.

Rosalyn Carson-DeWitt, M.D.

FURTHER READING

Feldman, Mark, Lawrence S. Friedman, and Lawrence J. Brandt, eds. *Sleisenger and Fordtran's Gastrointestinal and Liver Disease: Pathophysiology, Diagnosis, Management.* New ed. 2 vols. Philadelphia: Saunders/Elsevier, 2010. A comprehensive textbook of gastrointestinal diseases and physiology. Contains excellent endoscopic photographs.

Fuccio, L., et al. "Meta-analysis: Can *Helicobacter pylori* Eradication Treatment Reduce the Risk for Gastric Cancer?" *Annals of Internal Medicine* 151, no. 2 (2009): 121-128. A journal article exploring the question of reducing the risk of gastric cancer through the eradication of *H. pylori.*

Kapadia, Cyrus R., James M. Crawford, and Caroline Taylor. *An Atlas of Gastroenterology: A Guide to Diagnosis and Differential Diagnosis.* Boca Raton, Fla.: Pantheon, 2003. Provides a fully illustrated, nonspecialist understanding of myriad gastrointestinal diseases, including ulcers, heartburn, dyspepsia, diarrhea, irritable bowel syndrome, and pancreatitis.

Kirschner, Barbara S., and Dennis D. Black. "The Gastrointestinal Tract." In *Nelson Essentials of Pediatrics,* edited by Karen J. Marcdante et al. 6th ed. Philadelphia: Saunders/Elsevier, 2011. A chapter on the gastrointestinal tract in a respected text in pediatrics.

McColl, Kenneth E. L. "*Helicobacter pylori* Infection." *New England Journal of Medicine* 362 (2010): 1597-1604. An updated examination of *H. pylori* infection and its role in peptic ulcer disease.

National Digestive Diseases Information Clearing-house. "What I Need to Know About Peptic Ulcers." Available at http://digestive.niddk.nih.gov/ddiseases/pubs/pepticulcers_ez. A good introduction to peptic ulcers.

National Digestive Diseases Information Clearing-house. "*H. pylori* and Peptic Ulcers." Available at http://digestive.niddk.nih.gov/ddiseases/pubs/hpylori. A good introduction to the role of *H. pylori* in the development of peptic ulcers.

WEB SITES OF INTEREST

American College of Gastroenterology
http://www.acg.gi.org/patients

American Gastroenterological Association
http://www.gastro.org

Centers for Disease Control and Prevention
http://www.cdc.gov

Helicobacter Foundation
http://www.helico.com

National Digestive Diseases Information Clearinghouse
http://digestive.niddk.nih.gov

National Institute of Diabetes and Digestive and Kidney Diseases
http://www.niddk.nih.gov

See also: Antibiotics: Types; Diverticulitis; Duodenal ulcer; Enteritis; Gastritis; *Helicobacter; Helicobacter pylori* infection; Intestinal and stomach infections; Norovirus infection; Peritonitis; Viral gastroenteritis.

Pericarditis

CATEGORY: Diseases and conditions
ANATOMY OR SYSTEM AFFECTED: Cardiovascular system, heart

DEFINITION

Pericarditis is the irritation and swelling of the pericardium, the two-layered sac that envelops the heart. Pain is caused when the inflamed layers rub together or against the heart. The inflammation may in turn cause fluids to build up within the sac. Complications include cardiac tamponade (excessive fluid buildup that squeezes the heart) and constrictive pericarditis (scarring and stiffening of the pericardial sac).

Causes

Most often, pericarditis is caused by a viral infection such as influenza, meningitis, mumps, infectious mononucleosis, intestinal tract disorder, or complications from acquired immunodeficiency syndrome. Bacterial pneumonia, meningitis, or influenza; other bacterial infections such as empyema, tuberculosis, or skin and wound diseases; and fungal infections can also spread to the pericardium and cause inflammation. Pericarditis may also be related to cancer, chest trauma (including surgery), kidney failure, autoimmune disease, and radiation therapy. Often the cause is unknown.

Risk Factors

Anyone can develop pericarditis; however, the condition is most common in men age twenty to fifty years. Children younger than four years of age are more apt to develop bacterial pericarditis. After an acute episode, 15 to 30 percent of people will have a recurrence; some will develop chronic pericarditis.

Symptoms

Pericarditis caused by a virus typically comes on suddenly and is short-lived, whereas bacterial pericarditis may develop gradually. Sharp chest pain is the most common symptom, although some people report dull pain or pressure; chronic episodes can be painless. The neck, left shoulder, back, and abdomen may also be affected, and pain may worsen with deep breathing and coughing or when lying flat; the pain may ease when sitting upright or bending forward. Shortness of breath is also common, as is a dry cough, fatigue, an increased heart rate, and a fever. In cases of constrictive pericarditis, the legs and ankles may swell; with cardiac tamponade, blood pressure levels may drop.

Screening and Diagnosis

The affected person's symptoms, especially from any recent flulike infections, are important in the diagnosis. During the physical examination, the clinician will use a stethoscope to listen for the scratchy sound of the pericardium rubbing against the heart and for other signs of fluid buildup. A chest radio-graph, echocardiogram, and computed tomography scan can confirm fluid buildup or other signs of pericardial damage. Cultures of the blood and pericardial fluid can detect bacterial or fungal infections.

Treatment and Therapy

Treatment generally depends on the underlying cause. Pericarditis caused by a virus usually resolves within three weeks; affected persons are advised to rest and are given medications to relieve pain and reduce inflammation. Persons who do not respond to this regimen may be given corticosteroids or colchicine. Antibiotics or antifungal medications are also prescribed for bacterial pericarditis. Those with fluid buildup or other complications are typically hospitalized for observation and further testing. Fluids may be drained from the pericardial sac, which requires local anesthetic. For persons with chronic or constrictive pericarditis, part or all of the pericardium may be surgically removed.

Prevention and Outcomes

Untreated bacterial pericarditis can be life-threatening. Prompt medical treatment and follow-up can help to prevent complications or a second attack.

Judy Majewski, M.S.

Further Reading

Berger, John. "Pericarditis, Bacterial." Available at http://emedicine.medscape.com/article/891369-overview.

Spodick, David H. *The Pericardium: A Comprehensive Textbook.* New York: Marcel Dekker, 1997.

Sydell and Arnold Miller Family Heart and Vascular Institute. *Pericarditis Guide.* Cleveland, Ohio: Cleveland Clinic, 2009. Available at http://my.cleveland-clinic.org/documents/heart/pericarditis_treatment_guide.pdf.

Zipes, Douglas P., et al., eds. *Braunwald's Heart Disease: A Textbook of Cardiovascular Medicine.* 7th ed. Philadelphia: Saunders/Elsevier, 2005.

Web Sites of Interest

American Heart Association
http://www.heart.org

National Heart, Lung, and Blood Institute
http://www.nhlbi.nih.gov

See also: Bacterial endocarditis; Bacterial infections; Endocarditis; Infection; Inflammation; Mycotic aneurysm; Myocarditis; Pleurisy; Viral infections.

Peritonitis

CATEGORY: Diseases and conditions
ANATOMY OR SYSTEM AFFECTED: Abdomen, digestive system, gastrointestinal system, intestines, stomach, tissue

DEFINITION

Peritonitis is an inflammation or infection of the peritoneum, a thin tissue lining that covers the inside of the abdominal cavity. The peritoneum also covers the outside of the intestines and other abdominal organs. The types of peritonitis are primary, secondary, and peritoneal-dialysis-related. Peritonitis is a serious condition that requires immediate treatment. If not promptly treated, it can be fatal.

CAUSES

Primary peritonitis occurs when there is a buildup of fluid in the abdomen. This fluid buildup is called ascites. It is caused by chronic liver disease, among other conditions. Secondary peritonitis is caused by bacteria that enter the abdominal cavity. Secondary peritonitis also can be caused by an injury or a condition, such as a ruptured appendix. Dialysis-related peritonitis is caused by bacteria that enter the peritoneal cavity during or after peritoneal dialysis (a treatment for kidney disease).

RISK FACTORS

Risk factors for peritonitis include abdominal penetration or trauma, compromised immunity, blood in the abdomen, ruptured appendix, peptic ulcer, colitis, diverticulitis, gangrene of the bowel, pancreatitis, pelvic inflammatory disease, inflamed gallbladder, recent surgery, tubes or shunts in the abdomen, and cortisone drugs.

SYMPTOMS

Symptoms of peritonitis may include severe pain or tenderness in the abdomen, pain in the abdomen that is worse with motion, bloating of the abdomen, constipation, fever, nausea and vomiting, weakness or dizziness, shortness of breath, rapid pulse or breathing rate, and dehydration (signs of dehydration include dry skin and lips and decreased urine production).

SCREENING AND DIAGNOSIS

A doctor will ask about symptoms and medical history and will perform a physical exam. Tests for peritonitis may include blood tests, analysis of fluids from the peritoneum, abdominal X rays (to look for signs of inflammation), and laparotomy (surgery to open and examine the abdomen).

TREATMENT AND THERAPY

Treatment for peritonitis, which depends on the cause, may include surgery to repair openings in the skin surface or to remove damaged tissue, antibiotics to treat infection, and the replacement of fluids.

PREVENTION AND OUTCOMES

There are no guidelines for preventing peritonitis.
Michelle Badash, M.S.; reviewed by Rosalyn Carson-DeWitt, M.D.

FURTHER READING

Conn, Harold O., Juan Rodés, and Miguel Navasa. *Spontaneous Bacterial Peritonitis: The Disease, Pathogenesis, and Treatment.* New York: Marcel Dekker, 2000.

Feldman, Mark, Lawrence S. Friedman, and Lawrence J. Brandt, eds. *Sleisenger and Fordtran's Gastrointestinal and Liver Disease: Pathophysiology, Diagnosis, Management.* New ed. 2 vols. Philadelphia: Saunders/Elsevier, 2010.

Icon Health. *Peritonitis: A Medical Dictionary, Bibliography, and Annotated Research Guide to Internet References.* San Diego, Calif.: Author, 2004.

Kapadia, Cyrus R., James M. Crawford, and Caroline Taylor. *An Atlas of Gastroenterology: A Guide to Diagnosis and Differential Diagnosis.* Boca Raton, Fla.: Pantheon, 2003.

Townsend, Courtney M., et al., eds. *Sabiston Textbook of Surgery.* 18th ed. Philadelphia: Saunders/Elsevier, 2007.

Yamada, T., et al. *Textbook of Gastroenterology.* 4th ed. Philadelphia: Lippincott Williams & Wilkins, 2003.

WEB SITES OF INTEREST

American College of Gastroenterology
http://www.acg.gi.org

American Gastroenterological Association
http://www.gastro.org

Canadian Association of Gastroenterology
http://www.cag-acg.org

National Digestive Diseases Information Clearinghouse
http://digestive.niddk.nih.gov

See also: Antibiotic-associated colitis; Appendicitis; Bacterial infections; Cholecystitis; *Clostridium difficile* infection; Diverticulitis; Enteritis; Gastritis; Infection; Infectious colitis; Inflammation; Intestinal and stomach infections; Norovirus infection; Pancreatitis; Pelvic inflammatory disease; Peptic ulcer.

Pertussis. *See* Whooping cough.

Pharyngitis and tonsillopharyngitis

CATEGORY: Diseases and conditions
ANATOMY OR SYSTEM AFFECTED: Pharynx, throat, tissue, tonsils, upper respiratory tract
ALSO KNOWN AS: Sore throat, throat infection

DEFINITION

Pharyngitis is the swelling and inflammation of the pharynx. The pharynx is the back of the throat, including the back of the tongue. Tonsillopharyngitis is the swelling of the pharynx and the tonsils. The tonsils are soft tissue that make up part of the throat's immune defenses. Both pharyngitis and tonsillopharyngitis are commonly called a sore throat. Sore throats are easily treated.

CAUSES

Pharyngitis and tonsillopharyngitis can be caused by infection with a virus, such as the viruses that cause influenza (the flu) and the common cold; infection with bacteria, such as the bacteria that cause strep throat; mucus from sinuses that drains into the throat; smoking; breathing polluted air; drinking alcoholic beverages; hay fever or other allergies; acid reflux from the stomach; allergies; food debris collecting in

small pockets in the tonsils; and infectious mononucleosis.

RISK FACTORS

Almost every person will get a sore throat some time in his or her life, but the following risk factors increase the chance of getting a sore throat: age (children, teenagers, and people age sixty-five years and older); exposure to someone with a sore throat or any other infection involving the throat, nose, or ears; situations that cause stress, such as traveling, working, or living in close contact with others; exposure to cigarette smoke, toxic fumes, industrial smoke, and other air pollutants; having medical conditions that affect the immune system; stress; and hay fever or other allergies.

SYMPTOMS

The symptoms depend on the cause of the condition but generally include a sore throat, pain or difficulty when swallowing, difficulty breathing, fever, and enlarged lymph nodes in the neck.

SCREENING AND DIAGNOSIS

A doctor will perform a physical exam and will look closely at the mouth, throat, nose, ears, and the lymph nodes in the neck. This physical exam may include using a small instrument to look inside the nose, ears, and mouth; gently touching the lymph nodes (glands) in the neck to check for swelling; and taking one's temperature. The doctor will ask about any recent exposure to someone with strep throat or any other infection of the throat, nose, or ears. Other tests include rapid strep test or throat culture using a cotton swab to touch the back of the throat, blood tests to identify conditions that may be causing the sore throat, and a mono spot test (if mononucleosis is suspected).

TREATMENT AND THERAPY

Treatment depends on the cause of the sore throat and includes medications such as antibiotics for strep throat; drugs to reduce sore throat pain, including ibuprofen (Motrin or Advil), acetaminophen (Tylenol), and aspirin. Aspirin, however, is not recommended for children or teens with a current or recent viral infection because of the risk of Reye's syndrome. One should consult a doctor about medicines that are safe for children.

Other treatment options include a numbing throat

spray for pain control; decongestants and antihistamines to relieve nasal congestion and runny nose, vitamin C (if recommended by the doctor), throat lozenges, and corticosteroids (used in combination with antibiotics for severe cases).

One should also drink increased amounts of water; gargle with warm salt-water several times a day; drink warm liquids (tea or broth) or cool liquids; avoid irritants that might affect the throat, such as smoke from cigarettes, cigars, or pipes, and cold air; and avoid drinking alcohol.

PREVENTION AND OUTCOMES

To reduce the chance of getting a sore throat, one should wash hands frequently, especially after blowing one's nose or after caring for a child with a sore throat. If someone at home has a sore throat, their eating utensils and drinking glasses should be kept separate from those of other family members. These objects should be washed in hot, soapy water. One should also wash the toys of infected toddlers who have been sucking on their toys.

Furthermore, one should immediately dispose of used tissues and then wash hands. Persons with hay fever or another respiratory allergy should consult a doctor and should avoid substances that cause the allergy or allergies.

Jennifer Lewy, M.S.W.;
reviewed by Elie Edmond Rebeiz, M.D., FACS

FURTHER READING

EBSCO Publishing. *DynaMed: Streptococcal Pharyngitis.* Available through http://www.ebscohost.com/dynamed.

Ferrari, Mario. *PDxMD Ear, Nose, and Throat Disorders.* Philadelphia: PDxMD, 2003.

Hayward, G., et al. "Corticosteroids for Pain Relief in Sore Throat: Systematic Review and Meta-Analysis." *British Medical Journal* 339 (2009).

National Library of Medicine. "Pharyngitis." Available at http://www.nlm.nih.gov/medlineplus/ency/article/000655.htm.

Perkins, A. "An Approach to Diagnosing the Acute Sore Throat." *American Family Physician* 55 (1997): 131-138, 141-142.

Vincent, M. T., N. Celestin, and A. N. Hussain. "Pharyngitis." *American Family Physician* 69 (2004): 1465-1470.

WEB SITES OF INTEREST

American Academy of Pediatrics
http://www.healthychildren.org

Canadian Society of Otolaryngology—Head and Neck Surgery
http://www.entcanada.org

Clean Hands Coalition
http://www.cleanhandscoalition.org

National Institute of Allergy and Infectious Diseases
http://www.niaid.nih.gov

Public Health Agency of Canada
http://www.phac-aspc.gc.ca

See also: Adenovirus infections; Common cold; Coxsackie virus infections; Cytomegalovirus infection; Epstein-Barr virus infection; Fever; Herpes simplex infection; Herpesvirus infections; HIV; Hygiene; Infection; Inflammation; Influenza; Laryngitis; Mononucleosis; Nasopharyngeal infections; Orthomyxoviridae; Parotitis; Parvovirus infections; Respiratory syncytial virus infections; Rhinovirus infections; Saliva and infectious disease; Strep throat; Streptococcal infections; Thrush; Viral infections; Viral pharyngitis; Viral upper respiratory infections.

Picornaviridae

CATEGORY: Pathogen

DEFINITION

Picornaviruses, specifically rhinoviruses and other enteroviruses, are major causes of infections in the developed world. More than sixty types of nonpoliomyelitis enteroviruses, including three different polioviruses, can cause disease. Common examples of the genera affecting humans include *Enterovirus* (coxsackie virus, echovirus, poliovirus, rhinovirus), *Hepatovirus* (hepatitis A virus), and *Parechovirus* (respiratory tract viruses).

NATURAL HABITAT AND FEATURES

The Picornaviridae family comprises small, sensitive, single-stranded, ribonucleic acid (RNA) viruses whose genomes are surrounded by sixty copies of

---

Taxonomic Classification for Picornaviridae

Order: Picornavirales
Family: Picornaviridae
Genera: *Enterovirus, Hepatovirus, Parechovirus*
Species:
Coxsackie virus A, B
Echovirus
Poliovirus
Rhinovirus
Hepatitis A virus
Human parechovirus
Ljungan virus

---

each of the four structural proteins. *Enterovirus* is the most important genus of the picornaviruses, and there are at least ninety-two serotypes known; they are divided into four groups. For the poliovirus, humans are the only likely hosts.

Enteroviruses are acquired usually through fecal contamination; occasionally through respiratory droplets or other secretions such as sputum, saliva, or nasal mucus; and primarily through direct contact with an infected person or through indirect contact with contaminated objects (fomites) or surfaces such as telephones, cell phones, and drinking glasses.

PATHOGENICITY AND CLINICAL SIGNIFICANCE

Replication of Picornaviridae pathogens occurs entirely in the cytoplasm, and the cycle is rapid—between five and ten hours, with eight hours as the norm. The pathogens feature different cellular receptors (such as poliovirus CD155 and rhinovirus ICAM-1) and the RNA enters the cell through the membrane at the center of the penton; this occurs after one of the viral proteins has enclosed itself in the cell's membrane. A secondary viremia may occur when symptoms are present.

The spread of the virus goes into the gastrointestinal (GI) tract, whereby the secondary viremia starts ten days or so after the initial infection. This action leads to a cell-mediated and humoral immune response. It rapidly limits the replication of the virus in all tissues except the GI tract. A picornavirus induces disease depending on its viral genetics and how it adapts to the host cells.

Enteroviruses can damage many organs and systems in the body, including the heart, liver, kidney, pancreas, lungs, muscles, skin, and central nervous system (CNS). The damage is caused by local necrosis and the inflammatory response of the host. CNS infections are connected many times with mononuclear pleocytosis (increased cell count) of the cerebrospinal fluid, consisting of macrophages and activated T lymphocytes; this increase causes a meningeal inflammatory response.

Every person is at risk for contracting a picornavirus infection. Infants, children, and teenagers are at a higher risk because they are unlikely to have developed an adequate immune response to infection. Among adults, pregnant women have a higher risk of serious illness, especially if they do not have antibodies from earlier exposures. The nonpolio enteroviruses, which usually occur the United States in the fall and summer months, are common and second in prevalence to the common cold viruses. The rhinoviruses are the most common viruses among humans. Enteroviruses cause an estimated 10 to 20 million infections each year in the United States alone.

DRUG SUSCEPTIBILITY

Viral replication is a major problem that limits the effectiveness of antiviral therapy for a Picornaviridae-caused infection. Pleconaril, a newer drug, inhibits viral growth by blocking the viral uncoating and viral attachment to the host cell. This drug has shown potent, broad-spectrum, activity against the rhinovirus, according to one study.

Vaccines are a major preventive measure against viruses. Highly effective vaccines have almost eradicated poliomyelitis worldwide. No vaccines exist, however, for the coxsackie virus and other enteroviruses. These viruses are not considered life-threatening, although older or immune-compromised persons may acquire serious infections that can be life-threatening. Continued research for new vaccines is ongoing because the genetics of virulence phenotypes of picornaviruses needs further study to be understood.

Marvin L. Morris, M.P.A.

FURTHER READING

Cherry, James D. "Enteroviruses and Parechoviruses." In *Feigin and Cherry's Textbook of Pediatric Infectious Diseases*, edited by Ralph D. Feigin et al. 6th ed. Philadelphia: Saunders/Elsevier, 2009. Introduces enteroviruses and parechoviruses. Explains how they are grouped and discusses their similar characteristics and the many diseases they cause.

Modlin, John. "Introduction to Picornaviridae." In *Principles and Practice of Pediatric Infectious Diseases*, edited by Sarah S. Long, Larry K. Pickering, and Charles G. Prober. 3d ed. New York: Churchill Livingstone/Elsevier, 2008. Introduces the picornaviruses, their classification, and the different types.

Santti, J., et al. "Molecular Epidemiology and Evolution of Coxsackievirus A9." *Journal of General Virology* 81 (2000): 1361-1372. Examines the relationship between thirty-five clinical isolates of coxsackie virus A9 (CAV9) collected for five decades from different geographic locations. Twelve CAV9 genotypes were identified. They discuss isolates patterns in different regions.

WEB SITES OF INTEREST

Big Picture Book of Viruses
http://www.virology.net/big_virology

International Committee for Taxonomy of Viruses
http://www.ictvdb.org

Virus Pathogen Database and Analysis Resource
http://www.viprbrc.org/brc

See also: Antiviral drugs: Types; Coxsackie virus infections; Echovirus infections; Enterovirus infections; Fecal-oral route of transmission; Pathogens; Picornavirus infections; Poliomyelitis; Rhinovirus infections; Viral infections.

Picornavirus infections

CATEGORY: Diseases and conditions
ANATOMY OR SYSTEM AFFECTED: All

DEFINITION

Picornaviruses are single-stranded RNA (ribonucleic acid) viruses that belong to the Picornaviridae family. This family has twelve genera, although some of these are unique either to plants or to animals. Common examples of the genera affecting humans include *Enterovirus* (coxsackie virus, echovirus, poliovirus, rhinovirus), *Hepatovirus* (hepatitis A virus), and *Parechovirus* (respiratory tract virus). Picornaviruses are common and have worldwide prevalence, with the exception of poliovirus, which has been virtually eliminated in most countries.

CAUSES

Picornaviruses are most commonly transmitted by the fecal-oral route or by the respiratory route. They also may be sexually acquired, as with hepatitis A, or during pregnancy through the placenta or labor and delivery. Also, many enteroviruses are often spread in hospitals because of improper handwashing or through contaminated equipment.

RISK FACTORS

Immunocompromised persons are at greatest risk. Enterovirus infections may occur at any age, but the younger the person, the higher the risk. Hepatitis A infections increase with age, sexual contact with the virus, or illicit drug use. Additional risk factors include occupational exposure, such as in a day-care or hospital setting, and poor living conditions. Seasonal variations also may be observed and differ among virus type.

SYMPTOMS

Symptoms depend on the type of picornavirus diagnosed. Many infections are asymptomatic. Common findings include a flulike fever, upper respiratory tract infection, lethargy, irritability, poor feeding, and rash. More severe findings are inflammation of the liver (hepatitis), pancreas (pancreatitis), heart (myocarditis), and brain (encephalitis or meningitis), which place a person at an increased risk for long-term complications such as liver dysfunction or neurological deficits. The greatest risk for morbidity and mortality exists with hepatitis and poliomyelitis.

SCREENING AND DIAGNOSIS

Testing is performed by sampling through serum, throat, or rectal swab; stool sample; or cerebrospinal fluid. The diagnosis is confirmed by isolating the virus in cell culture. Reverse transcriptase polymerase chain reaction (RT-PCR) is also available with the benefit of a shorter turnaround time. Prenatal diagnostic tests such as amniocentesis may be available for specific types of enteroviruses.

TREATMENT AND THERAPY

The majority of affected persons have mild symptoms that do not require treatment, as many infections independently resolve within one week. Antiviral therapy is not available for most infections. Thus, medical care is provided based on specific symptoms. Possible avenues of treatment include medication for cold and flu symptoms, hospitalization, immunoglobulins, diet modification, or liver transplantation in the case of hepatitis.

Prevention and Outcomes

No method exists to prevent all picornavirus infections. However, recommendations for some include routine vaccination for poliovirus and hepatitis. Universal hygiene practices such as handwashing, avoiding contact with contaminated items, and safer sexual practices may reduce the spread of picornaviruses.

Janet Ober Berman, M.S., CGC

Further Reading

Holmes, Robert L., and Larry I. Lutwick. "Picornavirus: Overview." Available at http://emedicine.medscape.com/article/225483-overview.

Rotbart, Harley, and Frederick Hayden. "Picornavirus Infections: A Primer for the Practitioner." *Archives of Family Medicine* 9 (2000): 913-920.

Tebruegge, M., and N. Curtis. "Enterovirus Infections in Neonates." *Seminars in Fetal and Neonatal Medicine* 14 (2009): 222-227.

Web Sites of Interest

Big Picture Book of Viruses
http://www.virology.net/big_virology

Centers for Disease Control and Prevention
http://www.cdc.gov

Virus Pathogen Database and Analysis Resource
http://www.viprbrc.org/brc

See also: Coxsackie virus infections; Echovirus infections; Enterovirus infections; Fecal-oral route of transmission; Infection; Opportunistic infections; Picornaviridae; Pregnancy and infectious disease; Puerperal infection; Respiratory route of transmission; Rhinovirus infections; Viral hepatitis; Viral infections.

PID. *See* Pelvic inflammatory disease.

Piedraia

CATEGORY: Pathogen
TRANSMISSION ROUTE: Direct contact

Definition

Piedraia is a genus of fungi of which one species, *P. hortae*, causes black piedra, an infection of hair on the scalp.

Taxonomic Classification for *Piedraia*

Kingdom: Fungi
Phylum: Ascomycota
Class: Euascomycetes
Family: Piedraiaceae
Genus: *Piedraia*
Species:
P. hortae
P. quintanilhae

Natural Habitat and Features

Piedraia is found in soils worldwide but most often in humid tropical regions of Central America, South America, Southeast Asia, and Africa. The highest concentration is in South America. In Brazil, it is found almost exclusively in regions with a mean average temperature of 78.8° Fahrenheit (26° Celsius), average yearly rainfall of 99 inches (30 meters), and average humidity of 80 percent. International travel and migration have led to reports of isolated detection and sporadic outbreaks of infection in nontropical areas.

Piedraia is a saprotrophic mold, meaning it lives on decaying material and dead tissue. It is also found in organisms in stagnant water and on crops.

There are two species of *Piedraia*. *Quintanilhae* has been isolated from the hair of chimpanzees in central Africa, but no cases of human infection have been reported. *Hortae* causes an infection of human scalp hair and can occur anywhere on the scalp. It occurs most often on the front and top of the scalp, near the forehead. Infection of hair elsewhere on the body, such as beard, moustache, or pubic hairs, almost never occurs.

Transmission of *hortae* and its infection between persons occurs primarily through the use of shared hair-care tools and products. In the tropics of Brazil, some indigenous people use plant oils to dress the hair, which can introduce *hortae* to the scalp and encourage its transmission. Infection is most common among young adults, with a slightly higher preponderance among males.

In persons infected with *hortae*, the scalp reveals small, firm, tightly packed, irregular (oval or elongated), dark brown to black nodules that are composed of fungal matter attached to the sides and tip of hairs. The genus name derives from the Spanish word *piedra*, which means "stone." The nodules look and feel like tiny stones. Each infected hair contains from four to eight or more nodules, each 0.03 to 0.07 inches (1 to 2 millimeters) in diameter. Infected hair may have a gritty feel or give off a metallic sound when brushed. The fungus remains on the hair surface without penetrating the hair. Unlike other fungal scalp infections, such as tinea capitis, *Piedraia*-infected hairs usually do not break off.

Hortae is cultured in a standard media such as Sabouraud's agar at room temperature for two to three weeks. The colonies are distinguished by thick-walled, branched, dark-colored septate hyphae. The front is folded and velvety with a flat margin. A colony may remain glabrous (smooth and hairless) or become covered with short, light, airy hyphae. From the reverse, the colony is black.

Under microscopic examination, colonies of *hortae* reveal packed masses of dark septate hyphae (segmented filaments). Also seen are asci, which are thin-walled sacs that contain sexual spores called ascospores. The ascospores of *hortae* are hyaline (transparent), one-celled, and tapered toward both ends to form whiplike appendages. The ascospores of *quintanilhae* do not have these appendages.

PATHOGENICITY AND CLINICAL SIGNIFICANCE

Hortae is the cause of black piedra, an infection of scalp hair. White piedra, in contrast, is caused by five species of the fungus *Trichosporon* and infects hair on the scalp, face, and pubic regions. Black piedra does not cause itching or any other symptoms. Because of this, and because the nodules, although plentiful, are small, the infection may be under-reported. Persons may be infected for many years without seeking treatment.

DRUG SUSCEPTIBILITY

There is scant data on drug susceptibility of infection caused by *hortae*. No standard method for testing or comparison has been developed, although terbinafine has been shown to be effective. Shaving or clipping infected hair may resolve the infection, and it is the standard treatment of choice. In persons who are reluctant to have hair removed, a topical antifungal agent (cream, ointment, or solution) may be used instead. A topical agent may also be applied to the scalp in conjunction with hair removal. Common choices of topical agents are a salicylic acid preparation or an imidazole cream. Oral ketoconazole or terbinafine may also be used. Medical treatment without hair removal has a greater risk of relapse than does hair removal or combination therapy alone. In immunocompromised persons, infection may spread and produce purplish hemorrhagic nodules on the skin.

Ernest Kohlmetz, M.A.

FURTHER READING

Berger, T. G. "Dermatologic Disorders." In *Current Medical Diagnosis and Treatment 2011*, edited by Stephen J. McPhee and Maxine A. Papadakis. 50th ed. New York: McGraw-Hill Medical, 2011.

Richardson, Malcolm D., and David W. Warnock. *Fungal Infection: Diagnosis and Management*. New ed. Malden, Mass.: Wiley-Blackwell, 2010.

Schwartz, R. "Superficial Fungal Infections." *The Lancet* 364 (2004): 1173-1182.

WEB SITES OF INTEREST

American Academy of Dermatology
http://www.aad.org

Canadian Dermatology Association
http://www.dermatology.ca

Microbiology and Immunology On-line: Mycology
http://pathmicro.med.sc.edu/book/mycol-sta.htm

See also: Antifungal drugs: Types; Athlete's foot; Dandruff; Dermatomycosis; Dermatophytosis; Fungal infections; Fungi: Classification and types; Imidazole antifungals; Jock itch; *Malassezia*; Mycosis; Pityriasis rosea; Skin infections; Tinea capitis.

Pigs and infectious disease

CATEGORY: Transmission

DEFINITION

Transmission of infectious diseases from pigs to humans is rare and is usually a result of direct contact of humans with pigs. The infectious diseases transmissible from pigs to humans include erysipelas, leptospirosis, brucellosis, swine flu, and *Pasturella multocida*. Of these infectious diseases, swine flu is of primary concern. The food-borne disease salmonellosis is one exception to direct-contact transmission; it is caused by eating contaminated foods, including meat from pigs.

DIRECT CONTACT

The swine flu received its name because of similarities in the genetic makeup of the flu strain with a strain that lived in pigs. The World Health Organization declared a swine flu pandemic in 2009; however, there is no indication that humans contacted this strain from pigs. In fact, this strain has not been observed in pigs. To avoid using this rather misleading name, some have preferred to call swine flu the H1N1 virus, a name derived from the presence of two surface antigens on the virus. Although cross-species (pig to human and human to pig) infections have been known to occur, these infections were caused by direct contact of humans with pigs and have been limited to local areas.

The genetic code of influenza viruses consists of eight ribonucleic acid (RNA) segments. The H1N1 virus consists of one segment from a human flu segment, two from avian strains, and five from swine strains. This mixing of RNA segments occurs through a process called antigenic shift. If a pig is infected simultaneously by a pig and human flu virus, for example, segments from both species can be incorporated into a new virus with different surface antigens. The host species is then vulnerable to infections because its immune system does not recognize the different antigens. Pigs are particularly susceptible to cross-species infection.

The symptoms of swine flu are similar to other flu infections and include fever, lethargy, lack of appetite, and coughing. Other symptoms can include runny nose, sore throat, nausea, vomiting, and diarrhea.

Practical prevention methods include washing hands frequently; avoiding touching one's mouth,

---

Pig Facts

TAXONOMIC CLASSIFICATION

Kingdom: Animalia
Phylum: Chordata
Subphylum: Vertebrata
Class: Mammalia
Subclass: Theria
Order: Artiodactyla
Family: Suidae
Subfamily: Suinae
Genus: *Sus*

Geographical location: There are no true wild pigs in the Western Hemisphere, but there are feral hogs, except in Antarctica; the javelina, native to North and South America, is not a true pig
Habitat: Wide range, from swamps and rain forests to dry lands and mountains
Gestational period: A little less than four months (111-115 days)
Life span: Domestic pigs generally have a life span of six to ten years, with an occasional occurrence of more than twenty years
Special anatomy: Pigs have an excellent sense of smell and exceptional hearing, but their eyesight is weak

---

nose, and eyes; avoiding crowds, especially those in which people are coughing or sneezing; and avoiding drinking or eating foods touched by others. Swine flu vaccines are readily available, and can be administered either by injection or by nasal spray.

Four antiviral drugs are approved for treatment of swine flu; however, the virus has developed resistance to two, amantadine and rimantadine. The effective drugs, oseltamivir and zanamivir, should be taken within forty-eight hours of developing symptoms. One should get an official diagnosis of swine flu because taking the drugs will lead to having side effects.

Brucellosis is a serious disease in livestock and humans in many regions of the world, but it is now rare in the United States because of veterinary control measures. Humans contract the disease through direct contact with domestic species, especially cattle, sheep, goats, and swine, or through dairy products or

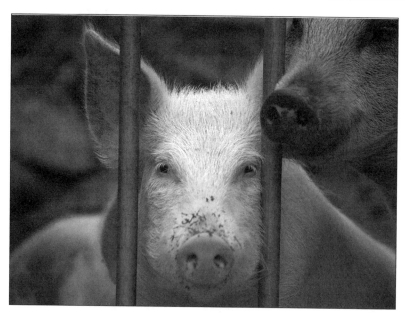

Pigs, rarely, can transmit disease to humans. (©Dreamstime.com)

meat derived from them. Brucellosis can be chronic or acute and is characterized by intermittent fever, malaise, anorexia, and prostration.

Pasturella multocida causes respiratory disease in swine, and infection in humans is rare. Although respiratory infection from *P. multocida* has been reported in pig farmers and others who work with pigs, most human cases come from dog or cat bites.

Erysipelas is caused by group A beta-hemolytic streptococci. It is spread to humans only by direct contact with affected pigs by farmers, butchers, or veterinarians. The bacterium typically enters through a person's wound while that person is handling an infected animal. The disease causes classic fiery-red plaques on the face, although the legs are most often affected. Death is very rare. The disease is typically restricted to isolated cases and has declined in importance since the mid-twentieth century.

Leptospirosis is caused by several *Leptospira* species. Although swine and other domestic animals can transmit the disease, wild animals are the most important reservoirs. Leptospirosis is spread by contact with the urine of infected animals or with the food, water, or other substances contaminated by the urine of infected animals. The organisms have flagella that allow them to burrow through the skin or mucous membranes. Most cases of leptospirosis are asymptomatic

or mild. Although a variety of symptoms can occur, the most serious is a type of meningitis with a severe headache and a stiff neck. A more severe form with multiple organ failure occurs in 5 to 10 percent of cases. The disease is now rare in the United States, and the U.S. Centers for Disease Control and Prevention estimates that between one hundred and two hundred cases are identified each year.

FOOD-BORNE DISEASES

Salmonella infection (salmonellosis) is caused by eating foods contaminated with *Salmonella* organisms. Poultry and eggs are most commonly implicated, although other meats, including that from pigs, and some fruits and vegetables, can also cause salmonellosis. Many species of *Salmonella* can cause the infection, whose symptoms include severe diarrhea, nausea, and abdominal pain. Cleanliness is essential to prevention and includes handwashing after handling raw foods.

IMPACT

Most of the diseases transmitted from pigs to humans are also transmitted from other animals, both domestic and wild. Likewise, most of the diseases described are of low incidence and have little impact on the population of the United States. Some diseases affect only workers who have direct contact with swine or swine meat. Food-borne illness and influenza outbreaks are the exceptions.

David A. Olle, M.S.

FURTHER READING

Center for Food Security and Public Health. "Brucellosis." Available at http://www.cfsph.iastate.edu/Factsheets/pdfs/brucellosis.pdf. Provides a complete discussion on all aspects of brucellosis.

_____. "Leptospirosis." Available at http://www.cfsph.iastate.edu/Factsheets/pdfs/leptospirosis.pdf.

Centers for Disease Control and Prevention. "2009 H1N1 Flu." Available at http://www.cdc.gov/H1N1flu. This news report is updated frequently.

Davis, Charles. "Swine Flu (Swine Influenza A [H1N1] Virus)." Available at http://www.medicinenet.com/swine_flu/article.htm.

Hendrickson, Susan, et al. "Animal-to-Human Transmission of *Salmonella typhimurium* DT104A Variant." *Emerging Infectious Diseases* 10, no. 12 (December, 2004): 2225-2227.

National Library of Medicine. "*Salmonella* Enterocolitis." Available at http://www.nlm.nih.gov/medlineplus/ency/article/000294.htm.

WEB SITES OF INTEREST

Center for Food Security and Public Health
http://www.cfsph.iastate.edu

Clean Hands Coalition
http://www.cleanhandscoalition.org

U.S. Department of Agriculture, Food Safety Information Center
http://foodsafety.nal.usda.gov

See also: Brucellosis; Cysticercosis; *Erysipelothrix* infection; Food-borne illness and disease; Parasites: Classification and types; Parasitic diseases; Taeniasis; Tapeworms; Worm infections; Zoonotic diseases.

Pilonidal cyst

CATEGORY: Diseases and conditions
ANATOMY OR SYSTEM AFFECTED: Skin
ALSO KNOWN AS: Pilonidal abscess, pilonidal sinus

DEFINITION

A pilonidal cyst is a fluid-filled defect found at the base of the spine, or tailbone area. The different stages of the disease process are referred to by the terms "cyst" (not infected), "abscess" (pocket of pus), and "sinus" (an opening between a cyst or other internal structure and the outside).

When a pilonidal cyst is infected, it forms an abscess, eventually draining pus through a sinus. Pilonidal cysts are harmless until they get infected. At this point they form an abscess that causes pain, a foul smell, and drainage. This is more likely to occur in young Caucasian men with a large amount of hair in the region of the tailbone. This condition is not serious, but because it is an infection similar to a boil or carbuncle, it can enlarge and become uncomfortable.

CAUSES

A pilonidal condition may be congenital or acquired. If congenital, it probably began as a defect that existed when the person was born. Sometime later, the defect allowed an infection to develop. An acquired pilonidal condition may be caused by the enlargement of a simple hair follicle infection or by a hair penetrating the skin and causing an infection.

RISK FACTORS

The factors that increase the chance of developing a pilonidal abscess are personal or family history of similar problems (such as acne, boils, carbuncles, folliculitis, or sebaceous cysts), large amounts of hair in the region, a tailbone injury, horseback riding, and cycling.

SYMPTOMS

The symptoms that indicate a pilonidal abscess that needs to be treated by a doctor are painful swelling over the sacrum (just above the tailbone), a foul smell, and pus draining from the area.

SCREENING AND DIAGNOSIS

A doctor will ask about symptoms and medical history and will perform a physical exam. The infected person will then be referred to a surgeon for treatment. No diagnostic tests are required.

TREATMENT AND THERAPY

The choice of treatment will depend on the extent of the condition and the person's general, overall health. As with all localized infections under the skin, hot water soaks will draw out the infection. This will not completely cure the condition, but it will help.

Another treatment option is incision and drainage, in which the abscess is sliced, the pus is drained, and the wound is packed with sterile gauze. This helps the wound heal from the inside out. However, this usually does not cure the problem because abnormal tissue remains. To completely cure the condition, all affected tissue needs to be removed. This is an extensive surgical procedure that involves more than simple incision and drainage. The surgical wound may be closed with sutures or left open to heal from the inside. Also, reports suggest that laser hair removal in the area may be effective treatment for pilonidal cysts.

PREVENTION AND OUTCOMES

To reduce the chance of getting a pilonidal abscess, one should keep the area clean and dry, avoid sitting for long periods of time on hard surfaces, and remove hair from the area.

Ricker Polsdorfer, M.D.;
reviewed by Ross Zeltser, M.D., FAAD

FURTHER READING

Humphries, Ashley E., and James E. Duncan. "Evaluation and Management of Pilonidal Disease." In *Anorectal Disease*, edited by Scott R. Steele. Philadelphia: Saunders, 2010.

Icon Health. *Abscess: A Medical Dictionary, Bibliography, and Annotated Research Guide to Internet References.* San Diego, Calif.: Author, 2004.

Sadick, N. S., and J. Yee-Levin. "Laser and Light Treatments for Pilonidal Cysts." *Cutis* 78 (2006): 125-128.

Velasco, Alfonso L., and Wade W. Dunlap. "Pilonidal Disease and Hidradenitis." In *Skin Surgery and Minor Procedures*, edited by Frederick Radke. Philadelphia: Saunders/Elsevier, 2009.

Weedon, David. *Skin Pathology.* 3d ed. New York: Churchill Livingstone/Elsevier, 2010.

WEB SITES OF INTEREST

American Academy of Dermatology
http://www.aad.org

Canadian Dermatology Association
http://www.dermatology.ca

Pilonidal Support Alliance
http://www.pilonidal.org

See also: Abscesses; Acne; Anal abscess; Boils; Hordeola; Methicillin-resistant staph infection; Skin infections.

Pinkeye. *See* Conjunctivitis.

Pinta

CATEGORY: Diseases and conditions
ANATOMY OR SYSTEM AFFECTED: Skin
ALSO KNOWN AS: *Azul, carate, mal de pinto*

DEFINITION

Pinta is a rare, endemic, treponemal bacterial infection characterized by chronic skin lesions that occur primarily in young adults. Pinta, with yaws and endemic syphilis, are the three chronic granulomatous diseases that constitute the group of pathogenic nonvenereal (nonsexual) treponematoses in humans.

CAUSES

Pinta is caused by the spirochete bacterium *Treponema pallidum carateum*. The disease is contagious and spread from person to person through close, prolonged, nonsexual contact involving skin or mucous membranes.

RISK FACTORS

Pinta occurs in scattered foci in remote rural areas of Central America and South America where poor hygiene and crowded conditions exist, primarily among disadvantaged persons. The exact prevalence of the disease is unknown. A few hundred cases are reported each year (from Brazil, Venezuela, Colombia, Peru, Ecuador, Mexico, and countries of Central America).

Pinta affects children and adults of all ages, but the peak age of incidence is fifteen to thirty years. Women and men are equally affected, and the disease is frequently spread to family members. Economically underprivileged peoples with frequent skin trauma, limited protective clothing, and little or no access to health care are at increased risk.

SYMPTOMS

Pinta is classified into an early stage (with initial and secondary lesions) and a late stage (latent phase and tertiary stage). The initial skin lesion usually appears after an incubation period of two to three weeks. It begins as one or more erythematous papule most frequently found on exposed parts of the body (legs, dorsum of the foot, forearm, and hands). The lesion slowly enlarges and becomes pigmented and hyperkeratotic. It may be accompanied by regional lymphadenopathy.

The secondary lesions appear between one and twelve months of the primary lesion. They vary in size and location, become pigmented with age, may change colors; several colors may exist within the same lesion. Late or tertiary pinta usually begins several years after the onset of the disease and is characterized by disfiguring achromic and atrophic lesions. Pinta is the most benign among the spirochetal diseases because it has skin manifestations only.

Neurologic, bone, or cardiac manifestations do not occur, and no congenital form of the disease exists. Pinta is not a fatal disease, but it is a disfiguring one that often leads to social ostracism.

SCREENING AND DIAGNOSIS

Diagnosis is based on the lesions' appearance and on microscopical examination. Also available is serologic testing for *T. carateum* antibodies.

TREATMENT AND THERAPY

The treatment of choice is benzathine penicillin. Adults are treated by a single intramuscular administration in two injection sites. Children are treated with a single dose. After this treatment, lesions become noninfectious in twenty-four hours. Alternative therapies for persons who are allergic to penicillin include tetracycline and erythromycin.

The prognosis for persons with pinta is good. Primary and early secondary lesions may take four to six months to disappear. Late secondary lesions heal slowly, within six to twelve months. Pigmentary changes in late lesions may persist.

PREVENTION AND OUTCOMES

Good personal hygiene is the main preventive measure. Children should avoid physical contact with persons who have skin lesions caused by pinta. Improvement of sanitation, access to antibiotics in endemic rural areas, and campaigns against infection are essential for the eradication of this infectious disease.

Katia Marazova, M.D., Ph.D.

FURTHER READING

Antal, George M., Sheila A. Lukehart, and Andre Z. Meheus. "The Endemic Treponematoses." *Microbes and Infection* 4 (2002): 83-94.
Feigin, Ralph D., et al., eds. *Textbook of Pediatric Infectious Diseases.* 6th ed. Philadelphia: Saunders/Elsevier, 2009.
Klein, Natalie C. "Pinta." Available at http://emedicine.medscape.com/article/225576-overview.
Nassar, Naiel N., and Justin David Radolf. "Nonvenereal Treponematoses: Yaws, Pinta, and Endemic Syphilis." In *Kelley's Textbook of Internal Medicine,* edited by H. David Humes et al. 4th ed. Philadelphia: Lippincott Williams & Wilkins, 2000.

WEB SITES OF INTEREST

Centers for Disease Control and Prevention
http://www.cdc.gov/parasites

Neglected Tropical Diseases Coalition
http://www.neglectedtropicaldiseases.org

Virtual Museum of Bacteria
http://www.bacteriamuseum.org

See also: Bacterial infections; Developing countries and infectious disease; Skin infections; Syphilis; *Treponema*; Tropical medicine; Yaws.

Pinworms

CATEGORY: Diseases and conditions
ANATOMY OR SYSTEM AFFECTED: Gastrointestinal system, genitalia, intestines
ALSO KNOWN AS: Enterobiasis, pinworm infection, roundworm

DEFINITION

Pinworms are common parasites that live in the intestine. Pinworms are most active at night, two to three hours after bedtime. The female worm comes out of the body through the anus and deposits eggs in the perineal area. The perineal area is between the thighs and runs from the anus to the genitals.

Pinworms are visible to the naked eye. They are about the size of a staple, are yellow-white, and look like an actively moving piece of thread.

CAUSES

A small white worm called *Enterobius vermicularis* causes pinworm infection. A separate species (*E. gregorii*) reportedly caused infection in England. Pinworms are spread when a person accidentally ingests

Roundworm (Pinworm) Facts

TAXONOMIC CLASSIFICATION

Kingdom: Animalia
Subkingdom: Bilateria
Phylum: Nematoda
Classes: Adenophorea (having no phasmids, mostly aquatic, free-living species, some plant and animal parasites); Secernentea (having phasmids, mostly terrestrial, free-living species, some plant and animal parasites)
Orders: Adenophorea–Chromadorida and Enoplida; Secernentea–Rhabditida, Strongylida, and Oxyurida

Geographical location: Found worldwide
Habitat: Soil, freshwater, and salt water; extreme habitats such as decaying cacti and vinegar malts; several species are plant or animal parasites
Gestational period: Varies with species
Life span: Varies with species; specialized dauer larvae are dormant stages resistant to drying and can survive for months under adverse environmental conditions
Special anatomy: External cuticle made of collagen; cylindrical bilaterally symmetrical organisms with a psuedocoelom; exchange of oxygen and carbon dioxide occurs across the body wall

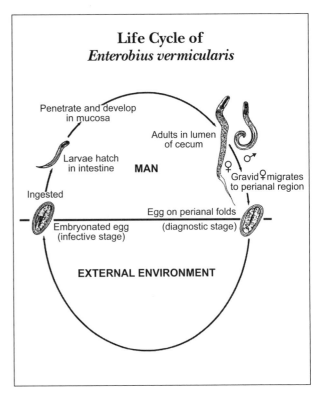

The cycle of infection by the pinworm Enterobius vermicularis. (CDC)

the eggs of the pinworm found on infected clothing, bedding, or toys, or in the stool of an infected person (such as through a stool in diapers).

RISK FACTORS

The risk factors for pinworm are contact with an infected person (usually a child or family member of an infected child); contact with contaminated clothing, bedding, or other object; and regular exposure at schools, day-care centers, and other places where pinworms may be present. Also at higher risk are children ages five to fourteen years.

SYMPTOMS

Symptoms of pinworm may include an itchy perineal area, disturbed sleep, and irritability. Symptoms may be worse at night. While the itching caused by pinworms can be uncomfortable, pinworms do not otherwise cause serious illness. Many people infected with pinworms have no symptoms.

SCREENING AND DIAGNOSIS

When present, pinworms can be seen in stool or on the skin around the anus. If pinworm infestation is suspected but no worms are seen, then one could employ the so-called tape test. The tape test detects the presence of pinworms on three patient-supplied samples of clear adhesive tape that has been placed over the anus, pressed down, and removed (for a total of three samples). The doctor will have the samples examined for pinworms. Some laboratories supply special tape or "pinworm paddles" to use for this test. The best time to do this test is two to three hours after bedtime, or before bathing in the early morning.

TREATMENT AND THERAPY

Pinworm infections are most commonly treated with prescription medications such as Albenza (albendazole) or Vermox (mebendazole), though pyrantel pamoate may also be used. Pyrantel pamoate is available over-the-counter under several names, including Pin-X and PinRid. However, women who are or may become pregnant should not these medications and should consult a doctor about the best therapy.

Medication for pinworm is generally given in two or more doses, each separated by two weeks. To avoid reinfection, all members of the family should be treated. After each treatment, persons should change underwear, nightclothes, and sheets; wash all bedding every three to seven days for three weeks; wash underwear and pajamas daily for two weeks; and wash all clothing and toys to destroy remaining eggs.

PREVENTION AND OUTCOMES

To prevent pinworm infection, one should always wash hands thoroughly after using the toilet, after changing diapers, and before eating; change and wash underwear daily; bathe shortly after waking up to reduce egg contamination; and discourage nail biting and scratching of the anal area.

Michelle Badash, M.S.;
reviewed by David L. Horn, M.D., FACP

FURTHER READING

Centers for Disease Control and Prevention. "Pinworm Infection." Available at http://www.cdc.gov/parasites/pinworm.

Despommier, Dickson D., et al. *Parasitic Diseases.* 5th ed. New York: Apple Tree, 2006.

EBSCO Publishing. *DynaMed: Enterobiasis.* Available through http://www.ebscohost.com/dynamed.

Roberts, Larry S., and John Janovy, Jr. *Gerald D. Schmidt and Larry S. Roberts' Foundations of Parasitology.* 8th ed. Boston: McGraw-Hill, 2009.

WEB SITES OF INTEREST

American Academy of Pediatrics
http://www.healthychildren.org

Centers for Disease Control and Prevention
http://www.cdc.gov/parasites

National Institute of Allergy and Infectious Diseases
http://www.niaid.nih.gov

Public Health Agency of Canada
http://www.phac-aspc.gc.ca

See also: Amebic dysentery; Anal abscess; Ascariasis; Capillariasis; Cryptosporidiosis; Enterobiasis; Hookworms; Intestinal and stomach infections; Oral transmission; Parasites: Classification and types; Parasitic diseases; Pilonidal cyst; Roundworms; Skin infections; Trichinosis; Whipworm infection; Worm infections.

Pityriasis rosea

CATEGORY: Diseases and conditions
ANATOMY OR SYSTEM AFFECTED: Skin

DEFINITION

Pityriasis rosea is a common skin rash that occurs mainly in children and young adults. The scaly, reddish-pink rash first appears on the back, stomach, or chest. The rash can then spread to the neck, arms, and legs. Pityriasis rosea usually occurs in the spring and fall.

This condition may last several weeks. Although the lesions usually go away on their own after two to three months, one should contact a doctor if experiencing any of the symptoms listed here.

CAUSES

The cause of pityriasis rosea is unknown, although research suggests that it may be caused by viruses or certain medications, such as antibiotics or heart medications.

RISK FACTORS

Pityriasis rosea occurs most often in children older than age ten years and in adults up to the age of thirty-five years, although the condition can occur at any age. Also, the condition most often occurs in the spring and fall months.

SYMPTOMS

The symptoms of pityriasis rosea include feeling as if one is getting a cold, just before the rash appears, and having a "herald patch" (usually the first lesion to appear). This patch is a large, oval, scaly lesion that typically occurs on the back, stomach, armpit, or chest. After several days, more lesions appear on the body.

Lesions that are found on the back tend to form a Christmas tree pattern. The scale of pityriasis rosea is often described as trailing scale. It forms inside the leading pink edge of the lesions.

Mild to severe itching of the lesions can occur as well. The rash of pityriasis rosea is typically not itchy, but itching may occur in some persons. Itching worsens when the body overheats (such as during physical activities or after taking a hot shower). Other symptoms include skin redness or inflammation and feeling tired and achy. If symptoms last more than three months, one should consult a doctor.

SCREENING AND DIAGNOSIS

The doctor will ask about symptoms and medical history and will perform a physical exam, including an examination of the skin. The patient may be referred to a doctor who specializes in skin disorders (a dermatologist). A dermatologist can usually diagnose pityriasis rosea by examining the skin.

Because the condition can look like other skin disorders, including eczema, ringworm, syphilis, and psoriasis, other tests may be needed to confirm the diagnosis. Tests may include blood tests, a skin scrape, and a skin biopsy (removal of a sample of skin tissue from the lesion to test for pityriasis rosea).

TREATMENT AND THERAPY

There is no cure for pityriasis rosea. The rash will usually go away on its own after several weeks. The symptoms of pityriasis rosea, such as itching, can be relieved using different treatments. Treatment options include medications to relieve itching and inflammation caused by pityriasis rosea (antihistamine pills, steroid pills, steroid creams or ointments, calamine lotion).

One should avoid physical activities that can raise body temperature and worsen itching, and should avoid hot baths or showers to prevent the itching from worsening. Oatmeal baths, however, may soothe the itching. Exposure to sunlight or treatment with artificial ultraviolet light (by a doctor) may speed the healing process.

PREVENTION AND OUTCOMES

Because the cause of pityriasis rosea is unknown, there is no way to prevent it. It is not contagious and rarely recurs. There are no permanent marks left after the lesions disappear. However, persons with darker skin may experience skin discoloration that usually fades with time.

Marjorie M. Montemayor, M.A.;
reviewed by Ross Zeltser, M.D., FAAD

FURTHER READING

American Osteopathic College of Dermatology. "Pityriasis Rosea." Available at http://www.aocd.org/skin/dermatologic_diseases.

Icon Health. *Pityriasis Rosea: A Medical Dictionary, Bibliography, and Annotated Research Guide to Internet References.* San Diego, Calif.: Author, 2004.

National Library of Medicine. "Pityriasis Rosea." Available at http://www.nlm.nih.gov/medlineplus/ency/article/000871.htm.

Turkington, Carol, and Jeffrey S. Dover. *The Encyclopedia of Skin and Skin Disorders.* 3d ed. New York: Facts On File, 2007.

Weedon, David. *Skin Pathology.* 3d ed. New York: Churchill Livingstone/Elsevier, 2010.

WEB SITES OF INTEREST

American Academy of Dermatology
http://www.aad.org

American Osteopathic College of Dermatology
http://www.aocd.org

College of Family Physicians of Canada
http://www.cfpc.ca

See also: Acne; Chickenpox; Children and infectious disease; Dandruff; Erythema infectiosum; Erythema nodosum; Impetigo; Jock itch; Measles; Roseola; Rubella; Scabies; Scarlet fever; Skin infections.

Plague

CATEGORY: Diseases and conditions
ANATOMY OR SYSTEM AFFECTED: All
ALSO KNOWN AS: Black Death, bubonic plague, pharyngeal plague, pneumonic plague, septicemic plague

DEFINITION

Plague is a bacterial infection that can be deadly. The disease occurs naturally after a bite by an infected flea or from handling or eating an infected animal.

Governments have studied the use of the bacterium as a biological weapon. As a weapon, it would be released into the air.

There are several types of plague, depending on where the exposure and symptoms occur. These types are pneumonic (in the lungs), from breathing in droplets or as a progression of another type; bubonic (in the lymph nodes), occurring after a rodent or flea bite; septicemic (a systemwide infection), occurring after a rodent or flea bite; and pharyngeal (in the throat and nearby lymph nodes), caused by ingesting infected tissue or inhaling large droplets.

CAUSES

The bacterium *Yersinia pestis* causes the infection. It is spread by droplets in the air. A person can catch pneumonic plague after having face-to-face contact with someone who has the disease. Bubonic and septicemic plague, lacking respiratory complications, are rarely spread from person to person.

RISK FACTORS

Risk factors for plague include exposure to the bacteria, contact with rodents, and biological terrorism.

SYMPTOMS

Symptoms, which depend on the type of plague, occur in naturally acquired cases within two to eight days. Plague can progress within a few days and cause sepsis, meningitis, or death.

Experts expect the first symptoms after a biological attack would appear within a couple of days. People would likely die soon after the first symptoms occurred.

The following are symptoms of pneumonic plague: fever; chills; weakness; headache; cough, with bloody or watery secretions; difficult breathing; chest pain; and possible nausea, vomiting, and diarrhea. Symptoms of bubonic plague include fever; chills; weakness; headache; swollen, tender lymph nodes; skin appearing red and tight over affected lymph nodes; raised bumps or sores at site of flea bite; restlessness; lack of energy; possible agitation, confusion; and possible nausea, vomiting, and diarrhea. A symptom of pharyngeal plague is swollen lymph nodes. Symptoms of septicemic plague and progression of other forms include bleeding under the skin; black fingers, toes, or nose; abnormal clotting; difficulty breathing; shock; organ failure; and death.

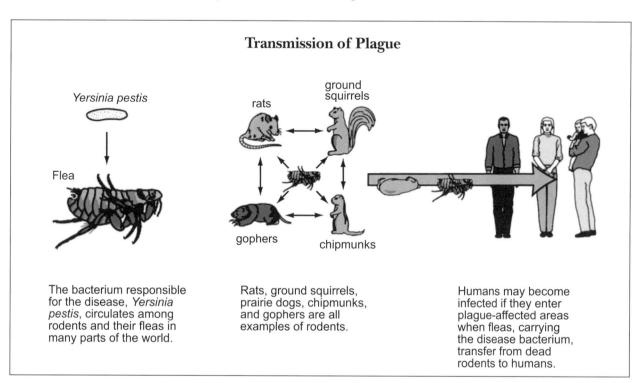

Transmission of Plague

Yersinia pestis

Flea

rats

ground squirrels

gophers

chipmunks

The bacterium responsible for the disease, *Yersinia pestis*, circulates among rodents and their fleas in many parts of the world.

Rats, ground squirrels, prairie dogs, chipmunks, and gophers are all examples of rodents.

Humans may become infected if they enter plague-affected areas when fleas, carrying the disease bacterium, transfer from dead rodents to humans.

Many small animals, particularly rodents, carry the flea that transmits the plague bacterium Yersinia pestis *to humans.*

SCREENING AND DIAGNOSIS

A doctor will ask about symptoms, medical history, and possible source of exposure, and will perform a physical exam. Other cases in the area may alert health care workers of the possibility of a bioterrorism attack. Tests for plague include a chest X ray, blood tests to look for indications of an infection, a blood test to detect antibodies to plague bacteria, an examination of body fluids using special techniques, and a culture of body fluids to check for bacteria.

TREATMENT AND THERAPY

Early treatment with antibiotics is essential. Any delay greatly increases the risk of death. The drugs are injected in a muscle or given through a vein. Later in treatment, some drugs can be given by mouth. A patient with lung symptoms will be placed in isolation to protect others. Caregivers and visitors should wear a mask, gloves, goggles, and a gown. Lymph nodes may require draining. Finally, all cases are reported to public health officials.

Any of the following antibiotics may be used: streptomycin (may be combined with a tetracycline), gentamicin, tetracycline or doxycycline, chloramphenicol, or ciprofloxacin. For persons with septicemic plague, health professionals will monitor the patient for changes in status and will take appropriate action. Maintaining adequate heart function, blood pressure, and oxygen supply are of prime importance.

PREVENTION AND OUTCOMES

Antibiotics may prevent infection following close contact with someone who has the disease and should be taken daily while in contact and for seven days after the last exposure. In addition, the caregiver and patient should wear masks.

Antibiotics may be ordered in the event of a terrorism exposure. People may be placed on the drugs after developing a cough. There would be no warning systems to alert authorities that plague bacteria had been released. The success of an attack would depend on the bacteria's quality and strain, the way they were produced, and weather conditions at the time of release. A vaccine does not exist for pneumonic plague.

Measures to prevent naturally occurring plague include avoiding dead rodents or sick cats, using insecticides and eliminating rat habitats around residences, and keeping dogs and cats from roaming in areas where plague is common.

Reviewed by David L. Horn, M.D., FACP

FURTHER READING

Andreoli, Thomas E., et al., eds. *Andreoli and Carpenter's Cecil Essentials of Medicine.* 8th ed. Philadelphia: Saunders/Elsevier, 2010.

Inglesby, Thomas V., et al. "Plague as a Biological Weapon: Medical and Public Health Management." *Journal of the American Medical Association* 283 (2000): 2281-2290.

Mandell, Gerald L., John E. Bennett, and Raphael Dolin, eds. *Mandell, Douglas, and Bennett's Principles and Practice of Infectious Diseases.* 7th ed. New York: Churchill Livingstone/Elsevier, 2010.

Marquardt, William C., ed. *Biology of Disease Vectors.* 2d ed. New York: Academic Press/Elsevier, 2005.

Pickering, Larry K., et al., eds. *Red Book: 2009 Report of the Committee on Infectious Diseases.* 28th ed. Elk Grove Village, Ill.: American Academy of Pediatrics, 2009.

Rakel, Robert E., Edward T. Bope, and Rick D. Kellerman, eds. *Conn's Current Therapy 2011.* Philadelphia: Saunders/Elsevier, 2010.

WEB SITES OF INTEREST

Center for Biosecurity
http://www.upmc-biosecurity.org

Centers for Disease Control and Prevention
http://www.bt.cdc.gov/agent/plague

World Health Organization
http://www.who.int/topics/plague

See also: Airborne illness and disease; Anthrax; Bacterial infections; *Bartonella* infections; Biological weapons; Bioterrorism; Botulinum toxin infection; Botulism; Brucellosis; Bubonic plague; Cat scratch fever; Cats and infectious disease; Colorado tick fever; Dogs and infectious disease; Fleas and infectious disease; Hantavirus infection; Insect-borne illness and disease; Lyme disease; Lymphadenitis; Rat-bite fever; Respiratory route of transmission; Rocky Mountain spotted fever; Rodents and infectious disease; SARS; Tropical medicine; Tularemia; Vectors and vector control; *Yersinia*; Zoonotic diseases.

Plantar warts

CATEGORY: Diseases and conditions
ANATOMY OR SYSTEM AFFECTED: Feet, skin

DEFINITION

Plantar warts are growths on the soles of the feet. They are often mistaken for corns or calluses. The warts are different because they are caused by a virus. Warts grow in clusters and are usually flat. A plantar wart can often be distinguished by numerous black dots visible on its surface.

Although plantar warts are generally harmless, their location beneath the feet can make them tender. They also have a tendency to spread locally to other sites on the foot and elsewhere on the body.

CAUSES

Plantar warts, which are caused by the human papillomavirus (HPV), can be contracted by walking barefoot on unsanitary surfaces. Touching and scratching can cause the virus to spread.

RISK FACTORS

Factors that increase the chance for plantar warts include exposing one's feet to unsanitary surfaces. Plantar warts are more common in children and teens and in persons with atopic dermatitis (eczema) or with a suppressed immune system caused by AIDS, lymphoma, or the use of immunosuppressive drugs.

SYMPTOMS

Symptoms of plantar warts are hard, flat growths on the soles of the feet; heaped-up calluses surrounding the wart surfaces; and pain in the area of the warts.

SCREENING AND DIAGNOSIS

A doctor will ask about symptoms and medical history and will examine the patient's feet. Some doctors may wish to refer difficult cases to a specialist, such as a podiatrist, whose focus is on foot disorders, or a dermatologist, whose focus is on skin disorders.

TREATMENT AND THERAPY

There are many over-the-counter products available to treat warts. These therapies often contain a mild acid and can usually be applied when a wart first appears. Another popular and less expensive treatment is using duct tape to cover a wart for one week at a time. This is also done with weekly "sanding" of the wart with a pumice stone. A person should see a doctor if experiencing recurrent warts, if initial treatment fails, if over-the-counter therapies are not well-tolerated, and when the diagnosis is unclear.

After confirming the diagnosis of plantar warts, the doctor may use one or more of the following treatments: cryotherapy (freezing the warts to kill the virus), laser treatment (using a laser to kill the virus and destroy wart tissue), electrocautery treatment (burning the wart), surgical removal (cutting out the wart, with the patient under anesthetic), and immune therapy (application of substances that stimulate the immune system's response to the wart-causing virus).

PREVENTION AND OUTCOMES

The best way to prevent plantar warts is to keep one's feet from coming into contact with the virus that causes the warts. The following preventive measures are recommended: Avoid walking barefoot, except on sandy beaches; wear plastic sandals when showering in public bathrooms; change shoes and socks daily, and keep feet clean and dry; avoid direct contact with warts (of others or of one's own body). In addition, periodically checking for warts on children's feet may help prevent the warts from becoming larger and painful.

*Jennifer Hellwig, M.S., RD;
reviewed by Ross Zeltser, M.D., FAAD*

FURTHER READING

Al-Gurairi, F. T., M. al-Waiz, and K. E. Sharquie. "Oral Zinc Sulphate in the Treatment of Recalcitrant Viral Warts: Randomized Placebo-Controlled Clinical Trial." *British Journal of Dermatology* 146 (2002): 423-431.

Alexander, Ivy L., ed. *Podiatry Sourcebook.* 2d rev. ed. Detroit, Mich.: Omnigraphics, 2007.

Brodell, Robert T., and Sandra Marchese Johnson, eds. *Warts: Diagnosis and Management.* Washington, D.C.: Taylor & Francis, 2003.

Lorimer, Donald L., et al., eds. *Neale's Disorders of the Foot.* 7th ed. New York: Churchill Livingstone/Elsevier, 2006.

McCance, Dennis J., ed. *Human Papilloma Viruses.* New York: Elsevier Science, 2002.

Weedon, David. *Skin Pathology.* 3d ed. New York: Churchill Livingstone/Elsevier, 2010.

See also: Athlete's foot; Genital warts; Human papillomavirus (HPV) infections; Jock itch; Onychomycosis; Skin infections; Viral infections; Warts.

Pleurisy

CATEGORY: Diseases and conditions
ANATOMY OR SYSTEM AFFECTED: Chest, lungs, respiratory system
ALSO KNOWN AS: Pleuritis

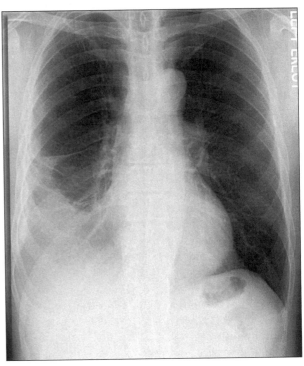

A chest X ray shows a region of prominent pneumonia and an associated pleural effusion, bottom left.

DEFINITION

Pleurisy is an inflammation of the pleura, the double-layered membrane that surrounds each lung and the rib cage. The double-layered pleura protects and lubricates the surface of the lungs as they inflate and deflate within the rib cage. Healthy pleura have a thin, fluid-filled space between the two layers that lets them glide gently across each other. When the pleura become inflamed, the diseased surfaces rub painfully together, causing a characteristic sound called friction rub.

Pleurisy cases are defined as having pleural effusion or as being dry. Pleural effusion, an accumulation of fluid in the pleural space, is more common, and is essentially a side effect of numerous diseases or trauma. Dry pleurisy refers to cases in which there is no fluid buildup. Pleural effusion is less painful because of the fluid forcing some separation of the membranes. However, the fluid puts pressure on the lungs, which can lead to respiratory distress and even lung collapse.

Pleurisy is a potentially serious condition that can have long-term effects. Persons should seek medical care as soon as possible. Doing so leads to a more favorable outcome.

CAUSES

There are several causes for either acute or chronic pleurisy. These causes include a viral infection (such as influenza or mumps); lung infections, such as tuberculosis (from bacteria) or amebiasis (from parasites); systemic lupus; asbestos-related illnesses; pancreatitis; rheumatoid arthritis; cancer metastasis; chronic liver and kidney disease; sickle cell disease; inflammatory bowel disease; Dressler's syndrome (sometimes follows a heart attack); heart failure; pulmonary embolism; chest injury; and drug reactions (such as to nitrofurantoin or procainamide).

RISK FACTORS

The following factors increase the chance of developing pleurisy: infection, injury, or tumor, or an underlying lung condition, such as pneumonia, tuberculosis, lung abscesses, or influenza. These are the most common causes; however, pleurisy can occur spontaneously.

SYMPTOMS

Symptoms of pleurisy include a sharp, stabbing pain toward the side and lower part of the chest, especially when lying down (and with relief by sitting up); pain along the shoulders, neck, and abdomen; aggravated pain during any movement of the chest, such as during breathing and coughing; dry coughing; weakness; headaches; loss of appetite; chills; fever; rapid pulse; and rapid and shallow breathing.

SCREENING AND DIAGNOSIS

A doctor will ask about symptoms and medical history and will perform a physical exam. The distinctive pain associated with pleurisy can be enough to diagnose the condition. The doctor will use a stethoscope to listen for abnormal chest sounds, such as those made by a friction rub. The next step is determining the illness that caused the pleurisy. Tests may include a chest X ray, a blood test, an EKG, a computed tomography (CT) scan (a detailed X-ray picture that identifies abnormalities of fine tissue structure), an ultrasound scan, and fluid analysis after thoracentesis. If a fluid analysis is not helpful, the physician may decide to perform a biopsy of the pleura with video-associated thoracic surgery (VATS).

TREATMENT AND THERAPY

Treatment options include pain management, in which analgesics and anti-inflammatory drugs, such as acetaminophen, ibuprofen, and indomethacin, are used to treat the pain. Some patients can reduce their pain by lying on the painful side, by holding a pillow tightly, or by wrapping the chest with elastic bandages. The physician may prescribe codeine-based cough syrup to treat a painful cough.

Another option is to treat the source of the infection. If pleurisy is the result of a bacterial infection, the physician can prescribe antibiotics. If it is the result of a viral infection, treatment is simply letting it run its course. If the cause is an autoimmune disease such as lupus, steroid treatment will quickly relieve pain.

PREVENTION AND OUTCOMES

To help reduce the chances of getting pleurisy, one should seek early medical attention for conditions that can cause pleurisy and should consider getting vaccinated for pneumonia, especially if one is elderly, has a chronic illness, or has weakened immunity.

Beth Walsh, M.A.; reviewed by Christine Colpitts, M.A., CRT

FURTHER READING

Fishman, Alfred, ed. *Fishman's Pulmonary Diseases and Disorders.* 4th ed. New York: McGraw-Hill, 2008.

Kass, S. M., and B. V. Reamy. "Pleurisy." *American Family Physician* 75 (2007): 1357-1364.

Levitzky, Michael G. *Pulmonary Physiology.* 7th ed. New York: McGraw-Hill Medical, 2007.

Mason, Robert J., et al., eds. *Murray and Nadel's Textbook of Respiratory Medicine.* 5th ed. Philadelphia: Saunders/Elsevier, 2010.

West, John B. *Pulmonary Pathophysiology: The Essentials.* 7th ed. Philadelphia: Wolters Kluwer/Lippincott Williams & Wilkins, 2008.

WEB SITES OF INTEREST

American Lung Association
http://www.lungusa.org

Canadian Lung Association
http://www.lung.ca

National Heart, Lung, and Blood Institute
http://www.nhlbi.nih.gov

Public Health Agency of Canada
http://www.phac-aspc.gc.ca

See also: Autoimmune disorders; Bacterial infections; Bronchiolitis; Bronchitis; Croup; Diphtheria; Empyema; Infection; Inflammation; Legionnaires' disease; *Pneumocystis*; Pneumocystis pneumonia; Pneumonia; Tuberculosis (TB); Vaccines: Types; Viral infections; Whooping cough.

Pneumococcal infections

CATEGORY: Diseases and conditions
ANATOMY OR SYSTEM AFFECTED: Lungs, respiratory system
ALSO KNOWN AS: Pneumococcal disease, *Streptococcus pneumoniae* infection

DEFINITION

Pneumococcal infection is caused by the encapsulated, gram-positive bacterium *Streptococcus pneumoniae*, also known as pneumococcus. The term "pneumococcus" was first used in the 1880's to describe this type of infection, because pneumococcus was considered the most common cause of bacterial pneumonia.

CAUSES

Pneumococcal disease is caused by an infection of the bacterium *S. pneumoniae*.

RISK FACTORS

Children younger than age two years are at greatest risk of pneumococcal disease. The next most commonly affected are adults age sixty-five years and older. Conditions that cause deficits in the immune system (such as human immunodeficiency virus infection, malignancy, and absence of the spleen) or conditions associated with decreased lung function (such as asthma, chronic bronchitis, and cigarette smoking) are associated with increased risk of pneumococcal disease. Absence of breast-feeding, day care attendance, and lack of vaccination can increase the risk of disease too. Native Alaskans, Navajo and Apache Indians, and African Americans are more commonly affected than other ethnic groups.

SYMPTOMS

Pneumococci bacteria can attack different parts of the body. When the bacteria attack the lungs, they cause pneumonia. When the bacteria invade the bloodstream, they cause bacteremia. Infection of the covering of the brain causes meningitis. Pneumococci may also cause middle-ear infection (otitis media) and sinusitis.

In adults, symptoms of pneumonia include chills, fever, shortness of breath or rapid breathing, chest pain that is worsened by breathing deeply, and a productive cough. Symptoms of meningitis include stiff neck, fever, mental confusion, and photophobia (visual sensitivity to light). Symptoms of bacteremia can include some of the symptoms of pneumonia and meningitis.

In children, symptoms of pneumonia include fever, cough, rapid breathing, and grunting. The symptoms of meningitis vary with age, but include diarrhea, vomiting, and fever. In older children, meningitis symptoms include headache, sensitivity to light, and a stiff neck. Bacteremia typically causes nonspecific symptoms, such as fever and irritability. Otitis media typically causes a painful ear and also may cause sleeplessness, fever, and irritability.

SCREENING AND DIAGNOSIS

If pneumococcal disease is suspected, Gram's stain and cultures are performed. Chest X rays are done if pneumonia is suspected. Additional tests include a complete blood cell count, erythrocyte sedimentation rate, and C-reactive protein.

TREATMENT AND THERAPY

Penicillin antibiotics are used to treat pneumococcal disease. However, pneumococcal strains have emerged that are resistant to these antibiotics. These resistant forms of pneumococcus are difficult to treat.

PREVENTION AND OUTCOMES

Vaccination is the best prevention strategy. There are two types of pneumococcal vaccine available: a polysaccharide vaccine and a conjugate vaccine. The pneumococcal polysaccharide vaccine protects against the twenty-three types of *S. pneumoniae* that are responsible for more than 90 percent of all cases of pneumococcal disease in adults. In children, the pneumococcal conjugate vaccine protects against 86 percent of the bacteria types that cause blood infections and 83 percent of those that cause meningitis.

Anita P. Kuan, Ph.D.

FURTHER READING

French, Neil. "Pneumococcal Diseases." In *Manson's Tropical Diseases*, edited by Gordon C. Cook and Alimuddin I. Zumla. 22d ed. Philadelphia: Saunders/Elsevier, 2009.

Hoffman-Roberts, H. L., E. Babcock, and I. F. Mitropoulos. "Investigational New Drugs for the Treatment of Resistant Pneumococcal Infections. *Expert Opinion in Investigational Drugs* 14 (2005): 973-995.

Surhone, L. M., M. T. Tennoe, and S. F. Henssonow, eds. *Pneumococcal Infection*. Saarbrücken, Germany: VDM, Mueller, 2010.

WEB SITES OF INTEREST

Centers for Disease Control and Prevention
http://www.cdc.gov

Immunization Action Coalition
http://www.immunize.org/pneumococcal-pcv

National Institute of Allergy and Infectious Diseases
http://www.niaid.nih.gov/topics/pneumococcal

National Institutes of Health
http://www.nlm.nih.gov/medlineplus/streptococcalinfections.html

See also: Asplenia; Bacteria: Classification and types; Bacterial infections; Bacterial meningitis; Children and infectious disease; Middle-ear infection; Pneumococcal vaccine; Pneumonia; Sepsis; Sinusitis; Streptococcal infections; *Streptococcus*.

Pneumococcal vaccine

CATEGORY: Prevention
ALSO KNOWN AS: Pneumococcal polysaccharide vaccine, *Streptococcus pneumoniae* vaccine

DEFINITION

The pneumococcal vaccine prevents disease caused by various types of *Streptococcus pneumoniae* bacteria (also known as pneumococcus), depending on the type of immunization administered. These diseases include pneumonia, middle-ear infection (otitis media), and sinusitis. Pneumococcal disease can spread quickly to the blood and spinal cord, resulting in bacteremia and meningitis, respectively, the effects of which can be devastating.

MECHANISM OF ACTION

The vaccine is made by taking the shell, or polysaccharide coating, of the *S. pneumoniae* bacterium and linking it to another protein. Injection of this safe combination incites the body to produce an immune response against this bacterial coating without actually causing the disease, thus protecting against future infection.

Eighty-five different types of *S. pneumoniae* bacteria exist. The polysaccharide coatings from the thirteen types that are most dangerous to children are those found in the Prevnar 13 vaccine. For the adult version of the vaccine, Pneumovax, the coatings from the twenty-three most commonly encountered types of *S. pneumoniae* are used.

VACCINE HISTORY

The first pneumococcal vaccine was licensed in 1977 and protected against fourteen different types of *S. pneumoniae*. The most recent 23-valent form of the

vaccine was released in 1983 under the name Pneumovax. In 2000, the 7-valent pediatric form of the pneumococcal vaccine was licensed under the name Prevnar, and routine administration to all children was recommended. The pediatric vaccine was further improved to provide broader coverage against pneumococcal disease with the 13-valent form of Prevnar released in 2010.

ADMINISTRATION

Medical experts recommend that children receive the 13-valent pneumococcal vaccine at two, four, six, and fifteen to eighteen months of age. The 23-valent pneumococcal vaccine is given as a separate immunization to all adults age sixty-five years and older and to children age two years and older who are at high risk of developing pneumococcal disease. Routine administration in adults between these age groups is also recommended if the person smokes cigarettes or has asthma.

IMPACT

Before the development of the pneumococcal vaccine, diseases caused by pneumococcus were rapidly becoming resistant to the antibiotics available, rendering them more virulent and difficult to treat. The introduction of the pneumococcal vaccine helped prevent these diseases, making antibiotic resistance less of an issue. However, these bacteria continue to be resistant, making prevention the primary focus of public health efforts.

New pneumococcal vaccines, with increasing protection against the different types of *S. pneumoniae*, are under development. In early 2010, a form of the pediatric vaccine with an extended spectrum of thirteen pneumococcus subtypes was released, giving children increased defense against the disease.

Jennifer Birkhauser, M.D.

FURTHER READING

Behrman, Richard E., Robert M. Kliegman, and Hal B. Jenson, eds. *Nelson Textbook of Pediatrics*. 18th ed. Philadelphia: Saunders/Elsevier, 2007.

Fisher, Margaret C. *Immunizations and Infectious Diseases: An Informed Parent's Guide*. American Academy of Pediatrics, 2006.

Harvey, Richard A., Pamela C. Champe, and Bruce D. Fisher. *Lippincott's Illustrated Reviews: Microbiology*. 2d ed. Lippincott Williams and Wilkins, 2006.

Loehr, Jamie. *The Vaccine Answer Book: Two Hundred Essential Answers to Help You Make the Right Decisions for Your Child.* Naperville, Ill.: Sourcebooks, 2010.

National Library of Medicine. "Pneumococcal Polysaccharide Vaccine." Available at http://www.nlm.nih.gov/medlineplus/ency/article/002029.htm.

Plotkin, Stanley A., Walter A. Orenstein, and Paul A. Offit. *Vaccines.* 5th ed. Philadelphia: Saunders/Elsevier, 2008.

WEB SITES OF INTEREST

About Kids Health
http://www.aboutkidshealth.ca

Centers for Disease Control and Prevention
http://www.cdc.gov/vaccines

Children's Hospital of Philadelphia, Vaccine Education Center
http://www.chop.edu/service/vaccine-education-center

See also: Asplenia; Bacteria: Classification and types; Bacterial meningitis; Children and infectious disease; Pneumococcal infections; Pneumonia; Sepsis; Sinusitis; Streptococcal infections; *Streptococcus*; Vaccines: Types.

Pneumocystis

CATEGORY: Pathogen
TRANSMISSION ROUTE: Direct contact, inhalation

DEFINITION

Pneumocystis is a fungus that lives in the lungs of mammals, including humans, in a parasitic relationship. It causes no disease and does no harm unless the mammal's immune system becomes suppressed by medications, age (very young and very old), disease (such as acquired immunodeficiency syndrome), pregnancy, malnutrition, chemotherapy, leukemia, or organ transplant.

NATURAL HABITAT AND FEATURES

Pneumocystis species are either oval or cup-shaped, and they have a thick cell wall. These larger cells usu-

---

Taxonomic Classification for *Pneumocystis*

Kingdom: Fungi
Phylum: Ascomycota
Order: Pneumocystidales
Family: Pneumocystidaceae
Genus: *Pneumocystis*
Species:
P. carinii
P. jirovecii
P. murina
P. oryctolagi
P. wakefieldiae

---

ally contain eight spores. The trophozoite cells are smaller and look like ameba. They have a thin cell wall. *Pneumocystis* cells blend in with the alveolar cells unless a stain is applied to the specimen. There is limited information about the appearance of *Pneumocystis* species cells.

Pneumocystis species require a host to live and reproduce. They cannot be grown in a culture medium. They do not appear to be present in the environment. Although hundreds of species of *Pneumocystis* are thought to exist, only five have been named: *jirovecii*, which lives in humans; *murina*, which lives in mice; *wakefieldiae* and *carinii*, which both can live in rats; and *oryctolagi*, which lives in rabbits. These species are found only in their related mammal and do not cross-contaminate other types of mammals.

Pneumocystis species find their way into the lungs of their respective mammal early in life. In humans, *jirovecii* inhabits the lungs of a child during his or her first year of life. In other mammals, such as the rat, *carinii* is found in the lungs of newborns within hours of delivery. Humans and other mammals do produce antibodies to their respective *Pneumocystis* species.

The life cycle of *Pneumocystis* species is not completely known. Most of the available information about *Pneumocystis* species has come from studying *carinii* in lab rats. It is thought that *Pneumocystis* reproduces by two means: mitosis and sexual reproduction. Trophic forms of the fungus reproduce by replicating their genetic material and then splitting into two. Trophic cells provide nutrition for other cells. In sexual reproduction, two haploid cells merge to produce a zygote or sporocyte. Haploid cells are cells that contain one-half of the necessary genetic material. The zygote produces four haploid nuclei by splitting its genetic material, and then, by mitosis, the zygote produces eight haploid nuclei. The zygote cell then packages the eight nuclei into eight double-walled spores. The spores are released from the zygote cell and are capable of both asexual and sexual reproduction. It is not known how the spores are released from the lung.

PATHOGENICITY AND CLINICAL SIGNIFICANCE

In the healthy, immune-competent mammal, *Pneumocystis* appears to be a benign parasite. There appears to be a delicate balance of normal host function and normal fungus replication as long as the host's immune system remains strong. The mammal's immune system does not attack the *Pneumocystis* because of its surface antigens, and the *Pneumocystis* does not invade its host. Airborne transmission of *Pneumocystis* does not generally cause disease. Disease arises from the *Pneumocystis* that already resides within the mammal.

When a *Pneumocystis* infection occurs, it almost always develops in the lungs. When the host's immune system becomes weakened, the *Pneumocystis* cells increase in number and are said to colonize the lung. Within the alveoli of the lung, the *Pneumocystis* trophic cells cling to the epithelial cells in the alveoli. The immune system of the host attempts to fight the emerging infection by instituting the inflammatory response, a mechanism for responding to cellular damage. In the inflammatory response, the area is flooded with white blood cells, particularly the neutrophils and lymphocytes, and the white blood cells called macrophages; tumor necrosis factor, which regulates immune cells, also plays a major role. The inflammatory response causes more damage to the alveoli than does the *Pneumocystis*. The inflammatory response damages the alveolar tissue and interferes with oxygen and carbon dioxide exchange in the lungs.

In the immune compromised person, the T cells may be absent or decreased, but still, the alveoli fill with thick, white fluid. Pneumocystis pneumonia is a serious condition with a mortality rate of between 30 and 50 percent. Sometimes, persons using immune suppressing drugs will be given a medication to prevent pneumocystis pneumonia.

DRUG SUSCEPTIBILITY

The treatment of choice for pneumocystis pneumonia is trimethoprim-sulfamethoxazole, which can be administered orally or intravenously. Other antibiotics or medications against protozoa, including *Pneumocystis*, include pentamidine, dapsone, primaquine plus clindamycin, and atovaquone. There have been some reports of *Pneumocystis* resistance to trimethoprim-sulfamethoxazole. Corticosteroids may be administered during the first seventy-two hours of pneumocystis pneumonia treatment to depress lung inflammation.

Christine M. Carroll, R.N.

FURTHER READING

AIDS InfoNet. "Pneumocystis Pneumonia (PCP)." Available at http://www.aidsinfonet.org.

Cushion, Melanie T. "Are Members of the Fungal Genus *Pneumocystis* (a) Commensals; (b) Opportunists; (c) Pathogens; or (d) All of the Above?" *PLoS Pathogens* 6 (September 23, 2010). Available at http://www.plospathogens.org.

Van Oosterhout, Joep J. G., et al. "Pneumocystis Pneumonia in HIV-Positive Adults, Malawi." *Emerging Infectious Diseases* 13 (2007): 325-328.

West, John B. *Pulmonary Pathophysiology: The Essentials.* 7th ed. Philadelphia: Wolters Kluwer/Lippincott Williams & Wilkins, 2008.

Wilkin, Aimee, and Judith Feinberg. "*Pneumocystis carinii* Pneumonia: A Clinical Review." *American Family Physician* 60 (October 15, 1999): 1699-1714. Also available at http://www.aafp.org/afp/991015ap/1699.html.

WEB SITES OF INTEREST

AIDSinfo
http://aidsinfo.nih.gov

American Lung Association
http://www.lungusa.org

Canadian AIDS Treatment Information Exchange
http://www.catie.ca

Microbiology and Immunology On-line: Mycology
http://pathmicro.med.sc.edu/book/mycol-sta.htm

See also: Airborne illness and disease; Atypical pneumonia; Fungi: Classification and types; *Histoplasma*; *Legionella*; Opportunistic infections; Pleurisy; Pneumocystis pneumonia; Pneumonia; Respiratory route of transmission.

Pneumocystis pneumonia

CATEGORY: Diseases and conditions
ANATOMY OR SYSTEM AFFECTED: Lungs, respiratory system

DEFINITION

Pneumocystis pneumonia (PCP) is a lung infection caused by the fungus *Pneumocystis jiroveci* (formerly called *P. carinii*). This preventable infection affects people who have a weakened immune system, and it is the most common serious infection among people with acquired immunodeficiency syndrome (AIDS).

CAUSES

Most scientists believe that *P. jiroveci* is spread in the air. It is not clear if it lives in soil or elsewhere. In healthy people, the fungus can exist in the lungs without causing pneumonia. However, in people who have a weakened immune system, PCP may cause a lung infection.

RISK FACTORS

People who are at increased risk for PCP include those who have AIDS or cancer and those who are being treated for cancer.

SYMPTOMS

Symptoms of PCP usually develop over the course of a few weeks or months. The main symptoms are shortness of breath, fever, dry cough, tightness in the chest, and weakness. One should consult a doctor immediately if experiencing any of these symptoms.

SCREENING AND DIAGNOSIS

A sample of the patient's sputum is examined under a microscope. Sputum is mucus from the lungs that is produced when one coughs. The doctor will collect samples by giving the patient a vapor treatment to induce coughing or through a bronchoscopy, an instrument that is inserted into the airway.

TREATMENT AND THERAPY

Treatment will depend on the seriousness of the infection. For mild cases, the patient will be given medication in pill form. For severe cases, the patient will probably be treated in a hospital and receive medication by IV (intravenously).

Several drugs are used to treat PCP, including trimethoprim-sulfamethoxazole (TMP-SMZ, Bactrim, Septra, Cotrim), which is available in pill and liquid forms; dapsone plus trimethoprim; primaquine plus clindamycin; atovaquone; pentamidine (given by IV); trimetrexate plus folinic acid; and corticosteroids, given in severe cases when blood oxygen pressure falls below a certain level. Most of these treatments have side effects. Even when treatment is given for PCP, the death rate is 15 to 20 percent.

PREVENTION AND OUTCOMES

Persons who are at risk for PCP may be given medicine to prevent the disease. In general, for those with human immunodeficiency virus (HIV) infection, preventing PCP with medication is recommended if that person's CD4 cell count falls below 200. Other conditions, such as having a temperature higher than 100° Fahrenheit that lasts for more than two weeks or getting a fungal infection in the mouth or throat, are reasons to start preventive therapy. Some of the same drugs used to treat an infection can be taken regularly to prevent the infection. These drugs include TMP-SMZ, dapsone, atovaquone, and pentamidine aerosol.

If a person gets PCP once, he or she is more likely to get it again. Each time one gets it, the PCP causes damage to the lungs. The body can suffer side effects from the drugs.

Pneumonia vaccine only protects against a different kind of pneumonia. It will not keep a person from getting PCP.

Julie J. Martin, M.S.;
reviewed by Christine Colpitts, M.A., CRT

FURTHER READING

AIDS InfoNet. "Pneumocystis Pneumonia (PCP)." Available at http://www.aidsinfonet.org.

American Academy of Family Physicians. "Pneumocystis Pneumonia (PCP) and HIV." Available at http://familydoctor.org.

Centers for Disease Control and Prevention, National Center for HIV, STD, and TB Prevention. "You Can

Prevent PCP: A Guide for People with HIV Infection." Available at http://www.cdc.gov/hiv.

Corrin, Bryan, and Andrew G. Nicholson. *Pathology of the Lungs.* 2d ed. New York: Churchill Livingstone/Elsevier, 2006.

EBSCO Publishing. *DynaMed: "Pneumocystis carinii" Pneumonia.* Available through http://www.ebscohost.com/dynamed.

Fan, Hung Y., Ross F. Conner, and Luis P. Villarreal. *AIDS: Science and Society.* 5th ed. Sudbury, Mass.: Jones and Bartlett, 2007.

Hughes, Walter T. *"Pneumocystis carinii" Pneumonitis.* 2 vols. Rev. ed. Boca Raton, Fla.: CRC Press, 1987.

West, John B. *Pulmonary Pathophysiology: The Essentials.* 7th ed. Philadelphia: Wolters Kluwer/Lippincott Williams & Wilkins, 2008.

Web Sites of Interest

AIDS Treatment Data Network
http://www.atdn.org/access

AIDSinfo
http://aidsinfo.nih.gov

American Lung Association
http://www.lungusa.org

Canadian AIDS Treatment Information Exchange
http://www.catie.ca

Canadian Lung Association
http://www.lung.ca/pneumonia

Centers for Disease Control and Prevention
http://www.cdc.gov/hiv

Centers for Disease Control and Prevention, National Prevention Information Network
http://www.cdcnpin.org

National Institute of Allergy and Infectious Diseases
http://www.niaid.nih.gov

See also: AIDS; Airborne illness and disease; Atypical pneumonia; Bronchiolitis; Bronchitis; Croup; Cryptococcosis; Diagnosis of fungal infections; Diphtheria; Fungal infections; Fungi: Classification and types; Histoplasmosis; HIV; HIV vaccine; Infection; Legionnaires' disease; Nocardiosis; Opportunistic infections; Pleurisy; *Pneumocystis*; Pneumonia; Respiratory route of transmission; Tuberculosis (TB); Vaccines: Types; Whooping cough.

Pneumonia

CATEGORY: Diseases and conditions
ANATOMY OR SYSTEM AFFECTED: Lungs, respiratory system
ALSO KNOWN AS: Bronchopneumonia, community acquired pneumonia

Definition

Pneumonia is an infection of the lungs. It affects the lower respiratory tract, including the small bronchi (airways) and air sacs in the lungs.

Facts: Pneumonia

• Leading cause of death in children worldwide.

• Kills an estimated 1.6 million children every year, more than acquired immunodeficiency syndrome, malaria, and tuberculosis combined.

• Caused by viruses, bacteria, or fungi.

• Can be prevented by immunization, by adequate nutrition, and by addressing environmental factors.

• Can be treated with antibiotics, but less than 20 percent of children with pneumonia receive the antibiotics they need.

Source: World Health Organization.

Causes

There are three main types of pneumonia: bacterial, caused by bacteria, most commonly *Streptococcus pneumoniae*; viral, caused by a virus (and responsible for one-half of all pneumonias); and atypical bacterial, often called walking pneumonia, which can cause a more serious or potentially fatal pneumonia. Other causes of pneumonia include fungal infections such as pneumocystis pneumonia (PCP), an infection that is common in people with acquired immunodeficiency syndrome (AIDS), and pneumonia defined by where the pneumonia was acquired or by how a person was exposed to it. These types include community acquired pneumonia, which is acquired in a community setting (such as at school, at work, or in a gym); nosocomial pneumonia, acquired during hospitalization; and aspiration pneumonia, which occurs when foreign matter (often the contents of the stomach) is inhaled.

Risk Factors

Factors that increase the chance of pneumonia include influenza or other respiratory illness; chronic illness, such as heart or lung disease; stroke (which causes aspiration pneumonia because of difficulty swallowing); a weakened immune system caused by having AIDS or by undergoing chemotherapy; chronic bronchitis; malnutrition; pregnancy; alcohol or drug abuse; smoking; and chronic exposure to certain chemicals (during, for example, construction or agricultural work). Also at higher risk are infants, young children, and adults age sixty-five years or older.

Symptoms

Symptoms for bacterial, viral, and atypical pneumonia include the following: fever, often low-grade; chills; a cough that produces green, yellow, or rust-colored mucus; a dry cough; a violent cough that produces white mucus; chest pain; headache; nausea or vomiting; profuse sweating; muscle pain; weakness; bluish color to the nails or lips caused by diminished oxygen in the blood; and a confused mental state.

Screening and Diagnosis

A doctor will ask about symptoms and medical history and will perform a physical exam. Diagnosis is based on symptoms and listening to the patient's chest. Tests may include a chest X ray (a test that uses radiation to take pictures of structures inside the body); a computed tomography (CT) scan (a detailed X-ray picture that identifies abnormalities of fine tissue structure); blood tests; a bronchoscopy (the direct examination of the airways); a sputum culture (tests mucus coughed up from deep in the lungs); a pulse oximetry (measures the amount of oxygen in the blood); and an arterial blood gas test (measures oxygen, carbon dioxide, and acid in the blood).

Treatment and Therapy

Treatment of pneumonia depends on the type of pneumonia and the severity of symptoms. Common treatment approaches include antibiotics for bacterial pneumonia; antiviral medicines, which may be prescribed for young children and for people with weakened immune systems, for viral pneumonia (antibiotics are ineffective for treating viral pneumonia); and antibiotics for atypical pneumonia.

One should take all medicine that is prescribed, as stopping medicine early may cause a relapse. Doing so may also lead to the creation of a strain of drug resistant bacteria. General treatment includes getting extra rest, drinking increased amounts of fluids, and eating a healthy diet that includes fruits and vegetables. Those who suspect that they do not get enough vitamin C in their diet should consult a doctor about possibly taking a vitamin supplement (up to 1,000 milligrams per day). Other treatments used are over-the-counter medicines to reduce fever, aches, and cough, and, in severe cases, hospitalization.

Prevention and Outcomes

Certain vaccines may prevent pneumonia. These include a flu shot, for people at high risk, particularly the elderly, because pneumonia may be a complication of the flu. Another vaccine that may prevent pneumonia is a pneumococcal vaccine, which is recommended for people age sixty-five years and older; for those who have a chronic illness, such as diabetes or sickle-cell disease; and for children two years of age or younger.

Other preventive measures include avoiding smoking, because smoke weakens the lungs' resistance to infection; avoiding close contact with people who have the cold or flu; washing one's hands often (especially after contacting infected people); protecting oneself on jobs that can affect the lungs; eating a healthy diet; getting adequate rest; and exercising regularly.

Michelle Badash, M.S.;
reviewed by Rosalyn Carson-DeWitt, M.D.

Further Reading

Fishman, Alfred, ed. *Fishman's Pulmonary Diseases and Disorders.* 4th ed. New York: McGraw-Hill, 2008.

Fleming, C. A., H. U. Balaguera, and D. E. Craven. "Risk Factors for Nosocomial Pneumonia: Focus on Prophylaxis." *Medical Clinics of North America* 85 (2001): 1545-1563.

Hemila, H., and P. Louhiala. "Vitamin C for Preventing and Treating Pneumonia." *Cochrane Database of Systematic Reviews* (2009): CD005532. Available through *EBSCO DynaMed Systematic Literature Surveillance* at http://www.ebscohost.com/dynamed.

Levitzky, Michael G. *Pulmonary Physiology*. 7th ed. New York: McGraw-Hill Medical, 2007.

Mason, Robert J., et al., eds. *Murray and Nadel's Textbook of Respiratory Medicine*. 5th ed. Philadelphia: Saunders/Elsevier, 2010.

Niederman, M. S. "Recent Advances in Community-Acquired Pneumonia: Inpatient and Outpatient." *Chest* 4 (April, 2007): 1205-1215.

_____. "Review of Treatment Guidelines for Community-Acquired Pneumonia." *American Journal of Medicine* 117, suppl. 3A (2004): 51S-57S.

West, John B. *Pulmonary Pathophysiology: The Essentials*. 7th ed. Philadelphia: Wolters Kluwer/Lippincott Williams & Wilkins, 2008.

Web Sites of Interest

American Academy of Family Physicians
http://familydoctor.org

American Lung Association
http://www.lungusa.org

Canadian Lung Association
http://www.lung.ca

Public Health Agency of Canada
http://www.phac-aspc.gc.ca

See also: Antiviral drugs: Types; Atypical pneumonia; Bacterial infections; Bronchiolitis; Bronchitis; Croup; Diagnosis of fungal infections; Diphtheria; Empyema; Fungal infections; Histoplasmosis; Hospitals and infectious disease; Iatrogenic infections; Infection; Influenza vaccine; Legionnaires' disease; Nocardiosis; Pleurisy; Pneumococcal vaccine; Pneumocystis pneumonia; Seasonal influenza; Streptococcal infections; Tuberculosis (TB); Vaccines: Types; Viral infections; Whooping cough.

Polio vaccine

Category: Prevention

Definition

There are two types of polio vaccine: inactivated and oral, first available in 1955 and 1962, respectively. The vaccines provide immunity to poliomyelitis, or polio, a viral disease that damages nerve cells. The virus enters through the mouth and replicates in the intestines. It then enters the bloodstream and crosses into the central nervous system, where it attacks the nerve cells.

The first signs of polio are fatigue, headache, nausea, neck stiffness, and fever. Eventually, the nerves no longer send out electrical impulses to move muscles, and the body can become paralyzed; paralysis, however, is uncommon. The arms and legs are affected first, and in serious cases, the chest muscles are affected, resulting in respiratory failure.

Types

The inactivated polio vaccine (IPV), developed by Jonas Salk in the early 1950's, was the first polio vaccine available (1955). Salk based his vaccine, which is injected, on a then-new premise, that only the outer shell of the virus was needed to confer immunity. At the time, all vaccines were manufactured from live but weakened viruses.

In the late 1950's, Albert Sabin produced an oral form of the polio vaccine. Sabin's oral polio vaccine (OPV), first administered in 1962, used a weakened form of the live poliovirus to stimulate antibody production. Decades earlier, Sabin proved that polio resides in the intestines rather than the nervous system, laying the theoretical groundwork for an orally administered vaccine. Once introduced, OPV quickly became the dominant polio vaccine because it was so easy to administer and it quickly conferred immunity.

The unique advantage of OPV is the use of live poliovirus. The virus, although weakened, is shed in feces from recently vaccinated persons. An unvaccinated person who comes in contact with the shed virus from a recently vaccinated person, for example, a parent who recently changed a baby's diaper, may contract the weakened poliovirus and thus become passively vaccinated. This ability of OPV to confer immunity to persons not directly vaccinated helped spread immunity and helped eliminate outbreaks of polio.

Side Effects

Although the live virus contained in OPV is weakened, it is still a live virus that can cause infection. In rare cases, OPV causes vaccine-associated paralytic poliomyelitis, or VAPP. People vaccinated with OPV shed

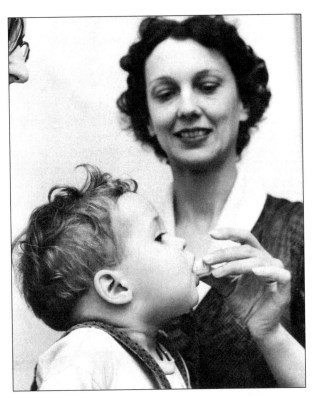

A nurse administers oral polio vaccine to a toddler in 1959. (AP/Wide World Photos)

the weakened poliovirus up to six weeks after each dose. Caregivers or others with a weakened immune system, such as those who have had organ transplants or who have human immunodeficiency virus (HIV) infection, may develop VAPP if they come in close contact with newly vaccinated children.

The most common adverse events associated with IPV is soreness at the injection site. Allergic reactions, including respiratory difficulties, increased heart rate, hives, dizziness, or swelling of the throat, are rare.

IMPACT

Polio has no cure and can be prevented only through vaccination. Together, IPV and OPV eradicated polio from most of the world. Polio has become so rare in the United States that the small risk of VAPP associated with OPV is now greater than the benefit of passive immunization. IPV is now the recommended vaccine for all children. Recommendations require three injections for infants at two, four, and six months of age, between six and eighteen months of age, and booster shots between four and six years of age.

Cheryl Pokalo Jones

FURTHER READING

Bruno, Richard L. *The Polio Paradox: Understanding and Treating "Post-Polio Syndrome" and Chronic Fatigue.* New York: Warner Books, 2002.

Naden, Corinne J., and Rose Blue. *Jonas Salk: Polio Pioneer.* Brookfield, Conn.: Millbrook Press, 2001.

Offit, Paul A. *The Cutter Incident: How America's First Polio Vaccine Led to the Growing Vaccine Crisis.* New Haven, Conn.: Yale University Press, 2005.

Strauss, James, and Ellen Strauss. *Viruses and Human Disease.* 2d ed. Boston: Academic Press/Elsevier, 2008.

Wagner, Edward K., and Martinez J. Hewlett. *Basic Virology.* 3d ed. Malden, Mass.: Blackwell Science, 2008.

WEB SITES OF INTEREST

Centers for Disease Control and Prevention: National Immunization Program
http://www.cdc.gov/nip

Emerging and Reemerging Infectious Diseases Resource Center
http://www.medscape.com/resource/infections

Global Polio Eradication Initiative
http://www.polioeradication.org

Immunization Action Coalition
http://www.immunize.org

See also: Developing countries and infectious disease; Emerging and reemerging infectious diseases; Poliomyelitis; Vaccines: History; Vaccines: Types; Viral infections.

Poliomyelitis

CATEGORY: Diseases and conditions
ANATOMY OR SYSTEM AFFECTED: All
ALSO KNOWN AS: Polio

DEFINITION

Poliomyelitis, commonly known as polio, is a contagious viral infection. The infection can lead to paralysis. Now extremely rare in the Western world because of effective vaccination programs, polio remains a significant problem in parts of Africa and Asia.

CAUSES

Polio is caused by the poliovirus. A person can get the virus from contact with an infected person, infected saliva or feces, or contaminated water or sewage. The virus enters the body through the mouth and travels to the intestines, where it reproduces quickly. The virus then travels through the blood and the lymph fluid and attacks and destroys areas of the nervous system.

RISK FACTORS

The factors that increase the chance of developing polio are lack of vaccination or incomplete vaccination, travel to countries where polio is still common (areas of Africa and Asia), pregnancy, strenuous exercise, recent tonsillectomy or dental procedure, and immunodeficiency. At higher risk are preschool children with immune disorders, who are exposed to a live poliovirus through vaccination; young adults exposed to poliovirus through contact with persons recently vaccinated; and the elderly.

SYMPTOMS

If a person experiences any of the following symptoms, he or she should not assume the symptoms are caused by polio. These symptoms may be caused by other, less serious health conditions. One should, however, contact a physician if experiencing these symptoms, which indicate a minor illness: headache, fever, and sore throat that lasts about one week.

One should contact a physician if experiencing the following symptoms, which indicate a major illness: fever, headache, nausea and vomiting, diarrhea, stiff neck, neck pain, severe muscle pain, muscle spasms, muscle weakness, paralysis (usually asymmetric, affecting each side to varying amounts, or only affecting a single side), flaccid (loose, floppy) muscles (legs more commonly affected than arms), paralysis of muscles required for breathing, and urinary retention. Decades later, previously stable muscle weakness may worsen because of postpolio syndrome.

SCREENING AND DIAGNOSIS

A doctor will ask about symptoms and medical history and will perform a physical exam. Tests may in-

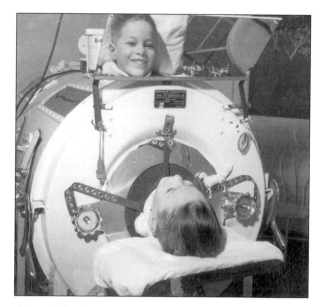

A boy with polio rests in a mechanical ventilator, commonly known as an iron lung, circa 1955. (NMLM)

clude throat swabs, rectal swabs, stool samples, or cerebrospinal fluid to look for the virus; a spinal tap (removal of a small amount of cerebrospinal fluid to check for the virus); and immunological tests to show whether the body has responded to the presence of poliovirus by producing antibodies designed to fight the virus.

TREATMENT AND THERAPY

There are no treatments available to get rid of the virus. Treatment is designed to be supportive and therapeutic. Bed rest is necessary for patients during fever (this is in the initial phase of illness). Medications can be prescribed to lower the fever and decrease muscle pain. These medications include acetaminophen (such as Tylenol) and nonsteroidal anti-inflammatory drugs (such as ibuprofen).

If the breathing muscles become too weak or paralyzed, the patient may require time on a mechanical ventilator. This machine will take over the work of breathing.

The virus can cause contractures, a tightening of tissue around a joint. The patient may need to be fitted with splints, which will keep the joints from becoming too stiff. The patient may also receive physical therapy, during which the patient's limbs will be moved through what are called passive exercises. After the fever passes, exercises and therapy will help the patient regain mobility and improve muscle strength.

PREVENTION AND OUTCOMES

Two types of vaccines are available to prevent polio. Oral polio vaccine is given by mouth and uses weakened live viruses. Injected vaccine is in shot form and uses killed viruses. There is a small chance of actually acquiring polio from exposure to the live viruses in the oral polio vaccine. Therefore, the Centers for Disease Control and Prevention (CDC) recommends that only injected vaccine be used.

The following are updated immunization recommendations from the CDC: Children should receive a series of four immunization injections: at age two, four, and six to eighteen months, and at age four to six years. Adults who have never been immunized should receive a series if they are at high risk of contracting polio. Risk is increased in adults who travel to areas where poliovirus is still common, who care for persons with polio, or who work in laboratories where poliovirus is handled.

Rosalyn Carson-DeWitt, M.D.; reviewed by David L. Horn, M.D., FACP

FURTHER READING

Bear, Mark F., Barry W. Connors, and Michael A. Paradiso. *Neuroscience: Exploring the Brain.* 3d ed. Philadelphia: Lippincott Williams & Wilkins, 2007.

Centers for Disease Control and Prevention. "Polio Disease." Available at http://www.cdc.gov/vaccines/vpd-vac/polio/dis-faqs.htm.

Howard, R. S. "Poliomyelitis and the Postpolio Syndrome." *British Medical Journal* 330 (2005): 1314.

Silver, Julie K. *Post-Polio Syndrome: A Guide for Polio Survivors and Their Families.* New Haven, Conn.: Yale University Press, 2002.

Strauss, James, and Ellen Strauss. *Viruses and Human Disease.* 2d ed. Boston: Academic Press/Elsevier, 2008.

Wagner, Edward K., and Martinez J. Hewlett. *Basic Virology.* 3d ed. Malden, Mass.: Blackwell Science, 2008.

WEB SITES OF INTEREST

American Academy of Pediatrics
http://www.healthychildren.org

Centers for Disease Control and Prevention
http://www.cdc.gov

Global Polio Eradication Initiative
http://www.polioeradication.org

Post-Polio Health International
http://www.post-polio.org

World Health Organization
http://www.who.int

See also: Contagious diseases; Developing countries and infectious disease; Encephalitis; Enterovirus infections; Fecal-oral route of transmission; Intestinal and stomach infections; Oral transmission; Polio vaccine; Saliva and infectious disease; Viral infections; Waterborne illness and disease.

Polyene antifungals

CATEGORY: Treatment

DEFINITION

Polyene antifungals, which were derived from *Streptomyces* species in the 1950's, were the first antifungal agents available to reliably treat deep-seated fungal infections. The polyenes were named for the alternating conjugated double bonds that are part of their macrolide ring structure.

MECHANISM OF ACTION

Polyene antifungals are membrane disruptors. They function by inserting themselves into sterol-containing cell membranes and by then forming channels. Important intracellular components such as calcium, sodium, and potassium cations can then leak, leading to cell death. Polyenes have a much higher affinity for ergosterol, the predominant lipid in fungal cells, than they do for cholesterol, which is more prevalent in mammalian cell membranes. Polyenes have no significant activity in bacterial, viral, or protozoan infections, but they work against yeast and yeastlike fungi.

DRUGS IN THIS CLASS

Three drugs are available in this class, and they have very different uses. Nystatin (Mycostatin) is considered first-line therapy for mild oral candidiasis (thrush) and is given as either a suspension or a lozenge. The lozenges should be allowed to dissolve slowly and the suspension should be held in the mouth for as long as possible before swallowing to allow adequate contact time with the infected area. The drug is not absorbed orally, so it cannot be used to treat systemic infections; a tablet is available, however, to treat fungal infections of the gastrointestinal tract. In this case, the drug does not need to enter the bloodstream and is already available at the site of action. The most common adverse effects of nystatin are rash, nausea, vomiting, diarrhea, and gastrointestinal upset. Nystatin is too toxic to be formulated for systemic use.

Amphotericin B (Fungizone) is a broad-spectrum injectable agent that must be used with caution. It has serious adverse effects that include infusion reactions (fever, chills, and hypotension), low potassium levels, and renal toxicity. Even with this side effect profile, amphotericin B is the drug of choice for a number of life-threatening systemic fungal infections, including those involving *Candida* species, *Cryptococcus neoformans*, and *Aspergillus* species. Because of poor water solubility, the drug has been formulated as a complex with deoxycholic acid. This allows the drug to be formulated as a solution for intravenous administration but does nothing to limit toxicity.

Formulation development has focused on limiting the kidney toxicity of the drug. Three available lipid-based formulations lead to selective delivery of the drug to organs in the reticuloendothelial system (liver, spleen, and lung). This protects the kidney from the drug. In cases in which the fungal infection is primarily in the liver or related organs, the lipid formulation will take the drug directly to the site of the infection. Two of the formulations are drug-lipid complexes (Abelcet and Amphotec), while the other is a liposome (AmBisome). These formulations, however, are not more effective than the conventional product and cost significantly more.

Natamycin (pimaricin) is active against yeasts and molds. It is available as an ophthalmic suspension for treatment of fungal infections of the eye.

IMPACT

Healthy persons can generally easily fight fungal infections, but in those persons with impaired immune systems, these infections can become life-threatening. Fungal infections are most serious in persons with acquired immunodeficiency syndrome (AIDS) or in persons who have undergone organ transplant or chemotherapy.

Karen M. Nagel, Ph.D.

FURTHER READING

Allen, L. V., N. G. Popovich, and H. C. Ansel. "Novel Dosage Forms and Drug Delivery Technologies." In *Ansel's Pharmaceutical Dosage Forms and Drug Delivery Systems*. 9th ed. Baltimore: Lippincott Williams & Wilkins, 2011.

Griffith, R. K. "Antifungal Drugs." In *Foye's Principles of Medicinal Chemistry*, edited by Thomas L. Lemke et al. 6th ed. Philadelphia: Lippincott Williams & Wilkins, 2008.

Murray, Patrick R., Ken S. Rosenthal, and Michael A. Pfaller. "Antifungal Agents." In *Medical Microbiology*. 6th ed. Philadelphia: Mosby/Elsevier, 2009.

Webster, John, and Weber, Roland. *Introduction to Fungi*. New York: Cambridge University Press, 2007.

WEB SITES OF INTEREST

British Mycological Society
http://fungionline.org.uk

Centers for Disease Control and Prevention, Division of Foodborne, Bacterial, and Mycotic Diseases
http://www.cdc.gov/nczved/divisions/dfbmd

DoctorFungus
http://www.doctorfungus.org/thedrugs/antif_pharm.htm

Microbiology and Immunology On-line: Mycology
http://pathmicro.med.sc.edu/book/mycol-sta.htm

Systematic Mycology and Microbiology Laboratory
http://www.ars.usda.gov

See also: Antifungal drugs: Mechanisms of action; Antifungal drugs: Types; Diagnosis of fungal infections; Echinocandin antifungals; Fungal infections; Fungi: Classification and types; Imidazole antifungals; Immune response to fungal infections; Infection; Mycoses; Prevention of fungal infections; Thiazole antifungals; Treatment of fungal infections; Triazole antifungals.

Polymerase chain reaction (PCR) method

CATEGORY: Diagnosis

DEFINITION

Polymerase chain reaction (PCR) is a rapid technique that enables the copying of desired deoxyribonucleic acid (DNA) molecules. This technique consists of three steps: denaturation, annealing, and extension, repeated in a cyclical fashion.

In step one of PCR, the reaction is exposed to temperatures as high as 194° to 201° Fahrenheit (90° to 94° Celsius). The high temperature helps to separate the two strands of the DNA template by breaking the hydrogen bonds that hold the two strands together. This melting of the DNA duplex is called denaturation.

The second step in PCR is called annealing or hybridization and requires short single-stranded DNA sequences called primers. The reaction uses two primers, one complementary to each strand of the original DNA duplex. The primers bind to their complementary sequences (or anneals) on the template DNA and provide the free 3'OH (hydroxyl) group that DNA polymerase needs to copy the DNA. This sets the stage for the last step in PCR, extension. During extension, the DNA polymerase uses deoxyribonucleotides (dNTPs) to build the complementary strand on the template DNA.

The foregoing set of three processes (making up a cycle) is typically repeated several times, about twenty to twenty-five cycles, to allow for an exponential increase in copies of the target gene. A simple formula can be used to calculate the yield (number of copies of the DNA or gene template). According to this formula, the number of gene copies after n cycles of PCR is $2n$. For example, if a person starts with a single copy of the gene, the yield will be 225 at the end of a PCR reaction with twenty-five cycles.

BACKGROUND

PCR was discovered by Kary Mullis in 1983 while trying to develop a method that would allow the sequencing of single nucleotide polymorphisms (SNPs). SNPs are variations produced in DNA by alterations to a single nucleotide and, therefore, serve as the absolute genetic marker. Specifically, Mullis was trying to devise a rapid clinical assay for genetic disorders such as sickle cell disease that are caused by a single nucleotide polymorphism. DNA research in the 1980's faced two major challenges: not enough DNA and no easy way to separate a gene's DNA from the genomic DNA (1 milligram of DNA contains about 200,000 copies of a person's target gene). PCR offered a solution to both of these problems; one could amplify DNA rapidly and could obtain as many copies as needed of the target gene alone.

THE PCR REACTION

A PCR reaction, which is typically around 50 milliliters, requires the following: DNA template or target gene (10 femtograms to 10 milligrams), primers (0.1-1.0 millimolars each), dNTPs (200 millimolars each), DNA polymerase (0.2-2 units) and Tris buffer (pH8.0). Also, a PCR reaction requires $MgCl_2$ (magnesium chloride), which is a cofactor for DNA polymerase. The DNA polymerase used in PCR is unique in that it can withstand high temperatures such as those used for melting DNA during the denaturation step. Before thermostable polymerases such as Taq and Vent were discovered, fresh polymerase had to be added after each round of PCR.

DNA in the cell is typically bound to packaging proteins such as histones. For a successful PCR reaction, the DNA template must be free of any inhibitory molecule (such as these packaging proteins) and thus easily accessible to the primers and polymerase. Therefore, once the DNA has been extracted from the cell, it is typically purified using some kind of enzymatic, mechanical, or chemical purification technique.

Next in the PCR process is the design of primer (forward and reverse primers). PCR primers are chemically synthesized nucleotide segments called oligonucleotides (or oligos) and are typically 18 to 30 bases long. Because primers are short sequences, misalignment can occur, leading to erroneous amplification. To minimize nonspecific binding, primers are preferably 18 to 21 bases long. The length of the PCR product is determined by the distance between the annealing sites of the two primers. Also important in primer design are factors such as guanine-cytosine content, polypurine or polypyrimidine stretches (multiples of any one nucleotide), the secondary structure of the primer (mutually complementary sequences within the primer can form "hairpin" structures), and

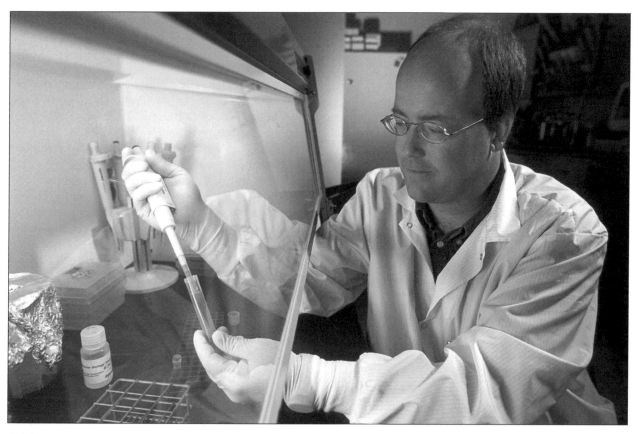

A laboratory scientist prepares a sample to be examined using the PCR technique.

the probability of a complementary sequence on the DNA residing anywhere except on the intended target gene (or region of amplification).

Once the PCR reaction is completed, the next important step is analysis of the PCR products with electrophoresis and various DNA intercalating dyes; this is followed by sequencing the amplimer (the amplified PCR product).

IMPACT

It is widely believed that since the discovery of the DNA double helix in the 1950's, few discoveries have transformed the field of biology as rapidly as PCR. This technique that allows the copying of millions of desired DNA beginning with minute DNA samples has accelerated progress in forensics and in medical diagnostics and has revolutionized biotechnology and biomedical research.

Several modifications of the original PCR technique have been developed to meet the diverse needs of biomedical research. One such modification, qPCR (quantitative PCR), is frequently used in drug discovery to look for and assess new putative drug target sites in humans. The qPCR method is also used to determine the number of working copies of a specific gene, and this measure of gene expression is important in analysis of genetic disorders. For example, in STEP (single target expression profiling), qPCR is used to compare active gene numbers in affected versus healthy (unaffected) persons, allowing for the study of the progression or development of genetic disorders.

Sibani Sengupta, Ph.D.

FURTHER READING

McPherson, M., S. G. Møller. *PCR (The Basics)*. New York: Taylor & Francis, 2006. This is an excellent resource for those learning to set up and run PCR experiments.

Rabinow, P. *Making PCR: A Story of Biotechnology*. Chicago:

University of Chicago Press, 1996. A great description of how the PCR technique has evolved since its development.

Van Pelt-Verkuil, E., A. van Belkum, and J. P. Hays. *Principles and Technical Aspects of PCR Amplification.* New York: Springer, 2008. A great resource for persons interested in furthering their understanding of PCR.

WEB SITES OF INTEREST

Biochemical Society
http://www.biochemistry.org

Protocolpedia
http://www.protocolpedia.com

Virtual Library of Biochemistry, Molecular Biology, and Cell Biology
http://www.biochemweb.org

See also: Acid-fastness; Bacteria: Classification and types; Bacteriology; Biochemical tests; Biostatistics; Diagnosis of bacterial infections; Diagnosis of viral infections; Gram staining; Immunoassay; Microbiology; Microscopy; Pulsed-field gel electrophoresis; Serology.

Pontiac fever

CATEGORY: Diseases and conditions
ANATOMY OR SYSTEM AFFECTED: Lungs, respiratory system
ALSO KNOWN AS: Legionnaires' disease, legionellosis

DEFINITION

Pontiac fever, an infectious disease produced by the bacterial genus *Legionella*, is a milder form of Legionnaires' disease (or Legion fever). Pontiac fever is a respiratory illness with flulike symptoms, but without the pneumonia that develops with Legionnaires' disease. Pontiac fever and Legionnaires' disease are referred to separately or collectively as legionellosis.

CAUSES

More than 90 percent of all cases of legionellosis are caused by the bacterium *L. pneumophila.* The bacteria are contracted by breathing mist that comes from a contaminated water source. It is not known to be transmitted from person to person.

RISK FACTORS

Contaminated water supplies constitute the primary risk factor for legionellosis. The *Legionella* species of bacteria can survive in warm water and moist air, such as that associated with hot tubs, showers, humidifiers, hot water tanks, and the air conditioning systems of large buildings, including hospitals.

Most infections occur in middle-aged or older people. The disease is typically less severe in children. Other risk factors include the use of medications that suppress the immune system, such as chemotherapy and steroids, and alcoholism, cigarette smoking, chronic lung disease, cancer, kidney failure, and diabetes.

SYMPTOMS

Typical symptoms associated with Pontiac fever are mild fever, muscle aches, coughing, runny nose, and sore throat, without pneumonia. For more severe infections, known as Legionnaires' disease, which produce pneumonia, the symptoms are high fever, chest pains, chills, coughing, penetrating muscle aches, headaches, tiredness, loss of appetite, coughing up blood, loss of coordination, and, sometimes, nausea and diarrhea.

SCREENING AND DIAGNOSIS

A medical history is taken to characterize the symptoms. Chest X rays are examined for lung inflammation. Blood samples determine complete blood count. As necessary, sputum samples are examined for *Legionella* bacteria, urine samples for *L. pneumophila* antigens, and blood samples (taken about three weeks apart) to be contrasted for *Legionella* antibody levels.

TREATMENT AND THERAPY

Symptoms of Pontiac fever typically disappear in a few hours to five days, often without the need for any treatment. Antibiotics are used to fight the infection as necessary. Antibiotics used to treat Legionnaires' disease are quinolones, such as ciprofloxacin and levofloxacin, and macrolides, such as azithromycin and erythromycin. Other treatments include fluid and electrolyte replacement and administration of oxygen through a mask or breathing machine. Timely therapy has dropped the mortality rate to less than 5 percent.

PREVENTION AND OUTCOMES

Water supply regulations and ordinances must be in place and enforced. Water delivery systems should be periodically tested and treated for *Legionella* bacteria. The removal of any slime in these water systems is a necessary control process.

Alvin K. Benson, Ph.D.

FURTHER READING

Frazier, Margaret Schell, and Jeanette Wist Drzymkowski. *Essentials of Human Diseases and Conditions.* 4th ed. St. Louis, Mo.: Saunders/Elsevier, 2009.

Mason, Robert J., et al., eds. *Murray and Nadel's Textbook of Respiratory Medicine.* 5th ed. Philadelphia: Saunders/Elsevier, 2010.

Neil, K., et al. "Increasing Incidence of Legionellosis in the United States, 1990-2005: Changing Epidemiologic Trends." *Clinical Infectious Diseases* 47 (2008): 591.

Shader, Laurel. *Legionnaires' Disease: Deadly Diseases and Epidemics.* New York: Chelsea House, 2006.

Uzel, Atac, and E. Esin Hames-Kocabas. *"Legionella pneumophila": From Environment to Disease.* Commack, N.Y.: Nova Science, 2010.

WEB SITES OF INTEREST

Centers for Disease Control and Prevention
http://www.cdc.gov/legionella

National Institute of Environmental Health Sciences
http://www.niehs.nih.gov

National Institutes of Health
http://www.nlm.nih.gov

See also: Airborne illness and disease; Antibiotics: Types; Atypical pneumonia; Bacterial infections; Bronchiolitis; Bronchitis; Infection; Influenza; *Legionella*; Leptospirosis; Melioidosis; Pleurisy; Pneumonia; Respiratory route of transmission; Soilborne illness and disease; Tuberculosis (TB); Waterborne illness and disease; Whooping cough.

Postherpetic neuralgia

CATEGORY: Diseases and conditions
ANATOMY OR SYSTEM AFFECTED: Peripheral nervous system, skin

DEFINITION

Postherpetic neuralgia (PHN) is a common, potentially debilitating complication that occurs in 10 to 18 percent of persons with herpes zoster infection, or shingles. PHN is characterized by pain and other unpleasant sensations that persist for months or years after the resolution of the shingles rash.

CAUSES

Shingles is a painful rash caused by a reactivation of the varicella zoster virus, which remains latent in nerve ganglia for years after a chickenpox episode. Most often, symptoms of active shingles last about one month. A subset of persons subsequently develops PHN and continues to feel pain long after. The proposed pathogenetic mechanisms underlying this phenomenon stem from the intense inflammation associated with this viral infection and include degeneration of neuronal axon and cell body, atrophy of the spinal cord dorsal horn, scarring of dorsal root ganglia, and loss of skin nerve supply in the affected region.

RISK FACTORS

The risk for developing this complication increases with advancing age, particularly in people age fifty and older, irrespective of other risk factors. The likelihood of suffering from PHN is also higher in persons who had severe pain or severe rash during the acute episode and in persons who experienced a prodrome of pain in the nerve distribution area, before the rash appeared.

SYMPTOMS

In PHN, persons experience constant or intermittent pain along cutaneous nerves for more than thirty days after the lesions have healed. Pain intensity ranges from mild to excruciating. Sometimes, the pain occurs in response to normally innocuous stimuli such as fabric touching the skin (allodynia). Consequently, the affected person's quality of life suffers. Sleep and daily activities are affected, often leading to social withdrawal and depression.

SCREENING AND DIAGNOSIS

Usually, the appearance of the rash and the characteristics of pain render the clinical diagnosis simple and straightforward.

TREATMENT AND THERAPY

Postherpetic neuralgia is usually managed by a primary care physician and most often resolves within a year. The affected person may be referred to a pain specialist if the neuralgia cannot be controlled rapidly and effectively in primary care.

The condition is difficult to treat because of its refractoriness to the usual analgesics. Early treatment may be more effective than delayed treatment. Persons may benefit from topical anesthetics, topical capsaicin, anticonvulsants, opioids, tricyclic antidepressants (TCAs), and stress reduction techniques.

Interventions such as nerve blocking injections and electrical stimulation may help. As a last resort, surgical sectioning of the affected nerve root can be performed, but surgery itself can induce pain, including a dreaded complication called anesthesia dolorosa.

PREVENTION AND OUTCOMES

No treatment appears to prevent PHN completely, but some approaches may shorten the duration or lessen the severity of symptoms. Aggressive, early treatment of shingles reduces the likelihood of complications. Studies have shown that administration of antiviral drugs (especially valaciclovir and famciclovir) attenuates the severity of the infection and the neural damage it causes, thereby reducing the incidence and duration of PHN. Amitriptyline (a TCA) also holds promise in reducing the pain prevalence after herpes zoster.

Mihaela Avramut, M.D., Ph.D.

FURTHER READING

Johnson, R. W., and R. H. Dworkin. "Treatment of Herpes Zoster and Postherpetic Neuralgia." *British Medical Journal* 326 (2003): 748-750.

Mounsey, Anne L., Leah G. Matthew, and David C. Slawson. "Herpes Zoster and Postherpetic Neuralgia: Prevention and Management." *American Family Physician* 72 (2005): 1075-1080.

Stankus, S., et al. "Management of Herpes Zoster (Shingles) and Postherpetic Neuralgia." *American Family Physician* 61, no. 8 (April 15, 2000): 2437-2444, 2447-2448.

Tyring, S. K. "Management of Herpes Zoster and Postherpetic Neuralgia." *Journal of the American Academy of Dermatology* 57, no. 6 (December, 2007): S136-S142.

Weaver, Bethany A. "Herpes Zoster Overview: Natural History and Incidence." *Journal of the American Osteopathic Association* 109 (2009): S2-S6.

Whitley, Richard J. "Varicella-Zoster Virus." In *Mandell, Douglas, and Bennett's Principles and Practice of Infectious Diseases*, edited by Gerald L. Mandell, John F. Bennett, and Raphael Dolin. 7th ed. New York: Churchill Livingstone/Elsevier, 2010.

WEB SITES OF INTEREST

American Academy of Dermatology
http://www.aad.org

College of Family Physicians of Canada
http://www.cfpc.ca

HealingChronicPain.org
http://www.healingchronicpain.org/content/neuralgia

National Institute of Neurological Disorders and Stroke
http://www.ninds.nih.gov/disorders/shingles

National Shingles Foundation
http://www.vzvfoundation.org

See also: Aging and infectious disease; Antiviral drugs: Types; Chickenpox; Herpes zoster infection; Immunization; Reinfection; Shingles; Skin infections; Viral infections.

Poxviridae

CATEGORY: Pathogen
TRANSMISSION ROUTE: Direct contact, inhalation

DEFINITION

Poxviridae is a family of double-stranded DNA (deoxyribonucleic acid) viruses that comprises two subfamilies: *Chordopoxvirinae* and *Entomopoxvirinae*. All poxviruses that cause disease in humans belong to *Chordopoxvirinae*. Infamous members of this subfamily include variola virus, which causes smallpox, and vaccinia virus, which was used to create the vaccine against smallpox. Other human diseases caused by poxviruses are molluscum contagiosum, monkeypox, cowpox, milker's nodes, orf, yabapox, and tanapox.

All poxvirus infections in humans are associated with skin lesions. Smallpox and molluscum contagiosum occur only in humans; the others are animal diseases that are occasionally transmitted to humans.

Taxonomic Classification for *Poxviridae*

Order: Unassigned
Family: *Poxviridae*
Subfamily: *Chordopoxvirinae*
Genus: *Molluscipoxvirus*
Species: *Molluscum contagiosum virus*
Genus: *Orthopoxvirus*
Species:
Variola virus
Vaccinia virus
Cowpox virus
Monkeypox virus
Genus: *Parapoxvirus*
Species:
Orf virus
Milker's nodule virus (paravaccinia)
Genus: *Yatapoxvirus*
Species:
Yaba monkey tumor virus
Tanapox virus

NATURAL HABITAT AND FEATURES

Poxvirus family members are the largest and most complex of all viruses. With a length of 220 to 450 nm (nanometers) long, they are large enough to be seen under a light microscope. The virions are oval or brick-shaped, which differs considerably from the highly symmetrical structure of other viruses. A dumbbell-shaped core contains linear double-stranded DNA that is 130 to 375 kilobase pairs in length. The viral core is surrounded by a core wall and a phospholipid-bilayer envelope. As infectious viral particles exit the cell, they gain a second envelope.

Poxviruses bind to one of several types of cell surface receptors and enter the cell through endocytosis or by direct fusion of the viral envelope with the plasma membrane. Poxviruses replicate in the cytoplasm of the host cell rather than in the nucleus. This distinguishes them from other DNA viruses and requires that they carry their own enzymes for replication. The poxvirus capsid contains more than one hundred different types of proteins, including dozens of enzymes required for transcription and translation of the viral genome.

PATHOGENICITY AND CLINICAL SIGNIFICANCE

Human history has been shaped by the devastating effects of variola, the smallpox virus. Smallpox has determined the outcome of wars, toppled civilizations, and killed countless persons on multiple continents. Smallpox also holds a unique place in history as the first disease to be eradicated worldwide. The last known case of smallpox was in Somalia in 1977.

Variola virus was one of the most pathogenic viruses known. With a mortality rate of 30 to 50 percent, it killed 300 to 500 million people during its existence. Molluscum contagiosum virus is the only other poxvirus that is found worldwide. In contrast to variola, molluscum contagiosum virus is a trivial pathogen. It causes painless, benign skin lesions and is not associated with systemic illness. It is most common in children, and it also can be transmitted sexually.

All other members of the poxvirus family that cause disease in humans are animal viruses that are transmitted to humans only rarely. Human-to-human transmission has not been seen. Human monkeypox, the only seriously pathogenic illness in this group, occurs in villages in the tropical rain forests of West Africa and Central Africa. Monkeypox virus is transmitted to humans through close contact with monkeys and squirrels and other rodents. The symptoms of monkeypox are similar to those of a mild case of smallpox, with a mortality rate of 10 to 15 percent.

Three different poxviruses can be transmitted from cows to humans during milking. Vaccinia virus, cowpox virus, and milker's nodule virus cause minor, localized infections, usually on the hands. Orf virus, which causes similar skin lesions, is acquired through direct contact with sheep or goats.

Yabapox and tanapox viruses occur only in tropical regions of Africa. Yabapox produces large, benign tumors and is transmitted to humans through monkeys. Tanapox is a somewhat common skin infection in regions of Kenya and Zaire. Systemic illness lasts about four days, with symptoms that include fever, headache, and backache. Skin lesions heal within several weeks.

DRUG SUSCEPTIBILITY

No pharmaceutical treatment exists for poxvirus infection. Nucleoside and nucleotide analogs have been investigated for use as anti-poxvirus agents. Vaccination remains the only weapon against smallpox. The smallpox vaccine also confers 85 percent protection against monkeypox virus. A recent rise in the number of monkeypox cases in the Democratic Republic of Congo has been attributed to the termination of smallpox vaccination programs following smallpox eradication.

Kathryn Pierno, M.S.

FURTHER READING

De Clercq, Erik, and Johan Neyts. "Therapeutic Potential of Nucleoside/Nucleotide Analogues Against Poxvirus Infections." *Reviews in Medical Virology* 14 (2004): 289-300. Presents evidence that this class of drugs may be effective in treating poxvirus infections.

Madigan, Michael T., and John M. Martinko. *Brock Biology of Microorganisms.* 12th ed. Upper Saddle River, N.J.: Pearson/Prentice Hall, 2010. A standard microbiology textbook for undergraduate college students, with detailed descriptions of cell structures and clear illustrations. Includes evolutionary perspectives and covers pathogenesis.

Mercer, Andrew, Axel Schmidt, and Olaf Weber, eds. *Poxviruses.* Basel, Switzerland: Birkhauser, 2007. Detailed discussions of each genus of poxvirus, including replication strategies, immune system interactions, and therapeutics.

Rimoin, Anne W., et al. "Major Increase in Human Monkeypox Incidence Thirty Years After Smallpox Vaccination Campaigns Cease in the Democratic Republic of Congo." *Proceedings of the National Academy of Sciences* 107 (2010): 37. Discusses a rapid increase in monkeypox cases and its relationship to smallpox vaccination.

WEB SITES OF INTEREST

Big Picture Book of Viruses
http://www.virology.net/big_virology

eMedicine: Poxviruses
http://emedicine.medscape.com/article/226239-overview

Viral Zone
http://www.expasy.org/viralzone

See also: Cowpox; Developing countries and infectious disease; Emerging and reemerging infectious diseases; Molluscum contagiosum; Monkeypox; Poxvirus infections; Smallpox; Smallpox vaccine; Tropical medicine; Viral infections; Zoonotic diseases.

Poxvirus infections

CATEGORY: Diseases and conditions
ANATOMY OR SYSTEM AFFECTED: Skin

DEFINITION

Poxvirus infections are infections with any organism from the family of viruses known as *Poxviridae.* These infections include variola (smallpox), vaccinia, monkeypox, cowpox, mousepox, and molluscum contagiosum. Smallpox and molluscum contagiosum are diseases of humans; the others are diseases of animals that occasionally occur in humans. Smallpox, which was one of the scourges of history, was eradicated through a worldwide vaccination campaign in the 1970's. Chickenpox, despite the similarity of name, is caused by a virus from another family.

The *Poxviridae* viruses are large, enveloped, brick-shaped viruses containing linear, double-stranded DNA (deoxyribonucleic acid). There are eight genus categories (subgroups) of *Poxviridae,* the most significant being orthopoxvirus, to which the smallpox virus belongs.

CAUSES

Smallpox was typically spread through the respiratory tract. Sneeze or cough droplets from infected persons were inhaled by others who had not had the disease and who had not been vaccinated. Though less common, smallpox could also be spread through contact with pustules.

In the vaccination process, healthy persons are cutaneously exposed to vaccinia virus. Molluscum contagiosum virus is spread through direct skin-to-skin contact or through contact with contaminated objects (fomites). Most often, however, the disease is spread through sexual contact.

There are many *Poxviridae* organisms, including cowpox and monkeypox viruses, whose principal reservoir is animals, making cowpox and monkeypox zoonotic diseases. These diseases occasionally are spread to humans through animal-human contact. Monkeypox is the most significant of these diseases; a monkeypox outbreak involving about fifty people occurred in the United States in 2003.

RISK FACTORS

The principal risk factors for smallpox were one's location (Africa and the Indian subcontinent) and one's vaccination status. (Smallpox vaccination programs were discontinued after the World Health Organization declared the disease eradicated in 1980.) Smallpox is now considered a possible biological weapon, and because few people have been vaccinated, most people would be vulnerable to attack. A risk factor now is contact with a recently vaccinated member of the military.

The risk factor for molluscum contagiosum is skin contact with an infected person. Persons with human immunodeficiency virus infection or with compromised immune systems are susceptible to more serious infections. The risk factor for zoonotic poxvirus infection is exposure to animals.

SYMPTOMS

Poxvirus infection typically begins with high fever and respiratory symptoms, but the hallmark symptom is the characteristic vesicular skin lesions that eventually form pustules. The resolution of the skin lesions typically involves significant scarring. The other poxviruses typically cause localized lesions only. Monkeypox is the exception, and its symptoms can be both generalized and severe.

SCREENING AND DIAGNOSIS

Smallpox can be differentiated from chickenpox by the simultaneous presentation of skin lesions (all lesions will be at the same stage, contrary to the lesions of chickenpox) and by the severity of general malaise.

TREATMENT AND THERAPY

No direct treatment for variola major, which has a mortality rate as high as 30 percent, was ever developed. Treatment involved supportive therapy for symptoms such as high fever and dehydration. Left untreated, molluscum contagiosum usually resolves within six months. Treatment options include surgical removal of the lesions; cryotherapy, which uses cold to freeze the lesions off of the skin (liquid nitrogen may be used for this treatment); and retinoid or imiquimod

cream, separately or in combination. No treatment exists for monkeypox, but the smallpox vaccine has been shown to help prevent and reduce the severity of the disease.

PREVENTION AND OUTCOMES

Two laboratory reservoirs of smallpox virus were retained after WHO declared smallpox to be eliminated worldwide. The challenge now is to balance the risks of vaccination complications (serious complications occur in about 1 in 1,000 persons) with the risks of a potential smallpox outbreak caused by bioterrorism.

To reduce the risk of exposure to the molluscum contagiosum virus, one should avoid contact with infected persons; avoid sharing towels, clothing, baths, and pools; and avoid sexual contact with infected persons. The smallpox vaccine is the best prevention against monkeypox. In high-risk areas, people should limit exposure to wild animals.

Cathy Frisinger, M.P.H.

FURTHER READING

Damon, Inger K. "Smallpox, Monkeypox, and Other Poxvirus Infections." In *Cecil Medicine*, edited by Lee Goldman and Dennis Arthur Ausiello. 23d ed. Philadelphia: Saunders/Elsevier, 2008.

Henderson, D. A. *Smallpox: The Death of a Disease—The Inside Story of Eradicating a Worldwide Killer.* Amherst, N.Y.: Prometheus Books, 2009.

Reed, Kurt D. "Monkeypox and Other Emerging Orthopoxvirus Infections." In *Emerging Infectious Diseases: Trends and Issues*, edited by Felissa R. Lashley and Jerry D. Durham. 2d ed. New York: Springer, 2007.

WEB SITES OF INTEREST

Big Picture Book of Viruses
http://www.virology.net/big_virology

eMedicine: Poxviruses
http://emedicine.medscape.com/article/226239-overview

Emerging and Reemerging Infectious Diseases Resource Center
http://www.medscape.com/resource/infections

PathInfo Project
http://ci.vbi.vt.edu/pathinfo

World Health Organization
http://www.who.int/mediacentre/factsheets/
smallpox

See also: Cowpox; Developing countries and infectious disease; Emerging and reemerging infectious diseases; Molluscum contagiosum; Monkeypox; *Poxviridae;* Smallpox; Smallpox vaccine; Tropical medicine; Viral infections; Zoonotic diseases.

Pregnancy and infectious disease

CATEGORY: Transmission

DEFINITION

Infections in pregnancy may cause maternal illness, fetal birth defects or disorders, postnatal medical concerns, and adverse pregnancy outcomes. Often, maternal symptoms are mild compared with the fetal effects. Infections are spread by vertical transmission, whereby the pregnant woman (or girl) passes an active infection to the fetus in pregnancy through the placenta or through the birth canal during delivery.

The timing of a maternal infection is important. In general, the earlier in pregnancy that a pregnant woman acquires an infection, the less likely the fetus is to acquire the infection through the placenta but the more likely the affected fetus is to have severe symptoms. Conversely, the later in pregnancy that a pregnant woman acquires an infection, the more likely her fetus is to acquire the infection but with less significant abnormal findings. For sexually transmitted diseases, the risk is greatest at time of contact with the vaginal canal during delivery.

After blood tests, urinalyses, or vaginal cultures have confirmed a maternal infection, additional studies of the fetus may be performed. Abnormal ultrasound findings suggest fetal infection but cannot confirm the diagnosis. Invasive prenatal diagnosis by amniocentesis may be available to confirm a fetal infection but cannot detect the severity of the infection. The prognosis, management, and treatment vary depending on the type of infection.

THE TORCH PANEL

Many infections may be screened using a TORCH ("toxoplasmosis," "other," "rubella," "cytomegalovirus,"

and "herpes") panel. "Other" includes infections such as hepatitis B, syphilis, coxsackie virus, parvovirus, and varicella. The TORCH panel is performed on maternal blood to confirm the presence of either a past or a primary (new) infection in the pregnancy. For many infections, past exposure makes it unlikely that a current pregnancy would be at risk because of maternal immunity.

Congenital toxoplasmosis. Toxoplasmosis is caused by *Toxoplasma gondii*, a common parasite that typically does not lead to illness in otherwise healthy persons. Those who are at highest risk are those who have outdoor pets (such as cats) who carry the parasite, those who garden, and those who ingest uncooked meat. An infected person may present with fever, fatigue, and sore throat. A primary infection confers a 40 percent risk of congenital toxoplasmosis and subsequent risk of miscarriage, stillbirth, or premature delivery.

Abnormal ultrasound findings may be seen in one-third of affected fetuses; examples of abnormalities include calcifications in the brain, water on the brain, and an enlarged or small head size. Newborns have symptoms that range from mild to severe, with little or absent signs of the infection at delivery. They develop inflammation of the retina, leading to visual loss, hearing loss, seizures, cerebral palsy, mental retardation, enlarged liver and spleen, feeding difficulties, and low birth weight. Antibiotics are given to reduce the chance of vertical transmission, although medications are not 100 percent effective.

Congenital rubella (German measles). Most females of childbearing age are immune to rubella because of childhood vaccinations. One to two percent of pregnant women are at risk for the virus. Pregnant women present with flulike symptoms and arthritis. If a woman acquires the infection within the first sixteen weeks of pregnancy, the risk is greatest (50 to 85 percent) for the fetus to have congenital rubella syndrome, which entails hearing loss, cataracts, heart defects, enlargement of the spleen, developmental delay, and diabetes. An infection acquired at sixteen to twenty weeks gestation places the pregnancy at a lower risk, and after twenty weeks, an infection does not increase the risk for birth defects. No treatments exist to prevent vertical transmission. The vaccine is recommended before but not during pregnancy.

Congenital cytomegalovirus. Cytomegalovirus is the most common congenital infection in the United States. All pregnant women are susceptible to the in-

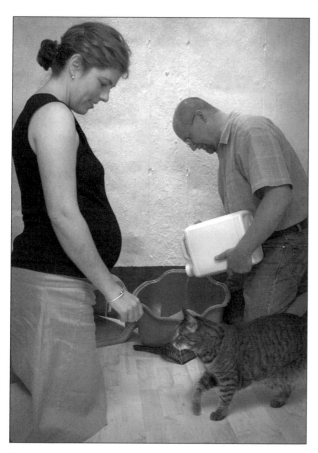

A pregnant woman refrains from cleaning her cat's litter box. Cat feces contain the parasite Toxoplasma gondii, *which can cause serious health complications for a pregnant woman and her fetus/child.* (CDC)

fection, although it is more prevalent in populations of low socioeconomic status. A primary infection occurs in 1 to 4 percent of pregnant women and puts the pregnancy at risk for vertical transmission. An infected woman might be asymptomatic or may show mild symptoms that include a fever and sore throat. Of these women, one-third will transmit the cytomegalovirus to the pregnancy.

Abnormal ultrasound findings include extra fluid around the fetus or in the fetal tissues, an enlarged heart or heart block, enlarged ventricles of the brain, and calcifications in fetal organs. Some newborns have transient symptoms such as jaundice or low birth weight. About 1 in 750 newborns will develop significant long-term complications such as hearing and vision loss, enlargement of liver and spleen, mental re-

tardation, and seizures. Not all findings are readily apparent at delivery. Approximately one-third of severely affected newborns do not survive.

Treatment for congenital cytomegalovirus is experimental. Initial studies of administering hyperimmunoglobulin to pregnant women are promising, with resolution of abnormal ultrasound findings and delivery of healthy babies. Randomized clinical trials are needed to confirm the efficacy.

Parvovirus. Human parvovirus B19 is a common virus that causes fifth disease (also called erythema infectiosum). Women who work in child care or who have an affected family member are at greatest risk for a primary infection. Many women remain asymptomatic or have mild flulike symptoms. A characteristic red facial rash with a "slapped cheek" appearance is often observed. The chance of vertical transmission in the pregnancy is approximately one-third. Risk of miscarriage and stillbirth exists, especially if the infection was acquired in the first twenty weeks of pregnancy. There is no increased risk for birth defects, but the fetus is at risk for a heart infection and anemia.

Abnormal ultrasound findings include extra fluid in the fetal tissues, an enlarged heart, and abnormal blood flow in the fetal brain. If the heart infection and anemia are severe enough, they may ultimately result in fetal death. The anemia might require blood transfusions through a percutaneous umbilical blood sampling. The extra fluid may conversely disappear and result in a normal outcome for the pregnancy. No other treatment or vaccines are available.

SEXUALLY TRANSMITTED DISEASES

Sexually transmitted diseases (STDs) are routinely screened for at a pregnant woman's initial prenatal visit. Most STDs are transmitted at delivery by newborn skin contact with secretions in the vaginal canal, although some may cross the placenta. Pregnant women should avoid sexual contact and should take appropriate precautions with partners who are untreated for STDs. Certain STDs are transmitted to the pregnancy through diagnostic procedures such as amniocentesis. Therefore, these procedures may not be recommended. Unlike the foregoing infections, this and the following category include infections that can recur and that require multiple courses of treatment.

Chlamydia. The bacterium *Chlamydia trachomatis* causes chlamydia infection, the most common bacterial STD in the United States. Seventy-five percent of women are asymptomatic; some have abnormal vaginal bleeding or discharge and pain with sexual intercourse. Antibiotics are prescribed, but when untreated, chlamydia may result in an ectopic pregnancy or a preterm delivery. If there is an untreated chlamydia infection at the time of delivery, vaginal wall contact places the newborn at risk for developing pneumonia and a severe eye infection that could cause eye damage and blindness.

Congenital syphilis. Syphilis is a bacterial infection caused by *Treponoma pallidum*. Primary syphilis is characterized by an open internal or external genital sore. Without medication, this progresses to secondary and tertiary syphilis with findings of fever, rash, sore throat, hair loss, and, eventually, blindness and dementia. Syphilis may be transmitted through the placenta to the fetus and result in a miscarriage, stillbirth, and premature delivery. Syphilis is also transmitted during both vaginal and cesarean sections, although the latter may reduce infection rates.

Newborns may not show immediate signs of congenital syphilis. Findings include oral and genital sores, rash, jaundice, and anemia. When untreated, children will develop mental retardation, vision and hearing loss, seizures, and bone and teeth damage; death can also occur. If syphilis is diagnosed before the sixteenth week of pregnancy, penicillin is effective in preventing congenital syphilis. After sixteen weeks, treatment is less successful.

Gonorrhea. Gonorrhea is caused by the bacterium *Neisseria gonorrhoeae*. It is the second most common bacterial STD. One-half of infected women are asymptomatic. Left untreated, it may lead to an ectopic pregnancy, miscarriage, premature delivery, and maternal infection after delivery. The fetal findings include decreased fetal growth. Neonatal effects result from contact with the vaginal wall and include eye or generalized infections and meningitis. Treatment is with antibiotics.

Hepatitis B and C. Newborns have a risk for vertical transmission of either hepatitis B or C, viruses that infect the liver, if a pregnant woman is a chronic carrier of the disease or if she has an acute infection. Risks to the fetus that are transient include jaundice, fatigue, and fever. Long term, a child is at risk for early onset cirrhosis of the liver and liver cancer. For hepatitis B, immunizations are provided in the newborn nursery and are 90 percent effective at preventing infection. A vaccine does not exist for hepatitis C.

Herpes simplex virus. Genital herpes may be caused by either herpes simplex types 1 or 2. The risk to the pregnancy includes a significant eye infection that may result in damage or blindness. The baby is at risk if the woman is having an active outbreak at delivery. In this circumstance, a cesarean section is often performed to avoid neonatal transmission during labor. Maternal infection is treated with oral antibiotics. Women may be on suppression therapy in the third trimester to prevent an outbreak at delivery. Eye drops are routinely administered after birth to prevent a neonatal eye infection.

Human immunodeficiency virus (HIV). HIV is the virus that causes acquired immune deficiency syndrome (AIDS). Vertical transmission of HIV may occur during pregnancy or at delivery. Without treatment, the risk to the fetus is 25 percent. With antiretroviral therapy, the risk is reduced to 2 percent. Certain medications for treating HIV may cause birth defects and disorders, so women are switched to safer medications during pregnancy. A cesarean section may be recommended if the woman has a large amount of virus detected, although this recommendation is controversial.

OTHER INFECTIONS

Bacterial vaginosis. Bacterial vaginosis (BV) is an imbalance of the beneficial and harmful vaginal bacteria that leads to an overgrowth of the latter. About 10 to 30 percent of pregnant women are diagnosed with BV, the cause of which is unknown. It is not a sexually transmitted disease, but sexual intercourse does increase the chance of BV. Women with a new partner or multiple sexual partners are at greatest risk. Often women are asymptomatic, but others have a grayish-white discharge with a fishy odor. This may cause a vaginal itch, pain, or a burning sensation. BV is associated with an increased risk for premature labor and delivery, miscarriage and low birth weight. Treatment includes oral antibiotics. Topical medications alleviate maternal symptoms but do not eliminate pregnancy complications.

Influenza. Influenza is an infection of the respiratory tract. Pregnant women are at increased risk for complications because of a decreased immune response. Symptoms include fever, chills, achy muscles, sore throat, and fatigue. Pregnant women often experience difficulty breathing. The greatest chance of acquiring the flu happens during the winter season (November through March). Data suggest an increased risk for pregnancy loss or premature labor and delivery. An increase in birth defects has not been observed. Maternal deaths have been reported.

Acetaminophen is given for fever control and antiviral medications are prescribed if flulike symptoms are reported. The Centers for Disease Control and Prevention recommends that all pregnant women receive the seasonal and H1N1 flu vaccines. The injected flu vaccine is an inactive form of the virus and does not place the pregnancy at increased risk for either influenza or birth defects. The nasal vaccine is not recommended during pregnancy because it contains live influenza virus.

Listeriosis. The bacterium *Listeria monocytogenes* causes listeriosis. Although the diagnosis is rare, pregnant women are much more likely to be diagnosed with listeriosis than are other persons.

Listeria may be found in uncooked or undercooked food. Pregnant women should avoid lunch meats or refrigerated meats unless these meats are heated to a safe temperature. Also, pregnant women should not consume unpasteurized milk and certain dairy products.

Listeriosis increases the risk of miscarriage, stillbirth, neonatal death and premature labor. Pregnant women report mild flulike symptoms, including fever, muscle aches, diarrhea, nausea, and vomiting. More severe symptoms appear if the infection spreads to the central nervous system; the severe symptoms include maternal seizures and cognitive disorientation.

Abnormal ultrasound findings include the possibility of an enlarged fetal heart and thickening of the gastrointestinal tract, where the bacteria typically resides. Fetal infection results in death in 20 to 30 percent of cases. Newborns may have significant findings such as breathing difficulties, fever, pneumonia, sepsis, and lethargy. Newborns are at greater risk of meningitis when acquiring the infection through vaginal delivery. Treatment for listeriosis includes antibiotics to prevent vertical transmission and is successful in decreasing the stillbirth and premature delivery rate.

Group B streptococcal infection. Group B *Streptococcus* (GBS) is a naturally occurring bacterium commonly found in up to 25 percent of otherwise healthy women. It lives in either the vagina or the rectum of asymptomatic pregnant women. Women are tested for GBS late in their third trimester of pregnancy by a vaginal or rectal swab. GBS is the most common cause of life-threatening infections of the newborn and is associated with stillbirth. A newborn may develop sepsis, meningitis, and pneumonia. Long-term complications include vision and hearing loss and a risk for developmental delay. Penicillin is given intravenously four hours before delivery to prevent vertical transmission.

Food-Transmissible Pathogens: Foods to Avoid During Pregnancy

Foods to avoid	Possible pathogen or pathogens
Soft cheeses made from unpasteurized milk, including brie, feta, queso blanco, and queso fresco	*E. coli, Listeria*
Raw cookie dough or cake batter	*Salmonella*
Raw or undercooked fish, such as sushi	various parasites, bacteria
Unpasteurized juice or cider, including fresh squeezed	*E. coli*
Unpasteurized milk	*Campylobacter, E. coli, Listeria, Salmonella*
Store-made salads such as ham salad, chicken salad, and seafood salad	*Listeria*
Raw shellfish, such as oysters and clams	*Vibrio* bacteria
Raw or undercooked sprouts, such as alfalfa, clover, mung bean, and raddish	*E. coli, Salmonella*

Source: U.S. Department of Health and Human Services

Urinary tract infection. Urinary tract infections (UTIs) are very common during pregnancy, with most women remaining asymptomatic. Therefore, urine cultures are performed on all pregnant women. If left untreated, an infection of the kidneys and ureters may occur. Symptoms include fever, back pain, anemia, and nausea and vomiting. Low birth weight and premature delivery result. Treatment is with antibiotics for the current infection and possible prophylactic antibiotics for women with recurrent UTIs.

Chickenpox. A primary maternal varicella infection is associated with the characteristic vesicular rash of chickenpox. More significant complications are maternal bacterial infections, inflammation of the lungs, and central nervous system involvement. During the first and second trimesters, fetal varicella syndrome findings consist of scarred skin, eye defects, underdeveloped limbs, small head size, and developmental delay; however, these findings occur in only 1 percent of all fetuses. During the third trimester, the fetus is at risk for severe symptoms and death. Pregnant women with a primary infection are isolated from other pregnant women and infants. Immunoglobulins, which are given when the diagnosis has been confirmed to reduce pregnancy and newborn complications, do not prevent vertical transmission.

IMPACT

Although many of the aforementioned infectious diseases have either preventive measures or possible treatments in pregnancy, the illnesses remain a significant cause of fetal and maternal morbidity and death. Many of the diagnoses are not detected until after the pregnant woman or the fetus has shown significant symptoms, often when it is too late for effective interventions. Overlapping symptoms also pose difficulties for determining the exact infection.

The impact of a preterm delivery or delivery of a child with multiple medical concerns is felt at the level of the patient and from a public health perspective. Increased long-term care puts a strain on the medical system. Proper patient education, and continuing drug and vaccine development, remain key components of reducing the incidence of infections in pregnancy.

Janet Ober Berman, M.S., CGC

FURTHER READING

Addler, Stuart P., et al. "Recent Advances in the Prevention and Treatment of Congenital Cytomegalovirus Infections." *Seminars in Perinatology* 31 (2007): 10-18. An overview of congenital cytomegalovirus and summary of data regarding newer prenatal treatment by hyperimmunoglobulin.

Al-Safi, Z. A., V. I. Shavell, and B. Gonik. "Vaccination in Pregnancy." *Women's Health* (London) 7 (2011): 109-119. Article argues for the importance of clinical discussions of vaccinations in pregnant women and of the risks to their fetuses.

Gratzl, R., et al. "Follow-up of Infants with Congenital Toxoplasmosis Detected by Polymerase Chain Reaction Analysis of Amniotic Fluid." *European Journal of Clinical Microbiology and Infectious Disease* 17 (1998): 853-858. A prospective longitudinal study of infants diagnosed prenatally with congenital toxoplasmosis and treated with antibiotics. Provides follow-up on the medical outcomes throughout the first year of life.

Khare, Manjiri. "Infectious Disease in Pregnancy." *Current Obstetrics and Gynaecology* 15 (2005): 149-156. An overview of the many infectious diseases of pregnancy, with discussion of their impact.

Yinon, Y., et al. "Cytomegalovirus Infection in Pregnancy." *Journal of Obstetrics and Gynaecology Canada* 32 (2010): 348-354. An updated examination of cytomegalovirus infection in pregnant women.

WEB SITES OF INTEREST

American Congress of Obstetricians and Gynecologists
http://www.acog.org

National Institutes of Health
http://www.nlm.nih.gov/medlineplus/infectionsandpregnancy

Organization of Teratology Information Specialists
http://www.otispregnancy.org

See also: Asplenia; Bloodstream infections; Breast milk and infectious disease; Childbirth and infectious disease; Children and infectious disease; Cytomegalovirus infection; Cytomegalovirus vaccine; Immunity; Neonatal sepsis; Ophthalmia neonatorum; Puerperal infection; Sexually transmitted diseases (STDs); Syphilis; Transmission routes; Vertical disease transmission; Women and infectious disease.

Prevention of bacterial infections

Category: Prevention

Definition

Bacterial infections are infections that are caused by microorganisms called bacteria. Common bacterial infections include urinary tract infection (UTI), strep throat, tuberculosis (TB), *Helicobacter pylori* infection, and methicillin-resistant *Staphylococcus aureus* (MRSA).

Types of Bacterial Infection

UTI is a bacterial infection of one or more parts of the urinary system. Most UTIs originate in the bladder or urethra, but they also can begin in the kidneys or ureters. Strep throat is an infection of the throat that is caused by the group *A Streptococcus* (GAS) bacterium. TB is a bacterial infection that affects the lungs. *H. pylori* is a bacterium that affects the intestinal tract. It causes chronic gastritis and duodenal and gastric ulcers, and it may contribute to the development of gastric cancer. MRSA is a staph infection that has become resistant to the antibiotics that are normally used to treat staph infections.

Prevention

UTIs most commonly occur when bacteria that normally live in the intestine enter the urethra. Other sources of bacteria that can cause UTIs are sexual intercourse, urinary catheters, and obstruction, such as kidney stones or prostate problems.

No vaccine exists for the prevention of UTI. However, one can take the following measures to reduce the risk for UTIs: Drink a minimum of eight glasses of water per day, urinate as soon as possible after intercourse, take showers instead of tub baths, wipe from front to back after urination or bowel movement, avoid spermicidal foams or jellies, and avoid feminine hygiene sprays or douches.

Strep throat is spread through droplets in the air when an infected person sneezes or coughs or by contact with infected objects. As with UTIs, no vaccine exists for the prevention of strep throat. One should take the following measures to reduce the risk of contracting strep throat: Wash hands frequently, especially before preparing or eating food; when possible, avoid contact with people who have strep infections; and avoid sharing personal items such as drinking glasses, eating utensils, and toothbrushes.

TB is spread through droplets in the air when an infected person sneezes or coughs. Although a vaccine has been developed for the prevention of TB, it is not commonly used in the United States. The TB vaccine, which is also known as the Bacillus Calmette-Guérin (BCG) vaccine, does not always protect against TB and could cause a false-positive result in people who are later tested for TB.

Even without the use of the BCG vaccine, there are still some things one can do to prevent the spread of TB. One method is to treat TB-infected persons before their disease becomes active. This involves regular testing of people who may be at risk. For persons who test positive for TB infection, certain medications can be prescribed by doctors to help prevent active disease. Other methods of preventing the spread of TB include covering the nose and mouth with a tissue when coughing or sneezing, opening windows to ventilate rooms if the weather permits, avoiding the workplace when sick, wearing a mask around others, and avoiding close contact with family members for the first few weeks of treatment.

It is not known how *H. pylori* infection is contracted, so there are no specific recommendations for prevention. However, to prevent complications of *H. pylori* infection, persons with symptoms of gastritis or gastric or duodenal ulcers are frequently tested for *H. pylori* and are treated if found to be infected.

MRSA can be acquired in hospitals and other health care settings, and in specific communities, such as nursing homes. MRSA infection is spread through contact with a contaminated person or object. In the health care setting, MRSA is frequently prevented through isolation of infected persons and through practicing standard precautions, such as handwashing and wearing protective gloves and clothing.

There are several measures that one can take to prevent the spread of MRSA in the community setting. These measures include covering wounds with clean, dry bandages until they have healed; frequent handwashing; not sharing personal items, such as towels, wash cloths, or razors; periodic cleaning of frequently touched surfaces with disinfecting wipes; and washing bed linens in hot water.

Impact

According to the National Institute of Diabetes and Digestive and Kidney Diseases, UTIs account for more than 8 million doctor visits each year in the United

States. UTI is more common in women, and one in five women will get a UTI at least once during her lifetime. The Centers for Disease Control and Prevention (CDC) reports that between 9,000 and 11,500 cases of invasive GAS disease occur each year in the United States, resulting in 1,000 to 1,800 deaths annually.

The World Health Organization estimates that one-third of the world's population is infected with TB at any given time, and that 5 to 10 percent of infected persons will develop active TB in the future. In 2009, about 1.7 million people died from TB.

The CDC estimates that approximately two-thirds of the world population is infected with the *H. pylori* bacterium, and that between 2 and 20 percent of those persons infected will develop ulcers. Furthermore, CDC statistics show that in 2005, more than 94,000 people developed a serious MRSA infection and more than 18,000 people died during a hospital stay related to these infections.

Julie Henry, R.N., M.P.A.

FURTHER READING

Brachman, Philip S., and Elias Abrutyn, eds. *Bacterial Infections of Humans: Epidemiology and Control.* 4th ed. New York: Springer, 2009.

Brogden, K., et al. *Virulence Mechanisms of Bacterial Pathogens.* 4th ed. Washington, D.C.: ASM Press, 2007.

Centers for Disease Control and Prevention. "*Helicobacter pylori*: Fact Sheet for Health Care Providers." Available at http://www.cdc.gov/ulcer/keytocure.htm.

Mayo Foundation for Medical Education and Research. "Tuberculosis." Available at http://www.mayoclinic.com/health/tuberculosis/DS00372.

_____. "Urinary Tract Infection." Available at http://www.mayoclinic.com/health/urinary-tract-infection/DS00286.

"Strep Throat." Available at http://www.webmd.com/oral-health/tc/strep-throat-topic-overview.

WEB SITES OF INTEREST

Centers for Disease Control and Prevention
http://www.cdc.gov

Mayo Foundation for Medical Education and Research
http://www.mayoclinic.com

Todar's Online Textbook of Bacteriology
http://www.textbookofbacteriology.net

See also: Antibiotic resistance; Antibiotics: Types; Bacteria: Classification and types; Bacteria: Structure and growth; Bacterial infections; Diagnosis of bacterial infections; Drug resistance; Epidemiology; *Helicobacter pylori* infection; Home remedies; Infection; Methicillin-resistant staph infection; Microbiology; Over-the-counter (OTC) drugs; Strep throat; Streptococcal infections; Treatment of bacterial infections; Tuberculosis (TB); Tuberculosis (TB) vaccine; Urinary tract infections.

Prevention of fungal infections

CATEGORY: Prevention

DEFINITION

A fungal infection is an infection that is caused by a fungus, an organism that lives by absorbing nutrients from its environment. Fungi include mildews, molds, mushrooms, rusts, smuts, or yeasts. Common fungal infections are athlete's foot, jock itch, ringworm, and vaginal yeast infection.

TYPES OF FUNGAL INFECTIONS

Athlete's foot, also known as tinea pedis, is a fungal infection of the foot. There are several types of fungi that can cause athlete's foot. The most common is *Trichophyton rubrum.*

Jock itch, also known as tinea cruris, is a fungal infection of the groin area. More than one fungus can cause jock itch, but the most common is *T. rubrum.*

Ringworm of the body, also known as tinea corporis, is a fungal infection of the skin. There are several types of fungi that can cause ringworm.

Vaginal yeast infection, also known as candidiasis or vaginitis, is an overgrowth of yeast cells that causes inflammation of the vagina. It is caused by the fungus *Candida.*

PREVENTION OF FUNGAL INFECTIONS

Athlete's foot is spread through contact with infected skin or contaminated surfaces, such as shower floors, locker room floors, swimming pools, towels, and shoes. The fungi that cause athlete's foot are normally found on the skin, but they can cause infection if given a warm, moist environment in which to grow. The following measures can help prevent the spread of athlete's foot: Avoid walking barefoot in public showers, locker rooms, or pool areas; wash feet daily with soap and water, and dry thoroughly; wear shoes that are well ventilated, such as sandals, when possible; alternate shoes daily to give each pair time to air out; avoid borrowing shoes from others; and wear cotton socks to absorb moisture.

Jock itch is spread by direct person-to-person contact during sexual intercourse or by contact with contaminated items (fomites), such as towels or clothing. The fungi that cause jock itch are normally found on the skin, but they can cause infection if given a warm, moist environment in which to grow. The following measures can help prevent the spread of jock itch: Avoid sharing towels, wash cloths, or clothing; wear clean, loose-fitting clothes; keep the genital area clean and dry; and avoid having sexual intercourse with someone who has jock itch until the infection has completely cleared.

Ringworm is spread by person-to-person contact, contact with infected animals, contact with infected objects, and contact with contaminated soil. The fungi that cause ringworm are normally found on the skin, but can cause infection if given a warm, moist environment in which to grow. The following measures can help prevent the spread of ringworm: Avoid sharing personal items, such as towels, wash cloths, or clothing; wear clean, loose-fitting clothes; avoid animals that have patches of missing fur; avoid walking barefoot in public showers, locker rooms, or pool areas; shower with soap and water after participating in contact sports; and keep skin clean and dry.

Vaginal yeast infection can be spread through oral-genital sexual contact. It also can be caused by the use of antibiotics, by increased estrogen levels, by uncontrolled diabetes, and by an impaired immune system. The fungi that cause vaginal yeast infection are normally found in the vagina, but they can cause infection if given a warm, moist environment in which to grow. The following measures can help prevent the spread of vaginal yeast infection: Avoid using douches, feminine sprays, or scented tampons or pads; wear cotton underwear and loose-fitting clothing; remove wet clothing as soon as possible; and avoid hot tubs and hot baths. If prone to vaginal yeast infections and before taking antibiotics, a woman should ask her doctor or other health care provider about using preventive antifungal medications.

IMPACT

Athlete's foot is the most common of the tinea infections and is more prevalent in men than in women. The medical literature suggests that about 70 percent of persons will have athlete's foot at least once in their lifetime. The incidence and prevalence of jock itch are unknown. It is most common in adolescent boys and men, particularly athletes.

According to the World Health Organization, no specific statistics are available on the incidence and prevalence of ringworm, but it is believed to be a frequent problem in most countries, particularly where hygiene is poor. Statistics from the Centers for Disease Control and Prevention show that most women will have a vaginal yeast infection at least once in their lifetimes, and approximately 50 percent will experience a recurrence.

Julie Henry, R.N., M.P.A.

FURTHER READING

American Academy of Family Physicians. "Tinea Infections: Athlete's Foot, Jock Itch, and Ringworm." Available at http://www.aafp.org/afp/980700ap/980700b.html.

National Institute of Allergy and Infectious Diseases. "Vaginal Yeast Infection." Available at http://www.niaid.nih.gov/topics/vaginalyeast.

Richardson, Malcolm D., and David W. Warnock. *Fungal Infection: Diagnosis and Management.* New ed. Malden, Mass.: Wiley-Blackwell, 2010.

Stewart, Elizabeth Gunther, and Paula Spencer. *The V Book: A Doctor's Guide to Complete Vulvovaginal Health.* New York: Bantam Books, 2002.

WEB SITES OF INTEREST

American Academy of Dermatology
http://www.aad.org

Centers for Disease Control and Prevention
http://www.cdc.gov

Microbiology and Immunology On-line: Mycology
http://pathmicro.med.sc.edu/book/mycol-sta.htm

See also: Antifungal drugs: Mechanisms of action; Antifungal drugs: Types; Athlete's foot; *Candida*; Candidiasis; Dermatomycosis; Dermatophytosis; Diagnosis of fungal infections; *Epidermophyton*; Fungal infections; Fungi: Classification and types; Fungi: Structure and growth; Jock itch; *Malassezia*; *Microsporum*; Mold infections; Mycoses; Ringworm; Skin infections; Treatment of fungal infections; *Trichophyton*; Vaginal yeast infection.

Prevention of parasitic diseases

CATEGORY: Prevention

DEFINITION

A parasitic disease is a disease caused by a parasite, an organism that feeds off a host (often a human) to survive. Common parasitic diseases include head lice, malaria, toxoplasmosis, giardiasis, and trichomoniasis.

TYPES OF PARASITIC DISEASES

Head lice infestation is an infestation of the hair, eyebrows, and eyelashes by the parasite *Pediculus humanus capitis*. Malaria is an infection of the red blood cells. It is caused by the parasite *Plasmodium*. Toxoplasmosis is an infection that may result in flulike symptoms. It can affect the brain, lung, heart, eyes, and liver. Toxoplasmosis is caused by the parasite *Toxoplasma gondii*. Giardiasis is an intestinal illness caused by the parasite *Giardia lamblia*. Trichomoniasis is a sexually transmitted disease (STD) caused by the parasite *Trichomonas vaginallis*.

PREVENTION

Head lice. Head lice are spread by direct contact with someone who is infested with head lice or by direct contact with infested items, such as clothing, bedding, combs, and brushes. One can take the following precautions to reduce the spread of head lice: avoid head-to-head contact, when possible; avoid sharing combs and brushes; avoid using furniture that has recently been used by an infested person; wash in hot water all bed linens, clothing, and towels that have been in contact with someone who is infested; and vacuum carpeting and furniture used by an infested person.

Malaria. Malaria is spread through the bite of an infected mosquito. There are some prophylactic medicines available that can help keep a person from contracting the disease. Persons who are planning to travel to a country where malaria is prevalent should talk to their doctors about whether or not they need a prophylactic medication, and they should do so a minimum of one month before traveling. Prophylactic malaria medications are not 100 percent effective, so it is important to take other precautions to reduce exposure to mosquitos.

In addition to taking prophylactic medications, one can take the following measures to reduce exposure to mosquitos, which will help prevent the spread of malaria: When possible, sleep in a screened-in room; sleep under mosquito netting when sleeping outdoors; spray clothing and skin with insect repellant that contains NN-diethyl metatoluamide (DEET); and wear long pants and long-sleeved shirts from dusk until dawn, when mosquitos are most active.

Giardiasis. Giardiasis is spread through contaminated water and by direct contact with someone who is infected. There is no vaccination or prophylactic medication for the prevention of giardiasis. However, one can take the following measures to prevent giardiasis infection: Use bottled water when camping or travelling to areas where the water supply may be contaminated; use water purification methods, such as boiling or filtering, before drinking water or before using it to brush one's teeth (when bottled water is not available); avoid raw fruits and vegetables when traveling to areas where the water may be contaminated; wash hands with soap and water before preparing or eating food and after using the toilet or changing a diaper; use an alcohol-based hand sanitizer when soap and water are not available; and use a condom when engaging in anal sex.

Toxoplasmosis. Toxoplasmosis is spread by contact with cat feces or by eating undercooked meat. There is no vaccination or prophylactic medication for the prevention of toxoplasmosis. However, one can take the following measures to help prevent transmission of the disease: Avoid undercooked meats; freeze meat at subzero temperatures for several days before cooking; avoid cleaning a litter box if pregnant; wear gloves when gardening or handling soil; wash hands with soap and water before eating or preparing food, and after handling raw meat; and cover children's sandboxes when not in use.

Trichomoniasis. Trichomoniasis is spread through sexual contact. There is no vaccination or prophylactic medication for the prevention of trichomoniasis. However, one can take the following measures to avoid becoming infected: Abstain from sex, use latex condoms when having sex, and engage in monogamous relationships only with persons who have recently been tested for trichomoniasis.

IMPACT

Head lice infestation is most common among preschool and elementary school children. The Centers for Disease Control and Prevention (CDC) estimates that between 6 and 12 million cases of head-lice infestation occur each year in the United States among children age three to eleven years.

The World Health Organization estimates that in 2008, there were 247 million cases of malaria and close to 1 million deaths from the disease. Most of the dead were African children. According to the CDC, an average of 1,500 cases of malaria are reported each year in the United States.

CDC statistics show that almost 2 percent of adults and between 6 and 8 percent of children in developed countries worldwide are infected with *Giardia*. Those same statistics show that almost 33 percent of people in developing countries have had giardiasis. In the United States, giardiasis is the most common intestinal parasitic disease in humans.

According to the CDC, more than 60 million people in the United States carry the *Toxoplasma* parasite, but most do not develop toxoplasmosis. However, toxoplasmosis is a leading cause of death related to food-borne illness in the United States. Trichomoniasis is the most common curable sexually transmitted disease in young, sexually active women. The CDC estimates that there are approximately 7.4 million new cases of trichomoniasis each year.

Julie Henry, R.N., M.P.A.

FURTHER READING

American Academy of Family Physicians. "How to Prevent Malaria." Available at http://familydoctor.org/online/famdocen/home/healthy/travel/384.html.

Centers for Disease Control and Prevention. "Head Lice: Prevention and Control." Available at http://www.cdc.gov/parasites/lice/head/prevent.html.

Fritsche, Thomas, and Rangaraj Selvarangan. "Medical Parasitology." In *Henry's Clinical Diagnosis and Management by Laboratory Methods*, edited by Richard McPherson and Matthew Pincus. 21st ed. Philadelphia: W. B. Saunders, 2007.

Mayo Foundation for Medical Education and Research. "Giardia Infection (Giardiasis)." Available at http://www.mayoclinic.com/health/giardia-infection/ds00739.

"Trichomoniasis." Available at http://www.webmd.com/sexual-conditions/guide/trichomoniasis.

WEB SITES OF INTEREST

Centers for Disease Control and Prevention
http://www.cdc.gov/parasites

Emerging and Reemerging Infectious Diseases Resource Center
http://www.medscape.com/resource/infections

Microbiology and Immunology On-line: Parasitology
http://pathmicro.med.sc.edu/book/parasit-sta.htm

Partners for Parasite Control
http://www.who.int/wormcontrol

See also: Antiparasitic drugs: Mechanisms of action; Antiparasitic drugs: Types; Children and infectious disease; Developing countries and infectious disease; Diagnosis of parasitic diseases; Emerging and reemerging infectious diseases; Giardiasis; Globalization and infectious disease; Head lice; Hosts; Immune response to parasitic diseases; Intestinal trichomoniasis; Malaria; Parasites: Classification and types; Parasitology; Pathogens; Toxoplasmosis; Treatment of parasitic diseases; Trichinosis; Tropical medicine.

Prevention of protozoan diseases

CATEGORY: Prevention

DEFINITION

A protozoan disease is a disease caused by a single-celled eukaryote known as a protozoan. Protozoa can be classified as amebas, sporozoans, flagellates, foraminiferans, or ciliates. Common protozoan diseases include amebiasis, giardiasis, malaria, trypanosomiasis, and toxoplasmosis.

TYPES OF PROTOZOAN DISEASES

Amebiasis is an intestinal illness. It is caused by the protozoan parasite *Entamoeba histolytica*. Giardiasis is an intestinal illness caused by the protozoan parasite *Giardia lamblia*. Malaria is an infection of the red blood cells caused by the protozoan parasite *Plasmodium*. Trypanosomiasis is an infection of the central nervous system caused by the protozoan parasites *Trypanosoma brucei rhodesiense* and *T. b. gambiense*. Toxoplasmosis is an infection that may result in flulike symptoms. It can affect the brain, lung, heart, eyes, and liver. Toxoplasmosis is caused by the protozoan parasite *Toxoplasma gondii*.

PREVENTION

Amebiasis. Amebiasis is spread through contaminated food or water and by direct contact with someone who is infected. There is no vaccination for the prevention of amebiasis. However, the following measures can help to prevent amebiasis infection: using bottled water when camping or when traveling to areas where the water supply may be contaminated (when bottled water is not available, one should use water purification methods, such as boiling or filtering, before drinking water or before using it to brush teeth); avoiding raw fruits and vegetables when traveling to areas where the water may be contaminated; washing hands with soap and water before preparing or eating food and after using the toilet or changing a diaper (if soap and water are not available, one can use an alcohol-based hand sanitizer); and using a condom when engaging in anal sex.

Giardiasis. Giardiasis is spread through contaminated water or by direct contact with someone who is infected. There is no vaccination for the prevention of giardiasis. However, the following measures can help to prevent contracting giardiasis: using bottled water when camping or when traveling to areas where the water supply may be contaminated (when bottled water is not available, one should use water purification methods, such as boiling or filtering, before drinking water or before using it to brush teeth); avoiding raw fruits and vegetables when traveling to areas where the water may be contaminated; washing hands with soap and water before preparing or eating food and after using the toilet or changing a diaper (if soap and water are not available, one can use an alcohol-based hand sanitizer); and using a condom when engaging in anal sex.

Malaria. Malaria is spread through the bite of an infected mosquito. There are some prophylactic medicines available that can help prevent contracting malaria. Persons who are planning to travel to a country where malaria is prevalent should consult a doctor (a minimum of one month before traveling) about whether or not they need a prophylactic medication. Prophylactic malaria medications are not 100 percent effective, so one should also take other precautions to reduce exposure to mosquitos.

In addition to prophylactic medications, the following measures can reduce exposure to mosquitos and, thus, help prevent the spread of malaria: When possible, one should sleep in a screened-in room; sleep under mosquito netting when sleeping outdoors; spray clothing and skin with insect repellant; and wear long pants and long-sleeved shirts from dusk until dawn, when mosquitos are most active.

Trypanosomiasis. Trypanosomiasis is spread through the bite of a tsetse fly. There is no vaccination; however, there are some measures one can take to reduce exposure to tsetse flies, which will help prevent the spread of the disease: wear long-sleeved shirts and pants in neutral colors, inspect vehicles for flies before entering, avoid bushes where flies may be hiding, and spray clothing and skin with insect repellant.

Toxoplasmosis. Toxoplasmosis is spread by contact with cat feces or by eating undercooked meat. There is no vaccination for the prevention of toxoplasmosis. However, the following measures can help keep people from contracting the disease: avoid undercooked meats; freeze meat at subzero temperatures for several days before cooking; avoid cleaning a litter box if pregnant; wear gloves when gardening or handling soil; wash hands with soap and water before eating or preparing food, and after handling raw meat; and cover children's sand boxes when not in use.

IMPACT

The World Health Organization (WHO) estimates that amebiasis causes more than 100,000 deaths per year worldwide. Statistics from the Centers for Disease Control and Prevention (CDC) show that almost 2 percent of adults and between 6 and 8 percent of children in developed countries worldwide are infected with *Giardia*. Those same statistics show that almost 33 percent of people in developing countries have had giardiasis. In the United States, giardiasis is the most common intestinal parasitic disease in humans.

WHO estimates that in 2008, 247 million cases of malaria worldwide led to the deaths of almost 1 million people. According to the CDC, an average of

1,500 cases of malaria are reported each year in the United States. Approximately 10,000 new cases of trypanosomiasis are reported to WHO each year. However, it is suspected that many cases are undiagnosed or not reported.

According to the CDC, more than 60 million people in the United States carry the *Toxoplasma* parasite, but most do not develop toxoplasmosis. However, toxoplasmosis is a leading cause of death that is related to food-borne illness in the United States.

Julie Henry, R.N., M.P.A.

FURTHER READING

American Academy of Family Physicians. "How to Prevent Malaria." Available at http://familydoctor.org/online/famdocen/home/healthy/travel/384.html. An overview of malaria and its symptoms and prevention.

Centers for Disease Control and Prevention. "Amebiasis." Available at http://www.cdc.gov/parasites/amebiasis/faqs.html. A question-and-answer sheet that includes a definition of amebiasis and information about symptoms, diagnosis, treatment, and prevention.

Chacon-Cruz, Enrique. "Intestinal Protozoal Diseases." Available at http://emedicine.medscape.com/article/999282-overview. This excellent article gives a complete overview of intestinal parasitic diseases.

Mayo Foundation for Medical Education and Research. "Giardia Infection (Giardiasis)." Available at http://www.mayoclinic.com/health/giardia-infection/ds00739. A detailed description of giardiasis that includes a definition of giardiasis and its symptoms, risk factors, complications, prevention, and treatment.

MedlinePlus. "Sleeping Sickness." Available at http://www.nlm.nih.gov/medlineplus/ency/article/001362.htm. An overview of trypanosomiasis, also known as African sleeping sickness, that includes discussion of its causes, symptoms, diagnosis, treatment, possible complications, and prevention.

WEB SITES OF INTEREST

Centers for Disease Control and Prevention
http://www.cdc.gov

World Health Organization
http://www.who.int

See also: Developing countries and infectious disease; Diagnosis of protozoan diseases; *Giardia*; Giardiasis; Immune response to protozoan diseases; Malaria; Malaria vaccine; Mosquitoes and infectious disease; Parasites: Classification and types; Parasitic diseases; Protozoa: Classification and types; Protozoa: Structure and growth; Protozoan diseases; Toxoplasmosis; Treatment of protozoan diseases; *Trypanosoma*; Trypanosomiasis; Trypanosomiasis vaccine.

Prevention of viral infections

CATEGORY: Prevention

DEFINITION

A viral infection is an infection caused by a virus, an intracellular parasitic organism that infects the cells of other organisms. Common viral infections include the common cold, influenza (the flu), chickenpox, and human immunodeficiency virus (HIV) infection.

TYPES OF VIRAL INFECTION

The common cold is an infection of the upper respiratory tract. It can be caused by several different types of viruses. Influenza is an upper respiratory tract infection that is caused by ribonucleic acid (RNA) viruses. Chickenpox is an infection that results in a skin rash. It is caused by the varicella-zoster virus. Acquired immunodeficiency syndrome (AIDS) is a chronic condition that is caused by HIV, a virus that attacks the immune system.

PREVENTION

Common cold. The common cold is spread through droplets in the air or by direct contact with infected surfaces. No vaccine exists for the prevention of the common cold. The best method of preventing the common cold is frequent handwashing, particularly before eating or preparing food.

Another way to help prevent the common cold is to periodically clean with antibacterial wipes common shared surfaces, such as telephones, computer keyboards, refrigerator handles, doorknobs, and toys. A third method for preventing the common cold is to teach children to drink from their own, rather than a shared, drinking glass or cup. A fourth method of prevention is to avoid close contact with people who have a cold or other respiratory tract infection.

Influenza. Influenza is spread through droplets in the air or by direct contact with infected surfaces. The best way to prevent the flu is to get a flu shot (influenza vaccination). The flu vaccine protects against the most common types of flu viruses: seasonal influenza and the H1N1 virus (swine flu). The Centers for Disease Control and Prevention (CDC) recommends that everyone who is six months of age or older be vaccinated, although there are some exceptions.

The following persons should not get a flu vaccine without first consulting a physician: those who are allergic to eggs, have had a previous allergic reaction to the flu vaccine, have Guillain-Barré syndrome, are younger than age six months, and are already sick and who have a fever. (Vaccination is okay after the person is no longer sick.)

In addition to being vaccinated, other preventive steps include frequent handwashing, using a tissue to cover the nose or mouth when coughing or sneezing, periodically cleaning shared surfaces, avoiding close contact with people who have symptoms of a cold or flu, not sharing drinking glasses, and not going to work when sick.

Chickenpox. The best method for preventing chickenpox is getting the varicella (chickenpox) vaccine. The CDC recommends that all children and adults who do not have evidence of immunity to varicella be vaccinated. The CDC defines "evidence of immunity" as any of the following: documentation of two doses of varicella vaccine, blood tests that show immunity, laboratory confirmation of prior varicella disease, a diagnosis of chickenpox or verification of a history of chickenpox from a qualified health care provider, or a diagnosis of herpes zoster (shingles) or verification of a history of herpes zoster (shingles) from a qualified health care provider.

Some people are given the chickenpox vaccine after exposure to help prevent them from contracting the disease. According to the CDC, the chickenpox vaccine is not recommended for persons who are allergic to gelatin, who have a moderate or serious illness (vaccination is okay after the illness), who are pregnant, who are immunocompromised because of illness (such as HIV infection) or treatment (such as chemotherapy) of an illness, who have received blood or blood products within the previous three to eleven months, or who have a family history of immune deficiency.

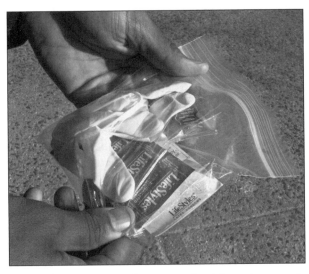

Viral infections such as those transmitted through sex can be prevented with the use of prophylactics, including condoms. (AP/Wide World Photos)

HIV. HIV is a sexually transmitted disease, but it also can be spread through contact with infected blood or from woman to fetus during childbirth. There is no vaccination for the prevention of HIV. The best way to prevent HIV is to avoid exposure to blood or body fluids of people who are or may be infected. One can do this by taking the following precautions: wash hands before and after eating, after using the toilet, and after contact with another person's blood or body fluids; wear disposable gloves when touching anything that may have come in contact with blood or body fluids, including wound dressings; avoid sharing personal items such as razors or toothbrushes; avoid sharing drug needles; and use latex condoms during sex. Health care workers should use universal precautions to avoid exposure to blood or body fluid.

IMPACT

According to the National Institutes of Health, more than one billion cases of the common cold occur in the United States each year. The World Health Organization (WHO) estimates that there are between 3 million and 5 million cases of severe influenza illness each year during seasonal epidemics, resulting in 250,000 to 500,000 deaths.

According to the CDC, before the varicella vaccine was developed in 1995, about 4 million cases of chickenpox occurred each year in the United States, averaging 10,600 hospitalizations and between 100 and 150 deaths. From 1995 to 2005, the United States saw a 90 percent decline overall in the incidence of chickenpox. In 2002, hospitalizations from chickenpox had decreased 88 percent from what they were in 1994-1995. Death rates dropped 66 percent from 1990 to 2001.

WHO estimates that 33.3 million people worldwide are living with HIV infection. In 2009, 2.6 million people were newly infected with the virus, and 1.8 million people died from AIDS-related complications.

Julie Henry, R.N., M.P.A.

FURTHER READING

Centers for Disease Control and Prevention. "Seasonal Flu: What to Do if You Get Sick." Available at http://www.cdc.gov/flu/whattodo.htm. Discusses influenza diagnosis, symptoms, medical treatment, recovery, and emergency warning signs.

Kane, Melissa, and Tatyana Gotovkina. "Common Threads in Persistent Viral Infections." *Journal of Virology* 84 (2010): 4116-4123. Examines how some viruses establish a permanent host relationship and recurrent infection by avoiding immune system actions.

Mayo Foundation for Medical Education and Research. "Common Cold." Available at http://www.mayoclinic.com/health/common-cold/ds00056. A detailed description of the common cold that includes a definition of the common cold and its symptoms, risk factors, complications, prevention, and treatment.

_____. "HIV/AIDS." Available at http://www.mayoclinic.com/health/hiv-aids/ds00005. An overview of HIV and AIDS that includes definitions, risk factors, symptoms, diagnosis, treatment, complications, and prevention.

MedlinePlus. "Chickenpox." Available at http://www.nlm.nih.gov/medlineplus/ency/article/001592.htm. An overview of chickenpox, including causes, symptoms, diagnosis, treatment, prevention, prognosis, and possible complications.

WEB SITES OF INTEREST

Centers for Disease Control and Prevention
http://www.cdc.gov

Universal Virus Database
http://www.ictvdb.org

See also: Antiviral drugs: Mechanisms of action; Antiviral drugs: Types; Chickenpox; Chickenpox vaccine; Common cold; Diagnosis of viral infections; HIV; Immune response to viral infections; Infection; Influenza; Influenza vaccine; Pathogenicity; Pathogens; Transmission routes; Treatment of viral infections; Vaccines: Types; Virology; Virulence; Viruses: Structure and life cycle; Viruses: Types.

Primary infection

CATEGORY: Transmission

DEFINITION

A primary infection is the initial manifestation of a new illness. Primary infections affect people of all ages and can occur in the perinatal period, during which the fetus has not yet formed antibodies and can thus acquire infection. The human immune system responds to infection by building antibodies to a specific illness. These antibodies remain in the person's system.

A primary infection also can cause a cascade of secondary infections, as a new infection predisposes a person to acquiring other illnesses because of that person's now-weakened immune system. Antibiotics and antiviral medications are often prescribed to treat the primary illness; but they are also prescribed to prevent the development of further illness, or secondary infection.

SYMPTOMS

The risk of transmitting an illness to other persons is highest in the period of primary infection. Although everyone is susceptible to new viral and bacterial illnesses, persons at greatest risk for developing a new infection are those who have a compromised immune system. Many primary infections are asymptomatic, but they typically cause more severe symptoms in immunocompromised persons.

Primary infections may lead to lifelong immunity against a particular illness, may predispose a person to future recurrences, or may cause chronic infections. An example of a resulting chronic infection is one caused by the human immunodeficiency virus (HIV). Primary infection of HIV is defined as the first phase of the illness and may last for a few weeks or months.

During this phase, persons are either asymptomatic or develop a rash or flulike symptoms. The infection will eventually enter a different phase, which results in the further progression of disease symptoms.

In contrast, one primary infection that results in recurrent episodes is herpesvirus infection, which includes herpes simplex and varicellovirus. Herpes simplex viruses will recur at sporadic times with symptoms that are similar to those of the initial infection, including oral and genital herpes. Primary varicellovirus infection causes chickenpox, to which the body then develops lifelong immunity. A recurrence, however, can lead to shingles. A primary infection may present differently than recurrent or chronic infections, with some illnesses remaining stable and some becoming progressively more severe.

PRIMARY INFECTIONS IN THE PERINATAL PERIOD

It is clinically important to distinguish between a primary infection and a recurrent or reactivated infection during pregnancy, as certain viral infections pose a risk to the fetus for congenital anomalies and also cause adverse pregnancy outcomes. Examples of viral infections include cytomegalovirus and toxoplasmosis. Pregnant women who have a past infection with these viruses are at a much lower risk of transmitting the illness to the fetus than are those who acquire a primary infection during pregnancy. Women who contract a primary infection during the first trimester of pregnancy are at low risk to transmit the illness to the fetus, but if the fetus is affected, it has a high likelihood of showing significant abnormal findings.

Newborns may also be diagnosed with a primary infection, either during labor and delivery or shortly after delivery. Such an illness is defined as a primary infection of the newborn. With neonatal herpes infection, for example, the risk to the newborn is greatest when a pregnant woman gives birth with a primary infection and during an outbreak of that infection during vaginal delivery.

DIAGNOSIS

Most infections are diagnosed by routine laboratory tests, including blood work, urinalysis, and cultures. However, the primary infection may not be detected immediately after infection occurs because of an incubation period and a conversion period, the time after the initial infection in which the immune system begins responding but has not yet made the antibodies that would be detected through laboratory analysis. For example, a primary infection with HIV leads to rapid replication of the virus and the immune system's subsequent response of a decreased white cell count. However, the HIV antibodies will not be detectable until one to three months after infection. Hence, a delayed detection time might consequently hinder the time to treat, which can be critical.

Serology screening of at-risk pregnant women may be performed to distinguish between a past or primary infection. Additionally, avidity testing may help distinguish a primary from a nonprimary infection for some viruses. Avidity testing measures the length of time passed since a person was first infected.

If a new infection is detected, prenatal diagnosis by amniocentesis is available. This invasive procedure can detect certain fetal infections by polymerase chain reaction on amniotic fluid.

IMPACT

The ability to rapidly diagnose and treat a primary infection is of great clinical importance. As the illness is most contagious during this time, proper education and treatment will allow for infection control. Although public health guidelines have set forth measures for prevention, such as using good hygiene technique, practicing safer sex or abstinence, and encouraging rapid medical care, the amount of primary infections in children and adults remains high and poses a significant health care and economic burden.

Janet Ober Berman, M.S., CGC

FURTHER READING

Crucerescu, Elena, and Diana Rodica Lovin. "Study on Specific IgG Avidity as a Tool for Recent Primary *Toxoplasma gondii* Infection Diagnosis." *Journal of Preventive Medicine* 10 (2002): 56-62.

Khare, Manjiri. "Infectious Disease in Pregnancy." *Current Obstetrics and Gynaecology* 15 (2005): 149-156.

Mandell, Gerald L., John E. Bennett, and Raphael Dolin, eds. *Mandell, Douglas, and Bennett's Principles and Practice of Infectious Diseases.* 7th ed. New York: Churchill Livingstone/Elsevier, 2010.

Pass, Robert, et al. "Congenital Cytomegalovirus Infection Following First Trimester Maternal Infection: Symptoms at Birth and Outcome." *Journal of Clinical Virology* 35 (2006): 216-220.

WEB SITES OF INTEREST

Center for Infectious Disease Research and Policy
http://www.cidrap.umn.edu

Centers for Disease Control and Prevention
http://www.cdc.gov

National Institutes of Health
http://www.nlm.nih.gov/medlineplus/infectionsandpregnancy

See also: Antibiotics: Types; Bacterial infections; Bacteriology; Bloodstream infections; Childbirth and infectious disease; Epidemiology; Fungal infections; Hospitals and infectious disease; Iatrogenic infections; Immunity; Infection; Microbiology; Opportunistic infections; Parasitic diseases; Pathogens; Pregnancy and infectious disease; Public health; Secondary infection; Superbacteria; Viral infections; Virology; Wound infections.

Primates and infectious disease

CATEGORY: Transmission

DEFINITION

Human primates can infect or be infected by nonhuman primates through a complicated and not completely understood process of pathogenic (parasitic, fungal, bacterial, viral) transmission from animal to human or human to animal. The widely similar physiologic and genetic characteristics shared by the two species support a susceptibility that can lead to cross-species transmission.

NONHUMAN-TO-HUMAN-PRIMATE TRANSMISSION

In ancient times, the contamination of humans by nonhuman primates through hunting or the sharing of water carried a threat to humankind that was quite small compared with the relatively recent pandemic of human immunodeficiency virus (HIV) infection, which leads to AIDS (acquired immune deficiency syndrome). Beginning about one hundred years earlier in Cameroon, Africa, HIV was transmitted, in the form of a chimpanzee virus, to the blood of a hunter who butchered the animal and ate its meat. First rec-

ognized in 1981, AIDS has killed more than 25 million people worldwide. No cure exists.

The Ebola virus, although frequently reaching epidemic levels through accidental human contact or through unsanitary medical care, can be traced to individual contact involving hunting, butchering, or eating nonhuman primate bushmeat (meat from forest animals), which also is linked to monkeypox and simian foamy virus. However, the Ebola virus, unlike HIV, cannot establish itself through human transmission and dies after a few cycles.

Transmission also can occur between nonhuman primates and persons who care for them in zoo and related settings. Other persons in danger of infection are those who have nonhuman primate pets.

HUMAN-TO-NONHUMAN PRIMATE TRANSMISSION

As human and nonhuman primates share a pathogenic susceptibility that can lead to the transmission of nonhuman diseases to humans, this same susceptibility promotes the transmission of human diseases to nonhuman primates in the wild. As disease transmission from nonhuman primates to humans portends dire human health issues, the transmission of disease from human to nonhuman primates also exacts a heavy toll on the health of nonhuman primates; ill health also affects animal conservation.

Increased contact between human and nonhuman primates, accomplished largely through the rise in human populations, adds to the number of wild primates eliminated through the deadly diseases transmitted from humans. Poliomyelitis (polio), a human disease, is one of the most lethal to chimpanzees, as is a variant of human paramyxovirus, which causes respiratory diseases in humans and leads to death in chimpanzees. Ebola virus, yellow fever virus, intestinal parasites, and a respiratory virus linked to measles virus, all thought to be of human origin, kill apes. Mountain gorillas are especially vulnerable to respiratory diseases transmitted to them by a growing human population engaged in the habituation of apes for research and ecotourism (such as gorilla watching).

DEFORESTATION AND CLIMATE CHANGE

The shared habitat of nonhuman primates and humans that existed for centuries has changed. Home to wild primates, tropical forests are being destroyed by road-building and logging, for example, which increase the human population and devastate primate

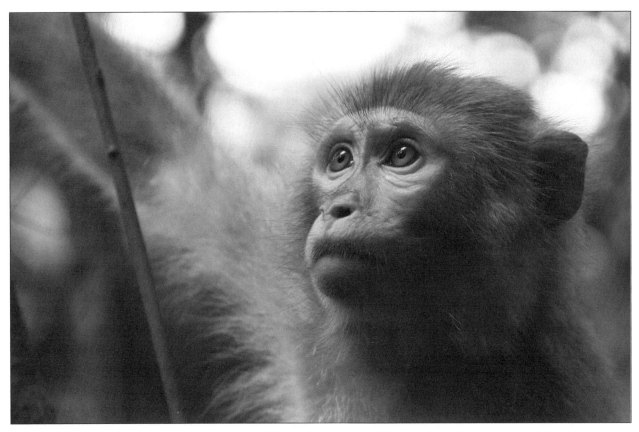

Diseases can be transmitted between human and nonhuman primates, such as this monkey. (©Dreamstime.com.)

populations, degrading the environment and natural primate habitats. The fragmented tropical forests and increased human populations in these habitats have widened the interface between primates and humans, creating increased health risks to both primates and humans.

Aided by these new logging roads, subsistence hunting, which had maintained indigenous peoples for centuries, is being replaced by the business of primate meat export. Hunters now supply bushmeat to local eateries, and primate meat is sold to distributors in cities, where the meat is sold at a premium. Cross-species transmission has become a special concern, as nearly thirty different species of primates are killed, butchered, and eaten. The enormous number of contacts with animal blood and bodily fluids easily promotes disease transmission. Also, widely accessible air travel provides a network of potentially infected persons, who move around the world and infect others.

IMPACT

Understanding the basis of primate transmission of infectious disease allows for the much-needed conservation of wild primates, educating persons about the consequences of butchering and eating primate meat, improvements to the health of primate communities in the grasp of human-made changes in land use (that threatens primate existence), and stopping pandemics before they begin.

Mary Hurd, M.A.

FURTHER READING

Fuentes, Augustin, and Linda D. Wolfe, eds. *Primates Face to Face: Conservation Implications Between Human-Nonhuman Primate Interconnections.* New York: Cambridge University Press, 2002.

Huffman, Michael, and Colin Chapman, eds. *Primate Parasite Ecology: The Dynamics and Study of Host-Parasite Relationships.* New York: Cambridge University Press, 2009.

Nunn, Charles, and Sonia Altizer. *Infectiousness Diseases in Primates: Behavior, Ecology, and Evolution.* New York: Oxford University Press, 2006.

Pedersen, A. B., and T. J. Davies. "Cross-Species Pathogen Transmission and Disease Emergence in Primates." *Ecohealth* 4, no. 4 (2009): 496-508.

Redmond, Ian. *The Primate Family Tree: The Amazing Diversity of Our Closest Relatives.* Buffalo, N.Y.: Firefly Books, 2008.

Romich, Janet A. *Understanding Zoonotic Diseases.* Clifton Park, N.Y.: Thomson Delmar, 2008.

WEB SITES OF INTEREST

American Society of Primatologists
https://www.asp.org

Bushmeat Crisis Task Force
http://www.bushmeat.org

See also: Bacterial infections; Bats and infectious disease; Birds and infectious disease; Cats and infectious disease; Developing countries and infectious disease; Dogs and infectious disease; Ebola hemorrhagic fever; Emerging and reemerging infectious diseases; Epidemiology; HIV; Monkeypox; Mosquitoes and infectious disease; Paramyxoviridae; Parasitic diseases; Pigs and infectious disease; Poliomyelitis; Reptiles and infectious disease; Rodents and infectious disease; Transmission routes; Tropical medicine; Viral infections; Zoonotic diseases.

Prion diseases

CATEGORY: Diseases and conditions
ANATOMY OR SYSTEM AFFECTED: All
ALSO KNOWN AS: Transmissible spongiform encephalopathies

DEFINITION

Prion diseases, also called transmissible spongiform encephalopathies (TSEs), are rare and relentlessly progressive and fatal neurodegenerative diseases affecting both humans and animals. The term "spongiform" refers to the spongelike vacuoles (Swiss-cheese-like holes) found in the cortex and cerebellum of the brain postmortem. In humans, there are sporadic and infectious forms of TSE, the most common of which is

Creutzfeldt-Jakob disease (CJD). Inherited forms are caused by defects in the PRNP gene. In animals, there are forms of TSE affecting sheep and goats (scrapie), deer and elk (chronic wasting disease, or CWD), and the well-known form affecting cattle, bovine spongiform encephalopathy (BSE, or mad cow disease).

CAUSES

TSEs are devastating yet fascinating diseases because they can be caused either by infection or by genetic mutation. However they are acquired, the cause is attributed to the misfolding of the prion protein PrPc, a normal cellular protein found primarily on the surface of neurons in the brain. Misfolding causes the protein to change shape, transforming it into the pathological isoform PrPsc. This isoform constitutes the prion, an infectious agent unlike any other living cell because it contains no genetic material and can transmit disease from cell to cell and from species to species by invading other PrPc proteins and converting them to prions. In turn, the prions invade other PrPc proteins, continuing the process until enough accumulate in the brain and disease sets in. Prions form tiny bubbles inside brain cells, causing them to gradually die off, resulting in a brain full of holes, the hallmark sign of prion disease.

The prion disease scrapie has been known for hundreds of years. (The "sc" in PrPsc stands for "scrapie.") Scrapie can be transmitted either by sheep ingesting pasture infected with prion-carrying placental tissue or by direct sheep-lamb transmission. It appears to be genetic and infectious and can be prevented through selective breeding. No reports of scrapie or CWD being transmitted to humans have ever been recorded.

BSE, the prion disease affecting cattle, captured world attention when an outbreak occurred in the United Kingdom in the 1990's and caused near-panic in the medical community, the food industry, and in the personal care industry, which uses animal proteins in its products. The epidemic peaked in 1993 with reports of one thousand cases per week. First recognized in the 1970's, BSE is believed to have originated from feedstock contaminated with infected products taken from a cow with a sporadic case of BSE and given to cattle, after which BSE spread throughout the United Kingdom.

The primary infectious forms of human prion diseases are sCJD, which accounts for 85 to 90 percent of cases, and the newly identified disease designated

The Discovery of Prions

In 1972, Stanley B. Prusiner, then a resident in neurology at the University of California School of Medicine in San Francisco, lost a patient to Creutzfeldt-Jakob disease, and resolved to learn more about the condition. Prusiner read that it and related diseases, scrapie and kuru, could be transmitted by injecting extracts from diseased brain into the brains of healthy animals. At the time, the diseases were thought to be caused by a slow-acting virus, but that virus had not been identified. Prusiner was intrigued by a study from the laboratory of Tikvah Alper that suggested that the scrapie agent lacked nucleic acid. When he started his own lab in 1974, Prusiner decided to pursue the nature of the infectious agent.

Prusiner and his associates determined to purify the causative agent in scrapie-infected brains. By 1982, they had a highly purified preparation. They subjected it to extensive analysis, and all of their results indicated that it indeed lacked DNA (deoxyribonucleic acid) or RNA (ribonucleic acid) and that it consisted mainly, if not exclusively, of protein. The infectivity was lost when treated with procedures that denatured protein, but not when treated with those detrimental to nucleic acids. He named the agent a "prion," meaning "proteinaceous infectious particle."

Shortly afterward, Prusiner showed that the prion consisted of a single protein. This was a highly unorthodox discovery because all pathogens studied to date contained nucleic acid. Skeptics were convinced that a very small amount of nucleic acid must be contaminating the prion, although the limits on detection showed that it contained fewer than one hundred nucleotides and would have to be smaller than any known virus.

Prusiner and his collaborators subsequently learned that the gene for the prion protein was found in chromosomes of hamsters, mice, humans, and all other mammals that had been examined. Furthermore, most of the time these animals make the prion protein without getting sick–a startling observation. Prusiner and his team subsequently showed that the prion protein existed in two forms, one harmless and the other leading to disease. The latter proved to be highly resistant to degradation by proteolytic enzymes and accumulated in the brain tissue of affected animals and humans.

In infectious disease, the harmful form of the prion appears to convert the harmless form to the harmful form, although the mechanism is not understood. In inherited disease, mutations in the prion may cause it to adopt the harmful form spontaneously or after some unknown signal, leading eventually to the disease state. While questions remain, research since the 1980's has established the involvement of prions in various spongiform encephalopathies.

In 1997, Prusiner was awarded the Nobel Prize in Physiology or Medicine for his pioneering discovery of prions and their role in various neurological diseases. The Nobel Committee also noted his perseverance in pursuing an unorthodox hypothesis in the face of major skepticism.

James L. Robinson, Ph.D.

---

vCJD. sCJD can be acquired either spontaneously for no known reason or acquired externally from prion-contaminated objects, such as neurosurgical instruments, or from infected tissue implants or blood. vCJD surfaced in 1996 and has been attributed to human consumption of BSE-infected beef products. This unsettling consequence of the BSE outbreak occurred at a time consistent with the long incubation periods for human prion diseases. The outbreak generated considerable concern in Europe and the United States because the elusive nature of the infectious agent and the known latency period made it nearly impossible to accurately assess the threat and predict the number of cases. vCJD and kuru, an obscure prion disease caused by cannibalism, are acquired prion diseases.

Despite being genetic, the inherited prion diseases are nonetheless infectious, although not in the tradi-

tional sense; rather, they are infectious on the basis of a protein-only hypothesis of infectivity proposed by scientists. The rationale is that the misfolding of the prion protein itself is sufficient to generate the infectious agent. Mutations associated with familial prion disease produce infectivity by generating a self-templating form of the protein that increases the likelihood of repeated misfolding events. Familial CJD, Gerstmann-Sträussler-Scheinker syndrome, and fatal familial insomnia are inherited forms of prion disease.

RISK FACTORS

The risk of anyone contracting CJD is extremely low, but it increases with age. In sCJD, the overall rate is 1 to 2 per one million people; for persons age fifty years and older, the rate is 3 to 4 per one million people. Fewer than three hundred cases are reported each year in the United States. In familial forms, age of onset varies according to type of mutation. People at risk for acquired vCJD are those who have had exposure to British beef products or who have had a transfusion exposure to bovine insulin.

Symptoms

Although clinical symptoms may vary somewhat, prion diseases all involve progressive loss of brain function leading to death, characterized by irreversible dementia and ataxia with worsening cognitive, neuropsychiatric, and motor dysfunction. When symptoms become visible, death is imminent. Before succumbing, patients are in a state of global cognitive dysfunction, urinary incontinence, profound ataxia, and complete dependency; just before death, they are bedridden, rigid, unable to speak, and totally unresponsive.

Screening and Diagnosis

The presence of the misfolded prion protein constitutes a definitive diagnosis of prion diseases. This diagnosis can be made only postmortem (at autopsy), when deposits of PrPsc and spongelike vacuoles and neuronal loss (and occasionally Alzheimer's-like amyloid plaques) are observed in the brain after death. Clinical symptoms and characteristics of neural lesions vary somewhat between different prion diseases. For instance, vCJD can be distinguished from CJD by clinical presentation (painful sensory disturbance or psychiatric symptoms), cerebral imaging, and neuropathologic changes. The clinical course of other acquired CJDs depends on the mode of infection. Diagnostic criteria for sCJD include rapidly progressive dementia; myoclonus (electrical-shock-type movements), which occurs in 80 percent of cases; and a characteristic periodic electroencephalogram.

Treatment and Therapy

No viable treatment or therapy exists for prion diseases. The median survival period for sCJD is four to six months; for vCJD, it is thirteen to fourteen months. Although there is no known cure for these diseases, scientists around the world are working to develop treatments. Hundreds of candidate molecules that may be able to prevent the formation of the abnormal prion protein have been identified and are being studied in animals.

Prevention and Outcomes

The U.S. Food and Drug Administration has taken preventive steps to minimize the risk of acquired prion diseases, stating that these safety measures should be sufficient to eliminate prion infection. A TSE-specific advisory committee has been set up to review and evaluate available scientific data concerning the safety of at-risk products. In May, 2010, the committee issued a revised industry guide with preventive measures for CJD and vCJD. Finally, the inherited forms of prion diseases cannot be prevented.

Barbara Woldin, B.S.

Further Reading

Mead, Simon, Sarah Tabrizi, and John Collinge. "Prion Diseases of Humans and Animals." In *Infectious Diseases*, edited by Jon Cohen, Steven Opal, and William Powderly. 3d ed. St. Louis, Mo.: Mosby/Elsevier, 2010. Discusses the types of TSE, its epidemiology, and its pathology.

Prusiner, Stanley B. "The Prion Diseases." *Scientific American* 272, no. 1 (January, 1995): 48-57.

_____, ed. *Prion Biology and Diseases*. 2d ed. Cold Spring Harbor, N.Y.: Cold Spring Harbor Laboratory Press, 2004. Two important sources on prion diseases.

Ridley, Rosalind M., and Harry F. Baker. *Fatal Protein: The Story of CJD, BSE, and Other Prion Diseases*. New York: Oxford University Press, 1998. An intriguing, comprehensive account of all aspects of prion diseases, written especially for nonspecialists.

Safar, J. R., et al. "Diagnosis of Human Prion Disease." *Proceedings of the National Academy of Science* 102 (2005): 3501-3506.

Spencer, Charlotte A. *Mad Cows and Cannibals: A Guide to the Transmissible Spongiform Encephalopathies*. Upper Saddle River, N.J.: Prentice Hall, 2004.

Yam, Philip. *The Pathological Protein: Mad Cow, Chronic Wasting, and Other Deadly Prion Diseases*. New York: Copernicus Books/Springer, 2003. This book's story format weaves a fascinating tale of prion disease horrors without sacrificing scientific data.

Web Sites of Interest

Centers for Disease Control and Prevention
http://www.cdc.gov/ncidod/dvrd/prions

Creutzfeldt-Jakob Disease Foundation
http://www.cjdfoundation.org

Genetic and Rare Diseases Information Center
http://rarediseases.info.nih.gov/gard

National Institute of Allergy and Infectious Diseases
http://www.niaid.nih.gov/topics/prion

National Institute of Neurological Disorders and Stroke:
 Transmissible Spongiform Encephalopathies
http://www.ninds.nih.gov/disorders/tse

National Organization for Rare Disorders
http://www.rarediseases.org

National Prion Disease Pathology Surveillance Center
http://www.cjdsurveillance.com

See also: Creutzfeldt-Jakob disease; Encephalitis; Fatal familial insomnia; Food-borne illness and disease; Gerstmann-Sträussler-Scheinker syndrome; Guillain-Barré syndrome; Kuru; Prions; Subacute sclerosing panencephalitis; Variant Creutzfeldt-Jakob disease.

Prions

CATEGORY: Pathogen
TRANSMISSION ROUTE: Blood transfusion, bone marrow, gastrointestinal, gene mutation, contaminated surgical instruments or biologics, tissue transplants

DEFINITION

The prion is an infectious agent resulting from a misfolding event in the normal PrPc prion protein (a normal cellular membrane protein found in the brain), whereby the alpha-helix structure of PrPc is transformed into a beta-sheet structure, forming PrPsc. This pathogenic (disease-causing) isomer is responsible for causing a group of rare, universally fatal neurodegenerative disorders affecting both humans and animals.

According to the International Code of Virus Classification and Nomenclature, prions are not classified as viruses but are assigned an arbitrary classification, one that seems useful to workers in particular fields. According to the International Committee of Tax-

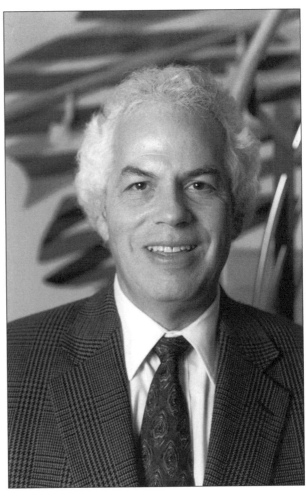

Stanley B. Prusiner. (AP/Wide World Photos)

onomy of Viruses, prions are classified as subviral agents/satellites.

NATURAL HABITAT AND FEATURES

PrPc was discovered by neurologist and biochemist Stanley B. Prusiner, who won the Nobel Prize in Physiology or Medicine in 1997 for his work in this area. He coined the term "prion" some twenty years after researchers had proposed that an aberrant form of a host protein could be the infectious agent in scrapie, a long-known and fatal disease affecting sheep.

PrPc is anchored to a glycolipid linker molecule, then synthesized in the rough endoplasmic reticulum (the "cellular assembly plant"); it then crosses the Golgi apparatus (distribution organelle) and is dispersed throughout the plasma membrane onto the surface of neurons. Though most PrPc remains concentrated in lipid rafts, some is transported to pitlike areas coated with cell-adhesion cadherins, engulfed by endocytic vesicles, and then recycled. PrPc has 209 amino acids and one disulfide double bond, a alpha-helix structure at its C-terminal half, and is unstructured at its N-terminal half.

The precise functionality of PrPc is not entirely understood, although its location predisposes it to being a membrane receptor, adhesion molecule, or transporter, and to having a role in cell-to-cell communication and synaptic function. PrPc appears to be neuroprotective and is protease sensitive (receptive to enzyme breakdown).

As an isomer, PrPsc is chemically identical to its parent protein PrPc but differs in conformation. (In inherited PrPsc, its amino acid sequencing also differs.) Misfolding of PrPc is thought to begin in postsynaptic membranes. On conversion, most of the alpha-helix structure of the host is lost to a large beta-helix that forms and then converts to fibrils (lengths) of beta sheets. This misfolded conformation, the beta-sheet model, constitutes the PrPsc molecule.

The infectious portion of the molecule, designated rPrPsc, is protease-resistant and able to form larger-order aggregates. rPrPsc is thought to propagate by polymerizing and forming amyloidlike fibrils within neurons that deposit as stable aggregates in plasma membranes, inducing conversion of more PrPc. This continuing process causes eventual death to neurons, which are overcome by accumulating aggregates and replaced with large vacuoles (holes).

PrPsc propagation and infectivity pathways are not fully elucidated, leading to much debate over exact mechanisms. The protein-only hypothesis proposed by Prusiner has long been held by scientists as the most plausible theory. This hypothesis maintains that rPrPsc is both toxic and infectious because it is insoluble and forms aggregates that interfere with nerve-cell function. The aggregates break down to release fragments, or "seeds," that become conformational templates for other prion proteins to adopt. Protein misfolding cyclic amplification, a process using in vitro purified misfolded protein, supports Prusiner's theory. Other interesting theories have been postulated, but the complex nature of the prion protein and the mechanisms of its infectivity remain elusive.

PATHOGENICITY AND CLINICAL SIGNIFICANCE

Collectively, prion diseases are a group of transmissible spongiform encephalopathies (TSEs) that affect mammals. They are characterized by the spongelike vacuoles (hence, the term "spongiform") found in the cortex and cerebellum of the brain postmortem and are the hallmark signs of TSE disease.

Among the best-known TSEs are scrapie, bovine spongiform encephalopathy (BSE, or mad cow disease), and Creutzfeldt-Jacob disease (CJD). Scrapie (the sc in PrPsc stands for "scrapie") is transmitted by ingestion of infected pasture or transmitted directly from sheep to lamb. Scrapie appears to be genetic and infectious. Chronic wasting disease (CWD) is a TSE that affects deer and elk. No incidence of scrapie or CWD being transmitted to humans has ever been reported.

BSE acquired notoriety in the 1990's when an outbreak occurred in the United Kingdom; up to one thousand cases were reported at its peak, leading to public outcry and political repercussions. First recognized in the 1970's, BSE is believed to have spread from the practice of feeding cattle meat-and-bone meal, which at some point became contaminated with by-products taken from an infected animal.

A chilling consequence of the BSE outbreak was the transmission of the disease to humans. In 1996, a variant of classic CJD (called vCJD) was identified and linked to human consumption of BSE-infected beef products. The link was made because the timing of the outbreak was consistent with known incubation periods for human forms of TSE. European and U.S. authorities were especially concerned because they were unable to make predictions about disease prevalence or incidence.

Prion diseases in humans can be acquired or inherited. There are three types of CJD: sporadic (sCJD), variant (vCJD), and familial (CJD). The sporadic or classic form occurs spontaneously for no known reason or is transmitted by prion-contaminated materials (such as neurosurgical instruments, tissue implants, and blood). A disease called kuru is also an acquired form of prion disease. Kuru was spread by New Guineans who practiced cannibalism until the 1950's. Its long incubation period meant that cases were still being reported up to the 1990's.

Inherited forms of TSE include familial CJD, Gerstmann-Sträussler-Scheinker syndrome (GSS), and fatal familial insomnia (FFI) and are caused by defects in the PrNP gene encoding the prion protein. Twenty such mutations have been identified, involving either amino acid substitutions or repeats of a twenty-four-base pair segment.

GSS is caused by mutations at codons 102, 117, or 198, and is characterized by progressive cerebellar dysfunction (worsening ataxia, motor problems, and dementia). GSS does not usually become symptomatic until the person is age forty to fifty years, and it lasts for several years before death.

FFI is caused by a mutation of asparagine for aspartate at codon 178. Patients have intractable insomnia and lack REM (rapid eye movement) sleep and have sympathetic hyperactivity and other characteristics of CJD.

DRUG SUSCEPTIBILITY

There is no cure for TSEs and no viable treatment. Researchers have identified hundreds of potential inhibitors of PrPsc that may someday reduce infectivity or prevent the onset of disease.

Barbara Woldin, B.S.

FURTHER READING

Bosque, Patrick J., and Kenneth L. Tyler. "Prions and Prion Diseases of the Central Nervous System (Transmissible Neurodegenerative Diseases)." In *Mandell, Douglas, and Bennett's Principles and Practice of Infectious Diseases*, edited by Gerald L. Mandell, John F. Bennett, and Raphael Dolin. 7th ed. New York: Churchill Livingstone/Elsevier, 2010. This chapter describes both human and animals forms of TSE and their modes of transmission.

Caughey, Byron. "Prion Protein Conversions: Insight into Mechanisms, TSE Transmission Barriers, and Strains." *British Medical Bulletin* 66 (2003): 109-120. A thorough, expert analysis of prion chemistry.

Mead, Simon, Sarah Tabrizi, and John Collinge. "Prion Diseases of Humans and Animals." In *Infectious Diseases*, edited by Jon Cohen, Steven Opal, and William Powderly. 3d ed. St. Louis, Mo.: Mosby/Elsevier, 2010. Discusses the types of TSE, its epidemiology, and its pathology.

Prusiner, Stanley B. "The Prion Diseases." *Scientific American* 272, no. 1 (January, 1995): 48-57. Prusiner's landmark work on prions and associated diseases.

_____, ed. *Prion Biology and Diseases*. 2d ed. Cold Spring Harbor, N.Y.: Cold Spring Harbor Laboratory Press, 2004. A comprehensive text on the biology of prions and prion diseases.

Rowland, Lewis P., and Timothy A. Pedley, eds. *Merritt's Textbook of Neurology*. 12th ed. Philadelphia: Lippincott Williams & Wilkins, 2010. An essential text for studies of neurological disorders, including those caused by prion diseases.

Sadowski, Martin, Ashok Verma, and Thomas Wisniewski. "Infections of the Nervous System: Prion Diseases." In *Neurology in Clinical Practice*, edited by Walter G. Bradley et al. 5th ed. Philadelphia: Butterworth Heinemann/Elsevier, 2008. This chapter covers types of prion diseases, epidemiology, pathogenesis, and more. Relatively technical.

WEB SITES OF INTEREST

Centers for Disease Control and Prevention
http://www.cdc.gov/ncidod/dvrd/prions

Creutzfeldt-Jakob Disease Foundation
http://www.cjdfoundation.org

Genetic and Rare Diseases Information Center
http://rarediseases.info.nih.gov/gard

National Institute of Allergy and Infectious Diseases
http://www.niaid.nih.gov/topics/prion

National Institute of Neurological Disorders and Stroke, Transmissible Spongiform Encephalopathies Information Page
http://www.ninds.nih.gov/disorders/tse

National Organization for Rare Disorders
http://www.rarediseases.org

National Prion Disease Pathology Surveillance Center
http://www.cjdsurveillance.com

See also: Creutzfeldt-Jakob disease; Diagnosis of prion diseases; Encephalitis; Fatal familial insomnia; Gerstmann-Sträussler-Scheinker syndrome; Immune response to prion diseases; Kuru; Pathogens; Prion diseases; Subacute sclerosing panencephalitis; Treatment of prion diseases; Variant Creutzfeldt-Jakob disease; Vertical disease transmission.

Progressive multifocal leukoencephalopathy

CATEGORY: Diseases and conditions
ANATOMY OR SYSTEM AFFECTED: Brain, central nervous system
ALSO KNOWN AS: Progressive multifocal leukodystrophy

DEFINITION

Progressive multifocal leukoencephalopathy (PML) is a rare subacute disease characterized by a widespread loss of myelin, the fatty material that covers nerve fibers in the white matter of the nervous system. Seen almost exclusively in persons with defective cellular immunity, PML causes multifocal neurologic deficits and has in most cases a fatal course.

CAUSES

The disorder results from the reactivation, in immunocompromised persons, of the JC virus (JCV). This ubiquitous human polyomavirus is typically acquired during childhood and remains latent in the kidneys and possibly other sites. It is unclear whether PML develops when a virus residing in the brain is reactivated or when the activated virus seeds the nervous system through white blood cells or in free form.

In the brain, glial cells support viral replication. The reactivated virus has an affinity for oligodendrocytes, the cells that produce myelin, and presumably destroys them.

RISK FACTORS

Most persons with PML have impaired cell-mediated immunity because of acquired immunodeficiency syndrome (AIDS), the most common risk factor, or other conditions (such as leukemia, lymphoma, sarcoidosis, and Wiskott-Aldrich syndrome). In AIDS, the risk increases with increasing human immunodeficiency virus (HIV) loads.

Rarely, PML occurs as a complication of chemotherapy, monoclonal antibody therapy (natalizumab, rituximab) for disorders such as multiple sclerosis and Crohn's disease, or antirejection medication (tacrolimus, mycophenolate mofetil) in transplant recipients.

SYMPTOMS

Because of the high variability in lesion localization and extent, clinical manifestations are diverse and insidious. Clumsiness may appear early. Cognitive impairment, aphasia, hemiparesis, weakness, and visual disturbances occur frequently. Cerebellar and brain stem deficits may be present. The disease progresses gradually and relentlessly. For 80 percent of affected persons, the disease culminates in death within nine months of onset. Spontaneous recovery, however, has been reported.

SCREENING AND DIAGNOSIS

The disorder is suspected in persons with unexplained progressive brain dysfunction, especially in those with impaired cell-mediated immunity. Provisional diagnosis is made by contrast-enhanced magnetic resonance imaging (MRI), which shows single or multiple white-matter lesions. Cerebrospinal fluid is analyzed for JCV antigen using polymerase chain reaction (PCR) amplification. A positive result, corroborated with compatible neuroimaging findings, is nearly pathognomonic. Pathologic examination of brain biopsy provides a definitive diagnosis. The biopsy will show multiple areas of myelin loss (demyelination), mostly in the subcortical white matter but also in the cerebellum, brainstem, and spinal cord.

TREATMENT AND THERAPY

No established treatment exists for PML. Providing supportive care and, if possible, improving immune function are essential.

Antivirals have failed to provide significant benefit. In persons with AIDS, however, highly active antiretroviral therapy (HAART) has improved outcomes and survival rates. Immune modulating (or immunomodulatory) agents such as interferon-alpha have been used experimentally, with promising results. Withdrawal of immunosuppressants or removal of monoclonal antibody by plasma exchange may also result in clinical improvement.

PREVENTION AND OUTCOMES

Timely initiation of HAART therapy and judicious use of immunomodulatory medication constitute important prophylactic measures. Several studies have reported that certain antipsychotic drugs block JCV entry into the cell and may prevent PML development.

Mihaela Avramut, M.D., Ph.D.

FURTHER READING

Antinori, A., A. Cingolani, and P. Lorenzini. "Clinical Epidemiology and Survival of Progressive Multifocal Leukoencephalopathy in the Era of Highly Active Antiretroviral Therapy." *Journal of Neurovirology* 9 (2003): 47-53.

Bradley, Walter G., et al., eds. *Neurology in Clinical Practice*. 5th ed. Philadelphia: Butterworth Heinemann/Elsevier, 2007.

Jubelt, Burk. "Progressive Multifocal Leukoencephalopathy." In *Merritt's Neurology*, edited by Lewis P. Rowland. 11th ed. Philadelphia: Lippincott Williams & Wilkins, 2005.

Marzocchetti, A., et al. "Determinants of Survival in Progressive Multifocal Leukoencephalopathy." *Neurology* 73 (2009): 1551-1558.

WEB SITES OF INTEREST

Genetic and Rare Diseases Information Center
http://rarediseases.info.nih.gov/gard

National Institute of Neurological Disorders and Stroke
http://www.ninds.nih.gov/disorders/pml

See also: Acute cerebellar ataxia; AIDS; Bacterial meningitis; Creutzfeldt-Jakob disease; Encephalitis; Encephalitis vaccine; Gerstmann-Sträussler-Scheinker syndrome; Guillain-Barré syndrome; Opportunistic infections; Poliomyelitis; Subacute sclerosing panencephalitis; Viral infections.

Prostatitis

CATEGORY: Diseases and conditions
ANATOMY OR SYSTEM AFFECTED: Genitourinary tract, glands, reproductive system
ALSO KNOWN AS: Prostadynia

DEFINITION

Prostatitis is inflammation of the prostate gland. The prostate is a walnut-sized gland in males that surrounds the urethra. The prostate produces a fluid that is part of semen.

There are four types of prostatitis: categories 1 through 4. Category 1, or acute bacterial, is the least common of the four types but is the most common in

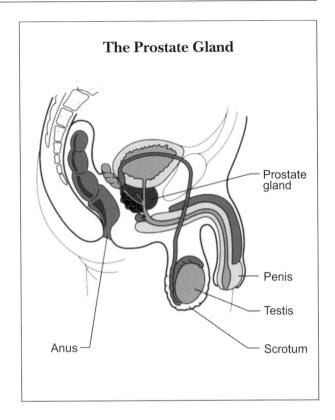

The Prostate Gland

Prostate gland

Penis

Testis

Scrotum

Anus

men age thirty-five years and younger. Category 2, or chronic bacterial, is not common but affects mostly men between the ages of forty and seventy years. Category 3, or chronic nonbacterial/prostadynia, is the most common type and causes chronic pelvic pain, or prostadynia. (Prostadynia is also known as chronic pelvic pain syndrome, or CPPS, a condition that has similar symptoms to those of chronic nonbacterial prostatitis. However, CPPS has no evidence of prostatic inflammation.) The final type of prostatitis is category 4, or asymptomatic inflammatory prostatitis.

CAUSES

Acute and some chronic bacterial prostatitis are caused by bacteria that infect the prostate gland. The bacteria usually come from the urinary tract or rectum. The causes of nonbacterial prostatitis can be difficult to identify, but some believe it may be caused by pathogens such as *Mycoplasma*, *Chlamydia*, a virus, or a fungus.

The causes of prostadynia can be even more difficult to identify. However, the condition can be associated with stress or disorders (or both) of pelvic floor muscle tension or conditions such as interstitial cystitis. Asymptomatic inflammatory prostatitis is found during a prostate biopsy. The cause is not clearly understood.

RISK FACTORS

Risk factors include medical procedures that involve inserting a catheter or other tubing into the urethra or rectum; anal intercourse; a recent bladder infection; abnormalities in the anatomy of the urinary tract; diabetes; a suppressed immune system; and obstruction of the bladder, such as by a tumor, a kidney stone, or an enlarged prostate gland.

SYMPTOMS

Symptoms of prostatitis can appear slowly or suddenly, and they can be mild or quite severe. In nonbacterial prostatitis, symptoms often come and go. Symptoms may include needing to urinate frequently or urgently, or both, especially at night; pain or burning while urinating; difficulty urinating; blood in the urine; psychological stress; lower abdominal pain or pressure; rectal or perineal discomfort; lower back pain; fever or chills; painful ejaculation; and impotence, because of inflammation around the gland.

SCREENING AND DIAGNOSIS

A doctor will ask about symptoms and medical history and will perform a physical exam. Diagnosis of prostatitis is usually based on the symptoms and on massaging the prostate gland. In this test, the doctor places a lubricated, gloved finger into the rectum to feel the back wall of the prostate. In prostatitis, the prostate is usually tender and soft. Other tests include bladder function tests and an analysis of urine and prostate fluid expressed after massaging the prostate gland.

TREATMENT AND THERAPY

Treatment depends on the type of prostatitis. Acute bacterial prostatitis is treated with oral antibiotics for one to two weeks. The commonly used drugs include quinolones (norfloxacin, ciprofloxacin, and levofloxacin) or trimethoprim, and in severe cases, treatment with intravenous antibiotics may be necessary. Chronic bacterial prostatitis is also treated with oral antibiotics, but for four to twelve weeks. Other medications include stool softeners, anti-inflammatory medications, other analgesics or pain medications, alpha-blockers such as Flomax, and 5-alpha reductase inhibitors such as Proscar or Avodart.

For noninfectious prostatitis, patients are often initially given a course of antibiotics in case an infectious cause was missed during diagnosis. Other treatments include alpha-blockers such as Flomax, 5-alpha reductase inhibitors such as Proscar or Avodart, anti-inflammatory medications such as ibuprofen, pain killers, warm sitz baths, and repeated prostate massages.

PREVENTION AND OUTCOMES

There are no guidelines for preventing prostatitis.
Rick Alan; reviewed by Adrienne Carmack, M.D.

FURTHER READING

Komaroff, Anthony, ed. "Prostate Gland." In *Harvard Medical School Family Health Guide*. New York: Free Press, 2005.

Propert, K. J., et al. "A Prospective Study of Symptoms and Quality of Life in Men with Chronic Prostatitis/Chronic Pelvic Pain Syndrome: The National Institutes of Health Chronic Prostatitis Cohort Study." *Journal of Urology* 175 (2006): 619-623.

"Prostate Disorders." In *The Merck Manual Home Health Handbook*, edited by Robert S. Porter et al. Whitehouse Station, N.J.: Merck Research Laboratories, 2009.

Walsh, Patrick C., et al., eds. *Campbell-Walsh Urology*. 4 vols. 9th ed. Philadelphia: Saunders/Elsevier, 2007.

WEB SITES OF INTEREST

National Kidney and Urologic Diseases Information Clearinghouse
http://kidney.niddk.nih.gov

Prostatitis Foundation
http://www.prostatitis.org

UrologyHealth.org
http://www.urologyhealth.org

See also: Acute cystitis; Bacterial infections; Bloodstream infections; Chlamydia; *Chlamydia*; Epididymitis; Gonorrhea; Inflammation; Kidney infection; Men and infectious disease; *Mycoplasma*; Urethritis; Urinary tract infections.

Prosthetic joint infections

CATEGORY: Diseases and conditions

ANATOMY OR SYSTEM AFFECTED: Blood, bones, joints, musculoskeletal system, tissue

ALSO KNOWN AS: Artificial joint infection, infectious arthritis of prosthetic joint, septic arthritis of prosthetic joint

DEFINITION

Prosthetic joint infections are illnesses caused by the contamination of an artificial (prosthetic) joint by an infectious microorganism such as a bacterium or fungus. These infections occur in 0.5 to 3 percent of all cases of joint replacement and are most common in persons with an artificial hip or knee. Infections can occur early in the course of recovery from joint replacement surgery (within the first two months) or much later.

CAUSES

Joint replacement is a surgical procedure designed to alleviate pain and to improve mobility in a person with damaged joints. A surgical team replaces a hip, knee, or shoulder with a prosthetic joint.

Prosthetic joint infections are caused by the growth of bacteria or fungi around a surgically implanted artificial joint. Most often, the infectious organisms reach the artificial joint during joint replacement surgery or from an infected wound after the surgery. These are called local infections and are most often caused by organisms such as coagulase-negative staphylococci, gram-negative bacilli, and *Staphylococcus aureus*. In other cases, the infectious organisms are present elsewhere in the body and travel through the bloodstream to affect the artificial joint. For example, the *Escherichia coli* bacterium that causes urinary tract infection can travel through the blood to infect a replaced hip joint. These types of infections are called hematogenous infections, and they involve a variety of organisms, including *S. aureus*, gram-negative rods, and anaerobes.

RISK FACTORS

An increased chance of becoming affected by a prosthetic joint infection can be related to a number of factors, including personal health behaviors, medical history, surgical conditions during joint replacement, and the healing process following surgery. Per-

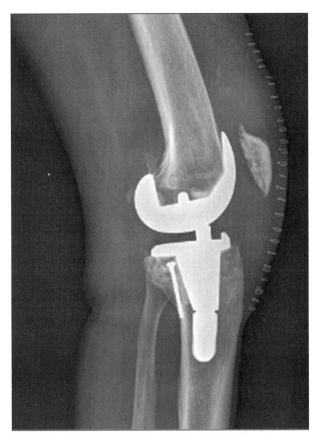

A side-view X ray of a knee fitted with a prosthetic joint. Infection can occur with such prosthetics.

sonal risk factors include a prior infection in the same joint, earlier joint replacement or revision surgery in the same joint, the use of tobacco products, rheumatoid arthritis, obesity, cancer, diabetes, poor nutrition, psoriasis, advanced age, and a weakened immune system. Surgical conditions that increase the risk of prosthetic joint infection include replacement of two joints at the same time and operations lasting more than two and one-half hours. After surgery, the risk for a prosthetic joint infection is increased with complications and other health issues, such as difficulties with wound healing, heart arrhythmia (such as atrial fibrillation), heart attack, and infection.

SYMPTOMS

The most commonly reported symptom of a prosthetic joint infection is joint pain. The pain may be of sudden onset or of more gradual onset. Other general symptoms include fever, chills, joint swelling, redness, elevated white blood cell counts, and drainage from the surgical wound.

Symptoms can vary depending on the timing of the infection, that is, whether infection comes immediately after joint replacement surgery or later. Infections that develop soon after surgery most frequently include symptoms of pain, redness, and swelling at the joint, and drainage from the wound. Later onset infections may have a more gradual onset of pain, without other signs of infection, such as fever or wound drainage.

Other than physical symptoms, further medical studies may reveal evidence of infection. This evidence includes translucent areas (periprosthetic lucencies) around the artificial joint, which can be shown through an X ray, and blood levels that show elevated C-reactive protein, interleukin-6, erythrocyte sedimentation rate, or white blood cells.

SCREENING AND DIAGNOSIS

For joint pain or other physical symptoms of a joint infection, screening tests can be used to suggest the diagnosis of a prosthetic joint infection. Laboratory testing of blood may include analysis for elevated C-reactive protein, interleukin-6 levels, erythrocyte sedimentation rate, or white blood cells. These blood studies are more effective in detecting hip infections but less effective in detecting shoulder or knee infections.

Imaging studies such as X rays can look for signs of infection such as radiolucencies around the prosthetic joint or changes in joint positioning. Other radiology exams include serial radionuclide scans, with agents such as technetium Tc 99m phosphate; a computed tomography (CT) scan; and a magnetic resonance imaging (MRI) scan. However, CT and MRI scans have extremely limited usefulness in the evaluation of prosthetic joint infections because the material that makes up the artificial joint can affect the image quality of the scans. None of these studies can positively diagnose a prosthetic joint infection.

The definitive diagnosis of a prosthetic joint infection can be difficult, but is most often made through a microbiological examination (culture) of tissue or fluid from around the artificial joint or from the joint's surrounding tissues. Obtaining and identifying the infectious organism from fluid or tissue found around the artificial joint often requires invasive procedures, such as joint aspiration or surgery.

TREATMENT AND THERAPY

Treatment for a prosthetic joint infection usually includes a long course of intravenous antibiotics and surgery to remove infected tissue. In many cases, the artificial joint must be removed, likely temporarily, to fight infection. The earlier the diagnosis and treatment of a joint infection are begun, the better the outcome. In an early diagnosed infection, the patient can often be given antibiotics that are tailored to treat the specific infectious agent and also a one-step surgical treatment to replace the infected tissue around the prosthesis. This is a procedure known as DAIR (debridement, antibiotics, and implant retention).

A longer duration infection may require two surgeries: removal of the infected joint (and a period of antibiotic treatment) and, once the infection is controlled, placement of a new prosthesis. In most cases, prosthetic joint infection can be treated and joint function can be preserved; however, in some cases, it is not possible to replace the prosthetic joint. In such cases, surgery to fuse the bones is recommended instead. In all cases, a team of specialists, including orthopedic surgeons, infectious disease physicians, microbiologists, and rehabilitation specialists, is needed for optimal diagnosis and treatment.

PREVENTION AND OUTCOMES

The prevention of prosthetic joint infections is not guaranteed by the use of a particular procedure or device; however, the risk for infection can be decreased. Given identified risk factors, infection risk can be reduced if artificial joint replacement surgery is performed by an experienced surgical team using sterile procedures in a nonemergency setting. Also, evidence shows that administering antibiotics, such as erythromycin, before the procedure decreases the risk of infection.

Dawn Laney, M.S.

FURTHER READING

Johannsson, Birgir, et al. "Treatment Approaches to Prosthetic Joint Infections: Results of an Emerging Infections Network Survey." *Diagnostic Microbiology and Infectious Disease* 66 (2010): 16-23. A large-scale study of infectious disease consultants and their medical management of prosthetic joint infections.
Lentino, Joseph R. "Prosthetic Joint Infections: Bane of Orthopedists, Challenge for Infectious Disease Specialists." *Clinical Infectious Diseases* 36 (2003):

1157. A useful discussion of prosthetic joint infection rates, risk factors, diagnosis, and treatment options.

Mayo Clinic. "Septic Arthritis Fact Sheet." Available at http://www.mayoclinic.com/health/bone-and-joint-infections/ds00545. Discusses joint infections and lists symptoms, causes, complications, and treatment of joint infections.

Peleg, Anton Y., and David C. Hooper. "Hospital-Acquired Infections Due to Gram-Negative Bacteria." *New England Journal of Medicine* 362, no. 19 (2010): 1804-1813. Examines hospital-acquired bacterial infections, including those of prosthetics.

Zimmerli, Werner, Andrej Trampuz, and Peter E. Ochsner. "Prosthetic-Joint Infections." *New England Journal of Medicine* 351 (2004): 1645-1654. A detailed review article about the diagnosis and treatment of prosthetic joint infections.

WEB SITES OF INTEREST

Arthritis Foundation
http://www.arthritis.org

Association for Professionals in Infection Control and Epidemiology
http://www.knowledgeisinfectious.org

National Institute of Arthritis and Musculoskeletal and Skin Diseases
http://www.niams.nih.gov/health_info/joint_replacement

See also: Bacterial infections; Blood-borne illness and disease; Bloodstream infections; Gangrene; Hospitals and infectious disease; Iatrogenic infections; Infection; Osteomyelitis; Pacemaker infections; Secondary infection; Sepsis; Septic arthritis; Staphylococcal infections; Wound infections.

Protease inhibitors

CATEGORY: Treatment

DEFINITION

Protease inhibitors (PIs) are a class of drugs that treat or prevent infection by viruses. They belong to a larger therapeutic category, antiretroviral drugs, and are used primarily to treat human immunodeficiency virus (HIV) infection and hepatitis C.

PHARMACOLOGY

Viruses that are blocked by protease inhibitors are prevented from maturing, infecting, or replicating. Protease inhibitors act on viruses at a very late stage of replication, stopping a cell's ability to incorporate proteins into viral particles.

RISK FACTORS

Protease inhibitors have dramatically improved the life expectancy of persons with HIV and hepatitis C, but PIs have a tendency to interact with other drugs, causing undesirable side effects. There is also a risk of drug-resistant mutated viruses. Persons who take PIs may experience kidney stones, nausea, diarrhea, and abnormal sensations around the mouth. Most of these side effects are not serious and tend to resolve rapidly.

Persons with acquired immunodeficiency syndrome (AIDS) who are taking PIs risk liver dysfunction, including hepatitis B and hepatitis C infections. Excess bleeding and blood clots are rare side effects. Persons taking PIs also report side effects such as high blood sugar, abdominal obesity, high triglycerides, fatty tissue disorders, insulin resistance, sexual dysfunction, and pancreatitis.

TREATMENT AND THERAPY

To reduce the risks of PI side effects and drug resistance, clinicians often implement combinations of drugs. For example, clemizole increases the effectiveness of PIs, enabling them to be used in smaller doses. Physicians have also had some success in treating persons with drug combinations that do not involve PIs. However, the research-based recommendation on this practice is to be cautious about removing a person from PI therapy if he or she has already done well on it. Preliminary studies are underway to see whether PIs might be used to treat cancer.

IMPACT

Pharmaceutical researchers developed the first protease inhibitors between 1989 and 1994. Additional drugs are under investigation, and a series of new PIs have been brought to market for treatment. PIs are the largest class of drugs in the fight against HIV infection. In terms of virology and immunology and clinical and survival issues, PIs offer patients a quality of life that was previously unattainable.

Merrill Evans, M.A.

FURTHER READING

Carr, Andrew, et al. "A Syndrome of Peripheral Lipodystrophy, Hyperlipidemia, and Insulin Resistance in Patients Receiving HIV Protease Inhibitors." *AIDS* 12 (1998): F51-F58.

Centers for Disease Control and Prevention. "Hepatitis C." Available at http://www.cdc.gov/hepatitis/hcv.

John, Mina, et al. "Hepatitis C Virus-Associated Hepatitis Following Treatment of HIV-Infected Patients with HIV Protease Inhibitors: An Immune Restoration Disease?" *AIDS* 12 (1998): 2289-2293.

Kilby, J. Michael. "Switching HIV Therapies: Competing Host and Viral Factors." *The Lancet* 375 (2010): 352.

Moatti, Jean-Paul, et al., eds. *AIDS in Europe: New Challenges for the Social Sciences.* New York: Routledge, 2000.

Villani, Paola, et al. "Antiretrovirals: Simlutaneous Determination of Five Protease Inhibitors and Three Nonnucleoside Transcriptase Inhibitors in Human Plasma." *Therapeutic Drug Monitoring* 23 (2001): 380-388.

Wit, Ferdinand W. N. M., Joep M. A. Lange, and Paul A. Volberding. "New Drug Development: The Need for New Antiretroviral Agents." In *Global HIV/AIDS Medicine,* edited by Paul A. Volberding et al. Philadelphia: Saunders/Elsevier, 2008.

WEB SITES OF INTEREST

AIDSinfo
http://aidsinfo.nih.gov

Canadian AIDS Treatment Information Exchange
http://www.catie.ca

Centers for Disease Control and Prevention
http://www.cdc.gov

Hepatitis Foundation International
http://www.hepfi.org

See also: AIDS; Antibodies; Antiviral drugs: Mechanisms of action; Antiviral drugs: types; Autoimmune disorders; Blood-borne illness and disease; HIV; Immunity; Integrase inhibitors; Maturation inhibitors; Quinolone antibiotics; Retroviral infections; Reverse transcriptase inhibitors; T lymphocytes; Treatment of viral infections; Viral infections.

Protozoa: Classification and types

CATEGORY: Pathogen

DEFINITION

Protozoa are members of an informal grouping of simple, usually unicellular, heterotrophic phyla that share similar characteristics. Some protozoa are pathogenic.

CLASSIFICATION

Traditionally, the kingdom Protista (also known as Protoctista) is made up of simple eukaryotic organisms that do not fit neatly into any of the other kingdoms. Often its members are more closely related to members of other kingdoms than to each other. For many years, this kingdom has been informally divided into three subgroups: the algae, which are photoautotrophs; the protozoa, which are ingestive heterotrophs; and the fungus-like protists, which are absorptive heterotrophs. These informal groupings sometimes break down, as among the euglenids and dinoflagellates, in which there are species that are photoautotrophs, species that are either absorptive or ingestive heterotrophs, and species that can switch between autotrophy and heterotrophy. Most taxonomists agree that the kingdom Protista is artificial (not monophyletic) and should be split into multiple kingdoms.

Like the taxonomy of the protists in general, the taxonomy of the protozoa is continually changing, as more species are subjected to rigorous cytochemical and genomic analysis. All protozoa are nucleated and are considered to be eukaryotic, although some may show both eukaryotic and prokaryotic characteristics. The normal classification hierarchy that starts with kingdom is often not used with Protista. The species are simply placed in taxa according to possible evolutionary and biochemical similarities without labeling the taxa.

CHARACTERISTICS AND HABITAT

Protists can live in fresh- or marine-aquatic habitats, in damp soil, or in other organisms such as parasitic or commensal organisms. All can reproduce asexually, while some, like the alveolates, can also reproduce sexually.

Most excavates reproduce asexually and have flagella, a cytoskeleton of microtubules, modified mitochondria, and a large ventral groove used in feeding. Diplomonads, like *Giardia* spp., have two haploid nuclei, multiple flagella, and a modified mitochondrion, the mitosome, that is unable to perform cellular respiration because it lacks electron transport. All are anaerobic with bacteria-like anaerobic metabolism, and some are parasitic in the guts of animals. The related parabasalids also have a modified mitochondria-like structure called a hydrogenosome. This double membrane structure produces hydrogen as a by-product of the oxidation of pyruvate, much like hydrogen-producing bacteria. Parabaslids also have a prominent Golgi body (or Golgi apparatus) called the parabasal body that is involved in protein synthesis. Parabasalids also have an undulating membrane thought to be involved in locomotion. Many digest cellulose in the guts of termites and ruminants, while others, such as *Trichomonas* spp., are commensal or parasitic in animals.

The euglenoid kinetoplastids have a single large mitochondrion with discoid inner membranes. The mitochondrial deoxyribonucleic acid (DNA) is enclosed in a structure called the kinetoplast. Kinetoplastids also have Golgi bodies and a haploid nucleus. Some are parasitic, such as *Trypanosoma* spp., *Leishmania* spp., and *Chrythidia* spp. Among the nonparasitic kinetoplastids are some of the few colonial protozoa.

Alveolates are recognized by their alveoli, the membrane-bound vesicles just inside the plasma membrane. Almost all have plastids of red algal origin. Among the heterotrophic dinoflagellates are no important human pathogens, although many photosynthetic dinoflagellates produce toxins that can affect humans and other animals. All apicomplexans, formerly called sporozoa, are nonmotile parasites, contain a modified plastid called the apicoplast, produce spores, and have sexual reproduction. The most prevalent protistan disease of humans, malaria, is caused by the apicomplexan *Plasmodium* spp. All ciliates, as the name implies, have cilia, either on the entire surface or clustered in tufts or rings. They also have two types of nuclei, macronuclei and micronuclei, and reproduce both sexually and asexually. All, except for the occasionally pathogenic *Balantidium*, are nonpathogenic.

Amebozoans all have lobe- or tube-like pseudopodia for locomotion and lack cilia or flagella at any stage of the life cycle. Most cannot reproduce sexually. The nucleus has a prominent nucleolar region called the endosome, and many can produce resting stages called cysts. Gymnamebas, like *Amoeba proteus*, are free-living, unicellular amoeba that produce multiple pseudopods. They usually are aquatic and feed on bacteria or detritus. *Entamoeba* spp. are also unicellular, produce a single pseudopod at a time, and are parasitic in animals.

IMPACT

Many protozoa are parasitic pathogens. They cause a number of diseases in humans and exact a huge toll on the peoples of developing countries. The various *Plasmodium* spp., for example, cause the different forms of malaria, a disease that has had a devastating effect on the developing world.

The protozoan *Giardia intestinalis* (also known as *G. lamblia*) causes diarrhea in hikers and backpackers, especially, and *Trichomonas vaginalis* causes vaginitis and urethritis. Trypanosomes are responsible for sleeping sickness (*T. brucei*) and Chagas' disease (*T. cruzi*), and because they can change their surface proteins, they often elude the host's immune system. *Leishmania* spp. most commonly cause cutaneous leishmaniasis, an ulcerative disease of the skin. *Toxoplasma gondii* can be transmitted to humans through cat feces and can cause toxoplasmosis. *Entamoeba hystolytica* is the only major amebic pathogen in humans and causes amebic dysentery.

Richard W. Cheney, Jr., Ph.D.

FURTHER READING

Katz, Laura, and Debashish Bhattacharya, eds. *Genomics and Evolution of Microbial Eukaryotes.* New York: Oxford University Press, 2008. A collection of articles about the modern evolutionary taxonomy of the protists.

Margulis, Lynn, and Michael Chapman. *Kingdoms and Domains: An Illustrated Guide to the Phyla of Life on Earth.* 4th ed. New York: Academic Press/Elsevier, 2009. Describes many protozoa, including their morphology and natural history.

Parker, Steve. *Protozoans, Algae, and other Protists.* Mankato, Minn.: Compass Point Books, 2009. Although written for middle-school students, this book provides good coverage for all general readers studying the basics of protozoa.

Rogers, Kara. *Fungi, Algae, and Protists*. New York: Britannica Educational Press, 2011. A middle- and high-school-level book with broad coverage of protozoa.

WEB SITES OF INTEREST

Catalogue of Life
http://www.catalogueoflife.org

Centers for Disease Control and Prevention
http://www.cdc.gov/parasites

Microbiology and Immunology On-line: Parasitology
http://pathmicro.med.sc.edu/book/parasit-sta.htm

See also: Diagnosis of protozoan diseases; Parasites: Classification and types; Parasitic diseases; Prevention of protozoan diseases; Protozoa: Structure and growth; Tropical medicine.

Protozoan diseases

CATEGORY: Diseases and conditions
ANATOMY OR SYSTEM AFFECTED: All

DEFINITION

The protozoa are a large and diverse group of often-pathogenic organisms that can cause a wide range of diseases in humans. Traditionally, these organisms have been described as single-celled eukaryotic microorganisms, but newer ultrastructural information challenges this uniform classification. The protozoan *Giardia lamblia*, for example, has been found to lack mitochondria and may be a transitional organism somewhere between the prokaryotic bacteria and eukaryotic protozoa.

Common protozoan diseases include travelers' diarrhea, malaria, trypanosomiasis (African sleeping sickness), and vaginitis. These diseases may best be classified by their mode of transmission, the most common of which are enteric, sexual, and arthropodal.

CAUSES

Enteric transmission is generally associated with intestinal illness in humans. Common protozoa that cause intestinal illness include the flagellate *G. lamblia*, the ameba *Entamoeba histolytica*, spore-forming organisms, and ciliates. Diseases caused by these groups begin with the ingestion of contaminated water or with fecal-oral transmission. *Toxoplasma* shares this group's route of oral-fecal transmission, but is not associated with gastroenteritis.

Sexually transmitted *Trichomonas vaginalis* infection is the most common type of pathogenic protozoan disease. *T. vaginalis* causes vaginitis in sexually active women who have multiple partners. Infection in men is usually asymptomatic. The organism survives in moist environments. Trichomoniasis may frequently coexist with other sexually transmitted diseases and may increase the risk of human immunodeficiency virus (HIV) transmission.

Arthropod-borne protozoa include the parasitic flagellate *Trypanosoma*, which is transmitted by the tsetse fly and causes trypanosomiasis. Malaria, the leading cause of death in tropical countries, is caused by four species of the protozoan *Plasmodium* and is transmitted by mosquitoes. Babesiosis is a tickborne illness caused by *Babesia microti*. Symptoms of babesiosis are similar to malaria. Infection with the protozoan *Leishmania* is caused by the bite of an infected sandfly.

RISK FACTORS

Risk factors for enteric transmission of protozoa are poor sanitary conditions and living or traveling to parts of the world where these conditions are endemic. Elderly persons and children may be at increased risk for these diseases. Giardiasis is more common in children than in adults and may be concentrated in child day-care centers. Pregnant women who are exposed to cat feces, undercooked meat, or unpasteurized milk are at increased risk for fetal transmission of toxoplasmosis. People with weakened immune systems are at higher risk from all the spore-forming protozoa. These risk factors include acquired immunodeficiency syndrome (AIDS), renal transplantation, cancer, and IgA deficiency.

The risk factor for tickborne babesiosis is living in areas where ticks are common. In the United States, this includes the coastal areas of New England and New Jersey and the Upper Midwest. The risk of being infected with *Plasmodium*, *Leishmania*, or *Trypanosoma* is directly related to living or traveling in tropical or subtropical parts of the world where these organisms are endemic.

Common Protozoan Diseases and Causal Parasites

Common Name	Scientific Name	Affected Body Part	Prevalence
Acanthamoeba	*Acanthamoeba* sp.	brain, eyes	worldwide
African sleeping sickness	*Trypanosoma brucei*	blood, central nervous system, lymphatic system	sub-Saharan Africa
Babesiosis	*Babesia* sp.	red blood cells	worldwide
Balantidiasis	*Balantidium coli*	intestinal mucosa	worldwide; common in Philippines
Blastocystitis	*Blastocystis hominis*	gastrointestinal tract	worldwide
Chagas' disease	*Trypanosoma cruzi*	blood, colon, esophagus, heart, muscles, nerves	Mexico, Central America, South America
Giardia	*Giardia lamblia*	small intestine	worldwide
Isosporiasis	*Isospora belli*	small intestine	worldwide
Leishmaniasis	*Leishmania* sp.	orifices, internal organs, skin	worldwide
Malaria	*Plasmodium* sp.	red blood cells	Tropical
Rhinosporidiosis	*Rhinosporidium seeberi*	nasopharynx, nose	India and Sri Lanka
Toxoplasmosis	*Toxoplasma gondi*	brain, eyes, heart, liver	worldwide
Travelers' diarrhea	*Dientamoeba fragilis*	lower gastrointestinal tract	worldwide
Trichomoniasis	*Trichomonas vaginal*	female urogenital tract	worldwide

SYMPTOMS

Symptoms of protozoan diseases vary greatly and can range from mild to severe. They can be grouped roughly by mode of transmission. Protozoan diseases that are transmitted by contaminated water or oral-fecal transmission and cause intestinal illness commonly lead to nausea, bloating, anorexia, weight loss, abdominal pain, diarrhea, colitis, and dysentery. Toxoplasmosis infection may cause symptoms of fever, body aches, headache, fatigue, and adenopathy. Infants infected with toxoplasmosis may be born with symptoms including seizures, jaundice, hepato or splenomegaly, and eye infection.

Common symptoms of arthropod-borne protozoan diseases include fever, chills, sweats, headache, myalgia, fatigue, anorexia, and weight loss. The visceral form of leishmaniasis causes symptoms similar to other arthropod-borne diseases. The cutaneous form of leishmaniasis causes symptoms that include skin bumps or nodules that may ulcerate and scab.

Trichomoniasis causes symptoms of copious, watery, vaginal discharge. Vulvovaginal irritation may be accompanied by dysuria, dyspareunia, and abdominal pain. Infection in men is usually asymptomatic but may also result in dysuria.

SCREENING AND DIAGNOSIS

The infected person's medical history and a physical examination are important for diagnosis, but symptoms of protozoan diseases may mimic many other diseases. Laboratory studies, then, are the most important screening and diagnostic tools. For all protozoa-related intestinal diseases, identification of the organism in a stool sample is the definitive method of confirming the diagnosis.

Other laboratory studies that may help in diagnosis include enzyme-linked immunosorbent assay antibody detection, electron microscopy, and polymerase chain reaction. Histology, imaging studies, and endoscopy may be used in selected cases. Diagnosis of arthropod-borne diseases frequently relies on serology, detection of underlying anemia, and identification of protozoa in blood or in a blood smear.

Trichomoniasis is frequently diagnosed by doing a wet mount of vaginal secretions. Immunoflourescent antibody staining and culture are more sensitive, but they could delay diagnosis. Skin scrapings from cutaneous leishmaniasis may be examined microscopically or may be cultured for diagnosis.

TREATMENT AND THERAPY

Treatment for most protozoan diseases requires specific antiprotozoal medication. In cases of intestinal protozoa causing dehydration, intravenous rehydration therapy is an important aspect of treatment. Nutritional status must also be addressed, especially in newborns and infants. Surgery may play a role in cases of necrotizing colitis or amebic liver abscess.

Some medications used in the treatment of intestinal protozoan infections include iodoquinol, paromomycin, metronidazole, tinidazole, quinacrine, furazolidone, tetracycline, nitazoxanide, and trimethoprim/sulfamethoxazole. Toxoplasmosis may be treated with the antimalarial medication pyrimethamine and the antibiotic sulfadiazine. Trichomoniasis responds to metronidazole and tinidazole. Babesiosis responds to quinine sulfate and clindamycin.

PREVENTION AND OUTCOMES

It is not possible to completely prevent the wide spectrum of protozoan diseases. Amebiasis is estimated to infect 10 percent of the world's population. *G. lamblia* is the most commonly isolated parasite in the world, infecting up to 40 percent of children in developing countries. The best hope for prevention is through education and through public heath efforts to provide safe water supplies. Arthropod-borne protozoal diseases may be prevented by avoiding endemic areas, by wearing protective clothing, by using insecticides, by sleeping in screened areas, and, in the case of malaria, by taking medications to prevent infection.

Christopher Iliades, M.D.

FURTHER READING

Chacon-Cruz, Enrique. "Intestinal Protozoal Diseases." Available at http://emedicine.medscape.com/article/999282-overview. This excellent article gives a complete overview of intestinal parasitic diseases.

McPhee, Stephen J., and Maxine A. Papadakis, eds. *Current Medical Diagnosis and Treatment 2011.* 50th ed. New York: McGraw-Hill, 2011. Chapter 35 of this classic reference text gives a complete review of the most common types of protozoan diseases.

Madigan, Michael T., and John M. Martinko. *Brock Biology of Microorganisms.* 12th ed. Upper Saddle River, N.J.: Pearson/Prentice Hall, 2010. A standard microbiology textbook for undergraduate college students, with detailed descriptions of cell structures and clear illustrations. Includes evolutionary perspectives and covers pathogenesis.

WEB SITES OF INTEREST

Centers for Disease Control and Prevention
http://www.cdc.gov/parasites

Microbiology and Immunology On-line: Parasitology
http://pathmicro.med.sc.edu/book/parasit-sta.htm

See also: Arthropod-borne illness and disease; Cholera; Developing countries and infectious disease; Diagnosis of protozoan diseases; Fecal-oral route of transmission; Food-borne illness and disease; Giardiasis; Hookworms; Immune response to protozoan diseases; Intestinal and stomach infections; Leishmaniasis; Malaria; Oral transmission; Parasites: Classification and types; Parasitic diseases; Prevention of protozoan diseases; Protozoa: Structure and growth; Sexually transmitted diseases (STDs); Toxoplasmosis; Travelers' diarrhea; Treatment of protozoan diseases; Trichomonas; Tropical medicine; *Trypanosoma*; Typhoid fever; Waterborne illness and disease.

Pseudomonas

CATEGORY: Pathogen
TRANSMISSION ROUTE: Direct contact, inhalation

DEFINITION

Pseudomonas is a member of the group of pseudomonads, which are gram-negative, rod-shaped, obligately aerobic, bacilli that include similar organisms in the genus *Burkholderia.*

NATURAL HABITAT AND FEATURES

The pseudomonads are commonly found in soil or water, where they play a significant role in the degradation of organic material. In humans, they are part of the normal skin flora and are found in intestinal and respiratory passages; they are generally considered to be harmless saprotrophs. Pseudomonads are distinguished from the enteric bacteria, which they physically resemble (as strictly aerobic and with a non-fermentative metabolism) and because they use the enzyme cytochrome oxidase in their respiratory pathways.

The pseudomonads produce a variety of water-soluble pigments, including the blue pigment pyocyanin and the red pigment pyorubin, and can be easily identified by the grapelike odor many types exhibit when grown on sheep's blood agar. Some species also produce the greenish pigment pyoverdin, which fluoresces in the presence of ultraviolet light.

PATHOGENICITY AND CLINICAL SIGNIFICANCE

Pseudomonas is considered a harmless organism in healthy persons. However, in persons with compromised immune systems, it becomes an opportunistic pathogen. It also becomes a pathogen if introduced into areas of the body that are generally sterile. *Pseudomonas* species, in particular *aeruginosa*, are problematic pathogens in persons with burns and other wounds to the skin. Under these conditions, the production of pigments by the bacterium results in a bluish-green pus.

Infections may be difficult to treat because the organism frequently exhibits resistance to antibiotics. The infection in adults has the potential to become severe, while in infants the danger significantly increases as the organism may pass into the bloodstream.

Aeruginosa is among the organisms commonly associated with nosocomial (hospital acquired) infections, in which bacteria are introduced into the body from respirators or through the use of catheters. The bacteria can develop a mucoid polysaccharide biofilm on catheters. The biofilm protects the bacterial cells from the body's immune defenses. Urinary tract infections too are not uncommon under these conditions, and as many as 15 percent of such nosocomial infections are caused by *Pseudomonas*.

A variety of factors are involved in the pathogenic properties of *Pseudomonas* once it is introduced into the body. Pili, protein extensions on the cell surface, allow the bacterium to attach to tissues. Once the bacterium has begun to colonize, it secretes several types of enzymes that are damaging to the host. These enzymes include an elastase, which is particularly damaging to respiratory epithelium; a cytotoxin, which can damage or kill white blood cells; and several hemolysins, which can break down red blood cells.

Aeruginosa also produces a toxin called exotoxin A, which acts in a manner similar to that of diphtheria toxin. It inhibits protein synthesis in cells that incorporate the toxin. The result is a potentially systemic disease, as the toxin may be released into the bloodstream.

The pigments produced by many *Pseudomonas* strains may also contribute to the potential virulence of the organism. Pyocyanin, a bluish pigment, impairs the normal functions of respiratory cilia and may also damage white blood cells. The pigment may also be modified by the bacterium, allowing it to increase the uptake of iron necessary for the bacterium's replication and growth.

Persons with underlying respiratory disease, such as those with compromised immune systems, chronic lung diseases, or cystic fibrosis, are at particular risk of *aeruginosa* infection. Because these infections are often caused by strains that produce mucoid layers on the bacterial cell surface, they are difficult to treat. Bacteremia and the dissemination of *Pseudomonas* may spread the organism to the heart (causing endocarditis) and to the central nervous system (causing meningitis).

A more common infection is that of otitis externa, an infection of the ear more commonly known as swimmer's ear, which may result from contaminated water. Swimmer's ear also may lead to an endogenous infection because *Pseudomonas* is commonly found among the microbiota already in the ear. Untreated middle- or inner-ear infections have the potential to develop into meningitis. An infection of the eye, keratitis, is less common but may become severe if the immune system has been compromised.

The species *fluorescens* exhibits many of the same features as *aeruginosa*. However, it grows poorly at body temperature (98.6° Fahrenheit, or 37° Celsius) and is rarely pathogenic.

DRUG SUSCEPTIBILITY

Pseudomonas is naturally resistant to most common antibiotics, largely because of its own efflux pumps, which efficiently prevent internalization of such drugs, and because of the type of outer membrane it produces on the surface of the cell. Many strains of *Pseudomonas* also possess resistance transfer factors in the form of plasmids, circular extrachromosomal pieces of deoxyribonucleic acid (DNA), which contain genes that confer the resistance to antibiotics.

These plasmids may also be passed to other bacteria, spreading the danger of antibiotic resistance.

Surface infections such as otitis externa may be treated with polymyxin. However, this antibiotic is too toxic for internal use. Most therapy for *Pseudomonas* infections utilizes combinations of drugs that act at different levels of metabolism. Although *Pseudomonas* is resistant to penicillin, combinations of the penicillin derivative piperacillin, which inhibits cell-wall formation, and the aminoglycoside tobramycin, an inhibitor of protein synthesis, have proven effective. Other antibiotics useful in the treatment of *Pseudomonas* infections include gentamycin, imipenem, aztreonam, and quinolones such as ciprofloxacin. Strains may differ in their susceptibility.

Richard Adler, Ph.D.

FURTHER READING

Brooks, George, et al. *Jawetz, Melnick, and Adelberg's Medical Microbiology.* 25th ed. New York: McGraw-Hill, 2010.

Forbes, Betty A., Daniel F. Sahm, and Alice S. Weissfeld. *Bailey and Scott's Diagnostic Microbiology.* 12th ed. St. Louis, Mo.: Mosby/Elsevier, 2007.

Murray, Patrick, et al., eds. *Manual of Clinical Microbiology.* 9th ed. Washington, D.C.: ASM Press, 2007.

Salyers, Abigail A., and Dixie D. Whitt. *Bacterial Pathogenesis: A Molecular Approach.* 2d ed. Washington, D.C.: ASM Press, 2002.

WEB SITES OF INTEREST

American Society for Microbiology
http://www.microbeworld.org

Todar's Online Textbook of Bacteriology
http://www.textbookofbacteriology.net

Virtual Museum of Bacteriology
http://www.bacteriamuseum.org

See also: Bacteria: Classification and types; Bacterial infections; Disinfectants and sanitizers; Hospitals and infectious disease; Opportunistic infections; *Pseudomonas* infections; Skin infections; Wound infections.

Pseudomonas infections

CATEGORY: Diseases and conditions
ANATOMY OR SYSTEM AFFECTED: All
ALSO KNOWN AS: Pseudomonal bacteremia

DEFINITION

Infections of skin, blood, bones, eyes, ears, the central nervous system, the heart, the lungs, the gastrointestinal system, wounds, and the urinary tract may all be traced to a infection with the bacterium *Pseudomonas*. Ranging from mild to life-threatening, *Pseudomonas* infection rarely affects healthy persons and is often the cause of hospital acquired, or nosocomial, infections. All infections are potentially curable, but infection with *Pseudomonas* is one of the most difficult types to treat. *Pseudomonas* is present in soil and water and also can be found on plants, animals, and healthy persons.

Taxonomic Classification for *Pseudomonas*

Kingdom: Bacteria
Phylum: Proteobacteria
Class: Gamma Proteobacteria
Order: Pseudomonales
Family: Pseudomonadaceae
Genus: *Pseudomonas*
Species:
P. aeruginosa
P. fluorescens

CAUSES

Pseudomonas infections are caused by the gram-negative *Pseudomonas* bacterium. The most prevalent is *P. aeruginosa*. Any body organ or part may be infected with *Pseudomonas*.

RISK FACTORS

Considered an opportunistic bacterium, *Pseudomonas* attacks debilitated persons, often those who are hospitalized or who have a disorder that weakens the immune system. Any break in the skin or the use of any medical device, such as a urine catheter, may provide an opportunity for the bacterium to enter the body and cause infection. Persons with diabetes or cystic fibrosis are at greater risk. Persons with human immunodeficiency virus (HIV) infection or cancer, and transplant recipients, are at increased risk because of their weakened immune systems, usually caused by the drugs they take to treat their diseases.

SYMPTOMS

P. aeruginosa may infect a variety of sites in the body, and symptoms depend on the site involved. External otitis, or swimmer's ear, causes pain and a discharge from the ear canal, whereas malignant external otitis seen in persons with diabetes has symptoms of fever, loss of hearing, and severe pain. Drainage is often seen in eye infections with *Pseudomonas*. Skin infections cause lesions or develop in open sores and may have a green-blue drainage with a fruity odor. Infection of the heart, or endocarditis, comes with a fever, a heart murmur, lesions, and an enlarged spleen.

Diarrhea and dehydration are the most common symptoms of gastrointestinal infections. Pneumonia with fever, difficulty breathing with a rattling sound, and lack of oxygen are symptoms of respiratory system infections. Fever, headache, and confusion are seen in persons with meningitis caused by *Pseudomonas* infection. Bacterial blood infection, or bacteremia, comes with jaundice, fever, rapid breathing, and a rapid heart rate. Lesions may occur with any *Pseudomonas* infection.

SCREENING AND DIAGNOSIS

The clinical site of the infection is cultured to determine the causative organism for the person's symptoms. Blood, wound drainage, body fluids, and tissue are sent to a laboratory for culture to determine the presence of *Pseudomonas* bacteria. Radiology or X-ray studies may show lesions within the body, but cultures are the only way to determine the actual organism causing problems.

TREATMENT AND THERAPY

Antipseudomonal antibiotics in combination are used to treat the infection. Supportive therapy, depending on the clinical condition of the infected person, is used. Hospitalization may be needed if symptoms are severe. Respiratory support, including the use of mechanical ventilation, may be indicated. Finally, the revision of wounds and the surgical removal of abscesses are options.

PREVENTION AND OUTCOMES

Good hygiene is the best prevention against *Pseudo-*

monas infection. Washing food carefully, drinking safe water, not tracking dirt from shoes into living spaces, and handwashing are helpful. In hospital settings, one should avoid the use of catheters, should change bandages often, and should clean equipment (such as ventilators, restrooms, and mops and other cleaning supplies) where moist conditions are commonly found.

Patricia Stanfill Edens, R.N., Ph.D., FACHE

FURTHER READING

Blaser, Martin J. "Introduction to Bacteria and Bacterial Diseases." In *Mandell, Douglas, and Bennett's Principles and Practice of Infectious Diseases*, edited by Gerald L. Mandell, John F. Bennett, and Raphael Dolin. 7th ed. New York: Churchill Livingstone/ Elsevier, 2010.

Salyers, Abigail A., and Dixie D. Whitt. *Bacterial Pathogenesis: A Molecular Approach*. 2d ed. Washington, D.C.: ASM Press, 2002.

St. Georgiev, Vassil. *Opportunistic Infections: Treatment and Prophylaxis*. Totowa, N.J.: Humana Press, 2003.

WEB SITES OF INTEREST

Centers for Disease Control and Prevention, Division of Foodborne, Bacterial, and Mycotic Diseases
http://www.cdc.gov/nczved/divisions/dfbmd

Todar's Online Textbook of Bacteriology
http://www.textbookofbacteriology.net

See also: Bacteria: Classification and types; Bacterial infections; Disinfectants and sanitizers; Hospitals and infectious disease; Opportunistic infections; *Pseudomonas*; Skin infections; Wound infections.

Psittacosis

CATEGORY: Diseases and conditions
ANATOMY OR SYSTEM AFFECTED: All
ALSO KNOWN AS: Ornithosis, parrot fever

DEFINITION

Psittacosis is an infection caused by the bacterium *Chlamydophila psittaci*. This infection causes fever, chills, dry coughing, headache, muscle aches, and sometimes pneumonia.

Causes

Humans get psittacosis from certain birds, including parrots, macaws, cockatiels, parakeets, turkeys, and pigeons. Some infected birds have symptoms such as the loss of feathers, a runny nose or runny eyes, changed eating habits, and diarrhea. Other birds appear well but can still spread the infection to humans. People usually become infected from breathing in dust from the dried droppings or the secretions of birds that are sick. The infection can also spread when a person touches his or her mouth to the beak of an infected bird. Even brief exposure to sick birds can lead to psittacosis. The infection rarely spreads from one person to another.

Risk Factors

Risk factors for psittacosis include owning a pet bird and working in occupations with exposure to birds, including as a veterinarian and as a worker in a zoo, laboratory, or poultry plant, or on a farm.

Symptoms

The symptoms of psittacosis begin one to four weeks after exposure to a sick bird. Symptoms include cough, chest pain, fever, chills, rash, headache, muscle aches, and pneumonia with severe breathing problems.

Screening and Diagnosis

A doctor will ask about symptoms and medical history and will perform a physical exam. Tests may include blood tests to check for the bacterium that causes psittacosis and a chest X ray to look for signs of pneumonia.

Treatment and Therapy

The main treatment for psittacosis is antibiotics, which one should continue taking for ten to fourteen days after the fever disappears. Persons with severe breathing problems may need to be hospitalized for oxygen and for intravenous antibiotics.

Prevention and Outcomes

Preventive measures include avoiding birds that appear to be sick; keeping one's mouth away from a bird's beak; buying pet birds from a dealer with an exotic bird permit; keeping bird cages apart; keeping new birds away from other birds for four to six weeks; and cleaning bird cages, food bowls, and water bowls every day and disinfecting them once a week with bleach or rubbing alcohol. One should take a sick or sick-appearing pet bird to a veterinarian promptly.

Diane W. Shannon, M.D., M.P.H.;
reviewed by David L. Horn, M.D., FACP

Further Reading

American Veterinary Medicine Association. "Psittacosis." Available at http://www.avma.org/pubhlth/psittacosis.asp.

Centers for Disease Control and Prevention. "Psittacosis." Available at http://www.cdc.gov/ncidod/dbmd/diseaseinfo/psittacosis_t.htm.

National Association of State Public Health Veterinarians. "Compendium of Measures to Control *Chlamydophila psittaci* Infection Among Humans (Psittacosis) and Pet Birds (Avian Chlamydiosis)." 2010. Available at http://www.nasphv.org/documents/psittacosis.pdf.

Schlossberg, D. "*Chlamydia psittaci* (Psittacosis)." In *Mandell, Douglas, and Bennett's Principles and Practice of Infectious Diseases*, edited by Gerald L. Mandell, John F. Bennett, and Raphael Dolin. 7th ed. New York: Churchill Livingstone/Elsevier, 2010.

Web Sites of Interest

American Veterinary Medicine Association
http://www.avma.org

Centers for Disease Control and Prevention: Healthy Pets Healthy People
http://www.cdc.gov/healthypets

See also: Avian influenza; Bacterial infections; Birds and infectious disease; *Chlamydophila*; Eastern equine encephalitis; Histoplasmosis; Respiratory route of transmission; Zoonotic diseases.

Psychological effects of infectious disease

Category: Epidemiology

Definition

Acquiring an infectious disease can affect perceptions of health, medical care, and quality of life. Indeed, some persons experience the social and emotional burdens of being sick as worse than the physical illness itself.

Infectious diseases are caused by pathogenic organisms, including viruses, bacteria, fungi, and parasites. Because these diseases are contagious, infected persons face powerful psychological disorders such as generalized stress, panic, posttraumatic stress, and depression. Health care workers face extra challenges in containing outbreaks with techniques such as vaccination or quarantine, which is stigmatizing.

THE PSYCHOLOGICAL SYMPTOMS

People with infectious diseases may experience a variety of depressive symptoms, such as fatigue, slowed motor action, anorexia, drowsiness, muscle aches, cognitive problems, and depressed mood. In studies, depressed mood and neurological impairments were reported by people with viral infections such as the common cold and influenza. People infected with herpesvirus, cytomegalovirus, Epstein-Barr virus, and the human immunodeficiency virus (HIV) also experienced depressed mood and neurological impairments.

Older persons who are HIV-positive are often at risk for social isolation and stress. HIV-positive persons in all age groups grapple with mental illnesses, especially depression. Persons with tuberculosis (TB) face the risks of delayed treatment or refusal of treatment. One study showed that 72 percent of persons with TB were worried, frustrated, or disappointed about their diagnosis, and that 28 percent did not initially believe their diagnosis. Persons also feared spreading the disease to others and feared the economic impact of their illness on their families.

A health-related quality-of-life tool evaluated the health status of those who are HIV-positive, who reported psychic trauma, low levels of social support, and lower quality of physical and mental health. Persons diagnosed with severe acute respiratory syndrome (SARS) reported posttraumatic stress disorder and depression.

THE SOCIAL AND CULTURAL SYMPTOMS

Persons in a tuberculosis study reported that they were afraid to inform employers about their illness, fearing the loss of their jobs. However, persons in the study who received transportation tokens and food vouchers, for example, were more willing to accept a diagnosis of TB; they were satisfied with the treatment and with their overall quality of life.

Another study of persons with tuberculosis found that some perceived respiratory isolation as peaceful; the majority, however, felt lonely, confined, and abandoned. In some cultures, TB is seen as a punishment for sins, with all family members implicated. This study concluded that persons with TB were more likely to accept their disease when cultural acceptance was common.

A study of infant diarrhea in Brazil showed the importance of respecting indigenous beliefs. If families do not trust medical staff, they will avoid treatment. Researchers in Nigeria found that traditional folk remedies were effective in slowing the development of parasites that cause malaria. Medical anthropologists can help break down communication barriers between cultures, in an effort to eradicate infectious disease. This has been most successful in the case of smallpox.

Infectious diseases such as plague and smallpox, along with viral and bacterial infections, have caused more deaths than wars, natural disasters, and noninfectious diseases combined. Because of their magnitude, epidemics of infectious diseases such as measles, influenza, and malaria have led to political, social, economic, and psychological disruptions. The most common contemporary response to epidemic is quarantine, a policy that may inflict psychological, emotional, and financial hardships on persons at risk. Persons under quarantine report feelings of isolation, depression, and posttraumatic stress.

During a SARS outbreak in Toronto, infected persons were quarantined at home, unable to leave or have visitors. They were instructed to wear masks when they were in a room with family members, had to avoid sharing any personal items, and had to wash their hands frequently. All persons quarantined experienced a sense of isolation.

When epidemics are being addressed, government health services should set the right tone in the discussion to gain citizen trust and cooperation. The disease in question should be presented as serious enough to warrant action but not so grave as to cause panic.

IMPACT

The psychological impact of an outbreak of infectious disease can be mitigated by modifying perceptions. Researchers and mainstream practitioners have reached a better understanding of the importance of a person's mental well-being in cases of infectious disease. Disturbances such as stress and depression can be minimized when warnings avoid panic, when treatment appears to be in accord with the person's belief systems, and when there is support from family and community.

Merrill Evans, M.A.

FURTHER READING

Chang, Betty. "Quality of Life in Tuberculosis." *Quality of Life Research* 13 (2004): 1633-1642. A study of the social and emotional burdens of persons with tuberculosis.

Gilman, Sander L. "The Art of Medicine: Moral Panic and Pandemics." *The Lancet* 375 (2004): 1866-1867. A historian looks at the social and cultural effects of infectious disease, focusing on moral panic and pandemics.

Glasser, Jordan B. "Infectious Diseases of Geriatric Inmates." *Reviews of Infectious Diseases* 12, no. 4 (1990): 683-692. This article discusses special risks faced by geriatric prison inmates with infectious diseases. These risks include depression, disorientation, and communication problems.

Hawryluck, Laura, et al. "SARS Control and Psychological Effects of Quarantine, Toronto, Canada." *Emerging Infectious Diseases* 10, no. 7 (2004): 1206-1212. An exploration of the benefits and adverse effects of using quarantine to control infectious disease.

Inhorn, Marcia C., and Peter J. Brown. "The Anthropology of Infectious Disease." *Annual Review of Anthropology* 19 (1990): 89-117. The role of infectious disease in human evolution, as examined by medical anthropologists.

Lovallo, William R. *Stress and Health: Biological and Physiological Interactions.* Thousand Oaks, Calif.: Sage, 2005. Explains links between stress, health, and disease, with attention to psycho-physiological response of the body to stress.

Perez, Isabel Ruiz, et al. "No Difference in Quality of Life Between Men and Women Undergoing HIV Antiretroviral Treatment: Impact of Demographic, Clinical, and Psychosocial Factors." *AIDS Care* 21, no. 8 (2009): 943-952. This research study concludes that social support is vital for sustaining health-related quality of life.

Wu, Ping, et al. "The Psychological Impact of the SARS Epidemic on Hospital Employees in China: Exposure, Risk Perception, and Altruistic Accep-

tance of Risk." *Canadian Journal of Psychiatry* 54, no. 5 (2009): 302-312. A discussion of the adverse effects of quarantine.

Yirmiya, R., et al. "Illness, Cytokines, and Depression." *Annals of the New York Academy of Sciences* 917 (2000): 478-487. A discussion of infectious diseases that are often associated with depressive symptoms.

WEB SITES OF INTEREST

American Psychological Association, Health Psychology
http://www.health-psych.org

National Institute of Mental Health
http://www.nimh.nih.gov

See also: Aging and infectious disease; Centers for Disease Control and Prevention (CDC); Children and infectious disease; Contagious diseases; Epidemiology; Infection; Men and infectious disease; National Institutes of Health; Outbreaks; Public health; Quarantine; Schools and infectious disease; Social effects of infectious disease; Stress and infectious disease; Women and infectious disease.

Pubic lice. *See* Crab lice.

Public health

CATEGORY: Prevention

DEFINITION

Public health is a practice that focuses on the promotion of physical, mental, and social health and well-being and on the prevention of disease and disability among groups of people. It differs from the practice of medicine because it focuses on prevention rather than cures and addresses the needs of people as a whole rather than as individual persons.

Public health is an evidence-based practice, which means that its professionals collect and analyze data to determine the health needs and risks of a population and then design programs to deliver services that will effectively address these needs and reduce risks.

AREAS OF SPECIALIZATION

Public health encompasses many specialized fields of study, including epidemiology, maternal and child care, environmental health, injury prevention and control, addiction, health education and promotion, and health program management and administration. These specialties evolved as the correlations between health and sanitation, safety, and behavior were better understood. Each specialization addresses the specific needs of a community.

EPIDEMIOLOGY

Epidemiology is the study of the relationship between causative agents and morbidity and mortality. This relationship may not be one of direct cause and effect, but the risk factors for a given illness are more likely to be identified. By determining the distribution of a public health concern, such as an infectious disease, within a population, commonalities may emerge that may then be tested for significance.

A classic example of epidemiology is the investigational work of John Snow, who looked into the source of a cholera outbreak in 1854 in central London. He began mapping the cases of cholera and found clusters in two areas. He interviewed the residents of these neighborhoods and found that they all had used the public water pump on one street. Direct examination of the water was inconclusive, but Snow's logic had convinced officials to remove the pump's handle, rendering it inoperable. Snow argued that the water company, Southwark and Vauxhall Waterworks, was delivering polluted water from the Thames River to this public well, which served areas that showed a high incidence of cholera. The cholera epidemic began to wane, although it could not be proven whether this occurred because of the pump's water supply being discontinued or because people had already left the area to escape the disease.

Snow used statistics and surveys to determine the distribution of the disease and to identify common factors, suggested a plausible causative agent, and proposed an effective solution. Similar, refined methods are used today in epidemiology. For example, when the incidence of hantavirus infection suddenly increased in the western and southwestern United States between 1993 and 2007, epidemiologists used morbidity and mortality statistics to identify the trend and the geographical distribution. They looked for common factors and found weather patterns, vegeta-tion, and rodents. Hantavirus was known to be transmitted when humans came in contact with the urine, feces, or saliva of infected rodents. The reason, however, for the sudden increase was not yet clear. When researchers began to study the relationships among common factors, they discovered that climate change (hotter, moister summers and warmer autumns) had nurtured increased vegetation, providing an increased food source (more seeds) for rodents. The rodents then had a greater survival rate in the winter months and multiplied at an accelerated rate. This increased rodent population propagated the hantavirus and shed it in greater quantities.

MATERNAL AND CHILD CARE

The primary goals of public health programs in maternal and child care are to reduce infant mortality, reduce the prevalence of child abuse and neglect, and extend the life expectancy of children. Studies indicate that for the first time, children in the United States may not live as long as their parents, primarily because of lifestyle choices and resultant chronic diseases rather than infectious diseases. Nearly one in three children is overweight or obese because of poor nutrition, excessive eating, and a lack of physical activity. Obesity can lead to diabetes and heart disease, both of which reduce a person's life expectancy.

Maternal and child health care begins with education in the schools about teenage pregnancy and providing access to prenatal care for all women. Although death during childbirth rarely occurs in the United States (13 deaths per 100,000 live births in 2004), women should have a safe, clean place in which to deliver with professional assistance. The rate of infant mortality is higher (679 deaths per 100,000 live births in 2004). Following birth, newborns need screening for diseases, disorders, and conditions so they can receive prompt and appropriate treatment and support. Newborns also benefit from breast-feeding and vaccinations. New mothers should also be screened for postpartum depression. Because mothers are still the primary caregivers, they must be taught about nutrition and healthy lifestyle choices for their children. In addition, they must have resources to care for children with special needs, such as autism, epilepsy, sickle cell disease, and hemophilia. Public health programs address these aspects of maternal and child health care, targeting at-risk populations such as teenagers, immigrants, and isolated rural residents.

ENVIRONMENTAL HEALTH

Environmental health involves the study of the human relationship with the surrounding world, or environment. Areas of study include outdoor air quality, water quality, waste management, agriculture, and chemical exposure. Environmental health professionals also inspect buildings for health hazards such as sick house syndrome, mold, radon, and infestations. They monitor climate changes because temperature and precipitation affect the spread of waterborne and food-borne diseases caused by bacteria, viruses, and parasites. Children are more sensitive than adults to their environment, so professionals also study allergies, asthma, chemical sensitivities, and secondhand smoke to improve pediatric health.

Environmental health specialists also influence a community's infrastructure. They determine access to public transportation for subsequent access to health care and similar resources; help create bike paths, hiking trails, and outdoor recreation areas for public exercise; and work on systems for emergency preparedness and response. Such emergencies include major collisions and explosions that result in mass casualties, chemical spills, radiation leaks, natural disasters and severe weather, and infectious disease outbreaks.

INJURY PREVENTION AND CONTROL

Injuries, which contribute to disability and death, are public health concerns. Injuries are like diseases because they have underlying causative factors, they have identifiable risk factors that increase their likelihood, and they have factors that make them preventable. Injuries may be divided into two categories: unintentional injuries and injuries caused by violence.

Unintentional injuries include motor vehicle collisions, falls, drowning, sports collisions (with other players or with equipment), burns and electrical injuries, and exposure to toxic chemicals. Public health addresses traffic safety (drinking and texting while driving and wearing seatbelts when driving), the regular use of protective equipment (motorcycle helmets, bicycle helmets, and athletic mouth-guards), chemical safety (medication interactions, binge drinking, and child-proofing home medicine cabinets), and identification of potential hazards in the home and workplace. The prevention of unintentional injuries reduces the expense of medical care, lowers the incidence and cost of long-term disability, and decreases the number of deaths from unnatural causes.

Violence is the intentional infliction of pain and injury and may result in death. Although it is usually perpetrated by one person against another, it may be carried out by a group of people or it may be self-inflicted. Public health programs address issues such as street gangs, domestic violence, child abuse, teen suicide, and self-mutilation. These can become epidemics depending on a community's socioeconomic status and access to professional resources with healthier alternatives.

SUBSTANCE USE, ABUSE, AND DEPENDENCY

Public health professionals are concerned with the use of substances that have detrimental health effects. These substances include tobacco, alcohol, and a variety of drugs. About 15 percent of adults worldwide have serious abuse problems with substances other than nicotine; this figure has remained constant for a minimum of twenty-five years. Nicotine addiction significantly contributes to heart disease and lung disease, making it the foremost lifestyle-related cause of death worldwide.

One goal of public health agencies is to educate people about the dangers of substance use, misuse, abuse, and dependency. Use is the habitual ingestion of and misuse is the use of a substance for which it was not intended, such as inhaling aerosol propellants to get intoxicated (or high). Substance abuse involves dangerous actions and continued use in the face of negative consequences. Dependency has a strong psychological component and physiological need.

Another goal of public health agencies is to promote substance abuse and dependency as diseases. Agencies seek to foster understanding from families and communities that will encourage users to seek treatment. Cessation programs begin with withdrawal or detoxification and continue with behavior modification therapy on an inpatient or outpatient basis.

Public health agencies may also seek to ameliorate the effects of substance abuse. For example, methadone clinics may be established to help people who are otherwise unable to give up illegal drugs. Clean needles may be distributed to reduce the spread of infectious diseases from sharing needles among intravenous drug users. Because sex is often "traded" for drugs, condoms may be distributed to reduce the spread of sexually transmitted diseases.

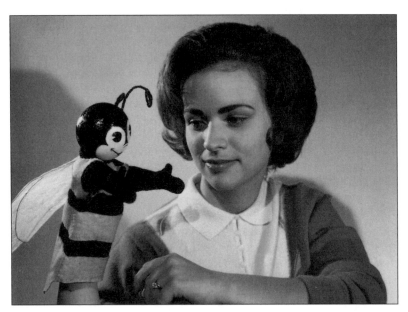

Public health campaigns often target children. In the early 1960's, for example, the Centers for Disease Control and Prevention's health symbol, Wellbee, promoted vaccination, handwashing, and other health practices. (CDC)

HEALTH EDUCATION AND PROMOTION

The first goal of health education and promotion is to improve the health of persons and families by providing accurate, timely, and understandable health information. One study found that 90 percent of adults have problems finding and using health information. Most adults (53 percent) have intermediate health literacy, meaning they can comprehend and apply some of the health information they read, but 14 percent have below-basic health literacy, meaning they can comprehend very little and apply almost none of the health information they read. Health information may be presented through brochures, posters, newspaper and magazine articles, and radio and television programs, and on Web sites. Many presentations are bilingual, depending, especially, on the region.

The second goal of health education and promotion is to create resources within the community to encourage and sustain a healthy lifestyle. These resources include school-based health centers; workplace programs such as stress management and smoking cessation (in support of a smoke-free environment); health fairs that showcase wellness resources such as yoga classes, massage therapists, and organic food shops; and community clinics for family planning, blood pressure monitoring, and flu shots.

The third goal of health education and promotion is to advocate for the public health needs of communities by educating politicians on the health issues that are affecting their constituents. Using the evidence-based approach, public health officials can statistically define a community's needs, propose well-established strategies for meeting those needs, outline the resources necessary to implement the strategies, and offer quantitative measures of the outcome. The desired results of such advocacy are effective legislation, such as health care reform acts, and appropriated funding for national, state, and local public health programs.

HEALTH PROGRAM MANAGEMENT AND ADMINISTRATION

Public health departments are found at the federal, state, and local levels. They maintain databases that include information on morbidity and mortality, births and deaths, and records of inspection of public places, such as restaurants and swimming pools. The departments operate laboratories for testing air, water, and soil samples and for investigating microorganisms. They conduct epidemiological surveillance and investigations into communicable diseases to prevent epidemics. They often work with other agencies, such as clinics, schools, businesses, and other government agencies.

Professionals in health program management and administration are frequently responsible for grant writing and reporting and for overseeing budgets and managing resources. Successful health programs depend on appropriate planning and design that are based on an accurate assessment of community needs. Measurable goals and objectives must directly arise from these data. The programs also depend upon timely implementation with adequate attendance by the target population. Finally, the programs depend on quantitative evaluation and plans for sustaining the results. Effective public health efforts must also consider the social, economic, and cultural characteristics of the communities they serve.

IMPACT

At the end of 2010, the U.S. Department of Health and Human Services released its Healthy People 2020 program, which includes national health goals and objectives through 2020. Several hundred objectives cover twenty-eight priority areas of public health. The focus of this program is not simply to reduce disease and death rates; its goal is to improve quality of life and increase the years of healthy living. Morbidity and mortality rates are easy to collect for specific populations and to analyze by cause. Life expectancy in the United States, however, has increased significantly since 1979, so these rates are less relevant than are reduced disability, premature death, and improvements in pain control and functional capacity.

A second focus of this program is to eliminate or, at minimum, greatly reduce health disparities for racial and ethnic minority groups, people with physical or mental disabilities, socioeconomically disadvantaged people, and the elderly. Disparities are pronounced in infant mortality, cardiovascular disease, diabetes, and human immunodeficiency virus (HIV) infection. Public health professionals believe that all members of a community should have access to health education, disease prevention information, and medical care, based on the ideal of social justice.

The effectiveness of public health initiatives has led to a shift in the major cause of death: from infectious diseases to chronic diseases. Although some future initiatives will continue to aim for the reduction of the incidence of infectious diseases, others will address lifestyle-related choices, such as obesity and cigarette smoking, which are controllable risk factors for chronic diseases.

Bethany Thivierge, M.P.H.

FURTHER READING

Clement, Jan, et al. "Relating Increasing Hantavirus Incidences to the Changing Climate: The Mast Connection." *International Journal of Health Geographics* 8 (2009): 1. An overview of the worldwide epidemiology of hantavirus, rodent carriers, and seasonal cycles, with an emphasis on plant growth and reproduction.

Kutner, Mark, et al. *The Health Literacy of America's Adults: Results from the 2003 National Assessment of Adult Literacy.* U.S. Department of Education. Washington, D.C.: National Center for Education Statistics, 2006. A statistical analysis report of health literacy among adults and its relationship to background variables such as highest level of education obtained and primary source of health information.

Scutchfield, F. Douglas, et al. *Principles of Public Health Practice.* 3d ed. Clifton Park, N.Y.: Delmar Cengage Learning, 2009. A respected textbook that examines the contemporary practice of public health.

Turnock, Bernard J. *Public Health: What It Is and How It Works.* 4th ed. Maynard, Mass.: Jones and Bartlett, 2008. This book discusses the public health system in the United States and its role in relation to the medical care system.

U.S. Department of Health and Human Services. *Healthy People 2010: Understanding and Improving Health.* 2d ed. Washington, D.C.: Government Printing Office, November, 2000. A document of national goals and objectives for public health from 2000 to 2010. A similar document for Healthy People 2020 is also available from the same source.

WEB SITES OF INTEREST

American Public Health Association
http://www.apha.org

Association of Schools of Public Health
http://www.asph.org

Centers for Disease Control and Prevention
http://www.cdc.gov

Partners in Information: Access for the Public Health Workforce
http://phpartners.org

Society for Public Health Education
http://www.sophe.org

U.S. Department of Health and Human Services
http://www.hhs.gov

See also: Biosurveillance; Centers for Disease Control and Prevention (CDC); Decontamination; Developing countries and infectious disease; Disease eradication campaigns; Emerging and reemerging infectious diseases; Emerging Infections Network; Endemic infections; Epidemics and pandemics: Causes and management; Epidemiology; Globalization and infectious disease; Hospitals and infectious disease; Immunization; National Institutes of Health; Outbreaks;

Tropical medicine; U.S. Army Medical Research Institute of Infectious Diseases; Vaccines: History; World Health Organization (WHO).

Puerperal infection

CATEGORY: Diseases and conditions
ANATOMY OR SYSTEM AFFECTED: Reproductive system, uterus
ALSO KNOWN AS: Peurperal fever

DEFINITION

Puerperal infection, a bacterial condition that occurs soon after childbirth, affects the birth canal and surrounding areas. Reported incidence rates in the United States range from 1 to 8 percent of postpartum women. However, the risk is up to ten times higher among women who deliver by cesarean section. The prognosis is good if treatment is initiated in a timely manner. If left untreated, puerperal infection can lead to more serious conditions, such as endometritis (infection of the uterine lining), peritonitis (inflammation of the peritoneum), and pelvic thrombophlebitis (inflammation of the pelvis, which is caused by a blot clot).

CAUSES

The most common cause of puerperal infection is a bacterial infection in the uterus. Organisms responsible for this infection include streptococci, *Escherichia coli*, coagulase-negative staphylococci, and *Clostridium perfringens*. Although such microbes are part of normal vaginal flora, they can trigger infection in the presence of predisposing factors, such as vaginal-membrane rupture, anemia, traumatic labor, or a labor period that is unusually long.

RISK FACTORS

The risk of puerperal infection and its predisposing factors is greatest for women of low socioeconomic status who have prolonged labor, who undergo cesarean section, or who experience rupture of membranes. Other risk factors include having sexual intercourse in the last week of pregnancy, not having adequate antenatal care, having comorbid diseases during pregnancy, and having a pelvic examination during pregnancy or labor.

SYMPTOMS

Symptoms of puerperal infection include headache, backache, abnormally high body temperature, vaginal discharge, foul-smelling lochia, and pain or tenderness in the abdominal region.

SCREENING AND DIAGNOSIS

The diagnosis is established on the basis of presenting symptoms and on confirmatory testing. Diagnostic assessments include complete blood count, urinalysis, pelvic examination, and cultures of lochia, uterine tissue, and incisional exudates (such as those from an episiotomy or cesarean incision). The white blood cell count usually is very high.

TREATMENT AND THERAPY

Broad-spectrum antibiotics, delivered intravenously, are the gold standard of treatment. Commonly used agents are gentamicin and clindamycin. For persistent cases, ampicillin may be added to the regimen. Once the fever has resolved, one should continue antibiotic treatment for an additional forty-eight hours. In cases of thrombophlebitis, heparin can be used to prevent blot clotting.

PREVENTION AND OUTCOMES

The best way to prevent puerperal infection is to ensure proper prenatal and antenatal care, including personal hygiene and regular obstetric visits. For women who undergo cesarean section, the prophylactic administration of antibiotics may ward off potential infectious bacteria.

Lynda A. Seminara, B.A.

FURTHER READING

Chen, C. L., et al. "Puerperal Infection of Methicillin-Resistant *Staphylococcus aureus*." *Taiwanese Journal of Obstetrics and Gynecology* 47 (2008): 357-359.

Gould, I. M. "Alexander Gordon, Puerperal Sepsis, and Modern Theories of Infection Control: Semmelweis in Perspective." *The Lancet Infectious Diseases* 10 (2010): 275-278.

Petersen, Eiko E. *Infections in Obstetrics and Gynecology: Textbook and Atlas*. New York: Thieme Medical, 2006.

WEB SITES OF INTEREST

Women's Health Matters
http://www.womenshealthmatters.ca

Women's Health.gov
http://www.womenshealth.gov

See also: Bacterial infections; Childbirth and infectious disease; Endometritis; Infection; Inflammation; Peritonitis; Pregnancy and infectious disease; Secondary infection; Women and infectious disease.

Pulsed-field gel electrophoresis

Category: Diagnosis
Also known as: Deoxyribonucleic acid (DNA) fingerprinting

Definition

Pulsed-field gel electrophoresis (PFGE) is a DNA fingerprinting technique that allows separation of large DNA fragments (of more than thirty kilo-base pairs) in an agarose gel by applying an alternating electric field among twelve pairs of electrodes. The DNA fragments ultimately form the distinctive pattern of bands in a column, or lane, in the gel. Small DNA fragments form bands at the bottom, and large DNA fragments form bands at the top of the gel. Genetic variation among strains causes fragments of differing sizes to be produced when DNA is digested with enzymes called restriction endonucleases. PFGE can thus detect differences in DNA as minor as one base change.

Genetic variations revealed after digestion with restriction endonucleases are referred to as restriction fragment length polymorphisms. The pattern of banding is analyzed visually then digitized and archived to determine the relatedness of biological samples.

Applications

PFGE is used, for example, in quality control of the genetic identity and stability of grapes and hops fermented for wine and beer and in quality control of the microbes used in food production. Cancer researchers use the technique to analyze damage to DNA caused by chemicals and radiation. Genetics research laboratories use the technique to map genetic defects routinely. Outbreaks of infectious diseases can be monitored to determine the similarity of the bacterial strains involved. While genetic matching does not ensure that isolates from two infected persons came

from the same source, epidemiologists can detect the rise in prevalence of a bacterial strain when an outbreak does occur. Microbes infecting hospitalized persons can be analyzed to determine if multiple patients are affected by the same strain, raising the possibility the hospital itself is the source of the infection.

Public Health

In 1992, an outbreak of food-borne illness occurred in the western United States. The bacterium *Escherichia coli* O157:H7 was implicated in the outbreak by using traditional microbiological techniques. The PFGE patterns of isolates from infected persons and from hamburger patties from the restaurant where those persons ate were the same. Scientists concluded that the infected persons had acquired the *E. coli* from that particular restaurant.

The Centers for Disease Control and Prevention (CDC) led the effort to develop a standardized protocol for PFGE for analysis of clinical isolates of *E. coli*. The materials, methods, and controls are now standardized and can be used to yield reliable results at a number of labs around the world. The protocol served as a platform for the development of PFGE typing of a host of microbial pathogens.

The CDC then developed PulseNet, a national network of public health and food regulatory agency labs. The labs perform PFGE fingerprinting of food-borne bacteria. In addition to *E. coli*, *Salmonella*, *Shigella*, *Listeria*, and *Campylobacter* are fingerprinted, and their patterns are entered into the CDC database. Member labs can access the database in real time and can compare clinical specimens.

Impact

Clusters of food-borne disease are identified far more quickly, in as little as a week, using PFGE and PulseNet. The origin of the infection can be identified and isolated, preventing further transmission. PFGE has also been used to trace the source and spread of antibiotic resistant tuberculosis. Epidemiologists learned that the infected persons had acquired the infection in the hospital.

Kimberly A. Napoli, M.S.

Further Reading

Brachman, Philip S., and Elias Abrutyn, eds. *Bacterial Infections of Humans: Epidemiology and Control*. 4th ed. New York: Springer, 2009.

Forbes, Betty A., Daniel F. Sahm, and Alice S. Weiss-feld. *Bailey and Scott's Diagnostic Microbiology.* 12th ed. St. Louis, Mo.: Mosby/Elsevier, 2007.

Tortora, Gerard J., Berdell R. Funke, and Christine L. Case. *Microbiology: An Introduction.* 10th ed. San Francisco: Benjamin Cummings, 2010.

WEB SITES OF INTEREST

Lab Tests Online
http://www.labtestsonline.org

Merck Manuals: Laboratory Diagnosis of Infectious Disease
http://www.merckmanuals.com/professional/sec14/ch168/ch168a.html

Protocolpedia
http://www.protocolpedia.com

See also: Acid-fastness; Bacteriology; Biochemical tests; Diagnosis of bacterial infections; Gram staining; Immunoassay; Microbiology; Microscopy; Pathogens; Polymerase chain reaction (PCR) method; Serology.